Issues and Choices in Clinical Nutrition Practice

ISSUES AND CHOICES IN CLINICAL NUTRITION PRACTICE

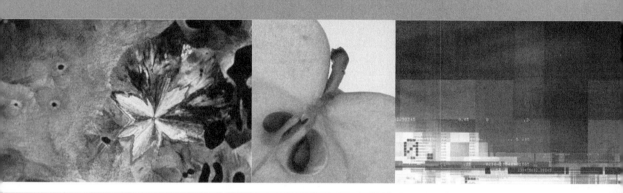

Edited by

Abby S. Bloch, PhD, RD, FADA
Vice President, Programs and Research
Dr. Robert C. Atkins Foundation
Formerly, Director of Clinical Nutrition
    Support Kitchen
Memorial Sloan-Kettering Cancer Center
Adjunct Assistant Professor, Department
    of Nutrition and Food Studies
New York University School of Education
New York, New York

Julie O'Sullivan Maillet, PhD, RD, FADA
Associate Dean for Academic Affairs and Research
Chairperson, Department of Primary Care
University of Medicine and Dentistry of New Jersey
Newark, New Jersey

Wanda H. Howell, PhD, RD
Professor, Nutrition Sciences
University Distinguished Professor
University of Arizona
Department of Nutritional Sciences
Tucson, Arizona

Marion F. Winkler, MS, RD, LDN, CNSD
Rhode Island Hospital
Department of Surgery/Nutritional
    Support Service
Brown University School of Medicine
Providence, Rhode Island

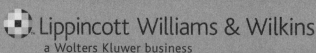
. Lippincott Williams & Wilkins
a Wolters Kluwer business
Philadelphia · Baltimore · New York · London
Buenos Aires · Hong Kong · Sydney · Tokyo

Acquisitions Editor: David B. Troy
Managing Editor: Linda G. Francis
Marketing Manager: Marisa O'Brien
Production Editor: Eve Malakoff-Klein
Designer: Wanda España/Wee Design Group
Compositor: Nesbitt Graphics, Inc.
Printer: Courier Corporation—Kendallville

351 West Camden Street
Baltimore, Maryland 21201-2436 USA

530 Walnut Street
Philadelphia, Pennsylvania 19106 USA

The publisher is not responsible (as a matter of product liability, negligence or otherwise) for any injury resulting from any material contained herein. This publication contains information relating to general principles of medical care which should not be construed as specific instructions for individual patients. Manufacturers' product information and package inserts should be reviewed for current information, including contraindications, dosages and precautions.

Printed in the United States of America

Library of Congress Cataloging-in-Publication Data

Issues and choices in clinical nutrition practice / edited by Abby S. Bloch ... [et al.].-- 1st ed.
    p. ; cm.
  Includes bibliographical references and index.
  ISBN-13: 978-0-7817-4846-9
  ISBN-10: 0-7817-4846-1
  1. Diet therapy. 2. Diet in disease. 3. Nutrition. I. Bloch, Abby S. II. Title.
  [DNLM: 1. Nutrition Therapy. 2. Dietetics--organization & administration. 3. Interprofessional Relations. 4. Nutrition. WB 400 I86 2007]
  RM216.I87 2007
  615.8'54--dc22
                                2005035383

The publishers have made every effort to trace the copyright holders for borrowed material. If they have inadvertently overlooked any, they will be pleased to make the necessary arrangements at the first opportunity.

To purchase additional copies of this book, call our customer service department at (800) 638-3030 or fax orders to (301) 223-2320. For other book services, including chapter reprints and large quantity sales, ask for the Special Sales department.

For all other calls originating outside of the United States, please call (301) 223-2300.

Visit Lippincott Williams & Wilkins on the Internet: http://www.lww.com. Lippincott Williams & Wilkins customer service representatives are available from 8:30 am to 6:00 pm, EST, Monday through Friday, for telephone access.

06 07 08 09 10
1 2 3 4 5 6 7 8 9 10

This book is dedicated to all of the dietitians who have advanced and who continue to advance the profession of dietetics, and to Dr. Maurice E. Shils, who has been an inspiration and mentor to so many and made such a difference in the field of nutrition and care of patients.

Many issues relating to science, education, professional advancement, and practice are critically important to dietetics professionals and healthcare providers. However, books and references frequently do not consider the complexities of care or the breadth of therapeutic options available. This publication examines selected clinical practice issues with the intention of raising awareness of practitioners and future practitioners who need to develop critical thinking skills rather than using a "cookbook" approach to practice. Many nutrition issues and controversies need to be examined as we move to evidence-based practice. Points of view that vary from the traditional approach of nutrition practice are raised in this publication. By confronting such issues, dietetic professionals will hopefully reevaluate their roles and practices within the broader healthcare setting. Additionally, the chapters will provide information on new advances in clinical nutrition and nutritional sciences.

Practitioners in various employment settings—including clinical care, community/public health nutrition, school/ food service management, education at all levels, research, health and wellness, consultation/private practice—as well as students who have some foundation in nutrition and dietetics should find outlined herein challenging issues and questions related to their practice or studies. Clinicians working in acute care and ambulatory/community-based care as well as alternate site care, third-party providers, and those offering home care should find this book provocative. Nurses, pharmacists, physicians, and other healthcare professionals interested in nutrition topics of current relevance to their practice should find this book challenging as well. Future practitioners will have an opportunity to understand the options and alternatives that exist in this field rather than a single focused, limited approach to a given topic.

Issues and controversies raised in each part of this book, which challenge and expand practices of dietetics professionals and present a variety of current and emerging views, allow readers to engage in thoughtful reasoning and dialogue with others prior to making practice decisions. Each part of this book provides the practicing healthcare professional in nutrition care with a number of broad analyses of professional policy and practice issues. New and emerging areas of nutrition science and research are discussed as they affect dietetic practice now and in the future. Most chapters include "Issues to Ponder," thus reinforcing the need for the reader to engage in critical thinking about the topic under discussion. The answers are not always available and will change over time.

This book is organized into four parts: The Dietetic Professional's Role in the Healthcare Setting; Clinical Practice Issues: An Evidence-Based Perspective; Effects of Emerging Science and Controversies on Dietetics Practice; and International Tables and Global Nutrition Standards, which includes tables and graphics presenting international recommended dietary intakes and dietary guidelines. Some repetition and overlapping of information occurs, but this is provided for continuity within a chapter and emphasis among chapters.

From beginning to end, Part I describes where dietetics is moving as a profession and why. The history of education, credentialing, and practice is integrated with the current and future challenges for the profession. The perspectives from other health professionals may improve your role on the team. As you read the section, determine how you personally or as part of an organization will move dietetics education, credentialing, and practice to a new level of performance that will ultimately improve the nutrition care of the public.

Part II encompasses nutrition screening, nutrition assessment, the measurement of nutrient intake, and research in the clinical setting. Readers will find a challenging approach to each of these topics in an effort to foster critical thinking, not the typical "how-to." The chapter entitled "Measuring Nutrient Intake" contains detailed information regarding existing tools and databases and examples of many dietary assessment forms. The nutrition care process, including examples of diagnostic codes, is discussed from the perspective of implementation and as a basis for conducting research in the practice setting.

Part III contains important new information as well as insights into controversies in the prevention and management of hypertension, coronary heart disease, obesity, diabetes mellitus, cancer, and food-drug interactions. The emerging areas of genomics and proteomics, as well as alternative/complementary nutrition therapies, are covered as part of the many unique features of this book. Nutrition care practitioners and educators will find this section to be particularly relevant to their advanced practice roles.

In Part IV, nutrient recommendations for numerous countries are presented for the reader to compare. Websites for international dietary guidelines illustrate the variation among countries. It is of interest to note the similarities as well as the differences among different populations and to wonder why any given country has established the recommendations published. Another provocative question raised is the concept of global food-based dietary guidelines: are they possible, desirable, and achievable? The possibility of defining one set of dietary guidelines is indeed attractive, considering the need for uniformity in the global village. Why should the optimal diet be different from one population to the next? These and other thought-provoking questions challenge the reader.

The editorial board of this publication reviewed a dozen or more of the most widely used nutrition texts around the country. None of those books approached nutrition topics by raising the issues and controversies found in everyday practice situations. Although many nutrition textbooks present theoretical research and practice information or "how-to" in assessing, evaluating, counseling, or managing a variety of dietary circumstances and needs, few facilitate critical thinking. It is our hope that readers will find the issues and controversies raised in the following chapters challenging and thought-provoking in relation to their current beliefs and practices.

Abby S. Bloch
Julie O'Sullivan Maillet
Wanda H. Howell
Marion F. Winkler

We are grateful for the diligence of the authors whose work appears in this book, as well as the professional associations and members who continue to move us all forward. Additionally, we are indebted to the friends and family members who have supported us throughout the process of compiling and editing of the book. Finally, we acknowledge the following reviewers for their insightful comments on the first draft:

Rachel E. Teneralli, MS, RD, CNSD
Clinical Dietitian
Newark Beth Israel Medical Center
Newark, New Jersey

B.J. Friedman, PhD, RD, LD
Professor and Chair
Texas State University
San Marcos, Texas

Jessie Pavlinac, MS, RD, CSR, LD
Clinical Nutrition Manager
Oregon Health and Science University
Portland, Oregon

CONTRIBUTORS

Patricia S. Anthony, MS, RD, CNSD
Manager, HealthCare Nutrition Support Services
Nutrition Strategic Business Division
Nestec, Ltd.
Vevey, Switzerland

Christina Biesemeier, MS, RD, LD, FADA
Assistant Director
Nutrition Services
Vanderbilt University Medical Center
Nashville, Tennessee

Jennifer Muir Bowers, PhD, RD, CNSD
Department of Nutritional Sciences
University of Arizona
Tucson, Arizona

Deborah D. Canter, PhD, RD, LD
Professor, Coordinated Program in Dietetics
Department of Hotel, Restaurant, Institution
Management and Dietetics
Kansas State University
Manhattan, Kansas

Pam Charney, MS, RD, LD, CNSD
PhD Candidate
School of Health Related Professions
University of Medicine and Dentistry of New Jersey
Newark, New Jersey

Robert S. DeChicco, MS, RD, LD, CNSD
Manager, Nutrition Support Dietetics
Nutrition Support & Vascular Access Department
The Cleveland Clinic Foundation
Cleveland, Ohio

Cecelia G. Echevarria, MS, RD, CNSD, RN
Professional Nurse I
Trauma Intensive Care Unit
Rhode Island Hospital
Providence, Rhode Island

Sylvia Escott-Stump, MA, RD, LDN
Dietetic Program Director
Department of Nutrition and Hospitality Management
East Carolina University
Greenville, North Carolina

Syed S. Haque, PhD
Professor and Chair
Department of Health Informatics
UMDNJ–School of Health Related Professions
Newark, New Jersey

Elvira Q. Johnson, MS, RD, CDE, LDN
Principal Consultant
EQJ Associates
North Reading, Massachusetts

Gail P. A. Kauwell, PhD, RN, LDN
Associate Professor
Department of Food Science and Human Nutrition
University of Florida
Gainesville, Florida

Robert F. Kushner, MD
Professor of Medicine
Medical Director, Wellness Institute
Northwestern University Feinberg School of Medicine
Northwestern Memorial Hospital
Chicago, Illinois

Beth Leonberg, MS, RD, FADA
Vice President, Nutrition Services
Sodexho Health Care Services
Washington Crossing, Pennsylvania

Laura E. Matarese, MS, RD, LD, FADA, CNSD
Clinical Instructor of Surgery
Director of Nutrition and Intestinal Rehabilitation
Thomas E. Starzl Transplantation Institute
University of Pittsburgh Medical Center
Pittsburgh, Pennsylvania

June H. McDermott, MS Pharm, MBA, FASHP, CPP
Program on Integrative Medicine
Physical Medicine and Rehabilitation
University of North Carolina School of Medicine
Chapel Hill, North Carolina

Esther F. Myers, PhD, RD, FADA
Director, Research and Scientific Affairs
American Dietetic Association
Chicago, Illinois

Adam Perlman, MD, MPH
Executive Director
Institute for Complementary and Alternative Medicine
University of Medicine and Dentistry of New Jersey
Newark, New Jersey

Diane Rigassio Radler, PhD, RD
Assistant Professor
Primary Care Clinical Nutrition
School of Health Related Professions
University of Medicine and Dentistry of New Jersey
Newark, New Jersey

Carol J. Rollins, MS, RD, PharmD, BCNSP
Clinical Associate Professor
Pharmacy Practice and Science
College of Pharmacy
University of Arizona
Tucson, Arizona

Phyllis J. Stumbo, PhD, RD, LD
General Research Nutritionist
Clinical Research Center
University of Iowa
Iowa City, Iowa

Cynthia A. Thomson, PhD, RD, FADA
Assistant Professor
Department of Nutritional Sciences
University of Arizona
Cancer Prevention and Control Program
Arizona Cancer Center
Tucson, Arizona

Riva Touger-Decker, PhD, RD, FADA
Associate Professor
School of Health Related Professions
University of Medicine and Dentistry of New Jersey
Newark, New Jersey

Ricardo Uauy, MD, PhD
Professor of Human Nutrition
Department of Public Nutrition
Institute of Nutrition and Food Technology (INTA)
University of Chile
Santiago, Chile
   Professor of Public Health Nutrition
   Department of Epidemiology and Public Health
   London School of Hygiene and Tropical Medicine
   University of London
   London, United Kingdom

Laura Heald Watson, MD, RD, CD
Region Director
Food and Nutrition Services
Utah Valley Regional Medical Center
Provo, Utah

Jane V. White, PhD, RD
Professor, Department of Family Medicine
University of Tennessee
Knoxville, Tennessee

Judith Wylie-Rosett, EdD, RD
Professor, Department of Epidemiology and
Population Health
Albert Einstein College of Medicine
Bronx, New York

CONTENTS

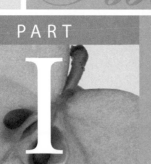

PART

I

THE DIETETICS PROFESSIONAL'S ROLE IN THE HEALTHCARE SETTING

Editor: Julie O'Sullivan Maillet

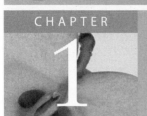

AN OVERVIEW OF THE DIETETICS PROFESSIONAL'S TRAINING AND OPPORTUNITIES IN HEALTHCARE

Robert S. DeChicco and Laura E. Matarese

The profession of dietetics is evolving and expanding, creating both challenges and opportunities for its practitioners. Dietetics professionals have established roles in all areas of healthcare, industry, government, education, sports, and wellness, from basic research to community nutrition; from advertising and marketing to academia. To meet the demands of these roles, dietetics professionals have developed new skills and increased their scope of practice. The profession continues to evolve in response to societal and economic forces, taking advantage of new opportunities and remaining at the forefront of healthcare. This chapter presents trends and emerging issues facing the dietetics professional in practice. Subsequent chapters examine some of the issues in more depth.

KEY TRENDS AFFECTING THE FUTURE OF DIETETICS

In 2002 the American Dietetic Association (ADA) conducted an environmental scan to determine important trends, issues, and events likely to influence dietetics professionals.[1] In that process, more than 100 such areas were identified. New opportunities for the dietetics profession over the next decade were derived from three broad factors: (1) greater public interest in diet and nutrition, (2) growth of the U.S. population, and (3) greater cultural and ethnic diversity of the U.S. population. These factors will affect the demand for dietetics services, how and to whom these services are provided, and how nutrition information is acquired and disseminated. From these three broad categories, seven key strategic challenges affecting dietetics professionals were identified (Table 1-1).

These challenges address concerns about (1) controlling the flow of information regarding the role of the diet in health and prevention of chronic disease and (2) providing dietetics services to an increasingly older and more diverse population. The goal is for dietetics professionals to be perceived by the public and other healthcare professionals as the most valued source of nutrition information. This will be made more difficult by the increasing number of alternative providers of nutrition information and the continued encroachment on dietetics professionals' scope of practice by other professions.

Information technology (IT) will become an increasingly integral part of the healthcare system and both benefit and challenge dietetics professionals. Methods of communication and the flow of information in healthcare will continue to evolve as more professionals and the public obtain access to IT. These factors will increase the availability of information and reliance on electronic communication. IT will provide networking opportunities with other professionals and decrease barriers to

TABLE 1-1	Key Strategic Challenges Affecting the Dietetics Profession[1]

Technological, social, political, global, and environmental forces are significantly reshaping the U.S. food system.

Keeping up with the relevant science and technology of food and health will be an increasing burden to dietetics professionals.

The competitive space of the dietetics profession is being seriously challenged.

Dietetics has to be relevant to more people, in more circumstances, at more life stages, and in more cultures.

Obesity is a "crisis opportunity" that the ADA and its members are uniquely prepared to address.

Although it may not have been a forefront issue in food and health, privacy will become a bigger and more important concern in dietetics.

More food, diet, and food-supply issues will be global, with the interchange of the standards and regulations.

the acquisition of knowledge by making the healthcare field a global community. On the other hand, there will also be more misinformation available, which will make the educational process more challenging.

Changes in the population will continue to have a significant impact on the market for dietetics services. The U.S. population is growing both larger and more ethnically and culturally diverse. This will increase the number and diversity of people who will require medical nutrition therapy (MNT). At the same time, the population is aging, which will result in a greater incidence of chronic disease. Preventive care can potentially slow the progression of certain chronic diseases,[2] but the demand for dietetics services will undoubtedly increase.

Family structure and lifestyle will continue to change. American families are smaller, with fewer children, and extended families living in the same household are becoming less common. This will result in fewer children and grandchildren available to assist in the care of elderly family members. Americans have become less physically active[3] and spend more hours at their places of work. Eating habits are changing, with more meals being consumed away from home or while engaged in another activity (e.g., working, reading, watching television). A larger percentage of women are in the workforce. Cooking skills have declined and less time is spent in food preparation. As a result, consumers are demanding foods that are convenient and easy to acquire, prepare, and consume.

Issues to Ponder

- How do we educate practitioners to work most effectively with individuals from varied cultural and ethnic backgrounds?
- How do you best educate clients on the selection of foods that are eaten out or prepared by others?
- What distinguishes registered dietitians (RDs) from other providers of nutrition information? How will the public know the difference?

The societal trend toward the consumption of more convenience foods and a more sedentary lifestyle favors continued increase in the prevalence of obesity. This will also increase the demand for dietetics services aimed at treating this disease and its comorbidities. The growing public health concern will provide opportunities for the profession, since dietetics professionals are uniquely qualified to address this issue on many levels.

EXPANDING THE SCOPE OF PRACTICE OF DIETETICS PROFESSIONALS

The American Dietetic Association (ADA) was founded during World War I to help the government conserve food and feed members of the military. From this beginning, the role of dietetics professionals has continued to evolve and expand in response to societal forces and trends. This expanding scope of practice has been the result of a science-based and diverse educational foundation, which allowed dietetics professionals to seize opportunities as they became available and help shape the future of the profession. This foundation comprises not only traditional academic education but also skills training in specialized areas. This multifaceted approach to education continues to serve the profession by preparing individuals with a wide variety of job skills, enabling them to perform multiple tasks.

The scope of a dietitian's practice is defined by a professional organization or society, by the institution where the individual dietetics professional is employed, by law in those states with practice acts, and by the individual practitioner. A review of the literature suggests a progressive expansion of the scope of dietetics practice over the years, particularly in specialty areas.[4–9] Dietetics professionals have moved from making general recommendations to performing many of the tasks that had previously been performed by other healthcare professionals. For example, dietitians have progressed from designing parenteral and enteral nutrition orders to actually writing the orders,[10] a task performed almost exclusively by physicians until the recent past.

Academic education has been the traditional avenue for acquiring knowledge, and dietetics professionals have one of the highest percentages of postgraduate degrees in the healthcare field. According to the ADA 2002 Dietetics Compensation and Benefits Survey,[11] 45% of registered dietitians (RDs) hold master's degrees, while 3% hold doctorates. These advanced degrees are in nutrition as well as related areas such as marketing, business administration, and education. Advanced degrees in nutrition are not limited to a master of science (MS) or doctorate of philosophy (PhD). A doctorate of clinical nutrition (DCN) is a new degree, which focuses on advanced clinical practice and requires completion of a clinical residency and research project. The value of this degree has yet to be determined, since it is not offered by many institutions and is clinically rather than academically oriented.[12] However, it does offer another option for dietetics professionals seeking additional educational opportunities. A dual degree is another means of diversifying an educational foundation by combining degrees in nutrition with medicine, nursing, pharmacy, exercise physiology, communications, or business.

Opportunities for academic education have dramatically increased with the advent of distance learning. Individuals can earn bachelor's, master's, or doctoral degrees without attending traditional bricks-and-mortar institutions. The majority of the course work is performed via the Internet. The institutions that provide these degrees vary from traditional universities offering courses from a single location to nationwide organizations with learning centers located in various cities. Another advantage of distance learning is that, since there are no traditional classes, course work can be performed at the student's convenience, which makes this option attractive to working professionals.

Skills training is another avenue for acquiring knowledge needed to perform a specific task; it can be obtained from a variety of sources such as workshops, seminars, conferences, the Internet, or on-the-job training. Skills can also be

TABLE 1-2	New Practice Activities for RDs[13]

Utilize the Internet as technical information resource.

Develop health education programs.

Utilize electronic media to communicate nutrition information.

Apply information technology to nutrition programs.

Develop quality management procedures.

Integrate nutrition services into complementary care.

Develop multimedia educational materials.

Teach self-monitoring of blood glucose.

Teach enteral nutrition techniques.

Teach in health-education programs.

Develop comprehensive obesity prevention and treatment programs.

Perform culinary demonstrations.

Conduct outcomes research.

Perform blood glucose monitoring.

acquired through self-education, which can be either formal or informal. These skills are usually related to a specific task and are more practical than academics, but both types of education can diversify an individual's foundation of knowledge. The types of skills that can be learned are varied. Table 1-2 lists tasks considered potentially new practice activities for RDs as determined by the Commission on Dietetic Registration (CDR) Practice Audit Committee.[13]

Dietetics internship programs, which combine academics with skills training, continually adjust their curricula to provide graduates with the skills necessary to compete in the job market. The Commission on Dietetic Education (CADE) establishes and updates quality standards for programs educating dietetics professionals based on practitioner and employer input, with the goal of matching competencies to future practice. The most recent standards were updated to include competencies in genetics, complementary care, supplements, and reimbursement to augment training in cultural diversity, counseling, communications, management, business, and leadership along with the traditional food and nutrition education.[14] (Competencies are available at http://www.eatright.org/ada/files/CADEHandbook.pdf.)

The acquisition of knowledge through academic education and skills training allows dietetics professionals to compete with other healthcare professionals by performing multiple tasks, commonly referred to as *multiskilling*. The development of multiskilling was spurred by the need to reduce healthcare costs by cutting operating expenses and the movement from department-focused to patient-focused healthcare. The goal of multiskilling is to improve productivity and cost-effectiveness. This enhances the continuity and quality of patient care by employing healthcare professionals who are able to perform multiple tasks both inside and outside their traditional scope of practice.

Multiskilling means more than simply acquiring additional clinical or technical skills. These expanded skills may be in the area of business, communications, writing, editing, or public speaking. They may involve developing leadership skills or becoming politically active to influence public policy. It is important for dietetics professionals to determine the appropriate skill set required to do a particular job or to achieve a particular goal and to eliminate, delegate, or streamline those skills that are less important or unnecessary.

Multiskilling is pervasive in all levels of healthcare. It is becoming more common for RDs, for example, to manage patients receiving parenteral nutrition—including writing daily orders, ordering intravenous replacements for fluid and electrolytes, and writing orders for insulin—in addition to traditional responsibilities such as performing nutrition assessments and nutrition education. To do this safely and effectively, dietetics professionals must possess skills that were previously considered out of the realm of clinical dietetics, such as performing physical examinations and reviewing microbiology, radiology, and pathology reports.

Multiskilling has always been practiced among managers owing to the nature of the managerial position. The trend, however, is toward having department heads manage multiple departments or multiple locations. Sixteen percent of respondents to a survey of members of the Management in Food and Nutrition Systems dietetics practice group of the ADA categorized themselves as multidepartment managers.[15] In addition to foodservice, other areas of responsibility were environmental services, administrative services, hospitality services, and patient care.

The downside to multiskilling is that as professional boundaries tend to become blurred because individuals are performing duties outside their traditional scope of practice, there will be resistance to this change, both from inside and outside the profession. Resistance may involve legal issues such as state licensure or liability or stem from other members of the healthcare team and their corresponding professional organizations wishing to protect their own scope of practice. Some dietetics professionals will

Issues to Ponder

- What checks and balances are needed as professional scopes of practice diversify and blur?
- How do we balance changing best practice, the value of the team approach, multiskilling, and cross training?

simply resist change. It is not clear how best to balance the expansion of roles for dietitians with protection from encroachment from other professions, but the value of multiskilling is likely to continue to increase as healthcare resources become scarcer.

INCREASING THE RECOGNITION OF DIETETICS PROFESSIONALS

Increasing the recognition of dietetics professionals as the most valued source of food and nutrition information by members of the public as well as other healthcare professionals is essential to the continued growth and development of the field. The increasing number and variety of sources of nutrition information and the amount of readily available misinformation, which can cause confusion among both the public and professionals, makes this task difficult. Efforts to increase recognition of dietetics professionals should use a multifaceted strategy that includes credentialing and certification, marketing, political activism, and outcomes research.

Credentials indicate that an individual possesses a certain level of education, achievement, or expertise. Credentials can include advanced academic degrees or specialty certification and usually reflect a level of practice beyond the standard for the field. Individuals seek credentials for a variety of reasons, including professional recognition, personal achievement, and opportunities to advance. Perhaps more importantly, specialty credentialing assures the public and other healthcare professionals that an individual possesses the educational background or skill sets to practice in a particular area. Specialty certifications measure knowledge and application in a particular area beyond formal education and experience. These credentials help to ensure minimal competence in a particular practice area as well as ensure patient safety. Further discussion of credentialing and certification appears in Chapter 3. A Certified Nutrition Support Dietitian (CNSD), for example, is required to pass an examination that conveys the possession of a basic body of knowledge in enteral and parenteral nutrition support. Recertification is required every 5 years to ensure that the individual maintains the necessary knowledge.

Advanced-level practice differs from specialty certification, although some specialty practitioners may also be functioning at an advanced level. Examples of advanced-level practice credentials include the Fellow of the American Dietetic Association (FADA) or the Fellow of the American College of Nutrition (FACN). These credentials recognize outstanding professional achievement and long-term commitment in the field as well as advanced level of practice.

Credentialing is not only associated with perceived value but also has been linked with actual cost savings for healthcare providers. Naylor and colleagues[16] reported that compared to discharge planners without credentials, discharge planners with master's degrees reduced admissions, lengthened time between discharge and readmission, and decreased costs for elderly subjects at high risk for poor outcomes after hospital discharge. The reasons for these results are not fully understood, but the authors suggest that advanced clinical experience and expertise in collaborating with physicians resulted in more timely interventions in the home, thereby preventing negative outcomes.

Marketing and public relations are increasingly important because of the growing number and variety of sources of nutrition information and the encroachment of other professionals and nonprofessionals into the dietetics professionals' scope of practice. Not surprisingly, the primary sources for nutrition information in the United States are television and magazines.[17] To combat this, it is necessary to promote dietetics professionals as the leading source of food and nutrition information. The objective is to build a "brand loyalty" among the public toward dietetics professionals much in the same manner that companies seek to have their products associated with qualities such as honesty and reliability. The ADA is attempting to do this through a multimedia approach that includes a public relations team, national and state spokespersons, its journal, and its website.

It is equally important to market dietetics to other healthcare professionals, particularly physicians. This can be accomplished by communicating directly with other professionals, building alliances through projects, research, and publications, and maintaining competency in areas of practice.[18] These steps help demonstrate that dietetics is a vital component of healthcare and make other disciplines more likely to seek the expertise of dietetics professionals.

Political activism is essential to promote dietetics because of the influence of the government on public policy. The goal is to ensure that federal agencies recognize nutrition as an essential component of healthcare and that dietetics professionals are the best source of nutrition information. The most visible group in dietetics is the ADA Political Action Committee (ADAPAC), which actively supports candidates

TABLE 1-3	ADA Strategic Goals for 2004–2008[20]
Build an aligned, engaged, and diverse membership.	
Influence key food, nutrition, and health initiatives.	
Impact the research agenda and facilitate research supporting the dietetics profession.	
Increase demand for and utilization of members' services.	
Empower members to compete successfully in a rapidly changing environment.	
Proactively focus on emerging areas of food and nutrition.	

and legislation consistent with the ADA's public policies. The ADA itself receives guidance in forming public policy from its Legislative and Public Policy Committee (LPPC). The LPCC has selected seven areas that they believe are the most important public policy issues to face dietetics professionals over the next decade. These areas are aging, child nutrition, Medicare Medical Nutrition Therapy (MNT) and Medicare reform, nutrition monitoring, nutrition research, obesity, and state government issues. The decision to include MNT for the elderly with diabetes and renal disease through Medicare is an example of a victory in the ongoing struggle to justify the cost-effectiveness of the services of dietetics professionals. The need for political activism will become increasingly apparent as dietetics professionals attempt to obtain reimbursement for other services while protecting their scope of practice from encroachment. The obesity crisis, for example, is an opportunity for the profession to gain prominence both politically and publicly by taking the lead in the prevention and treatment of what is essentially a preventable disease.

Outcomes research performed by dietetics professionals will increase recognition of the profession because of the potentially far-reaching impact of nutrition on health. Research involving nutrition and health can help society allocate its resources by identifying those strategies that will be most effective in achieving its goals and serving as the basis for continuous quality improvement.[19] The ADA believes that research is the foundation of the profession since it provides the groundwork for practice, education, and policy. In fact, facilitating research supporting the dietetics profession is one of the ADA's strategic goals for 2004–2008[20] (Table 1-3). At the same time, federal funding for research and development (R&D) continues to grow. The R&D budget for the National Institutes of Health (NIH), for example, increased by 15.5% in 2003, which nearly met the goal of doubling the NIH budget in the last 5 years.[21] This trend of increasing governmental funding of research is expected to continue, which will give dietetics professionals more opportunities to pursue outcomes research.

CAREER TRENDS

The current job market for dietetics professionals still centers on clinical dietetics in healthcare institutions. The 2004 Dietetics Professionals Needs Assessment[22] reported that

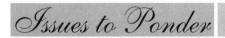

Issues to Ponder

- What factors would positively influence the compensation for dietetics practitioners?
- What are the consequences if this does not happen?

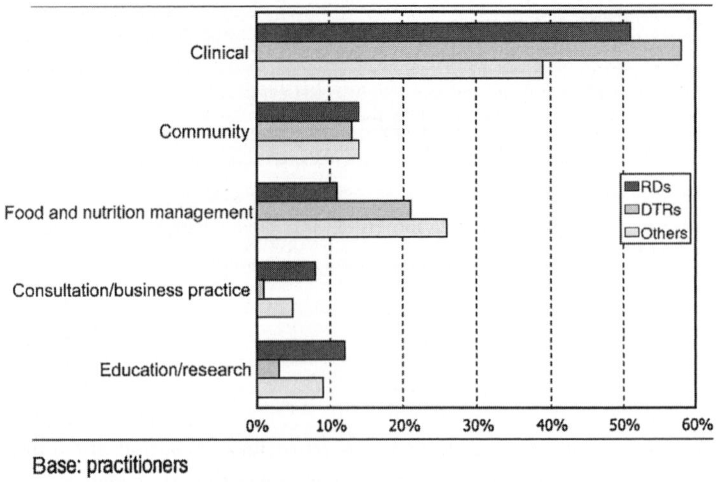

FIGURE 1-1 *Primary practice area for RDs, DTRs, and noncredentialed dietetics practitioners. Reprinted with permission from Report on the American Dietetic Association/ADA Foundation/Commission on Dietetic Registration 2004 Dietetics Professionals Needs Assessment. J Am Diet Assoc 2005; 105:1350.*

51% of RDs worked in clinical nutrition in an acute-care, outpatient, or long-term-care setting compared to 11% in foodservice management, 8% in consultation and business, and 12% in education and research (Figure 1-1). A similar percentage of dietetics technicians (DTRs) work in clinical nutrition (58%) compared to RDs, but more DTRs are employed in foodservice management (21%) and less in consultation and business (1%).

While most RDs and DTRs are employed in clinical dietetics, dietetics professionals are tending to move away from the traditional hospital-based setting as institutions reduce staff, being compelled to do so because of reduced lengths of stay and decreased reimbursement. Based on information gleaned from the ADA membership database and needs assessment survey, 42.4% of RDs and 46.8% of DTRs worked in hospitals in 1991, compared to 34.0 and 41.3% in 1997 and 28.0 and 35.0% in 2004[22,23] (Figure 1-2). This is likely the result of the emergence of subacute-care, long-term acute-care, and extended-care facilities, along with the growth of the home-care industry as more healthcare takes place outside the hospital. This trend should continue as the effort to control healthcare spending focuses on the delivery of services outside the hospital.

Regardless of the area of practice, compensation and job security remain primary concerns of dietetics professionals. These issues will remain at the forefront due to the constantly changing job market and the encroachment of other professions. It has always been difficult to compare wages and benefits nationally owing to the diversity of practice settings, job responsibilities, and job titles. Several factors are clearly associated with compensation for RDs. Years of experience, education level beyond a bachelor's degree, holding one or more specialty certifications, employment location, and area of practice were all associated with higher compensation and benefits.[11] For example, dietetics professionals employed in food and nutrition management, consultation and business, and research are compensated better than dietetics professionals employed in clinical or community nutrition settings. This disparity in salaries between practice areas has been documented since the early 1990s and continues to increase with time.[24]

Unfortunately, dietetics professionals are not compensated commensurate with their level of education and expertise as compared to other healthcare professions.

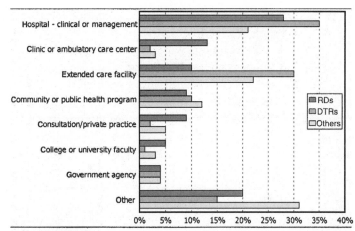

FIGURE 1-2 *Employment settings for RDs, DTRs, and noncredentialed dietetics professionals. Reprinted with permission from Report of the American Dietetic Association/ADA Foundation/Commission on Dietetic Registration 2004 Dietetics Professionals Needs Assessment. J Am Diet Assoc 2005;105:1350.*

According to the U.S. Bureau of Labor Statistics, dietitians and nutritionists earned less on average than pharmacists, physician assistants, registered nurses, audiologists, occupational therapists, physical therapists, and speech-language pathologists.[25] The reason for this disparity is multifactorial. In some instances, dietitians have been successful in negotiating salaries. But often, due to the heterogeneity of the profession, an employer may not recognize those individuals possessing advanced skill sets who are functioning at a high level. A solution would be to provide dietetics professionals with more detailed information on the salaries and benefits of others in the field, along with the negotiation skills needed to be able to bargain individually for better compensation packages.

A nontraditional approach to salary negotiation for dietitians is the formation of professional unions. Unions serve dietetics professionals by providing negotiations for salary and benefits as well as lobbying support for legislative activities. Unions represent a number of healthcare professions, including nursing, pharmacy, respiratory care, laboratory medicine, and radiology.

Future trends seem to favor job stability for dietetics professionals because of the steadily growing number of jobs in the field and the lower number of students entering the field. The U.S. Bureau of Labor Statistics projected a growth in employment for dietitians and nutritionists between 1998 and 2008 of 10,000 new jobs, or an increase of 19.1%, in addition to 11,000 jobs that will become available due to retirement, disability, or death, compared to an average annual net increase of approximately 2,200 RDs.[26] Concurrently, there has been a decrease in the number of students enrolled in dietetics programs and graduating as dietitians or dietetics technicians. Dietetics programs reported a 10% decline in enrollment in 2000 compared to 1999 and a 5% decrease in the number of graduates who completed the prerequisite course work for a dietetics internship or AP4 program during the same time period. Dietetics technician programs reported an 18% decrease in enrollment and a 19% decrease in graduates eligible for the registration examination in 2000 compared to 1999.[27]

Shortages of healthcare professionals in areas such as nursing and pharmacy will also affect the job market for dietetics professionals. The nursing shortage could open opportunities for dietitians to move into an area such as case management, which is dominated by nurses. Conversely, it may become more difficult to recruit students into dietetics as salaries and benefits in these other areas increase in response to the forces of supply and demand.[1]

Organizations will have to reconsider their recruitment and retention policies to compensate for the lack of growth in the number of dietetics professionals. One strategy is career laddering, by which individuals move up the organizational ladder based on education, experience, and expertise. Career laddering is an effective tool for retaining employees because it offers the opportunity to assume positions with more responsibility without having to leave one's organization. Many organizations, such as the Veteran's Administration, offer career laddering for dietetics professionals in both clinical nutrition and administration.

Population trends also favor job security for dietetics professionals. These trends include the growth and aging of the U.S. population, increases in life expectancy, and an increase in the prevalence of obesity. Adult obesity in the United States has increased by 60% since 1991 and affects approximately one-quarter of people 20 years old or older.[28] In 1991, only four states had an obesity prevalence above 15%, compared to 49 states in 2004.[29] These trends will increase the demand for MNT and perhaps change the focus more toward prevention rather than treatment of the disease.

Continuing professional education (CPE) and career planning are necessary for dietetics professionals to maintain competency and progress toward a career goal while remaining open to change directions due to personal choice or changes in the market. The Commission on Dietetic Registration (CDR) has implemented a system of CPE in which each member identifies the skills and knowledge needed for his or her individual professional competence and designs a personalized educational program to meet those needs. The CDR Professional Development Portfolio was implemented in 2001, with all RDs and DTRs using this system to maintain their credentials in 2006.

CAREER DEVELOPMENT

Dietetics professionals have many avenues through which they may advance their careers (Figure 1-3). These may include advancement in the job itself, committee participation, research activities, publications, and invited presentations. A dietitian's career generally begins in an entry-level position as a clinical or staff dietitian. With training, experience, and specialty certification, a dietitian can generally progress to an advanced practitioner role. Such an individual may then opt for a leadership role, perhaps as manager of a group of dietetics professionals, and eventually a director-level position. The truly innovative individuals possess global cognitive skills, which help them create opportunities; they also have the ambition and dedication to see that these opportunities come to fruition.

Dietitians may also expand their careers through committee participation. This often begins at their place of employment, such as a departmental or institutionwide committee. Eventually, the dietitian may opt to sit on committees at the local, state, national, and international levels. These types of activities are important to the individual, the institution he or she represents, and the profession as a whole. It provides opportunities for individuals to make professional contacts and learn skills that may not be part of their usual job responsibilities. The institution will benefit from increased recognition and from the employee's expanded skills. The profession will benefit from increased marketing of professional dietetics skills, particularly when it involves an interdisciplinary committee.

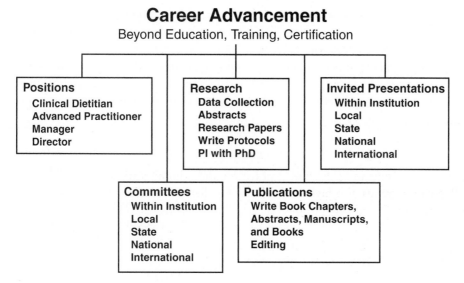

FIGURE 1-3   *Career avenues for dietetics professionals.*

Dietetics professionals can promote their careers and the profession through research. Outcomes research is highly regarded by all professions and in all areas of practice, whether it is clinical, administration, or education. This places the dietetics professional in the same arena as many of the other healthcare professionals. It brings a level of credibility and respect to the individual and the profession that is often difficult to obtain in any other manner. Those individuals who possess a terminal degree (e.g., PhD) may also enhance their credibility and respect by obtaining grant funding.

Dietetics professionals can also benefit through writing for publication and public speaking. Initial writing projects may be for smaller publications and limited audiences such as newsletters. With skill and persistence, dietitians can graduate to writing book chapters or review articles for national journals. If one's research skills have progressed as well, the publications may be in the form of abstracts or research manuscripts. Eventually, dietitians can progress to the point where they conceptualize the idea for a book, write the proposal and edit a contributed book, or become editor-in-chief for a national journal. Similarly, public speaking skills can be developed by dietitians and used to advance their careers. Initial presentations may be modest affairs involving small audiences, usually at the place of employment. Eventually, presentations can progress to larger audiences at the local, state, or national level. This may even lead to international speaking engagements once the dietitian's career has advanced to the point where he or she has been writing and lecturing extensively and has become a recognized expert in a particular area.

LEGAL ISSUES AFFECTING DIETETICS PROFESSIONALS

State laws regulate dietetics professionals and the practice of dietetics, much as such laws regulate the practice of medicine, nursing, pharmacy and other health professions. The purpose of these laws is to protect the public from harmful, incompetent, or negligent nutrition practices. The laws and level of protection vary from state to state. Those states that have *licensing* have statutes that include an explicitly defined scope of practice; it is illegal to perform work in the profession without first obtaining a license from the state. Some states have *statutory certification*, which limits use of particular titles to persons meeting predetermined requirements, while persons not certified can still practice the occupation or profession. *Registration* is the least restrictive form of state regulation. As with certification, unregistered persons are permitted to practice the profession. Typically, exams are not given and enforcement of the registration requirement is minimal.

Since professional licenses are issued by individual states, variability is found in the practice of dietetics as defined by state laws. In some states the practice of dietetics is defined as those duties performed by a licensed dietitian, and the scope of practice may be limited. For example, only a licensed dietitian may offer nutrition assessment, nutrition counseling, or education, and develop and evaluate nutrition care standards. The Practice Act requires that anyone who engages in these activities must be licensed as a dietitian or specifically exempt from licensure. The law may also define MNT and where it is to be practiced

Issues to Ponder

- What are the pros and cons of state licensure versus certification?
- What impact has licensure had on the profession?

(e.g., hospitals, extended-care facilities). In some states the title "dietitian" or "nutritionist" is protected, meaning that only persons holding this license can use one of these titles.

The degree of regulation is of little value if there is not an effective board to ensure that the laws are enforced. The board not only protects the public from unqualified individuals who attempt to infringe on the practice of dietetics but also polices its members to ensure that they are in compliance with the law.

Dietetics professionals are expected to practice according to a strict ethical code, abiding by all local, state, and federal laws. All healthcare professionals have standards of care that must be followed to provide quality patient care. Negligence occurs when there is a breach of these duties or standard of care.[30] Injuries occur as a result of this breach and damages result from these injuries. If all of these elements can be proven, the healthcare professional may be found negligent. In addition to practicing according to appropriate standards of care, it is important that the dietetics professional has a current license in those states requiring one and maintain all necessary certifications and registrations. Development and adherence to policies, procedures, and protocols will minimize liability risk. Informed consent must be obtained for all research protocols, to obtain additional patient-related information, or to share patient-related information.

FUTURE DIRECTIONS

The role of dietetics professionals is expanding and evolving. Dietitians are functioning at a higher level than they have in the past, with greater emphasis on cross training and multiskilling to acquire and practice new skills not traditionally taught in a dietetics program. Many dietitians have increased administrative responsibilities and some manage several departments, making them more attractive to prospective employers and providing cost benefits to the consumer. The quality of healthcare is improved by the dietitian's ability to view a problem from more than one vantage point. This ability also eliminates redundancy and serves to increase cross- and intra-department collaboration and cooperation.

Many of our current healthcare trends will persist. The healthcare field will continue to experience downsizing and cost containment as institutions struggle with economic constraints. Organizational restructuring and consolidation will continue as institutions attempt to maximize their assets and minimize their liabilities. At the same time, there will be an increased emphasis on quality management and outcome measures. The technological advances over the last several decades will continue and will affect how dietetics professionals practice. Clinically, research will continue in many areas—including obesity, diabetes, genetics, nutrient pharmacology, and complementary and alternative medicine—and the opportunities for dietetics professionals to participate in research will increase.

Dietitians need to remain abreast of and anticipate societal trends and changes in the provision of healthcare. It is vital for dietetics professionals to continue to acquire new skills in response to these changes so that they can take advantage of opportunities to further expand their roles. This will ensure that the profession will remain a vital component of the healthcare team and that dietetics professionals will continue to be recognized by the public and fellow healthcare professionals as the most valued source of nutrition information.

REFERENCES

1. Jarratt J, Mahaffie JB. Key trends affecting the dietetics profession and the American Dietetic Association. J Am Diet Assoc 2002;102:S1821–S1839.
2. Diet, nutrition and the prevention of chronic diseases. World Health Organization Technical Report Series. 2003;916: i–viii, 1–149.
3. Pate RR, Pratt M, Blair S, et al. Physical activity and public health: a recommendation from the Centers for Disease Control and Prevention and the American College of Sports Medicine. JAMA 1995;273:402–407.
4. Wade JE. Role of a clinical dietitian specialist on a nutrition support service. J Am Diet Assoc 1977;70:185–189.
5. Baird SC, Armstrong RVL. The ADA role delineation for the field of clinical dietetics. J Am Diet Assoc 1981;78:370–382.
6. Johnson EQ. The therapeutic dietitian's role in the alimentation group. J Am Diet Assoc 1973;62:648–650.
7. Schiller MR, Vivian VM. Role of the clinical dietitian. J Am Diet Assoc 1974;65:284–290.
8. O'Sullivan Maillet J, Skates J, Pritchett E. American Dietetic Association: scope of dietetics practice framework. J Am Diet Assoc 2005;105:634–640. Available at: http://www.eatright.org/member/policyinitiatives/83_21717.cfm. Accessed September 12, 2005.
9. Kieselhorst KJ, Skates J, Pritchett E. American Dietetic Association: standards of practice in nutrition care and updated standards of professional performance. J Am Diet Assoc 2005;105:641–645.
10. Mueller CM, Colaizzo-Anas T, Shronts EP, et al. Order writing for parenteral nutrition by registered dietitians. J Am Diet Assoc 1996;96:764–768.
11. Rogers D. Report on the ADA 2002 Dietetics Compensation and Benefits Survey. J Am Diet Assoc 2003;103:243–255.
12. Touger-Decker R. The new advanced clinical nutrition degree: the practice doctorate in clinical nutrition. Nutrition 2004;20:494–495.
13. Puckett RP. Education and the dietetics profession. J Am Diet Assoc 1997;97:252–253.
14. Maillet J, Oakley CB, Mitchell BE. Dietetics education today: dynamic, diverse and essential. J Am Diet Assoc 2002;102:1736.
15. Canter DD, Nettles MF. Dietitians as multidepartment managers in healthcare settings. J Am Diet Assoc 2003;103:237–240.

16. Naylor M, Brooten D, Campbell R, et al. Comprehensive discharge planning and home follow-up of hospitalized elders. JAMA 1999;281:613–620.
17. American Dietetic Association. Nutrition and You: Trends Survey. Chicago: American Dietetic Association, 2000.
18. Fuhrman MP. Issues facing dietetics professionals: challenges and opportunities. J Am Diet Assoc 2002;102:1618–1620.
19. Guthrie AF, Myers EF. USDA's Economic Research Service supports nutrition and health outcomes research. J Am Diet Assoc 2002;102:293–297.
20. American Dietetic Association. ADA Strategic Plan. Available at: http://eatright.org/Member/Governance/85_9457.cfm. Accessed October 15, 2003.
21. American Association for the Advancement of Science. In tight economic climate, R&D funding tops record. Available at: http://www.aaas.org/news/releases/2003/. Accessed July 25, 2003.
22. Report of the American Dietetic Association/ADA Foundation/Commission on Dietetic Registration 2004 Dietetics Professionals Needs Assessment. J Am Diet Assoc 2005;105:1348–1355.
23. Byrk JA, Soto TK. Report on the 1999 membership database of the American Dietetic Association. J Am Diet Assoc 2001;101:947–953.
24. Performance, Proficiency, and Value Tactical Workgroup. Performance, proficiency and value of the dietetics profession. J Am Diet Assoc 2002;102:1304–1315.
25. US Department of Labor, Bureau of Labor Statistics. National, state, and metropolitan area occupational employment. Available at: http://www.bls.gov/oes/2001/oes290000.html/. Accessed July 24, 2003.
26. Fullerton, HN. Laborforce projections to 2008: steady growth and changing composition. Monthly Labor Review 1999;122;19–32.
27. Commission on Accreditation for Dietetics Education. Trends in dietetics education. J Am Diet Assoc 2001;101:10–12.
28. US Department of Health and Human Services. Surgeon General's Call to Action to Prevent and Decrease Obesity and Overweight. Washington, DC: U.S. Government Printing Office, 2001.
29. Centers for Disease Control. Behavioral risk factor surveillance system. Available at: www.cdc.gov/needphp/dnpa/obesity/trend/maps/index.htm. Accessed October 3, 2005.
30. Ashley RC. Telemedicine: legal, ethical, and liability considerations. J Am Diet Assoc 2002;102:267–269.

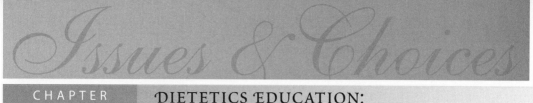

CHAPTER

2

DIETETICS EDUCATION:
PAST, PRESENT, AND FUTURE

Deborah D. Canter

In an article in the 1934 issue of the *Journal of the American Dietetic Association* (JADA), author Sarah Tyson Rorer, considered by many to be the first dietitian in this country, reminisced about her early days as a dietetics educator: "I was considered a very severe teacher by my pupils. It was not because I wanted to be severe, but because I wanted to send out pupils who knew how to do things. I believe in the education of hands and brains, working together."[1]

How much today's dietetics educators would agree with Ms. Rorer! Like her, we "believe in the education of hands and brains, working together." However, the sheer amount of knowledge and skills deemed essential for today's entry-level dietitian would amaze Ms. Rorer and her early colleagues.

The purpose of this chapter is to look back at the beginnings of dietetics education, chart the road to the present day, and pose some questions for the future. The journey is fascinating and reflects the exponential growth of knowledge encompassed by the field of dietetics. Figure 2-1 highlights key milestones.

IN THE BEGINNING: IT WAS ALL ABOUT FOOD

Sarah Rorer, opening her Philadelphia Cooking School in 1878, founded, at the request of several noted physicians, a diet kitchen where they could send a prescription and get, in return, "food well prepared for special diseases."[1] The curriculum included 10 classes on chemistry, 10 on cooking for the sick, and several on physiology and hygiene. Students were taught that diabetic patients had to avoid sugar and starches and that nephrotic patients must avoid protein. They learned about food values, proteins, and carbohydrates, as little was known at the time about calories or vitamins. As one of her students put it, "We were taught to cook, and to cook well."[2] Twelve students graduated from Ms. Rorer's cooking school each year for 33 years and graduates went on to become "superintendents of diet" in the kitchens of that day's leading hospitals.

THE AMERICAN DIETETIC ASSOCIATION AND ITS INFLUENCE ON DIETETICS EDUCATION

Around 1909, a small group of women interested in hospital dietetics joined with others from school lunchrooms, college dormitories, and other institutional food-service operations to form what was known as the Institution Administration Section of the American Home Economics Association (AHEA). In 1917, the United States

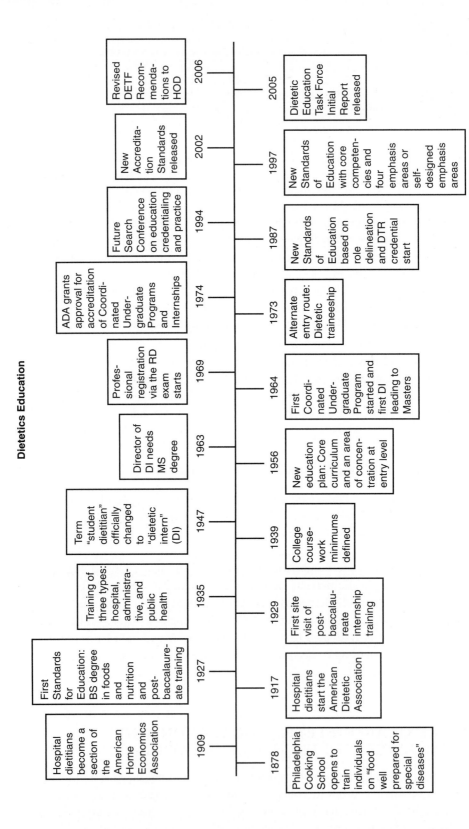

FIGURE 2-1 *Key milestones in dietetics education.*

was deeply involved in World War I; thus AHEA decided not to hold its annual meeting that year. However, those engaged in hospital foodservice and war-related food conservation efforts decided that they should meet because of the importance of their activities to the war effort. This group called a meeting in Cleveland, Ohio, for October 18 to 20 of that year. The culmination of that meeting was the birth of the American Dietetic Association on October 20, 1917.[3]

It did not take long for the dietitians' passion for education to surface. One of the first articles in JADA was "A Combination Theory and Practice Course for Student Dietitians," written by Florence A. Otis. The opening sentences of Ms. Otis's article show that, even then, there was a dichotomy between the foodservice management side of dietetics and the growing pull of the knowledge base in nutrition:

> At each annual meeting of the Dietetics Association, one cannot resist enthusiastic interest in the greater place being given to the rapid development of the study of diet in relation to disease and to the consequently greater responsibilities placed upon the hospital dietitian. She has been brought into closer contact with the medical departments because of the greater recognition given to food habits in the diagnosis of disease as well as the need of careful planning and supervision of special diets in their treatment, so many of which involve metabolic disturbances of such a nature that correction through food intake is possible. At the same time, the dietitian has not been released from the responsibility of the management of the whole dietary department—of buying equipment, supervising supplies, serving, and solving the "help" problem. Consequently, we who have a part in teaching students, whether in college or during their hospital training, must recognize the need of including institutional training in their course of study, and likewise scientific work that shall afford a usable knowledge of metabolic processes, normal and abnormal. The dietitian must merit the confidence of doctors, nurses, and patients, as well as the confidence of employees.[4]

Only a year later, in a March 1926 article, Agnes Fay Morgan suggested that the trend in dietetics education "will be toward the medical rather than the so-called practical side." As she indicated, "Further practice in large quantity cookery, marketing and recipe development is not likely to seem necessary." She believed that dietetics education should proceed along the path of medical training to include the study of symptoms of disease, pathology of diseased tissues and clinical experience in the recognition of these conditions. Ms. Morgan believed that such an educational path would emphasize the dietitian's close relationship to the "physician's end of the hospital and away from the nurse's."[5]

The definitive "Standard Course for Student Dietitians in Hospitals" was approved at the meeting of the American Dietetic Association in October 1927 and was published in the December issue of JADA.[6] The outline focused primarily on the hands-on, postbaccalaureate segment of dietetics training. Entrance requirements were relatively broad; the prospective dietetics intern had to be at least 21 years of age and have the minimum of a "bachelor's degree with a major in foods and nutrition from a college or university of recognized rank." The hospital sponsoring the dietetics course of study had to be a member of the American Hospital Association with all dietitians employed there eligible for membership in the ADA. The hospital had to have a capacity of 100 beds and the chief dietitian had to control all general and therapeutic diets, child feeding, infant formulas, private room service, and "personal dietaries."[6]

The internship was required to be at least 6 months in length, with a constant enrollment of at least two students working a minimum of 42 hours a week under the supervision of the dietetics staff. Interns were expected to attend weekly conferences, classes, or seminars. Experience was provided in administrative practice (for at least 2 months or longer); "dietotherapy" (for at least 2 months or longer); practice in the theory of teaching dietetics to student nurses; and an assortment of social service, medical clinic, metabolic ward, or laboratory assignments; field trips; rotations in housekeeping and laundry; and other affiliations that the preceptors felt would round out the internship experience.[6]

The March 1929 issue of JADA listed 33 hospitals as offering the standard course as approved by the ADA. The first site visits of programs were instituted late that year when ADA President Anna Boller said, "It is apparent that a method which depends entirely upon an individual's evaluation of her own work as a basis for approval is not entirely satisfactory." The chairman of the education section and the approval committee announced that a committee of three would visit each hospital on the approved list. The committee members were chosen for their ability in the educational field, their understanding of the hospital situation, and also on the basis of geography. The personnel of the committee were charged to "investigate and inspect the course."

Mary Northrop addressed the concept of developing professionalism in prospective dietitians in an article in the December 1929 issue of JADA. According to Ms. Northrop:

> We must take the college girl who comes to us and make her into a professional woman; that six months is too short a time in which to accomplish so complete a metamorphosis is obvious. It seems probable that we shall be forced either to increase the length of our courses or to demand that the colleges send us more mature and competent students. Another problem which we should be considering is giving our students an interest in their surroundings outside the limits of the dietary department. Many dietitians, engrossed in their own problems, fail to see their work in relation to the rest of the hospital and lack sympathy and appreciation for other groups who are also working for the well-being of the patients. The more we teach our students about the hospital as a whole and the dietary department in its relationship to the whole, the more successful they will be in working with other groups.[8]

Ms. Northrop also emphasized the need for teaching the code of ethics, the etiquette or protocol expected of a new dietitian, and the importance of maintaining a professional appearance. She stressed the need to have student dietitians who understood "dignity combined with courtesy, and friendliness combined with reserve" in working with other hospital staff.

THE 1930S: DEFINING AND REFINING THE ROLE OF THE DIETITIAN

JADA during the 1930s is replete with articles addressing various issues related to dietetics education. The commentaries reflect the growing diversity of dietetics practice and the concerns of dietetics educators regarding the goals and methods of the training programs of the time. A definite shift is seen from dietetics education and training as merely an apprenticeship under the tutelage of senior practicing professionals to a systematic approach with objectives and standards of education.

By 1932, the association's policy became that all dietetics education programs or "courses" would be inspected every 2 years; new courses applying for approval would be tentatively approved on the alternate year. Also in this year, the proposed "Outline for Administrative Student Dietitians" was published. The first program at The Women's Educational and Industrial Union in Boston was granted approval in 1933. In 1935, the executive committee accepted the outline for a proposed course for students interested in a food clinic or community nutrition and Frances Stern at the Boston Dispensary began the first course of this type. Thus, the three types of dietetics training—the hospital course, the administrative course, and the food clinic or public health course—were established; the legacy of that trilogy remains with us today.[7]

At the beginning of the 1930s, the role of nutrition in medicine and in medical education was a controversial subject. Few medical schools had any kind of course work in normal nutrition or the therapeutic use of foods.[9] Although the medical community of the time may have had mixed feelings about the role of nutrition, dietetics educators continued to prepare their young charges for what they believed was the growing role of the dietitian in medical care. Use of case studies was touted as a teaching tool, as a means to introduce the dietetics student to clinical practice. The prevailing belief was that "If a patient is not properly educated regarding his diet before he is discharged from the hospital, the dietitian has failed in her treatment."[10] Making sure that dietetics interns brought the right knowledge to the internship experience continued to be a subject of discussion.

Mary De Garmo Bryan, in a 1934 JADA article, brought to the ADA membership at large the issue of the rapidly growing nature of dietetics practice and its impact on dietetics education. Ms. Bryan stated that "courses for student dietitians should never become standardized," as the field of dietetics was developing so rapidly that new facts and new experiences could and should be added almost daily to the "curriculum." She discussed public health as a growing area of interest while at the same time reemphasizing the importance of the administrative role of the dietitian. She emphasized the increased pressure for the dietitian to carefully control the dietary department's budget, as food and the labor to prepare it was "the largest single item in the hospital budget." Bryan reiterated the importance of the postbaccalaureate hospital internship experience in the overall preparation of the entry-level dietitian and reported that 13 colleges had arranged for credit toward the master's degree for work during hospital training.[11]

Several articles in JADA during the 1930s dealt with the role of dietitians as teachers, particularly in nursing programs.[12,13] Lenna F. Cooper brought up the need for course work in educational methods, curriculum construction, and psychology as part of the academic preparation of the dietitian. Ms. Cooper bemoaned the problem of the dietitian-teacher trying to keep current with nutrition developments because, as she put it, "the essentials—even the fundamental principles of nutrition—have increased so remarkably in the last few years that it is almost impossible to discriminate without omitting certain essentials."[12]

In 1936, an editorial in JADA contrasted the definition of dietetics with the reality of dietetics practice at the time. Dietetics was defined by the Bureau of Vocational Information as the science of planning, calculating, and preparing diets based upon a scientific knowledge of digestion, metabolism, and excretion. Although the actual duties of a dietitian were largely determined by the institution where she worked, the major classifications were generally administrative and therapeutic. The nine duties most frequently cited as part of the dietitian's job description at this period were "(1) planning menus and meals; (2) planning regular and special diets; (3) consulting with doctors on diet therapy; (4) preparing and serving food; (5) ordering and purchasing supplies; (6) hiring and supervising help; (7) keeping records and inventories; (8) teaching student dietitians and nurses; and (9) teaching patients, a new innovation." This listing of duties shows the growing diversity of dietetics practice, branching out from the profession's roots in food preparation and foodservice administration. The editorial poses the still-unanswered question: "Are we asking dietitians to be superhuman? The great problem of directors of college home economics departments and of hospital training courses has been the time required to give the curriculum and training necessary for these varied responsibilities."[14] How much more is this dilemma true for 21st-century dietetics!

A classic article, which was a retrospective at the time of its publication, is "Pioneering in Dietetics," by Mary H. Philbrick, in the July 1936 JADA. This delightful article is a compilation of "I remember when I was a dietetics student" stories from various association leaders of the time. It should be required reading for today's dietetics students and interns. The author and others reminisce about the days "when a student was looked upon merely as a source of cheap labor and experience was gained solely in the training school of hard knocks." The last sentence of the article is a true "take-home message": "Every young dietitian should realize that each new experience, no matter how difficult, if properly met, is but a step up to a coveted place which may now seem unattainable."[15] The November 1936 JADA also provided some insightful statistics regarding dietetics students of the time. Analysis of data showed that in 1934 and 1935, some 313 dietetics students were in training and 262, or 84%, were employed by the end of 1935, 73% of them by hospitals. Student stipends for internship experiences ranged from a low of $35 to a high of $85 per month, with room and board included.[16]

In a 1938 JADA article, Florence Bateson asked the pointed question: "Should not the ultimate aim of the hospital training courses be the development of judgment?" She defined the essence of judgment to be the discriminating application of knowledge to the circumstances immediately at hand and made the case that it is not *what* is offered in the training programs but *how* it is offered that determines the success of the dietetics training experience. Ms. Bateson was concerned, as are educators today, over whether the training as delivered developed in students the qualities of leadership necessary to the continued advancement of dietetics as a profession.[17]

Another 1938 contribution outlined a "Questionnaire for the Would-Be Dietitian" that could very well be administered to today's aspiring dietitians. According to the questionnaire's designers, a high percentage of unfavorable answers to this questionnaire (Table 2-1) would suggest that the person answering needed an "attitude adjustment" or else should consider a change to another field of study![18]

The decade of the 1930s came to a close with an article discussing the college and university training of the dietitian. Although previous articles had focused almost exclusively on the hospital-based training program, this article finally ad-

TABLE 2-1	Questionnaire for the Aspiring Dietitian

How many food dislikes do you have?

Do you eat a wide variety of foods?

Do you like to eat?

Do you drink milk?

Do you follow the principles of good nutrition?

Do you have good health?

Do you like to cook?

Are you ever on the alert for new ideas in food preparation and service?

Are you interested in the use of leftovers?

Do you have a knack for making food attractive?

Are you interested in the food of different sections of this country?

Are you interested in the food of different nationalities?

Are you a good taster?

Are you cost-conscious?

Do you like to direct the work of others?

Do you object to long and irregular hour of work?

Do you like to teach others?

Do you have good sales resistance?

Are you calm in emergencies?

Do you meet people easily?

Are you familiar with the various possibilities for positions as a dietitian?

How many dietitians do you know?

Adapted with permission from Fleck.[18]

dressed the prerequisite college course work preceding the internship experience. At the time of this publication, there were 52 approved hospital courses, 4 administrative courses, and 1 food clinic course, making possible the training of 434 student dietitians in 1939.[19]

Ms. Gleiser, the author of this article, made the case that the college education of the prospective dietitian should be more than just a matter of ticking off the required courses in the physical and behavioral sciences, food, institution management, and nutrition. She put forth five suggestions. First, she believed that colleges should have a system of student counseling that nurtured the student from freshman to senior. She suggested that students should have a dietetics faculty counselor who could introduce the realities of dietetics practice, both pleasant and unpleasant. The second suggestion was the provision of an orientation course to help prospective students decide whether they had the qualities necessary for successful dietetics practice. One quote is especially telling regarding intern selection procedures of the day: "It is cited that some dietitians will not select a young woman who is less than 5 feet 2 inches tall. The short applicant, therefore, must have other qualifications to make up for this disadvantage."[19] Likewise, the underweight or overweight student was counseled to realize that she must learn to control her own weight if she were to run the gauntlet of admission to a hospital training course successfully.

The third practice proposed by Ms. Gleiser was the use of a "personality report," which she believed should be filed on every student by every instructor of a

home economics laboratory class, so that by the time the student was ready to graduate, there would be an average of 14 ratings from instructors who had seen the
student in varying situations and unrelated types of courses. Students were to be assessed on appearance and manner, poise, physical vigor, disposition (cheerful or
moody), voice quality, power of expression, character, refinement, tact, qualities of
leadership, judgment, initiative, industry, resourcefulness, attitude toward work,
self-confidence, willingness to cooperate, promise of growth, scholarship, technical
ability, and general ability. This sounds very reminiscent of the recommendation
form required today by every dietetics internship and coordinated program as part
of the application materials.

Fourth, the suggestion was made that the summer vacation between the jun-
ior and senior years of college be spent working in a hospital dietary department.
A member of the hospital's management department was encouraged to observe
the student, confer with dietitians who had worked with her, and then submit a
letter to the college administrator regarding the student's interests, abilities,
conduct, and overall attitude. Last, Ms. Gleiser suggested that in every dietetics-
related course, the student should be given the opportunity to show initiative,
power of organization, ability to solve problems and apply judgment, and independent thinking. She concluded by stressing the critical importance of cooperation between university faculty and dietitians in the field to best prepare students
for dietetics practice.[19]

The years 1938 and 1939 saw the introduction and revision of Outline 1 of required subjects for college students pursuing dietetics practice. Minimum course-
work and suggested additional requirements included courses in chemistry, biology,
social sciences, education, foods, nutrition, and institution management. New
courses recommended as additions to the curriculum included quantitative analytical chemistry and food chemistry, food economics or marketing, additional courses
in nutrition to include child nutrition, and at least 12 credit hours of institutional
management, including buying and accounting.[20]

THE 1940S: WORLD WAR II AND ITS IMPACT ON DIETETICS AND DIETETICS EDUCATION

The decade of the 1940s opened with the appointment of the first ADA educational
director, Gladys E. Hall. Her duties included the inspection of the established courses
and assisting in the development of new ones. As is still true today, having a full-time
professional overseeing the educational program was extremely valuable because of
the continuity provided. When Ms. Hall became the ADA's executive secretary in
1944, Lucille Refshauge succeeded her as educational director. During the war years
of the 1940s, these two women were instrumental in helping meet the dramatic increase in demand for dietetics services. The number of students in training doubled
from 500 to 1,000. An accelerated program for preparing students was developed
whereby a student would take 6 months of the regular course and then go into the
U.S. Armed Services as an apprentice dietitian for 6 months. Similar arrangements
were made to release students to civilian hospitals at the end of 9 or 10 months. The
accelerated program was discontinued in 1945, but the development and implementation of such a venture showed ADA's commitment to the war effort.[7]

In today's world of dietetics practice, we talk much about the importance of management skills and the ability to market one's expertise to administration. Obviously this is not a new concept, as evidenced by the opening paragraphs of this 1941 JADA article:

> The hospital dietitian is primarily an administrative officer. She is responsible for about one-fourth of the total expenditures of the hospital and for that reason the hospital administrator should be more interested in the effectiveness with which she manages her department than in the salary it is necessary to pay to secure and retain a fully qualified person. [21]

Dr. Warren Morrill, the author of this article, sounded the call to dietetics educators not to forget the importance of educating hospital dietitians in management skills, not in lieu of the allure of the therapeutic aspect of practice but in addition to those skills. As the country braced for the impending Second World War and organizations everywhere had to pursue new levels of efficiency, hospital administrators started looking for skilled administrative dietitians and found the available supply to be small. Dr. Morrill believed that administrative dietitians should be an integral part of the hospital management team. The development of critical thinking and problem-solving skills was encouraged as part of dietetics education, particularly in the internship. To quote Dr. Morrill:

> The basic course in dietetics is in the basic sciences and their application on a laboratory basis. No school has yet designed a course in the management of a sulky maid, a temperamental chef, a bull-headed butcher, a slick salesman or a "picky" patient. If the hospital is to have dietitians capable of meeting the everyday practical problems of dietetic management, it must train them itself. And it is the dietetics internship which solves the problem just as it is the medical internship that makes doctors out of recently graduated medical students.[21]

An August–September 1941 article posed questions as to the best curriculum to prepare future dietitians. Early research in dietetics education seemed to focus on asking graduates "What courses proved to be most helpful to you in your work as a dietitian?" The article's author believed that the "considered opinions of persons who are in the field are badly needed to help colleges shape the curriculum."[22] The article elucidated the early approach of designating course work to be taken rather than objectives to be achieved. However, the author pointed out that this approach was in direct contrast to the trend just starting in teacher-training programs, calling for focus on outcomes rather than process.

Evaluation of the effectiveness of the curriculum was made by studying the job specifications set up by employers of dietitians. Requirements showed that employers were looking for someone who "knew good food," was innovative, cost-conscious, pleasant, had good people skills, and who knew how to meet nutrition needs while maintaining high standards in foodservice.[22] There was a continuous demand for well-trained dietitians to work in hospitals, school lunchrooms, commercial foodservice, aviation and railroad services, state institutions, and army service.

Margaret Ohlson, in a 1941 article, voiced concerns about the pressure to meet ADA academic requirements while concurrently allowing students a truly broadening university education. Her concern might sound very familiar to today's university dietetics faculty, particularly in coordinated programs in dietetics where elective credits are virtually nonexistent:

> The struggle in the college to dovetail the subject matter requirements of the American Dietetic Association with the demands of the college administration for adequate prerequisite courses and some cultural background, results in a program with long hours of laboratory and very few elective credits during the college years. In other words, the college student majoring in dietetics is being pressed into a mold which guarantees a certain amount of theoretical, professional information but little spontaneous development of the individual. [23]

Ms. Ohlson concludes her article by saying that crowded college schedules encouraged superficial leadership as well as superficial learning and posed the challenge that it was time the dietetics profession scrutinized the recommended educational program for the flexibility needed by students in order to learn, grow, and develop the necessary leadership skills. An editorial in a 1942 issue of JADA echoed these sentiments, indicating that "a broad education should make a broad outlook, which is needed now (during wartime) more than ever before."[24]

A call for student dietitians appeared in the October 1944 issue of JADA. College graduates who had majored in dietetics were solicited for training as student dietitians in army and Veterans Administration (VA) hospitals. Student dietitians in the army were promised $720 a year and after 6 months would be advanced to apprentice dietitian at $1,752 per year. After another 6 months, they were eligible for appointment as second lieutenants in the army. The VA paid its student dietitians $1,752 a year. After 12 months of training as students, they were eligible for appointments as staff dietitians at $2,190 a year. Applicants between the ages of 20 and 40 were invited to apply.[25]

The breadth of experiences afforded the student dietitian continued to expand in the mid-1940s. By this time, 953 students were enrolled in the postbaccalaureate experience. There were 67 approved hospital courses with 865 students enrolled. Courses covered work in administration, therapeutics, community education, and professional education. About one-third of the time was devoted to some phase of administration. There were seven approved courses that focused on the administrative aspect of dietetics, offering highly specialized training in those areas not covered by the hospital or food clinic courses. Administrative courses offered opportunity for experience in more than one unit, with several types of foodservice, and with a variety of equipment and cost levels. Housekeeping administration was also included, including housekeeping methods, care of rooms, furnishings and equipment, cleaning procedures, study of cost and selection of new furnishings, equipment, supplies, and maintenance. There were 62 students enrolled in these specialized administrative courses. This need for dietitians to be experts in multiskilling is even more important today than in the 1940s. Today's administrative dietitians are often called upon to be multidepartment managers, using their administrative skills to oversee departments beyond food and nutrition services.

The food clinic course offered preparation, experience, and training in the dietetics treatment of the ambulatory patient and the teaching of professional and nonprofessional groups and the general public. Twenty-seven student dietitians opted for this specialization, which sounds similar to a community nutrition focus of today. Graduate credit was optional or required in 20 of the 75 courses described.[26]

In 1947, debate centered on what participants in the approved dietetics courses should be called. Directors of approved courses did not feel that the term "student dietitian" did justice to the type of graduate preparation being afforded in their three kinds of approved courses. On February 15, 1947, the executive board of ADA approved the term "dietetics intern" for official use by the Association.[27] Later in 1947, a new recruitment booklet entitled "A Bibliography of Dietetic Careers" was introduced to help draw women into the profession. It offered a list of approximately 175 magazine and journal articles, books, and pamphlets dealing with the occupational aspects of dietetics. The booklet was organized according to the various areas of dietetics practice and included sections entitled "Careers in Dietetics," "The Training of Dietitian," "The Dietitian in the Hospital," "The Dietitian in Government Service," "The Dietitian in a Food Clinic," "The Dietitian in Public Health Work," "The Dietitian in the School Lunchroom," "The Dietitian in Colleges and Universities," "The Dietitian in Industry," and "The Dietitian in Business."[28]

EXPANDING OUR HORIZONS: DIETETICS EDUCATION IN THE 1950S AND 1960S

The decreasing number of articles in JADA in the 1950s and 1960s related to dietetics education reflects not a lack of interest or concern about education but rather the growing maturity and breadth of dietetics practice. Education-related publications decreased in number while publications related to research and practice grew. Nonetheless, timely and provocative pieces continued to be published.

Gertrude Miller posed a "hot button" issue in the August 1950 issue of JADA. Her article brought up an interesting and thought-provoking issue. What is the common denominator that links all dietitians, no matter what their area of practice? Ms. Miller's article addressed the issue of segmentation, or specialization, within the profession. Her question echoes down the decades to us today: "Perhaps it is pertinent to ask whether, in the process of growth, we have changed so much that we no longer are what we are presumed to be; or whether we—all of us—still have major skills and knowledge in common."[29]

Her premise is that there is a common need for a sound knowledge of nutrition since it, as she put it, is "probably the *one* universal which binds us together," no matter what our area of dietetics practice. She goes on in the article to specifically address the importance of nutrition knowledge to the administrative dietitian and makes the point that the administrative person is still an integral part "of the medical team." Ms. Miller summarized her case by saying:

> Of the skills we hold in common, knowledge of nutrition is the most important because upon it we base our claim to professional status as one of the medical team; because it is expected of us by professional and lay groups; because when we put the patient into correct focus in relation to our work, we must have it; because it is inseparable from daily contacts; and, because it can be part of a significant administrative technique.[29]

The first educational requirements, released by the Association in 1927, had been adapted through the years by taking the basic requirement of a degree in foods and nutrition for everyone and adding 6 hours of institutional management in 1931. Specialized education for specialized areas of practice became a reality with Outline I, adopted in 1940. A new committee was appointed in 1952 to investigate and recommend changes. Their plan became known as Outline II, and it set forth requirements in four areas of knowledge, with students required to complete a specified number of hours in each of the four categories.[30] The "Current Comment" section in the February 1955 issue of JADA could have been dated today. The author, Dr. Ercel Eppright, said that "one of the principal problems in the undergraduate education of the dietitian is the ever-widening scope of subject matter envisioned as necessary to produce a good citizen, an educated person, a homemaker, and a dietitian."[31] He addressed the problem of "curricular inflation," where more and more courses are added, electives are squeezed out, and total credits for graduation are increased. Dr. Eppright proposed that the same objectives of dietetics education—that graduates would have technical knowledge, skill, judgment, vision, the spirit of service, the ability to get along well with people, and an urge for continued study and professional growth—are also the objectives of general or liberal education. A quote by Dr. Virgil Hanscher is pertinent for today's dietetics educators:

> We need to review our curricula often. We need to view them with a practical eye and to re-evaluate and eliminate and consolidate until we have only the fundamentals remaining. What we teach should be basic. It must lead the student out of those things which he can learn for himself, and it should be taught with that imagination and vision, that liberality of mind and spirit, necessary to assure that what the student learns will be learned in relation to the whole complex of modern knowledge and modern civilization. If this can be done, thousands of young men and women who otherwise might become merely narrow technicians will become not only able and effective citizens, but even their professional competence will be heightened because their eyes have been opened and their horizons widened to things beyond their childhood gaze.[32]

Dr. Eppright also discussed the phenomenon of colleges reducing laboratory time or eliminating it all together because of cost and difficulty of administration. He was especially concerned about the need to develop skills, particularly in food preparation and service. As Dr. Eppright pointed out, "With the public, the status of the dietitian rests heavily on her skill in planning and serving meals and in preparing foods. In fact, our profession loses prestige in the eyes of the public every time a qualified dietitian permits food of poor quality to be served."[32]

In 1956, a review was made of previous ADA academic plans, internship requirements, and ADA membership requirements. After two years of research, including discussions with faculty members in college programs, internship directors, the ADA House of Delegates (HOD), and ADA members, a new educational plan emerged which came to be known as Plan III. This plan contained a required core curriculum, one area of emphasis (food management, education, or business), and one area of concentration (general, administrative, or nutrition). Within this plan, students were allowed to choose courses that permitted specialized training in various areas of dietetics practice.[30]

As the decade of the 1960s opened, members of the ADA began talking about issues of licensure and registration. A questionnaire was distributed with the 1962 dues statement that included a question about the perceived need for legal licensing or certification.

New minimum standards for approval of a hospital dietetics internship were also introduced in 1963. One of the new requirements was that a dietetics internship director appointed after June 1, 1963, was required to hold a master's degree.[33]

One of the most exciting educational announcements came in 1964, when formal approval was given to the program in medical dietetics begun at the Ohio State University. This program integrated theory and practice by incorporating the internship into the degree program. Graduates of the program would be immediately eligible for ADA membership without having to go through a postbaccalaureate dietetics internship. This was the first of what later came to be known as a Coordinated Undergraduate Program (CUP).[34] Another educational innovation was the first internship leading to a master's degree. This program was introduced at the University of California, School of Public Health, Berkeley, and graduates earned a master of public health (MPH) degree along with qualifying for membership in the ADA.[35] Concern was expressed that more programs of this type were desperately needed to meet the growing need for food and nutrition professionals in the public health or community setting. Ms. Robinson also stressed the need for graduate education in business, but this was mentioned only for dietitians who were specialists in foodservice management. Graduate education was also indicated for those interested in dietetics consulting and in research. Another interesting comment in this article centered on the use of computers, which certainly reminds us of how much times have changed. Ms. Robinson said, "We do not need to learn how to operate computers, but we do need to know what we want the computer to tell us and how to evaluate and use the information we receive from it." In her summary, Ms. Robinson made a final statement that is reminiscent of recent debates within the ADA: "Continued development in our education patterns is also essential. In my opinion, this does not mean blind conformity to trends, but careful evaluation. We need opportunities for specialization. I think we need to give considerable thought to the further development of specialties. A single dietitian cannot be all things to all people."[36]

While distance education in dietetics is considered to be a relatively recent development, it is interesting to note Beatrice Donaldson's article in a 1968 issue of JADA. Dr. Donaldson discussed the development of the Articulated Instructional Media (AIM) Program at the University of Wisconsin, which enabled the faculty there to make graduate courses in foods, nutrition, and institution management available to dietitians enrolled at both the Madison and Milwaukee campuses. Courses were taught via telephone and were delivered at a time of day when dietitians who were working full time could attend. Dr. Donaldson concludes the article by saying:

To progress in our profession and as educators and learners, we need to accept every opportunity available for meeting the educational needs and challenges brought about by basic changes in society, to seek opportunities for using new technology, to recognize and make use of resources of specialists to implement new programs, and to continue improvement through experimentation and research.[37]

The 1960s ended with one of the pivotal happenings in the history of the profession. By vote of nearly 80% of the membership of ADA in February 1969, a system of national professional registration became a reality on June 1, 1969. The passage of registration had a major impact on dietetics education, for now graduates of university programs and dietetics internships or coordinated programs had to "prove themselves" on a written test. The first examination was given in January 1970 to 56 interns. All 56 passed the test.[30]

THE 1970S: COMPETENCY-BASED EDUCATION

Dr. Warren Perry, in an article in the 1970 JADA entitled, "Educating the Dietitian in a Changing World," alluded to the changing temperament of the time and the new kind of student seen on college campuses. The late '60s and early '70s were a time of great societal unrest, and Dr. Perry spoke of the questions posed by students of the day.

> Why is the curriculum so rigid? Why must a certain amount of time be spent on an internship? Why must a person who aspires to professional work follow such a specific path? Why is more of the didactic and clinical work not more relevant to the broader world of work? Why is the individual student not given more opportunity for choice and independent action?

Dr. Perry urged dietetics educators to listen to their students, discuss with them openly the issues involved in their questions, and include students on key committees for their internship experience. "As the consumers of our educational systems, they do have a right to be heard," said Dr. Perry, and collaboration is a positive thing.[38]

In the October 1971 issue of JADA, an ADA position paper entitled "Education for the Profession of Dietetics" was presented. The article addressed the "mushrooming knowledge base, unbelievable technologic advances, enlightening research results and endless resources confronting practitioners in the field of dietetics" and stresses that it is not feasible for the dietitian to be "all things to all people."[39]

The necessity of delineating limited areas of study and practice areas of specialization is discussed, with four specialty areas suggested: the generalist, the administrative dietitian, the clinical nutrition specialist, and the nutrition educator. The approach to educating dietitians was clearly outlined:

> The educational framework for preparation for the field will consist of an undergraduate program that integrates clinical experience with didactic training to provide knowledge of principles of nutrition, communication skill, conceptual thinking, research orientation, and the sciences. The practitioner at this level will preferably work under the guidance of a specialist. Career advancement will be to the level of a specialist through in-depth study leading to an advanced degree in a defined specialty area.[39]

As the new breed of dietetics student sought professional education and training, dietetics education programs continued to grow. There were 77 existing internships and 9 coordinated programs in dietetics and in 1972 alone, 5 new internships and 7 new coordinated programs were approved. The stated number-one priority of the dietetics internship board in 1971 was the identification of competencies for the entry-level dietitian, and this action set the tone for the decade of the '70s.[30]

In 1967, a decision was made by the Executive Board of the ADA to pursue a study of the profession of dietetics. Funded by the W. K. Kellogg Foundation, the study was designed to define the present and future roles of the dietitian and the educational needs appropriate for the dietitian of the future. The final report of the study was released in June 1972 and entitled "The Profession of Dietetics: The Report of the Study Commission on Dietetics."[40] Commonly known as "the Millis Report" after Dr. John S. Millis, who headed the study commission, the conclusions of this report had significant impact on the growth and development of coordinated undergraduate programs, dietetics education in general, and dietetics practice.[30]

In the 1973 JADA, an article by Marian Spears described the University of Missouri's coordinated undergraduate program in dietetics, and its emphasis in food-systems management. The University of Missouri was unique in that it sponsored two CUPs, one focused on food-systems management and another emphasizing medical dietetics. The author pointed to the benefits of the coordination achieved in such a program: "The quality of the integrated experience and its relationship to the didactic are considered the most sensitive and critical elements in a coordinated program."[41]

Also in 1973, the executive board of the ADA announced the requirements of dietetics traineeships. At that time, the number of openings in approved internships was insufficient for the number of graduates applying. Thus an alternate route, the traineeship, was developed. Traineeships provided for a minimum of 12 and no more than 24 months of training in a hospital or other eligible organization. Applicants to a traineeship had to have a bachelor's degree from an accredited college or university and had to meet the academic requirements of the association.[42]

The "essentials" or standards for dietetics education programs continued to undergo revision. The advent of coordinated undergraduate programs continued to affect the profession. By 1974, there were 23 approved coordinated undergraduate programs. Curriculum revision was widespread as educational institutions attempted to ascertain the best kinds of experiences and how to evaluate students. The "walls of the classroom" were expanded in new and exciting ways to medical centers, community agencies, commercial foodservice operations, and other innovative training sites. Curriculum revisions had to be completed by 1980, when only the newly released Plan IV, "Minimum Academic Requirements," would be in effect.[43]

Dr. Thomas E. Powers addressed the education and training of the dietetics technician in an article in the August 1974 JADA. The article outlined the typical program for a dietetics technician and differentiated this educational process from the "less-than-technician" educational offerings. It is interesting to note Dr. Thomas's hope that it would be possible for all the credits from the associate degree program to apply to the baccalaureate degree program, thus making it possible for the student to ultimately achieve professional stature as a dietitian.[44] Unfortunately, this dream is still largely unfulfilled in today's dietetics education scheme.

Immediately after the 1974 Annual Meeting, ADA was notified that the National Commission on Accreditation had accepted the application for accreditation of coordinated undergraduate programs (CUPs). During the November meeting of the ADA's executive board, approval of accreditation for dietetics internships was also received from the U.S. Office of Education. All dietetics students beginning their freshman year in the fall of 1975 were required to follow Plan IV academic requirements. The Plan IV document, which had officially become effective on July 1, 1972, outlined competencies to be held by the entry-level dietitian and focused less on completion of specific courses. Also in 1975, the Dietetic Internship Council (DIC) became known as the Section on Educational Preparation (SEP), so as to recognize the growing diversity of dietetics education programs, including internships, CUPs, baccalaureate degree programs, dietetics traineeships, dietetics technician programs, and dietetics assistant programs.[30]

SEP was relatively short-lived, as the group became known as the Council on Educational Preparation (CEP) with the advent of the new ADA bylaws in the mid-1970s. The group was charged to work closely with the Commission on Evaluation of Dietetic Education (CEDE), and the Council became "responsible for developing and approving standards for educational programs which prepare dietetics practitioners." Subgroups worked on the "Essentials" for each type of dietetics education program. Essentials for CUPs and internships were approved in 1976 and 1977 and Essentials for graduate, dietetics technician, and dietetics assistant programs were in progress.[45]

THE 1980S: DEFINING WHO WE ARE

Information was received from focus groups at the ADA's Annual Meeting in 1979, which was used to develop survey questionnaires to document the current state of dietetics practice. The questions to be answered were imposing: What is the business of our profession? Who are our clients? What *should* be the business of our profession? Who *should* be our clients? In 1979 a grant was also obtained to conduct a 15-month study to delineate the actual and appropriate roles and responsibilities of the entry-level dietitian. A further proposal was made in 1980 and extended the study to include foodservice systems management and community dietetics. Obviously the outcome of these actions would have a significant impact on dietetics education.[30]

In 1980, an article in JADA challenged the idea of competency-based education as the most appropriate method of producing competent entry-level dietetics practitioners. Author Wolfe Rinke concluded that dietetics educators should be aware of the pros and cons of competency-based education and recognize that it might not be the only or necessarily most appropriate educational paradigm to use for entry-level preparation of dietetics professionals.[46]

Another article that prompted much discussion was published in the February 1982 issue of JADA. Researchers Rinke, David, and Bjoraker investigated employer perceptions of the administrative skills and abilities of entry-level practitioners based on their educational route: internship, coordinated program, advanced degree, and traineeship. In their article, "The Entry-Level Generalist Dietitian," the authors concluded that all routes had room for improvement. Findings showed that the clinical (or supervised practice) component of dietetics education programs did not appear to provide for the attainment of uniform standards of quality in administration for the four routes investigated. The findings also revealed that graduates of the four routes had better preparation in technical aspects of practice than in human or conceptual administrative skills. Of the four routes investigated, employers rated internships as having the highest adequacy ratings, while CUP graduates received the lowest adequacy ratings. It must also be pointed out that the employers who were RDs favored graduates of the route which they themselves followed.[47]

The foodservice management role delineation study and the study in community dietetics were completed in 1983. The role verification for clinical dietetics was completed in 1984. Data from these studies were use to identify the major responsibilities for entry-level practitioners and the supporting skills and knowledge necessary for successful practice. A dietetics workforce demand study was also conducted and results published in JADA, which projected an increase in the total number of dietitians employed between 1982 and 1990.[48,49] Trend analyses revealed that hospitals would continue to be the major employer of dietitians, but with an increasingly diverse client population and practice in new settings.

In 1981, the ADA board of directors established a task force to consider the total place of education within the association and to make specific recommendations to the bylaws committee regarding the place of education in ADA's bylaws and structure. The final report of this task force was entitled "Promoting Quality Dietetic Education: A Report of The American Dietetic Association Task Force on Education." One outcome of this report was new Standards of Education, which were debated, revised, and finally implemented in the fall of 1987. The standards were the first validated quality assurance documents in dietetics history. The knowledge and performance requirements for the entry-level practitioner were closely aligned with actual dietetics practice because of the role-delineation studies.[30] With the advent of the Standards of Education, the numbering of the education plans was discontinued.

Although a variety of dietetics education–related articles appeared in JADA in the 1980s, the decade concluded with a push to emphasize critical thinking skills in dietetics education. In an April 1989 article in JADA, authors Judith Jackson and Mary Therese Hynak-Hankinson challenged dietetics educators to teach the vital skills of critical thinking to dietetics students so that they might become proficient managers in the competitive healthcare marketplace. Suggestions were made to incorporate conceptual thinking exercises such as brainstorming, brain teasers, and games in order to develop left and right brain and integrative thinking skills into dietetics curriculum.[50]

THE 1990S: PREPARING FOR THE NEW MILLENNIUM

The final decade of the 20th century found dietetics education programs growing and enrollments increasing. As of July 1991, there were 73 dietetics technician programs, 239 didactic programs, 58 coordinated programs, 92 preprofessional practice programs, and 94 dietetics internships. Enrollment approached 12,000. While enrollments were increasing, however, funding in general for higher education began to decline. The financing of educational programs was a major concern, and those who were in charge of dietetics education programs realized that they would have to respond to cost mandates by doing more with less.[51] Several articles in JADA in the early 1990s brought to the fore the issue of graduate education in dietetics. Rhoades and Franz addressed the issue of recruitment of graduate students in dietetics and alluded to the decrease in master's level individuals coming into dietetics when the master's plus 6 months of experience route was eliminated in the 1988 version of the Standards of Education.[52] The importance of introducing research and grant writing to undergraduates in dietetics was voiced by Oring and Goodwin[53] and by Gould and coworkers.[54]

One of the pivotal events of the 1990s was the 1994 Future Search Conference. The conference was attended by more than 125 participants from 25 different areas of dietetics practice. One of the outcomes of the conference was the challenge to dietetics education to change. Dietetics educators were urged to question the paradigms under which they had functioned and to develop new strategies for lifelong learning.[55] Emphasis was given to personal discovery, self-analysis, and self-responsibility for learning. New educational requirements were recommended by the Future Search Conference education workgroup. Priorities for immediate action included identifying core competencies for all dietetics practitioners and the development of a new matrix for more opportunities for concentration based on additional knowledge and skills; developing models for seamless education systems that include entry/re-entry points at various levels tied to job opportunities; using new methodologies to describe innovative, forward-looking models in all areas of dietetics practice; fostering collaborative practice-based research among dietetics practitioners, educators, and members of other disciplines; and identifying and using technology to develop self-paced, interactive learning opportunities.[56]

In November 1994, the association published a "Timely Statement of the ADA: Support of Dietetics Education Programs." This succinct statement was an important support to dietetics education programs, many of which were facing elimination as budget cuts continued to ravage colleges and universities.[57]

The phenomenon of distance education in dietetics saw rapid growth with the proliferation of computer technologies. Teleconferencing, e-mail, and the Internet began to be used with increasing regularity in dietetics education. For the first time, the 1995–1996 Directory of Dietetics Programs provided information about which programs were offering courses via distance education. An article in JADA by A. A. Spangler and colleagues encouraged dietetics educators to be knowledgeable about technology and aware of how technology could be used to educate students. Issues of faculty training, use of distance education in supervised practice, and the potential of distance education for continuing professional education were highlighted. The potential of using distance education to dialogue with international colleagues was also touted.[58]

Articles about competency-based education continued to appear in JADA. In 1996 and again in 1997, articles discussed the movement of dietetics students through the continuum of performance from novice to expert.[59,60] One of the outcomes of the 1994 Future Search Conference was the development of an educational competencies steering committee to study the feasibility of defining entry-level dietetics education in terms of expected competencies for practice. After extensive data collection and analysis, work groups of practitioners and educators convened to refine the identified competencies and determine the knowledge base needed to achieve them. The resulting foundation knowledge and skills for both dietetics and dietetics technician education were identified, as well as competencies for four emphasis areas: nutrition therapy, community, foodservice systems management, and business/entrepreneur. The option was also provided for dietetics programs to develop their own emphasis area based on the resources and needs of the program. The proposal for educating entry-level dietetics practitioners was presented to the ADA House of Delegates for comment at the October 1996 Annual Meeting and Exhibition. The final report and recommendations were approved by the Council on Professional Issues in December 1996 and forwarded to the Commission on Accreditation/Approval for Dietetics Education (CADE) for incorporation in the 1997 accreditation/approval standards.[60]

In her commentary in the same March 1997 issue of JADA, entitled "Education and the Dietetics Profession," Ruby Puckett threw down the gauntlet to dietetics education programs, insisting that change was imperative. Respondents to an informal survey she conducted of 33 dietetics practitioners, students, educators, administrators, and leaders in the foodservice industry agreed that "the education/competency of dietetics practitioners was not keeping pace with health care/industry changes." Ms. Puckett challenged dietetics educators to be more flexible, more practical, more in tune with the challenges faced by dietetics professionals in the workplace. She urged the inclusion of course work and experiences that would prepare graduates to work with an increasingly diverse employee and client population as well as to enhance management and business skills, including finance, entrepreneurship, human resource management, technology, economics, productivity measures, and quality improvement. She also urged that the view of education as a lifelong process and the need for continuing competence in practice be ingrained in dietetics graduates.[61]

The decade of the 1990s ended with a mixture of good news and bad news. Budgets in higher education were shrinking, competition for the "brightest and best" students was fierce, and the world of dietetics possibilities seemed to be growing exponentially. Never had dietetics faced more challenges as the new millennium dawned.

2000 AND BEYOND: THE FUTURE OF DIETETICS EDUCATION

The 2000 practice audit by the Commission on Dietetic Registration (CDR) identified the existing and emerging practice roles of dietetics professionals. In a 2002 issue of JADA, Bruening and colleagues made the following remarks:

> Results of the 2000 CDR Practice Audit showed that almost all practitioners, even those beyond entry level, are involved in many activities, with some supervising and little policy setting. RDs were involved primarily in nutrition care, teaching nutrition programs, and managing food and resources. The 2000 CDR Practice audit results support the need to prepare entry-level RDs for management supervisory and policy-setting roles. While RDs and DTRs have a sound technical base, employers suggested that dietetics practitioners need to enhance key business competencies (e.g., persuasive communication, negotiation skills, supervisory abilities, and financial knowledge) and professional characteristics (e.g., flexibility, creativity, and a customer-service focus).[62]

Revisions to the 1997 Standards were drafted and feedback was sought from a broad selection of stakeholders. The number of standards was reorganized from five to three. The standards were reformatted and the focus was shifted from a quantitative review to continuous quality improvement. All the required forms were eliminated, giving education programs the opportunity to present the information in the format that was most useful to their particular program. The rapid increase of distance education programs was considered and it was determined that the standards of accreditation for distance programs would be the same as traditional programs.

The approval of the 2002 Eligibility Requirements and Accreditation Standards by CADE in December 2001 and their unveiling and implementation in 2002 was an appropriate beginning for the new decade, the new century, and the new millennium.[62]

The start of a new millennium is the perfect time to look forward. ADA President Julie O'Sullivan Maillet, in a 2002 article in JADA, shared predictions of a group of leaders in dietetics on what the profession might be like in 2017, the 100th anniversary of the founding of the association. The clinical dietitian is predicted to become a nutrition therapist, reimbursed by third-party payers and writing diet orders based on well-established protocols. Dietetics professionals working with the foodservice industry are predicted to play a major role in shaping that industry to meet consumer demands and in providing an array of food and nutrition products/services to meet the ever-changing needs of the population. Management dietitians of the future are food-quality and food-safety experts, using technology and e-commerce to meet the needs of their clientele. Future dietetics researchers are helping unlock the secrets of obesity, diabetes, and other chronic diseases, while dietetics educators in 2017 are helping students and practicing professionals to meet their specific educational needs and goals. Community and public health dietitians of the next decade are leaders in creating healthy environments in communities, schools, work sites, homes, and playgrounds. Dietetics professionals in the 2017 food industry are working with nutraceuticals and biotechnology to meet the demands of a global market. Achieving this vision will rest in large part on dietetics educators of the present and their education programs, which must be ever-evolving and improving.[63]

As the normal ADA strategic planning process continued, the House of Delegates engaged in the 2002 Environmental Scan. An article, published in the trends supplement of the December 2002 issue of JADA, presented seven key strategic challenges:

- Technological, social, political, global, and environmental forces are significantly reshaping the U.S. food system.
- Keeping up with the relevant science and technology of food and health will be an increasing burden to dietetics professionals.
- The competitive space of the dietetics profession is being seriously challenged.
- Dietetics has to become relevant to more people, in more circumstances, at more life stages, and in more cultures.
- Obesity is a "crisis opportunity" that the ADA and its members are uniquely prepared to address.
- Although it may not have been a forefront issue in food and health, privacy will become a bigger and more important concern in dietetics.
- More food, diet, and food supply issues will be global, with the interchange of standards and regulations.[64]

What does all of this mean for the future of dietetics education? We are truly at a crossroads, a time in our history when crucial decisions must be made to take dietetics education to the next level. Recognizing this fact, the ADA House of Delegates (HOD), CADE, CDR, and ADA members came together to focus on the issue of the future of dietetics education. A "HOD Backgrounder" entitled "Dietetics Education and the Needs for the Future" acted as the starting point for a wide-ranging and provocative discussion of the issues at the 2003 ADA Food and Nutrition Conference and Exhibition in San Antonio, Texas. The HOD backgrounder raised the "mega issue" question to be addressed: "How will the demands of the marketplace reshape the entry-level dietetics practitioner and how will entry-level education need to evolve to prepare students for the future?"

To answer this question, many other questions also must be answered:

- What do we know about the needs, wants, and expectations of members, customers, and other stakeholders related to this issue?
- What do we know about the current realities and evolving dynamics of our members, marketplace, industry, and profession that is relevant to this decision?
- What do we know about the capacity and strategic position of the ADA in terms of its ability to address this issue?
- What ethical/legal implications, if any, surround the issue?

The backgrounder also cited the June 2003 CADE report to the ADA board of directors, which outlined challenges for dietetics education and the profession:

- Increasing practitioner involvement in accreditation review and education of students to close the gap between perception and reality.
- Increasing educators' understanding and use of outcomes assessment to improve education program quality between accreditation reviews.
- Determining the difference, if any, between entry-level and beyond entry-level knowledge and competencies based on current and future customer needs.
- Realizing that it may not be possible for education programs to further expand knowledge/competencies within the confines of the baccalaureate/900-hour supervised practice education process (RD) and associate degree/450-hour supervised practice education process (DTR). Does this "education process" dating back to 1927 for the dietitian and 1974 for the dietetics technician reflect current and future needs?
- Determining if there is a relationship between the baccalaureate/900-hour supervised practice education process and the number of dietetics majors who do not become RDs, and the impact on the profession.[65]

The spring 2004 House of Delegates also had a dialogue session about the future of management in dietetics. The question posed was, "How can the profession promote and strengthen the practical and theoretical management skills for both students and practitioners to ensure success? Ancillary questions posed included these:

- What can be done to strengthen the awareness and commitment of practitioners in all practice environments to employ more effective management and business skills?
- What skills are essential that are not currently easily acquired, either at the undergraduate or practitioner level?

- What should be done to strengthen the awareness and commitment of students at the undergraduate level to acquiring effective management and business skills?

The issue of education of practitioners was addressed in the management task force report. The suggestion was made for collaboration between CADE and the Dietetic Educators of Practitioners Dietetics Practice Group (DEP DPG) to identify and promote best practices for educating students regarding management, to develop a packet of exercises and tool kits to assist educators for use in management-related learning activities to be incorporated into class work, to address the issues of university staffing for management courses within the dietetics education programs, and to offer educational sessions to dietetics educators that are conducted by CADE/DEP DPG during DEP area meetings or at the ADA Food and Nutrition Conference and Exhibition (FNCE) meeting.[66]

In 2004 the House of Delegates appointed the Dietetic Education Task Force, charged to use a "clean-slate approach" to create a new plan for educating and credentialing RDs and DTRs based on a review of the roles of the RD and DTR and future practice needs. The Task Force examined all aspects of dietetics education and credentialing, both for RDs and DTRs. Questions to be addressed included the following:

- Is there a relationship between quality of dietetics practice at entry-level and the academic degree that the profession requires for entry-level practice?
- Given trends in health care requiring increased competence in clinical practice and outcomes research and given the global movement toward health promotion and disease prevention, should our profession rethink current requirements for knowledge and performance competencies in foodservice management, nutrition, counseling, outcomes research, and business? Should areas of educational program emphasis be revisited?
- What changes, if any, should be made in the way the profession educates and/or credentials dietetics technicians?

After months of fact-finding, focus groups, and intense debate and discussion, the Task Force made the following recommendations:

Recommendation #1: The Task Force recommends for dietetics education and credentialing that:

1. CDR require a graduate degree for eligibility for the CDR registration examination for registered dietitians and professional entry into dietetics practice.
2. CADE require accredited programs preparing students for RD credentialing to have a seamless educational system providing both the academic preparation and supervised practice necessary for credentialing in one graduate-degree-granting program.
3. CADE require accredited programs to provide opportunities for students of diverse educational backgrounds to enter the degree-granting programs and meet academic and supervised practice requirements for RD credentialing eligibility.

Recommendation #2: The Task Force recommends CADE, with input from the profession, reevaluate the core competencies for RD entry-level practice to allow more opportunity for CADE-accredited programs to emphasize a particular area of dietetics practice and to meet requirements for granting a graduate degree.

Recommendation #3: The Task Force recommends CADE include additional knowledge and performance competencies needed in the following content areas:

- Nutrition diagnosis/implementation of nutrition care process.
- Counseling and behavior management.
- General business management, e.g., managing staff/personnel and interdisciplinary teams, negotiations, generating revenues, communication skills.
- Practice management, e.g., ethical issues, cost-benefit/determining value of products and services, marketing, legal issues, reimbursement.
- Leadership.
- Food, e.g., cultural foods, product development, impact of food processing on nutrient value, environmental/agricultural issues.
- Outcomes research and evidence-based practice.
- Genetics.
- Others as needed to meet current and future needs for entry-level practice.

Recommendation #4: The Task Force recommends CADE expand the supervised practice hour requirements to allow sufficient time for students to acquire the depth and breadth of learning needed for dietetics practice now and in the future.

Recommendation #5: The Task Force expresses its support of education for advanced-level dietetics practice and recommends the House of Delegates develop a plan for accreditation of advanced-level education programs that include academic course work, supervised practice and research, and credentialing of advanced-level practitioners.

Recommendation #6: The Task Force recommends a gradual phaseout of the DTR credential and accreditation of DT education programs, with oversight by CDR, CADE, HOD, and the ADA board of directors, which will develop a plan for implementation.

Recommendation #7: The Task Force recommends ADA allocate resources to accomplish the Task Force's recommendations.[67]

When the Dietetics Education Task Force Report and Recommendations were released in February 2005, they were met with an onslaught of comment and controversy. Considerable time was devoted at the 2005 midyear HOD meeting to hearing testimony about the report and recommendations. The HOD decided to continue the work of the Task Force and offered a new charge to the group to continue working with the concerns expressed during the dialogue. The group was asked to further explore quality education alternatives to address the needs of the profession. All organizational units of ADA were to be kept informed of the Task Force's progress, to submit an update in October 2005, and to present a final report no later than May 2006.

Dietetics educators and practitioners alike eagerly awaited the extended Task Force's final report as the profession moved into 2006. Without a doubt, big changes are ahead for dietetics education.

LOOKING AHEAD: WHAT DOES THE FUTURE HOLD FOR DIETETICS EDUCATION?

The pioneering women who founded the profession of dietetics and the ADA would likely be both stunned and thrilled to see the scope of dietetics practice in today's marketplace. In speaking with prospective students, one of the great selling points

Issues to Ponder

- Since the 1920s we have been struggling with the "rapid development of the study of diet in relation to disease" and "the management of the whole dietary department." What direction should we promote today?
- What needs to be covered in the curriculum to teach "the development of judgment"? In 1941 terms, what "courses proved to be most helpful to you in your work as a dietitian?" What is the right balance of a broad university education and dietetics-specific course work?
- What does one need to know to be called a dietitian?
- What is the difference between "technical" and "professional" education?
- Should graduate degrees be required for entry-level practice or used to gain knowledge and skills in a specialty area?
- How do you teach "flexibility, creativity, and a customer-service focus"?
- How will the demands on the marketplace reshape the entry-level dietetics practitioner and how will entry-level education need to evolve to prepare students for the future?

for dietetics is its breadth and versatility. Any dietetics educator can recite the litany of areas of practice and all the exciting ways in which one might "ply one's trade" as a dietitian.

Although the breadth of the profession is indeed a blessing, it may also present one of the greatest challenges to today's dietetics educators. When we compare today's listing of "Foundation Knowledge and Skills" to the first "Standard Course for Student Dietitians in Hospitals," the exponential growth of what one must know and be able to do to qualify as an entry-level practitioner is astounding.

The questions about educational preparation that confront the profession and the ADA are complex and legion. The answers that must come will have far-reaching implications for our profession, for education programs, and for dietetics professionals of the future. Following are a few questions worthy of consideration:

- Can we teach it all? How do we prepare students for a profession that seems to know no limits? What is the best way to teach students information management and critical analysis/thinking in order to be effective lifelong learners?
- As we continue to identify more knowledge, skills, and abilities that must be demonstrated by graduates of our dietetics education programs, are we becoming vocational-technical in focus rather than graduating students with the broad-based, "classic" educational experience expected of a university graduate?
- Can we justify lengthening our educational programs or even requiring a master's degree for entry into the profession when salary levels are not commensurate and "respect" for our profession in some areas seems lacking?
- Is the day of the "generalist" dietitian over? Is now the time for specialization at the entry level? If so, what will those specialty areas be? What effect will this have on the flexibility and versatility we have always touted as a hallmark of our profession?
- What is the future of foodservice management in the profession of dietetics? Foodservice was the birthplace of the dietetics profession. The skills gained there—leadership, problem solving, decision making, fiscal accountability, customer service, human resources management, crisis management, and, yes, knowledge of good food and how to prepare and serve it—were the things that made our profession great and moved it to new levels of prominence and power.

Yet many dietetics students in today's programs are not interested in—and are often "turned off" by—their foodservice management rotations. Meanwhile, practicing dietetics professionals who work in the foodservice management area often feel disenfranchised from ADA and turn to other professional associations for continuing education and leadership opportunities. Will these two phenomena coalesce to the demise of this vital area of dietetics practice?

- With an ever-increasing breadth of knowledge and skills to bring to their students, can coordinated programs continue to survive? The concept of combining and coordinating theory with practice is a proven method of readying students for the real world of dietetics practice. However, accomplishing all that needs to be done in the span of 4 years—the original strong selling point for coordinated programs—is increasingly difficult if not impossible.

- Finding and maintaining high-quality supervised practice sites is increasingly challenging. Traditional facilities such as hospitals are often beset with extremely busy dietetics professionals who are increasingly asked to do more and more with fewer resources. Liability and patient confidentiality issues are making some organizations leery of accepting students. How can educators and facilities work together even more efficiently and effectively to produce a win-win situation?

- Finding dietetics faculty who have appropriate and recent practitioner experience is challenging. Students, faculty, and administrators in higher education programs value "real-world experience" in teaching faculty. From where will the next generation of dietetics faculty come?

- When and how will dietetics technicians find their rightful place in the dietetics world? Many areas of the country have no technician programs or DTRs in the marketplace. When will there be a critical mass of DTRs to work with and extend the abilities of the RD and truly become the dietetics team dreamed of by the visionaries who established the technician role?

- How will distance education affect the delivery of dietetics education and continuing education for dietetics professionals?

- Rather than always reacting and responding to change, CADE and dietetics education programs should be reading the trends and leading the change in dietetics practice. How can we move dietetics education ahead to be on the cutting edge of dietetics practice?

In 1919, Lenna Frances Cooper said it all: "A discussion of training for dietitians bring us to a point about which we could discuss indefinitely. Can a dietitian be trained properly in four years? Sometime I think we ought to spend half our lives getting ready for the rest of it."[68]

ACKNOWLEDGMENT

Special thanks to Karla Kepley, senior dietetics student at Kansas State University, for her assistance in the research for this chapter.

REFERENCES

1. Rorer ST. Early dietetics. J Am Diet Assoc 1934;10:289–295.
2. Byerly MG. A chapter in the history of dietetics. J Am Diet Assoc 1926;11:166–167.
3. Cooper LF. The dietitian and her profession. J Am Diet Assoc 1938;14:751–758.
4. Otis FA. A combination theory and practice course for student dietitians. J Am Diet Assoc 1925;1:138–140.
5. Morgan AF. College education and the food specialist. J Am Diet Assoc 1926;1:174–178.

6. Section on Education, the American Dietetic Association. Outline for standard course for student dietitians in hospitals. J Am Diet Assoc 1927;3:183–186.

7. Johnson KM. Evolving standards of training for the dietitian. J Am Diet Assoc 1949;25:504–509.

8. Northrop MW. The training of student dietitians. J Am Diet Assoc 1929;5:208–211.

9. Houghton HS. Nutrition training in the clinical years of the medical course. J Am Diet Assoc 1931;7:17–21.

10. Duckles D. Case studies: an outline for the student dietitian. J Am Diet Assoc 1933;9:207–211.

11. Bryan MDG. Progress in approved courses for student dietitians. J Am Diet Assoc 1934;9:377–381.

12. Cooper LF. The teaching of foods, nutrition and diet therapy to student nurses. J Am Diet Assoc 1935;11:211–216.

13. Hains A. One effective measure in the teaching of student nurses and dietitians. J Am Diet Assoc 1936;12:225–230.

14. Editorial Comment. Educational trends in the field of dietetics. J Am Diet Assoc 1936;12:248–250.

15. Philbrick MH. Pioneering in dietetics. J Am Diet Assoc 1936;12:130–135.

16. Tilt J. Professional Education Section: chairman's summary. J Am Diet Assoc 1936;12:346–347.

17. Bateson FE. What should be the ultimate aim of the hospital training courses? J Am Diet Assoc 1938;14:528–533.

18. Fleck HC. A questionnaire for the would-be dietitian. J Am Diet Assoc 1938;14:815–816.

19. Gleiser FW. The college and university training of the dietitian. J Am Diet Assoc 1939;15:558–563.

20. Hall GE. Professional education section: chairman's summary. J Am Diet Assoc 1940;16:1016–1018.

21. Morrill WP. Training hospital dietitians. J Am Diet Assoc 1940;16:240–243.

22. Godfrey G. Problems in the college training of the dietitian. J Am Diet Assoc 1941;17:639–643.

23. Ohlson MA. The student dietitian: an experiment in cooperative education. J Am Diet Assoc 1941;17:644–649.

24. Editorial. The long view of professional education. J Am Diet Assoc 1942;18:308.

25. U.S. Civil Service Commission. Student dietitians needed. J Am Diet Assoc 1944;20:601.

26. Refshauge LM. The wide scope of work offered in courses for student dietitians. J Am Diet Assoc 1945;21:94–94.

27. Anon. Term "dietetic intern" approved for student dietitian in approved courses. J Am Diet Assoc 1947;23:232.

28. A bibliography on dietetic careers. J Am Diet Assoc 1947;23:894.

29. Miller GE. Current comment: is dynamic knowledge of nutrition essential for every dietitian? J Am Diet Assoc 1950;26:600–606.

30. Cassell JA. Carry the Flame: The History of The American Dietetic Association. Chicago: The American Dietetic Association, 1990.

31. Eppright ES. Current comment: our responsibilities to the dietetic intern. J Am Diet Assoc 1955;31:152–155.

32. Hanscher M. Liberal education in professional curricula. Address given before the Association of Land-Grant Colleges and Universities, Columbus, OH, November 11, 1953.

33. Robinson WF. Educating the dietetic intern. J Am Diet Assoc 1964;45:26–28.

34. Wilson MA. Undergraduate education in dietetics. J Nutr Ed 1972;4:132–133.

35. Robinson WF. Programs in approved dietetic internships. J Am Diet Assoc 1964;45:29–34.

36. Walsh HE. The changing nature of public health. J Am Diet Assoc 1965;46:93–95.

37. Donaldson B. Extending educational opportunities for dietitians. J Am Diet Assoc 1968;53:329–333.

38. Perry JW. Educating the dietitian in a changing world. J Am Diet Assoc 1970;56:387–391.

39. The American Dietetic Association Position Paper on Education for the Profession of Dietetics. J Am Diet Assoc 1971;59:372–373.

40. The Profession of Dietetics: The Report of the Study Commission on Dietetics. Chicago: The American Dietetic Association, 1972.

41. Spears MC. The first year of a coordinated undergraduate program in food systems management. J Am Diet Assoc 1973;62:417–420.

42. Wenberg BG. Report of a dietetic traineeship conference in Michigan. J Am Diet Assoc 1973;63:549–550.

43. Hart ME. Dietetic education—past, present, and future. J Am Diet Assoc 1974;64:612–615.

44. Powers TF. The dietetic technician: paraprofessional as knowledge worker. J Am Diet Assoc 1974;65:130–137.

45. Hansen JR, Wenberg BG. The president's page. J Am Diet Assoc 1978;72:525–526.

46. Rinke WJ. Competency-based education. J Am Diet Assoc 1980;76:247–251.

47. Rinke WJ, David BD, Bjoraker WT. The entry-level generalist dietitian. J Am Diet Assoc 1982;80:132–147.

48. Fitz PA, Posner BM, Baldyga WW. Demand for dietitians: taking control of the future. J Am Diet Assoc 1983;83:68–73.

49. Fitz PA, Baldyga WW. Estimates of the future demand for dietetic services: results of the dietetic manpower demand study. J Am Diet Assoc1983;83:186–190.

50. Jackson J, Hynak-Hankinson MT. Incorporating hard boxes and soft bubbles into the dietetics curriculum. J Am Diet Assoc 1989;89:528–533.

51. Wood OB. ADA advances: Council on Education—visions and opportunities. J Am Diet Assoc 1991;91:1129–1130.

52. Rhoades PK, Franz, M. Market research to recruit graduate students in dietetics. J Am Diet Assoc 1993;93:920–922.

53. Oring KE, Goodwin JK. Integrating research and grant writing in an undergraduate dietetics curriculum. J Am Diet Assoc 1993;93:1293–1295.

54. Gould R, Shanklin CW, Canter DD, Miller JL. Stimulating research among dietetics students. J Am Diet Assoc. 1994;94:1103.

55. Parks SC, Babjak PM, Fitz PA, Maillet JO, Mitchell BE. President's page: Future Search Conference helps define new directions in practice, education, and credentialing. J Am Diet Assoc 1994;94:1046–1047.

56. Parks SC, Fitz PA, Maillet, JO, Babjak P, Mitchell B. Challenging the future of dietetics education and credentialing—dialogue, discovery, and directions: a summary of the 1994 Future Search Conference. J Am Diet Assoc 1995;95:598–606.

57. ADA. Timely statement of the American Dietetic Association: support of dietetics education programs. J Am Diet Assoc 1994;94:1316.

58. Spangler AA, Spear B, Plavcan PA. Dietetics education by distance: current endeavors in CAADE-accredited/approved programs. J Am Diet Assoc 1995;95:925–929.

59. Chambers DW, Gilmore CJ, Maillet, JO, Mitchell BE. Another look at competency-based education in dietetics. J Am Diet Assoc 1996;96:614–617.

60. Gilmore CJ, Maillet JO, Mitchell BE. Determining educational preparation based on job competencies of entry-level dietetics practitioners. J Am Diet Assoc 1997;97:306-316.

61. Puckett RP. Education and the dietetics profession. J Am Diet Assoc 1997;97:252–253.

62. Bruening KS, Mitchell BE, Pfeiffer MM. 2002 accreditation standards for dietetics education. J Am Diet Assoc 2002;102:566-577.

63. Maillet JO. Dietetics in 2017: what does the future hold? J Am Diet Assoc 2002:102;1404–1406.

64. Jarratt J, Mahaffie JB. Key trends affecting the dietetics profession and the American Dietetic Association. J Am Diet Assoc 2002;102:S1821–S1839.

65. HOD Backgrounder: dietetics education and the needs for the future. Available at: http://www.eatright.org/Member/85_17558.cfm. Accessed October 2003.

66. House of Delegates Management Task Force Report. Available at: http://www.eatright.org/Member/85_19540.cfm. Accessed June 2004.

67. Dietetics Education Task Force Report and Recommendations. February 2005. Available at: http://www.eatright.org/ada/files/FINALDIETEdTaskForceReport22105.doc. Accessed March 1, 2006.

68. Proceedings of Annual Meeting, The American Dietetic Association, 1919. Chicago: American Dietetic Association,1919.

CHAPTER 3

ADVANCED-LEVEL AND SPECIALTY PRACTICE: HOW NECESSARY OR BENEFICIAL ARE THEY FOR PRACTITIONERS?

Julie O'Sullivan Maillet and Wanda H. Howell

From Chapter 2, on dietetics education, it is obvious that dietetics started as a broad-based profession. Consider the definition of dietetics as a profession framed by the American Dietetic Association (ADA): "The integration and application of principles derived from the sciences of food, nutrition, management, communication, and biological, physiological, behavioral, and social sciences to achieve and maintain optimal human health."[1] This diversity is a positive attribute of the profession but also creates difficulty in achieving competency across the continuum of the profession. The difficulty of achieving this broad spectrum of competencies has been addressed throughout the history of the profession, as Chapter 2 so clearly illustrates. The topic is again under discussion by the 2004–2006 ADA Task Force on Dietetic Education. This Task Force is examining entry and setting a direction for advanced-level practice in the profession. The implications of the final recommendation once accepted by the ADA House of Delegates will shape the future of dietetics.

This chapter discusses entry, specialty, and advanced-level practice in dietetics, with an emphasis on the credentialing processes and the scope of practice for dietetics professionals. A detailed discussion of the 2005 ADA Scope of Dietetics Practice Framework is beyond the scope of this chapter. The framework well illustrates the development process, from entry through advanced-level practice, and the relationship of the Code of Ethics, the Standards of Professional Performance, the educational core competencies of the Commission on Accreditation of Dietetic Education programs, and the Standards of Nutrition Care. Figure 3-1 shows the interconnectivity.[2] With these tools, the practitioner should be able to engage in self-assessment and to determine whether a task is within his or her individual scope of practice considering entry-level education, licensure regulations, institutional standards, and personal competence obtained and observed. This process recognizes that while entry-level practice may be similar, continuing development is individualized.

THE ENTRY-LEVEL DIETITIAN

The knowledge, skills, and competencies needed by the entry-level dietitian continue to evolve. Over the almost 80 years since the establishment of educational standards, the profession has required a baccalaureate degree and 6 to 12 months of supervised practice. The profession has modified the standards of dietetics programs, so at times they have reflected a stronger emphasis or concentration in one type of practice. At other times programs did not declare an emphasis, although individuals knew the subject-matter strengths of individual programs. The debate over an entry-level generalist versus an entry-level person with more skills in one type of practice has chal-

American Dietetic Association
Scope of Dietetics Practice Framework

Block One: Foundation Knowledge

Definition of Dietetics as a Profession: "The integration and application of principles derived from the sciences of food, nutrition, management, communication, and biological, physiological, behavioral, and social sciences to achieve and maintain optimal human health" within flexible scope of practice boundaries to capture the breadth of the profession.

5 Characteristics of the Profession	Professionals Who Demonstrate This Characteristic...	Core Professional Resources	
Code of Ethics	Follow a Code of Ethics for practice	Code of Ethics	Ethics Opinions
Body of Knowledge	Possess a unique theoretical body of knowledge and science-based knowledge that leads to defined skills, abilities, and norms	Philosophy and Mission: • Research Philosophy and Diagram	Research, Position Papers, Practice Papers, Published Literature
Education	Demonstrate competency at selected level by meeting set criteria and passing credentialing exams	CADE (Core Competencies and Emphasis Areas)	CDR Certification (RD, DTR)
Autonomy	• Are reasonably independent and self-governing in decision-making and practice • Demonstrate critical thinking skills • Take on roles that require greater responsibility and accountability both professionally and legally • Stay abreast of new knowledge and technical skills	The CDR Professional Development Portfolio Process offers a framework for credentialed professionals to develop specific goals, identify learning needs, and pursue continuing education opportunities. This may encompass certificates (such as weight management), specialty certificates (such as CSR), advanced practice certification, or advanced degrees.	
Service	Provide food and nutrition care services for individuals and population groups and other stakeholders. Additional functions may include: • Manage food and other material resources • Market services and products • Teach dietitians and other professionals or students • Conduct research • Manage human resources • Manage facilities	Nutrition Care Process and Model	Nationally developed guidelines ADA Evidence-Based Guides for Practice
		Practice Based Evidence • Dietetics Practice Outcomes Research • Dietetics Practice Audit	

The Framework consists of three building blocks with flexible boundaries. The blocks describe the full range of responsibilities, roles, and activities that dietetics professionals are educated and authorized to perform. The flexible boundaries allow for new roles to emerge. Because of the complexity of our profession, it is impossible to present this information as a list of isolated activities that are parceled out at different levels. Rather, a stepped algorithmic approach is needed to capture the breadth of the profession, allow individual practitioners to draw from the full range of resources, and lend our scope of practice the flexibility it needs to evolve as new research in dietetics and practice emerge.

From an individual perspective, whether an activity is within your scope of practice is influenced by every level of the Framework – our Foundation Knowledge, Code of Ethics, Standards of Practice and Standards of Professional Performance, as well as by licensure and certification laws, research, guides for practice and expert opinion, new research, etc.

Block Two: Evaluation Resources

The evaluation resources listed here are intended for use in conjunction with relevant state, federal and licensure laws. Together with the laws, they serve as a guide for ensuring safe and effective dietetics practice. Practitioners can use them to determine whether a particular activity falls within their legitimate scope of practice, evaluate their performance, make hiring decisions, and as a basis for initiating regulatory reform. The core standards are based on the Nutrition Care Process and Model (NCPM) and Commission on Accreditation for Dietetics Education (CADE) educational core competencies.) Specialty and advanced standards can evolve for specific practice areas.

Code of Ethics	DTR Standards of Practice in Nutrition Care RD Standards of Practice in Nutrition Care ↓ RD Specialty or RD Advanced Standards of Practice	Standards of Professional Performance for Dietetics Professionals ↓ RD Specialty or RD Advanced Standards of Professional Performance

Block Three: Decision Aids

The healthcare environment in which we work is highly diverse and evolving. The resources listed here are intended to help dietetics professionals respond to new demands. By using the Decision Tree and Decision Analysis Tool, professionals can fully consider whether a new role or activity falls within their legitimate scope of practice, and thereby grow their practice to encompass new areas. This is particularly helpful when state, federal, organizational and educational guidelines have not yet expanded to address a need. The other resources can be applied to seek guidance when making such decisions, or when effecting change at the local or national level to reflect emerging trends and needs.

The arrows reflect the flexible, dynamic nature of the Framework. At both the individual practitioner level and our collective professional level, developments in one area of the Framework influence others. For example, as new trends in dietetics practice emerge, education, certification, and standards of practice and professional performance will change to address them. Likewise, as a practitioner tailors his or her individual scope of practice through experience and training, this will influence the resources utilized at every level.

Decision Analysis Tool	Decision Tree	Definition of Terms
Supporting Documentation for use with Decision Tree And Decision Analysis Tool		

Licensure/ Certification/Credentials Examples include: State Licensure, CDR Credentials, Specialty Certificates, Advanced Practice Certification, or Advanced Degrees. **Organizational Privileging** **Individual CDR Professional Development Portfolio** *Portfolio* Learning Plan and Learning Activities Log	**Evidence Based Practice** • Existing Research and Literature • ADA Position and Practice Papers, Ethics Opinions • Nationally-Developed Guidelines and ADA Guides for Practice **Practice Based Evidence** • Dietetics Practice Outcomes Research

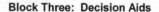

FIGURE 3-1 *Scope of dietetics practice framework. Used with permission.*[2]

lenged or plagued the profession since the 1940s. One of the hallmarks of the profession has been the stated advantage of being able to obtain and shift into a diversity of job roles. The interconnectedness of all of the elements of dietetics suggests the need for the traditional generalist.

The question is: What could be eliminated?

- Food? No, although emphasis on food science has been decreased, we may need to increase it as society incorporates more genetically modified foods, and we will continue to teach food preparation techniques.
- Nutrition? No, it is the heart of dietetics. But how much of the focus should be on prevention versus medical nutrition therapy? How much about enteral and parenteral nutrition should be taught? Which phases of our life span?
- Management? No, the profession started in management and currently does not cover enough. The dietitian's advancement is tied to management. How about foodservice systems?
- Communication? No, dietetics practitioners are counselors and work in teams, so communication is essential.
- Biological, physiological, behavioral, and social sciences? No, dietetics is grounded in chemistry and biology. Practitioners work with people to change behavior, so they need psychology and sociology.

With no topics to eliminate, the question of how to educate dietitians becomes a major discussion. Yet, throughout the past three decades, the entry-level positions tend not to be primarily for generalists but rather for broad specialty areas such as clinical, community, business, and foodservice systems and only secondarily for the occasional generalist. The ADA survey of primary practice areas does not even list "generalist" as a choice.[3]

Thus a number of questions should be raised about the profession:

- Should and can all entry-level practitioners be competent in each of the areas (clinical, community, food and nutrition management, consultation/business, and education/research), or is exposure to all areas sufficient? Indeed, most advanced practitioners would say that entry-level practitioners are not competent in consultation/business practice and education/research.
- Can the emphasis be on knowing how to think critically and to look at evidence and assess/measure competency at entry level and then pursue continuing professional education to facilitate moving through various dietetics careers?

The 2005 Scope of Dietetics Practice Framework is based on the premise that a dietitian cannot know everything about all aspects of dietetics, so each dietitian must assess his or her personal ability to perform a task or activity. The decision tree in Figure 3-2 is designed to help determine whether a given activity is within an individual's scope of practice.

Changes in the delivery of healthcare and therefore the work setting for the entry-level practitioner may influence the needed education and competency of new practitioners. Historically, the new registered dietitian worked in a hospital, whether clinically or administratively, under the direction of another RD. During this novice phase of development, the guidance of supervisors/mentors and other colleagues provided the reinforcement of learning needed to enhance entry-level

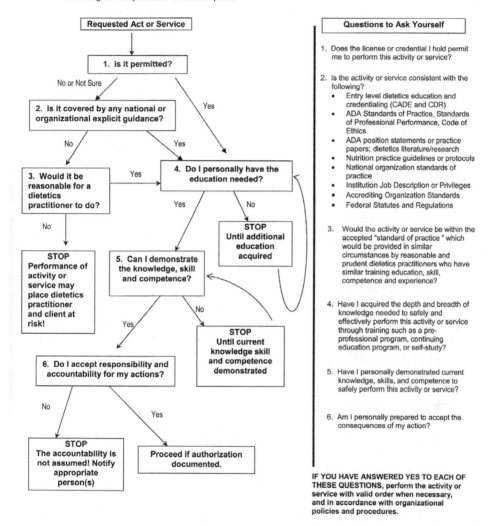

American Dietetic Association
Scope of Dietetics Practice Framework
Decision Tree

When to use the Decision Tree: Use this tool when trying to determine whether a specific activity or service (such as assuming responsibility for instructing patients with diabetes on insulin pump usage or ordering nutrition related labs) falls within your individual scope of practice.

Instructions for Use:
Start on the left side of the diagram and match numbered boxes with each "Question to Ask Yourself" on the right of the diagram. Fully consider all decision points.

Requested Act or Service

1. Is it permitted?

No or Not Sure

Yes

2. Is it covered by any national or organizational explicit guidance?

No   Yes

3. Would it be reasonable for a dietetics practitioner to do?   Yes

No

STOP Performance of activity or service may place dietetics practitioner and client at risk!

4. Do I personally have the education needed?

Yes   No

STOP Until additional education acquired

5. Can I demonstrate the knowledge, skill and competence?

Yes   No

STOP Until current knowledge skill and competence demonstrated

6. Do I accept responsibility and accountability for my actions?

No   Yes

STOP The accountability is not assumed! Notify appropriate person(s)

Proceed if authorization documented.

Questions to Ask Yourself

1. Does the license or credential I hold permit me to perform this activity or service?

2. Is the activity or service consistent with the following?
   • Entry level dietetics education and credentialing (CADE and CDR)
   • ADA Standards of Practice, Standards of Professional Performance, Code of Ethics
   • ADA position statements or practice papers; dietetics literature/research
   • Nutrition practice guidelines or protocols
   • National organization standards of practice
   • Institution Job Description or Privileges
   • Accrediting Organization Standards
   • Federal Statutes and Regulations

3. Would the activity or service be within the accepted "standard of practice " which would be provided in similar circumstances by reasonable and prudent dietetics practitioners who have similar training education, skill, competence and experience?

4. Have I acquired the depth and breadth of knowledge needed to safely and effectively perform this activity or service through training such as a pre-professional program, continuing education program, or self-study?

5. Have I personally demonstrated current knowledge, skills, and competence to safely perform this activity or service?

6. Am I personally prepared to accept the consequences of my action?

IF YOU HAVE ANSWERED YES TO EACH OF THESE QUESTIONS, perform the activity or service with valid order when necessary, and in accordance with organizational policies and procedures.

FIGURE 3-2 *Decision tree for determining whether an activity is within a dietetics professional's scope of practice. Used with permission.*[2]

competence. Also, historically, the new practitioner could ease into a full workload, thus having extra time to provide service or assess patients and provide care. Today, although the initial work environment remains the acute-care setting for about one-third of entry-level RDs, the settings are more diverse and the likelihood that the RD will be working without supervision by another RD has increased. This increased autonomy suggests that self-evaluation of competence is critical and that more in-depth knowledge of a given area may be needed. In addition, the luxury of slowly building up a workload is reduced in a cost-sensitive system that is accountable for the quality of care of all patients.

Another pivotal question is whether the current educational system and credentialing examination prepare entry-level practitioners well for the diversity of positions they enter when they begin to practice. There is no straightforward answer to this question, as illustrated by the focus group responses to the Dietetic Education Task Force.[4] Dietetics programs evaluate the success of their graduates partially by credentialing results and employer surveys. Credentialing results appear acceptable, and most educators obtain positive feedback from their alumni and employers. Both suggest that current education is accomplishing its mission. Yet the discussions among the practitioners of the profession often indicate that entry-level practitioners are not competent enough in each one of the areas of practice. This may be true or the profession may not clearly separate what is competency (minimal or acceptable) for entry practice versus superior practice or proficiency or specialty or advanced practice.

Sorting through whether the profession can and should remain very broad-based is an important debate. These discussions will assist in making the decision to leave some or all of entry-level practice to the baccalaureate degree or to move the profession to a master's degree at entry. Here are some of the pertinent questions:

- Does the diversity of skills at entry level strengthen or dilute the profession?
- Does the current structure help or diminish individuals' interest in entering the profession?
- Does the breadth assist, diminish, or confuse the view of the profession to the employers and the clients served?
- Even assuming that the current model has been the best, will it continue to be the best in a decade with the growing depth of knowledge in each aspect of dietetics?
- What scenario will make the dietitian the most valued source of food and nutrition information?

CREDENTIALING

The establishment of education requirements for entry-level dietetics practice began in the 1920s. It was 1969 before a credentialing program was developed for the dietetics internship graduate, the RD examination. Credentialing requires review, verification, and evaluation of an individual's competence against a standard, not just successful completion of a program. A credential may be given to allow someone to practice independently, generally at an entry level, or a credential may be earned after practicing in the profession to show proficiency, specialty, or advanced practice. Any credential is only as good as its foundation and the ultimate purpose of the credentialing process is to protect the public by distinguishing qualified from unqualified practitioners.

The Commission on Dietetic Registration (CDR) was established in 1969. In 1970, it started to offer the RD examination, and in 1987, the Dietetic Technician Registered (DTR) examination. CDR is recognized by the National Commission for Certifying Agencies (NCCA), the accreditation body of the National Organization for Competency Assurance. This accredited certification means that CDR examinations are psychometrically sound examinations that have the ability to distinguish qualified from unqualified practitioners. Throughout its history, CDR has relied on the didactic education program, supervised practice, and the examination as the

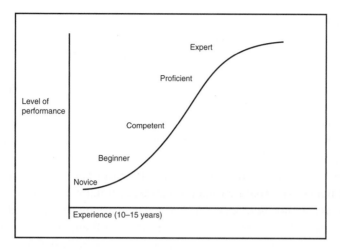

FIGURE 3-3 *Schematic representation of the stages in professional growth. Adapted with permission from Chambers et al.[6]*

three-tier system to assure competency. The development of the CDR entry-level examinations and the accredited educational programs is based on periodic practice audits/role delineations that provide the empirical data describing what dietetics practitioners do in practice as well as what future changes in practice may be anticipated. The practice audit is completed by practitioners at entry and beyond entry practice as well as by employers of practitioners. As described further on, the foundation credential for the practice of dietetics is the RD credential. It is generally regarded as necessary for entry-level practice and is a generalist examination.[5]

THE BEYOND-ENTRY-LEVEL DIETITIAN

What exactly is a "beyond-entry" dietitian? The ADA and others use this term to describe an individual who has been credentialed as an RD or DTR for more than 3 years, with entry level being described as the first 3 years of practice. It is used to measure how dietitians' knowledge, attitudes, and/or responsibilities change as they work in the profession. It also may be a transition phase from entry level to specialty practice. Figure 3-3 illustrates the educational spectrum for dietetics practitioners.[6]

THE SPECIALTY OR ADVANCED PRACTITIONER

Over time or upon employment, dietitians begin to work in one practice arena. The Professional Portfolio Self-Evaluation system, required after achieving RD status, is built on the premise that there are many aspects of practice and that individuals shall select and describe how they want to develop over the ensuing 5 years and then create and implement an education plan to achieve this. The opportunity to retake the RD examination rather than fulfill this continuing education requirement is rarely taken, because upon entry into practice, practice generally narrows.

A specialty practitioner is an individual "who concentrates on one aspect of the profession of dietetics. This specialty may or may not have a credential and additional certification, but it often has expanded roles beyond entry level practice."[2] On the other hand, an entry-level person without additional knowledge may be in a specialty role. This is unlikely, however, because of experience, educational opportunities, and professional ethics.

The specialty practitioner, even if a generalist, is considered an advanced practitioner when he or she has "acquired the expert knowledge base, complex decision-making skills and clinical competencies for expanded practice, the characteristics of which are shaped by the context in which she/he practices."[2] Advanced practitioners may have expanded or specialty roles or both. Advanced practice may or may not include additional certification. Generally the practice is more complex, and the practitioner has a higher degree of professional autonomy.[2] Often, one knows an advanced practitioner when interacting with one, but the characteristics are difficult to describe.

In the early 1990s the ADA developed an empirical research model to describe specialty practice and advanced-level practice.[7,8] The results of the research allowed the CDR to create specialty credentials in pediatrics as well as renal and metabolic care.[7]

The results of the advanced practice analysis conducted by the ADA/CDR in the early 1990s did not allow for a description of advanced practice, but the results illustrated the characteristics and attributes of an advanced-level individual. The Fellow of the American Dietetic Association (FADA) credential was established to recognize these individuals.[8] In 2005, Annalynn Skipper conducted structured interviews with known "experts"/advanced-level practitioners and confirmed and refined the Bradley model.[11] From 2002 to 2005, as the Scope of Dietetics Practice Framework[2] was being developed, the Standards of Practice for Nutrition Care[9] were also being developed. Both documents were published in May 2005 and describe what the dietitian and dietetics technician do and how to measure their performance. Concurrently, a task force for the Diabetes Care and Education practice group of the ADA developed and published Standards of Practice and Standards of Professional Performance for RDs at the generalist, specialist, and advanced levels.[10] The generalist in the model is the "entry-level dietitian practicing in part in diabetes." The standards reflect the Nutrition Care Process and Model (see Chapter 9) and cover the services of RDs in inpatient, outpatient, and community settings. Other specialty practice groups are in the process of defining levels of practice in their specialty areas. In addition to increased specialty descriptions, hopefully practice audits to validate these consensus documents will occur over the next decade.

THE SPECIALTY CREDENTIALS

Specialty credentials in dietetics were introduced in the early 1980s. Table 3-1 lists the generally agreed-on credible credentials for specialty and advanced practice, the organization developing and providing the credential, when the credential started, and the requirements for becoming credentialed and maintaining the credential. The information was obtained from each organization's website.[5,12,13]

Two entry-level or beyond entry-level credentials are available, depending on one's perspective, in two specialty areas of practice: the Certified Diabetes Educator

| TABLE 3-1 | Credentials for Specialty and Advanced Practice |

CREDENTIAL	INITIATED	ORGANIZATION	QUALIFICATION TO TEST EXAMINATION	RECERTIFICATION PROCESS
Registered dietitian (RD)	1969	Commission on Dietetic Registration	• Minimum of a baccalaureate degree or foreign equivalent • Completion of a Commission on Accreditation of Dietetics Education (CADE) accredited <u>Didactic Program in Dietetics</u> • Completion of an accredited dietetics internship or coordinated program	<u>Professional Development Portfolio Guide</u> submitted every 5 years; approximately 75 hours of planned education or advanced degree or specialty certification
Certified specialist pediatrics (CSP) or certified specialist renal (CSR)—board certification as a specialist in pediatric or renal nutrition	1993	Commission on Dietetic Registration	• Current RD, and • Three years minimum length of RD status, and • 4,000 hours of practice as an RD in the specialty within the last 5 years, and successful completion of the Board Certification as a Specialist in Dietetics examination	
Fellow of the American Dietetic Association (FADA)		Commission on Dietetic Registration	• RD credential • Master's or doctoral degree • At least 8 years of work experience • Multiple professional roles with diverse and complex responsibilities and functions • Dispersed professional contacts • Demonstrated an approach global, to practice that reflects a intuitive and evolving perspective; creating problem solving	Originally 10-year; now lifetime; moratorium since 2001
Certified diabetes educator (CDE)	1986	National Certification Board for Diabetes Educators	• RD credential or other license in the health professions • Professional practice experience: – A *minimum* of 2 years of professional practice experience in diabetes self-management training – A *minimum* of 1,000 hours of diabetes self-management training experience • Current employment in a defined role as a diabetes educator a minimum of 4 hours per week or its equivalent at the time of application	75 hours of diabetes continuing education or taking examination again after 5 years; starting in 2009, also 1,000 hours of practice

(Continued next page)

TABLE 3-1   Credentials for Specialty and Advanced Practice *(cont)*

CREDENTIAL	INITIATED	ORGANIZATION	QUALIFICATION TO TEST EXAMINATION	RECERTIFICATION PROCESS
Certified nutrition support dietitian (CNSD)		National Board of Nutrition Support Certification	• RD certification • Recommended candidates have at least 2 years of experience in specialized nutrition support	Every 5 years must retake and pass the Certification Examination for Nutrition Support Dietitians in order to retain certification
Board certified–advanced diabetes management (BC–ADM)	2000	American Nurses Credentialing Center	• RD certification, registration by the Commission on Dietetic Registration, RN, or licensed pharmacist • Master's or higher degree in a clinically relevant area of study • Practiced a minimum of 500 hours in advanced clinical diabetes after professional licensure and within 48 months prior to applying for certification	75 hours, with 51% of this in specialty area in a 5 year period
Certified nutrition specialist (CNS)	1995	Certification Board for Nutrition Specialists (CBNS)	• For professional nutritionists, an advanced degree (master's or doctoral level) from a regionally accredited institution in the field of nutrition or a field allied to nutrition and relevant to the practice of nutrition or other licensed health professionals a. 1,000 hours of supervised professional experience in nutrition or related activities or b. 4,000 hours of independent experience as a professional nutritionist in a professional setting but not part of degree program	Recertify every 5 years through 75 hours of continuing education

Developed from websites in references 5, 12, and 13.

(CDE) and the Certified Nutrition Support Dietitian (CNSD). These credentials are recommended for practice in diabetes and nutrition support, respectively. Both of these credentials, as with the entry-level CDR credential, rely on multiple-choice examinations that test knowledge and application to practice. Both credentials are about 15 years old. The CNSD has about 2,000 credentialed practitioners with about 50% of those recertifying holding a master's degree or higher and about 30% of those initially certifying having a master's degree or higher.[14] The CDE credential had about 5,000 RDs in 2003 and about 8,500 other health professionals, predominantly RNs.[12] Both credentials are designed to measure minimum knowledge to practice appropriately in the specialty and are thereby promoting quality care.[12,13] Both credentials also validate the individual's knowledge against national standards, which allows for accountability. The CDE website has a policy statement approved in June 1993; it says: "Passing the examination verifies certain basic knowledge in the field of diabetes. It does not confer to the CDE any permission to manage diabetes beyond the limitations of the individual's professional practice."[12]

This then leads RDs back to the Scope of Dietetic Practice Framework to assess whether an activity is within their scope.

In 1986, the ADA/CDR studied the potential for certification in "subspecialties" (subdividing clinical into renal, pediatrics, metabolic care) and the development of a system to "recognize advanced levels of practice."[15] The questions used to define what constitutes specialty and/or advanced-level practice are still applicable:

- Are there measurable and identifiable differences in knowledge and skills between entry-level and advanced-level practitioners?
- How do advanced-level and specialty practice interact?
- Is generalist practice actually a type of specialty practice and can the generalist practice at the advanced level?
- Is a reasonable pool of practitioners needed in the specialty? How would certification in the area improve quality of patient care or advance the science and practice of dietetics?[7]

As a result of these studies, the CDR offers two specialty certifications: board-certified specialist in pediatric nutrition (Certified Specialist Pediatrics, or CSP) and Board certified specialist in renal nutrition (Certified Specialist Renal, or CSR). Originally, a third certification in metabolic nutrition was available but it was discontinued in 1997. These certifications started in 1993. Role-delineation studies in 1989 and 1991 first identified the job functions of these professionals. These studies were updated in 1997 and they documented activities performed and the criticality of the activities to patient/client health.[2] In keeping with the ultimate purpose of credentialing, the board-certified examinations covered only activities that are critical to the health of the public served. Therefore, although items such as monitoring patient satisfaction and conducting research are critical to good professional practice, they are not on the examinations.

Each of these specialty credentials is based on being an RD and each can be used to fulfill the 5-year-period portfolio assessment to maintain the RD credential. In 2004, there were 141 CSRs and 150 CSPs; slightly more than 50% had a master's degree or higher (personal communication, C. Reidy, CDR, December 15, 2005). The credential is not needed for entry into the specialty practice but rather is used by employers and clients to document a level of specialized experience and knowledge necessary for competent practice, for career laddering, and for compensation. In a study of diabetes practitioners, practitioners were found to function at entry, specialty, and advanced levels independent of credentialing, although those credentialed were more likely to function at specialty and advanced levels.[16]

ADVANCED CREDENTIALS

As described above, the FADA was designed to assess the individuals' ability to have a global approach to practice and a creative problem-solving, intuitive style of practice based on Bradley's data.[8] The credential has about 350 designees and close to the same number who meet the eligibility requirements but who did not pass the examination. In 2002 the Commission on Dietetic Registration placed a moratorium on the credential. Discussions within the ADA continue to evolve on how to recognize those practicing at an advanced level. The original credential required a master's degree for eligibility.

The board-certified renal and pediatric credentials do not require a master's degree for eligibility, but many of those credentialed (53.8%) have a graduate degree (versus 31.3% with only a bachelor's degree).[17] Interestingly, of these board-certified individuals, more than 50% indicated also having other certifications beyond the entry level, such as the CDE and CNSD. The Board Certified–Advanced Diabetes Management credential (BC–ADM) that was introduced in 2000 does require a master's degree.

Quoting from the American Nurses Credentialing Center website:

> The Advanced Diabetes Management Practitioner has an advanced degree and is able to (1) perform complete and/or focused assessments, (2) recognize and prioritize complex data in order to identify needs of patients with diabetes across the life span, and (3) provide therapeutic problem-solving, counseling, and regimen adjustments. The scope of advanced diabetes practice includes management skills such as medication adjustment, medical nutrition therapy, exercise planning, counseling for behavior management and psychosocial issues. Attaining optimal metabolic control may include treatment and monitoring of acute and chronic complications. The depth of knowledge and competence in advanced clinical practice and diabetes skills affords an increased complexity of decision making, which expands the traditional discipline specific practice. Research, publications, mentoring, and continuing professional development are expected skill sets.[18]

The requirement for and use of this credential will evolve over the next decade.

ADVANCED DEGREES

The question of whether advanced degrees are a sign of or are needed for specialty or advanced practice has been discussed over the past 20 years. It is clear that some practitioners without advanced degrees practice at the advanced level. The question is whether they are the exception or the norm. Much more research is needed in this area.

The trend in most allied health disciplines, including dietetics, is toward higher levels of education prior to entry-level practice. This is due to the expanding body of knowledge in the professions and the increase in autonomous decision making within the professions. The referral models of care are also changing. While historically physicians referred patients to allied health practitioners, the community-based prevention model of healthcare is altering the referral patterns. The patient may see a dietitian, physical or occupational therapist, or nurse practitioner who provides care and makes referrals/suggestions to see a primary care provider. In short, many of the allied health disciplines are evolving into true professions with an independent body of knowledge, a code of ethics, autonomy, educational standards, and a distinct service to provide.

Within the past decade, the number of clinical practice or professional doctorates has grown within many allied health and nursing programs. There is variation as to whether the practice doctorate is for entry into the profession or for advanced practice. What most professions have determined is that the complexity of healthcare issues, research skills, management skills, interprofessional collaboration, and policy issues that are part of advanced practice extend beyond a traditional master's degree. Thus, the professional doctorate is one answer. An important question that must be addressed as dietetics progresses is: What role will clinical residencies and clinical practice doctorates play?[19,20]

HOW NECESSARY OR BENEFICIAL ARE ADDITIONAL CREDENTIALS FOR PRACTITIONERS?

As with most such questions, it depends. As numerous specialty and advanced practice levels are defined by experts and then validated, the possibility exists that the common denominators for specialty and advanced practice will be determined and credentialing can be in a broad area such as clinical dietetics. Especially at the subspecialty levels, however, there may not be enough core competencies or enough practitioners to allow broad-based competency assessment. The specialist in nutrition support, for example, can study, review literature, and become a specialist in pediatric critical care with reasonable effort. An important question to be addressed is how and what do specialists do to prove competency in a new area? Do they need dual credentials? Will competency assurance include continuing education, formal education, competency testing, and/or residency programs? Will institutions pay for the credentials as their measurement of competency assessment?

The ability to shift from one area of practice to another is essential to the dietetics profession. The question is how. Dietetics, as a relatively small profession, has to assess how it will recognize specialties, especially small specialties such as inborn errors of metabolism, rehabilitation, or even more narrow areas such as eating disorders or autism. Within specialties having small numbers of practitioners, formal methods of recognizing specialty skills are difficult to implement. High costs generally preclude specialty examinations; the limited numbers of students preclude educational programs focusing in very narrow areas. Moreover, individuals will not want to take specialty examinations as their practices evolve.

New specialties will continue to emerge, such as the dietitian-chef and the lifestyle coach. Chapter 5 describes many evolving areas of practice. The questions are: What are the competencies? Can they be defined and generalized? Is a credential valuable to the professional or to protect the public? Is there a large enough critical mass of individuals to maintain the credential?

So the profession is at a crossroads again. The profession is defining practice areas at the specialty and advanced levels. By 2010, many of the large specialties should be defined and hopefully validated at each of the levels of practice. The specialties with enough practitioners to support specialty credentials will continue to do so. The question remains whether the credential will influence/control what the scope of

Issues to Ponder

- Do we specialize at the entry or beyond-entry level? What are the implications of each?
- If specialty credentials are optional, what is their value to the public? To the healthcare team? To the dietetics profession?
- Are the CDE and CNSD credentials entry-level or beyond-entry credentials?
- Is an advanced degree needed to be an advanced practitioner?
- If the RD is already at the MS level, what education is needed for specialty or advanced practitioners?
- How do you move from an entry-level position to a specialty and on to an advanced practitioner?
- What is the role of education and experience in this transition?
- How will the Scope of Dietetic Practice Framework affect the evolution of the profession?
- How do the number of RDs and the diversity of practice affect the availability of specialty and advanced credentials?

TABLE 3-2	Proposed Model for Advanced Level Medical Nutrition Therapy Practice[11]
DIMENSION	**CRITERIA**
Education	• 3- to 5-years clinical experience following dietetic registration and before enrolling in the practice doctorate degree program, or • A practice doctorate degree followed by completion of 500 hours of supervised advanced practice
Expertise	• Mastery of the pharmacologic, physiologic, psychosocial, and nutrition knowledge, skills, abilities, and knowledge of current research literature necessary to order, perform, and interpret the results of nutrition related tests, procedures, and treatments • Has a comprehensive, evidence-based approach to assessment, diagnosis, and cost-effective management of complex nutritional problems of individuals, groups, or communities • Uses clinical information, distilling complex concepts to simplicity, but supplying synthesis, analysis, and enhancement as needed
Initiative	• Initiates, modifies, and develops medical nutrition therapy for patients and groups • Functions as an autonomous medical nutrition therapy provider within scope of practice • Employs intellectual curiosity to resolve the issues that produce complex questions
Collaboration	• Has working relationships with diverse network of professionals in and outside the work setting • Shares and seeks expertise to enhance own and others' practice • Provides efficient and effective consultation meeting the needs of the referring entity
Leadership	• Mentors the practice and professional development of others • Provides information to advance the profession through presentations, publications, and participation in professional organizations • Acts as a representative outside the profession concerning nutrition issues
Research	• Continually performs critical appraisal of new research findings and applies them to practice • Designs and conducts practice outcomes research using established research methods
Ethics	• Applies the highest ethical standards to practice, decision making, and interactions with others

Slightly adapted with permission. See reference 11.

practice is. Will we say that only a certified nutrition support specialist can do a task, such as tube placement? How will this impact the scope of practice of RDs without the credential but with the competency?

The next decade will also help us distinguish between specialty and advanced-level practice. Whereas specialty practices have a different body of knowledge, the attributes of advanced-level practice may be more similar. The Fellow of the ADA designation was created to differentiate advanced practice from other practice by identifying characteristics of advanced practitioners and then using essays to evaluate thinking patterns. Although this is a good attempt, the procedure seems to have too many false negatives, where the candidate met the criteria for advanced practice in the eyes of many but the essays did not reflect the criteria. The concept of credentialing the advanced-level practitioner needs to evolve as the measurement of performance improves. Can we adequately measure advanced practice and then give those individuals expanded functions? The Skipper model, Table 3-2, moves the medical nutrition therapy arm of the profession forward, but further validation is needed.[11]

We have many questions to explore as a profession. How do we train the practitioners of the future for entry, specialty, and advanced practice? What credentialing and licensure is needed as we differentiate practice? What is feasible with the size of the profession? What will best protect and improve the health of the public? How are we going to measure the impact of what we do? Will the model to collect data on effectiveness be enough evidence to support practice?

Create a great future. The profession and the public deserve it.

REFERENCES

1. American Dietetic Association definition re-affirmed by the Board of Directors, 2000. Scope of Practice Framework. Avaiable at: www.eatright.org. Accessed March 9, 2006.
2. O'Sullivan Maillet J, Skates J, Pritchett E. American Dietetic Association: scope of dietetics practice framework. J Am Diet Assoc 2005;105:634–640. Available at: http://www.eatright.org/member/policyinitiatives/83_2727.cfm. Accessed September 12, 2005.
3. Rogers D. Report on the American Dietetic Association/ADA Foundation/Commission on Dietetic Registration 2004 dietetics professionals needs assessment. J Am Diet Assoc 2005;105:1348–1355.
4. American Dietetic Association Dietetic Education Task Force Report. Available at: http://www.eatright.org/Member/Governance/85_21734.cfm. Accessed September 12, 2005.
5. Commission on Dietetic Registration. Available at: http://www.cdrnet.org. Accessed September 5, 2005
6. Chambers DW, Gilmore CJ, Maillet JO, Mitchell B. Another look at competency-based education in dietetics. J Am Diet Assoc 1996;96:614–617.
7. Bradley RT, Ebbs P, Young WY, Martin J. Specialty practice in dietetics: empirical models and results. J Am Diet Assoc 1993;93:203–210.
8. Bradley RT, Ebbs P, Young WY, Martin J. Characteristics of advanced-level dietetics practice: a model and empirical results. J Am Diet Assoc 1993;93:196–202.
9. Kieselhorst KJ, Skates J, Pritchett E. American Dietetic Association: standards of practice in nutrition care and updated standards of professional performance. J Am Diet Assoc 2005;105;641–645.
10. Kulkarni K, Boucher JL, Daly A, et al. American Dietetic Association: standards of practice and standards of professional performance for registered dietitians (generalist, specialty, and advanced) in diabetes care. J Am Diet Assoc 2005;105:819–824.
11. Skipper A, Lewis NM. Using initiative to achieve autonomy: a model for advanced practice in medical nutrition therapy. J Amer Diet Assoc 2006 (in press).
12. The National Certification Board for Diabetes Educators. Home page. Available at: http://www.nebde.org. Accessed September 5, 2005.
13. National Board of Nutrition Support Certification, Inc. Home page. Available at: http://www.nutritioncertify.org. Accessed September 5, 2005.
14. Schwartz DB. History and evolution of a successful certification program in nutrition support: the CNSD experience. J Am Diet Assoc 2003;103:736–741.
15. American Dietetic Association. Council on Practice Ad Hoc Specialization Committee, Motion from House of Delegates, October 1986 (unpublished).
16. Green DM, Maillet JO, Touger-Decker R, Byham-Gray L, Matheson P. Functions performed by level of practice of registered dietitian members of the Diabetes Care and Education Dietetic Practice Group. J Am Diet Assoc 2005;105:1280–1284.
17. Leonberg B, Rops MS. The current state of specialty practice in pediatric nutrition and renal nutrition. J Am Diet Assoc 1998;98:1339–352.
18. American Nurses Credentialing Center. Available at: http://www.nursingworld.org/ancc/certification/cert/exams/TCOs/ADM44_Diet_TCO.html. Accessed September 12, 2005.
19. Watters CA, Crozier L. Clinical nutrition residency programs. Support Line 2004;26:10–12.
20. Touger-Decker R. Online advance degree programs in dietetics: are they for real? Support Line 2004;26:13, 16–19.

CHAPTER

4

THE ECONOMICS OF DIETETIC PATIENT CARE

Elvira Q. Johnson, Chris Biesemeier, and Sylvia Escott-Stump

SECTION 1 Demonstrating Effectiveness of
Medical Nutrition Therapy Services

Elvira Q. Johnson

Coverage and appropriate reimbursement/payment for medical nutrition therapy (MNT) services has been a major concern for dietetics professionals for the last two decades. Owing to increased emphasis on accountability and shrinking resources in most areas of healthcare, the importance of defining MNT and documenting effectiveness to all customers—clients, payers, physicians, case managers, administrators, legislators, policy makers, etc.—continues to be a challenge. For many dietetics professionals, the availability of these data has become critical for retaining their job position in this era of cost-cutting measures in the healthcare field. Efforts over the past two decades resulted in limited Medicare coverage in 2002, but dietitians continue to work to expand and improve this benefit. This section focuses on the history of dietetics reimbursement, the current status, and the next steps for demonstrating the effectiveness of MNT.

BACKGROUND/HISTORY

Although dietitians have always been science and research oriented, few data were available on the specific impact they had on clinical outcomes or the effectiveness of their interventions until the early 1990s, when efforts to obtain reimbursement were paramount to the profession. Several states, driven by legislative, licensure, and reimbursement needs, compiled anecdotal data and testimonials from patients and leaders to support broader inclusion of nutrition services in payment and licensure efforts.[1-3] Although not rigorous scientific evidence, the information was used by individual states and the American Dietetic Association (ADA) to focus attention on the cost-effectiveness of MNT, which has been shown to save, on average, more than $8,000 per case, according to ADA's internal analysis of the studies. MNT saves money by reducing length of hospital stay, decreasing complications, decreasing the need for costly medications, and lessening the need for high-technology treatment. An analysis of nearly 2,400 case studies submitted by ADA members documented the per patient cost savings possible when MNT was provided for diseases and conditions for which such therapy is appropriate.[4] Several resources to assist dietitians in these efforts were also published.[5-7]

Simultaneously, ADA funded an outcome research project that was the first randomized, controlled clinical trial that provided scientific proof of the effectiveness of MNT in the treatment of non–insulin-dependent diabetes mellitus (NIDDM, now Type 2 DM)[8] and the search for evidence was under way. A notable study completed by the Lewin Group documented the positive impact registered dietitian (RD) interventions had on Medicare beneficiaries with cardiovascular disease or diabetes, resulting in reduced physician office visits and hospitalizations. They concluded that after an initial period of implementation, coverage for MNT could result in a net reduction in health services utilization and costs for at least some populations. In the case of persons age 55 and older, the savings in utilization of hospital and other services would actually exceed the cost of providing the MNT benefit.[9]

Several state and individual dietitians conducted larger studies that looked at the impact of MNT on diabetes and lipid management; this positive evidence contributed to the scientific basis for broader recommendations.[10–14] The federal government also committed funding to examine the impact of MNT. The Balanced Budget Act of 1997 called for studies on the expansion of preventive benefits in Medicare and specifically included MNT services. The National Academy of Sciences Institute of Medicine contracted with the Health Care Financing Administration to conduct such a study, called "The Role of Nutrition in Maintaining Health in the Nation's Elderly: Evaluating Coverage of Nutrition Services for the Medicare Population." The conclusion reached by the Institute of Medicine's committee was that nutrition therapy is "effective as part of a comprehensive approach to the management and treatment of many conditions affecting the Medicare population." It was also concluded that registered dietitians are "currently the single identifiable group of health care professionals with standardized education, clinical training, continuing education, and national credentialing requirements necessary to be directly reimbursed as a provider of nutrition therapy."[15]

In the spring of 2004, U.S. Department of Health and Human Services Secretary Tommy Thompson released a "Report to Congress on Medical Nutrition Therapy." The report was a further review of the research evidence of the effectiveness and efficacy of MNT.[16] The report "suggests that there may be a benefit from dietary modification using MNT for patients with hyperlipidemia and hypertension," although no specific recommendations were made to expand the benefit.

The research and healthcare climate were also changing. Several national reports emphasized the shortcomings of the U.S. healthcare system and the need for evidence-based practice and provider training in consistent care delivery.[17,18] The ADA was proactive in developing both practice guidelines and a defined Nutrition Care Process. Since 1996, standardized nutrition therapy protocols and guidelines had been developed by Dietetic Practice Groups (DPGs), the ADA Quality Management Committee, and staff.[19–21] Several of these were refined and made evidence-based[22–25] in 2002. In 2005 these guidelines were again updated, using a robust evidence-analysis process, and published on the ADA website.[26] These evidence-based MNT guidelines are the standards now used by Centers for Medicare and Medicaid Services (CMS) and many other insurers for defining MNT.[27]

In a continuing effort to improve quality and clinical effectiveness, the ADA developed and, in 2003, adopted, a Nutrition Care Process and Model (see Chapter 9) to assist members in practice. According to Lacey and Pritchett, "When providers of care, no matter their location, use a process consistently, comparable outcomes data can be generated to demonstrate value. A standardized nutrition care process effectively promotes the dietetics professional as the unique provider of nutrition care when it is consistently used as a systematic method to think critically and make decisions to provide safe and effective nutrition care"[28] ADA has also released a position statement that incorporates these concepts, "Integration of Medical Nutrition Therapy and Pharmacotherapy."[29] The ADA's position is that the application of MNT and lifestyle counseling as a part of the Nutrition Care Process is an integral component of the medical treatment for management of specific disease states and conditions, and should be the initial step in the management of these situations. If optimal control cannot be achieved with MNT alone and concurrent pharmacotherapy is required, then the ADA promotes a team approach to care for clients receiving concurrent MNT and pharmacotherapy and encourages active collaboration among dietetics professionals and other members of the healthcare team.[29]

A pilot study funded by the ADA Foundation assessed the impact of the RD as a care manager for obese patients with Type 2 diabetes. Improving Control with Activity and Nutrition (ICAN) was a 1-year randomized, controlled trial. Participants were randomized to case management (CM) or self-study (SS). CM involved 3 hours of individualized treatment, 6 hours of group classes, and monthly phone contact over 1 year by registered dietitians. The results indicate that the number of prescription medications, especially diabetes medications, decreased more in the CM group than in the SS group ($P = .13$).[30]

CURRENT STATUS: COVERAGE AND REIMBURSEMENT SUCCESSES

During the 1990s, more and more third-party payers (TPP) began to cover and reimburse for MNT by RDs. As the body of evidence supporting the efficacy and cost-effectiveness of MNT grew, so did coverage and reimbursement. In 2000, a survey of insurance companies showed that 52% were reimbursing for MNT.[31] Efforts to market MNT to managed care organizations and employers have resulted in MNT coverage within many insurance companies' plans.[32] Aetna US Healthcare provides MNT coverage nationally as defined in their MNT Coverage Policy Bulletin. The bulletin describes services provided, the number of visits, and treatment guidelines for a number of chronic diseases, including cardiovascular disease, diabetes mellitus, hypertension, kidney disease, eating disorders, gastrointestinal disorders, seizures (i.e., ketogenic diet), and other conditions based on the efficacy of diet and lifestyle changes in the treatment of these conditions.[33] Many of the Blue Cross Blue Shield (BCBS) insurance groups also include MNT as a benefit. BCBS of Massachusetts has based its nutrition coverage on the ADA's MNT protocols.[34]

Some employer groups also provide MNT benefits in an effort to improve employee health, reduce costs, and increase satisfaction.[35] A successful program at Texas Instruments in Dallas implemented MNT protocols and continuous improvement techniques to provide care; this effort resulted in a cost of less than $0.35 per member per month.[36] In 2002, the Medicare MNT benefit for beneficiaries with diabetes or renal disease was implemented.[37,38] Registered dietitians and nutrition professionals could now become Medicare providers.

CURRENT STATUS: CHALLENGES

The old adage "Be careful what you wish for, as you might get it" is especially fitting for dietitians who had hoped that Medicare coverage and reimbursement (MCR) would be a godsend. Although MCR is an important achievement, as many report increased exposure and visibility in their institutions as MCR providers, others are disenchanted with the limitations. Coverage is limited to only two diseases—diabetes and kidney disease—even though the Institute of Medicine report recommended coverage with a physician referral for all, and the research evidence is there for many other diagnoses. The reimbursement is also limited. As of March 2003, the national hourly averages of the total Medicare-approved payments were $60 per individual or $11.88 per participant in a group setting, including copayment. Since these rates are based on geographic factors, 1 hour of individual MNT ranges from a high of $86.56 in the San Francisco area to a low of $42.20 in Puerto Rico.[39]

In addition to low reimbursement rates, the administrative burden of meeting MCR regulations for tracking visits, referral, billing, and coordination add to the challenges for RD MCR providers. Although some dietitians may have the option of opting out of being providers, not all can do that. In Massachusetts, BCBS has instituted a new provider status for private practice RDs who were not covered previously by BCBSMA. They are required to become MCR providers, however, thus forcing them to accept the lower rates for beneficiaries (e-mail, Linda Greenan, April 9, 2003). Another troubling result is that in some states, several other insurers are lowering their reimbursement rates closer to Medicare rates. In Massachusetts, several private practice dietitians are struggling to maintain their current rates and are at a loss as to how to stem the reductions. Some have experienced more than a 30% drop in rates in 2003 alone (personal communication, M. Davis, D. Konkle, August 18, 2003).

Some hospitals, especially larger academic institutions, have been reluctant to add providers to staff, as that might entail teaching appointments at medical schools or other ramifications not dealt with before. Some have balked at the confusing and ever-changing requirements and billing issues and many question whether actual reimbursement is worth the effort.[40]

The changing fiscal climate is leading to increasing pressures to reduce costs in healthcare. With the decline in the economy hitting healthcare, many services, including nutrition and MNT, are increasingly being challenged. Faced with the continuing need to prove the value of MNT and the RD to changing administrations, providers, and payers, many experienced dietitians have become disenchanted, and relatively low salaries have discouraged those who might have considered entering the profession.

FUTURE: RESOURCES NEEDED

"The glass is still half full." With a foot in the door of MCR and the prospect that additional diagnoses may be covered in the near future, some RDs feel that the services and reimbursement for care are growing. The focus on quality care and reducing the cost of medications may still provide opportunities for RDs to practice in an outcome-focused manner in marketing and promoting their unique and effective services. Some dietitians who have participated in the Robert Wood Johnson

Foundation–funded experiment to improve care by implementing the chronic care model may be able to influence national policy for management of chronic diseases.[41–44]

Marketing directly to consumers may also prove effective, as they are the voters and drivers of many systems. Continued research efforts, especially related to the cost-effectiveness of MNT and customer satisfaction, are needed. The active support from national professional organizations in public policy, research funding, and development of necessary tools for dietitians is essential to this success.

The most important and essential component in this effort, however, are the dietitians themselves. The specific skill sets needed to be an effective nutrition therapist are being defined. Some believe that an advanced practice credential may be needed to enhance the entry-level RD's skills in behavior change, outcome management, marketing, and other competencies (for further discussion, see Chapter 3). These skills may also be required to break through the old image of the RD, who is still perceived as an inpatient ancillary provider who implements diet orders. The new image is a clinical provider, recognized by Medicare and others, with the academic training equivalent to a nurse practitioner and the skill sets to analyze data, make nutrition diagnoses, and implement appropriate nutrition therapy to achieve clinical outcomes appropriate to clients' diagnoses and lifestyle. In addition, measuring and monitoring changes and outcomes and comparing them to evidence-based standards will enable the dietitian to continuously improve care and outcomes. This is the practice standard that will enhance compensation. Additional business skills are also needed to be able to manage budget and resources, maintain data systems to manage outcomes, and then articulate to administrators the value and benefit of MNT services. Successful departments have been able to thrive and grow by implementing these techniques.

SECTION 2   Economic Considerations in
                              Healthcare Organizations
....
                              Chris Biesemeier

To practice at an advanced level, dietetics professionals must look beyond the basics of nutrition assessment and disease-specific nutrition interventions to the broader economic factors that affect and are affected by nutrition care and its delivery. This section describes economic considerations in the inpatient setting and defines ways that inpatient clinical dietitians can assist in achieving financial targets.

BUDGET

Each dietetics department operates within an annual budget that is part of the annual facility budget. Managers face ever-tightening limits on available resources. Departments within a facility are in competition with each other for their portion of the facility's total budget. Within dietetics departments, managers must establish priorities for use of allocated resources, monitor actual expenses against budgeted expenses, and be alert for ways to streamline and achieve further reductions in expenses while also maintaining established standards for quality.

In some instances, decisions made by dietetics managers affect the budgets of other departments. An example of this is the decision to implement a closed enteral nutrition support system. Not only the dietetics budget will be reduced by any cost changes resulting from purchasing products in ready-to-hang containers but also the budget of the department that currently purchases feeding bags and tube sets, if not the budget of the dietetics department as a whole. The amount of nursing time required for administering tube feedings will also be reduced—an important consideration for units that are experiencing shortages of staff nurses.

CHARGING FOR INPATIENT PRODUCTS AND SERVICES

In general, charging for nutrition products and services in the inpatient setting does not contribute additional revenue to the hospital's bottom line, although it may appear on paper that it does so. Departments use charges for nutrition products, such as tube feedings and supplements, and services—such as nutrition assessments, calorie counts, and diet education consults—as a way to track volumes and potentially evaluate services. Although product and service charges do appear as line items on patients' bills, hospitals receive fixed payments based on reimbursement schedules that are prospectively set and are often further discounted as a result of negotiated contracts with third-party payers. In theory, it is possible to increase the amount of the fixed payment by documenting malnutrition in the medical record and on the discharge diagnosis list. In recent years, however, medical record coding systems have become very sophisticated. As a result, while thorough documentation of nutrition issues in the medical record is important for analyses of services, it is unlikely that the addition of the diagnosis of malnutrition to the list of patients' discharge diagnoses will increase reimbursement.

PURCHASING FOOD AND SUPPLIES

Food purchasing and inventory control are important areas of resource management. Many facilities participate in buying cooperatives and have buying contracts that limit product choice to those of approved vendors to obtain substantial group buying discounts. Inventory control requires maintaining adequate but not excess quantities of needed items; monitoring the rate of inventory turnover; identifying atypical usage patterns in time to avoid running out; and reordering on a defined schedule to maintain established par levels. Some products (e.g., enteral feedings and specialty products) can be ordered directly from the manufacturer. More often, food and supplies are ordered through food distributors that maintain regional warehouses and make scheduled deliveries each week. Distributors have limited shelf space and often ask facilities to guarantee minimum volumes of product usage before agreeing to stock new items. Dietetics practitioners need to be aware that ordering products that are not on the buying contract or available through the food distributor increases costs. In addition, demand for products must be anticipated enough in advance to avoid the additional shipping costs that arise with overnight or express deliveries.

PATIENT FOODSERVICE

The type of food production system and patient menus a facility uses are major determinants of its food and labor costs. Many facilities have implemented systems for advance bulk food production, such as cook-chill systems. Cook-chill involves rapid chilling of food after preparation and storage at controlled temperatures for up to 5 days. With cook-chill systems, food production can be scheduled, thus promoting a more organized workflow, reducing reliance on staff to work early and late production shifts, and limiting the need for overtime when production staff do not report for work.

Patient menus define the food choices available to patients and are written in cycle or cafeteria formats. Cycle menus vary in length and either provide multiple options from which patients can choose (select menus) or are limited to one option in each food category (nonselect menus). Cafeteria menus offer patients a set of choices that provides variety, yet they usually remain the same from day to day. Generally, the longer the cycle and the larger the number and types of choices available, the greater the food storage and production facilities required to support a menu. With shorter lengths of stay, menus in either format are generally adequate to satisfy most tastes. However, patients with long lengths of stay—for example, those on oncology or transplant units—often tire of the available selections at some point and require additional food options from write-in lists or approved substitution lists.

Although some facilities use an on-demand system for tray delivery, most facilities deliver trays on a three-meal-a-day schedule, with options for between-meal nourishment. In these facilities, trays are assembled on a tray line either close to the time of service or in advance. Advance assembly requires the refrigeration of trays and rethermalization prior to service.

Clinical dietitians work directly with patients to assess their nutrition requirements and develop nutrition care plans to meet requirements. In this capacity, they observe how well patients eat their food and recommend alternative selections when food intake is inadequate. They also serve as links to food production and service for patients and other members of the healthcare team. As a result, it is important that they understand the systems in use, adhere to established procedures, and communicate information and feedback in a timely manner. Examples of clinical dietitians' involvement include the following:

- Food preferences: Procedures define which preferences can be honored, how preferences are to be communicated to the kitchen, and what to do when changes in preferences are identified during hospitalization. Staying within the limits that are set enhances patient satisfaction by avoiding unrealistic expectations. It also promotes budget compliance, since purchasing special foods can be costly and preparing additional foods requires extra effort.

- Meal and nourishment schedules: Cutoffs for diet orders, menu changes, and special requests are needed to allow advance preparation of food, assembly of trays, and adherence to delivery schedules. Changes in menus initiated after cutoff times result in extra work at several points in the production-delivery cycle and should be kept to a minimum. However, many changes that occur are unavoidable or are outside the control of clinical staff. Complying with cutoff times can also be a challenge in working with specific patient populations—for example, patients with cancer and children. Patients with cancer may find it difficult to know what foods they will be able to tolerate until immediately prior to a meal, making advance selection difficult. Likewise, children's food preferences and requests can change from one day to the next, especially in the case of children who are ill. Dietetics professionals should work with foodservice managers to devise systems that will meet the needs of patients with special feeding issues. Use of a hotel-style or room-service feeding system is one approach to increasing patient satisfaction and decreasing food waste. With this system, patients make their food selections close to meal delivery time and decide when to eat rather than having to depend on a predetermined meal schedule. The timing of meal and nourishment delivery can also affect medication schedules. Clinical dietitians should assess medication timing in relation to food consumption and communicate with unit staff about food or medication schedule changes that are necessary in order to avoid interactions.

- Cost control: Dietetics professionals are not expected to be the "food police" on the units. When possible, however, they should reinforce the established procedures to control food costs—for example, those for providing food to patients' families, delivering late trays, and sending duplicate trays. Late trays are for patients with diet-order changes after the cutoffs. Duplicate trays are prepared for patients who need a second tray—for example, when foods on the first tray served are not acceptable for one reason or another. Duplicate trays increase food costs owing to food waste. As noted above, use of a room-service system may reduce food waste, although personnel costs to support the system may be higher than those in facilities with more conventional systems.

- Feedback: Dietetics professionals gather information that can be very useful to foodservice managers. Their observations assist managers in defining the origins of problems—for example, a change in brand or vendor that results in the purchase of a product that does not meet quality standards, substandard preparation of a menu item on a particular day, and problems with the appearance of food or trays. Most facilities have a mechanism whereby dietetics professionals can communicate their observations.

CLINICAL DIETETICS STAFFING

Within the clinical dietetics unit, personnel costs are the primary expense. Benefit packages vary from one facility to another. At some facilities, registration fees, membership dues, and continuing education conference expenses are fully or partially paid. At other facilities, budget limitations preclude coverage of these fees and expenses.

Each department determines the number and type of clinical dietetics staff needed to accomplish the work of patient care, that is, the number of dietitians and dietetics technicians and whether they are full- or part-time employees. Determination of staffing needs takes careful consideration, and methods to do this have been described in detail elsewhere.[45] Since staffing needs change over time—for example, owing to the opening of a new patient-care unit or the addition of a new service—periodic evaluation is important.

Ideally, the workload is distributed after considering the nutrition acuity of patients, which is the number of patients at various levels of nutrition risk on different units within a facility, the intensity and type of nutrition care required, and the mix of dietetics professionals available to provide nutrition care. Staff can be assigned to patient care by location—for example, to specific units within a facility—or by patient service, such as the renal, geriatric, or oncology service.

At some facilities, dietetics professionals provide both inpatient and outpatient coverage for the same patient population. This coverage promotes continuity of care. It may also save time, since the registered dietitians (RDs) who work in the inpatient setting are already familiar with patients' nutrition needs when they transfer to the outpatient setting. When inpatient RDs cover outpatient areas, it is important to inform hospital administrators so as to avoid including the time that the RDs spend with outpatients on the Medicare cost report, especially if they generate charges to patients for their services. Failure to remove this RD time from the Medicare cost report gives the appearance of trying to obtain double payment for the same RD time. Table 4-1 gives an example of coverage of oncology and bone marrow transplant services across the care continuum.

Many factors related to clinical staffing and the use of dietetics professionals' time have economic implications:

- Staffing mix: In facilities that do not employ dietetics technicians, the RDs must perform all nutrition care activities, from basic to complex. Although care systems may run smoothly and all quality standards may be met, the opportunity cost can be significant. Low-complexity tasks can be performed at less cost by dietetics technicians without compromising quality

TABLE 4-1	Example of Coverage Across the Care Continuum: Oncology and Bone Marrow Transplant (BMT) Nutrition Program	
POSITION	**REGISTERED DIETITIAN**	**DIETETICS TECHNICIAN, REGISTERED**
Patients	• Oncology patients at high nutrition risk in the hospital and outpatient clinic • All BMT patients before and after transplant	• Oncology patients at moderate nutrition risk in the hospital
Duties	• Nutrition care process: Assesses nutrition needs, makes nutrition diagnoses, develops intervention plans, monitors effectiveness of plans, and revises plans as needed • Recommends and monitors nutrition support • Attends daily BMT bedside team rounds • Educates patients on diet guidelines, tube feeding regimen, symptom management, and food safety • Provides clinical oversight to the DTR	• Nutrition care process: Assesses nutrition needs, incorporates foods and supplements into menus to improve intake, monitors intake, and adjusts menus as needed • Interfaces with diet office and kitchen to ensure that patients' food preferences are met • Educates patients on home nutrition regimen • Communicates closely with registered dietitian
Full-time equivalents (FTE) allocated to acute-care oncology/BMT units	0.95 FTE	0.8 FTE
Full-time equivalents (FTE) allocated to outpatient BMT clinic	0.25 FTE	No time allocated
Full-time equivalents (FTE) allocated to outpatient oncology clinic	0.8 FTE	No time allocated

standards, thus freeing RDs to focus on more complex tasks or to expand into new or more advanced roles. More appropriate use of RD time also contributes to greater job satisfaction, which can translate into higher productivity and job retention.

■ Productivity and time use: Most facilities have systems in place to track productivity; that is, the volume of services produced using allocated resources. Facilities compare their productivity over time and may also participate in benchmarking programs to compare their productivity with that of similar external partner facilities. Evaluation of productivity and use of staff time can reveal opportunities to transfer some tasks to other more appropriate staff—for example, transferring responsibility for nutrition screening to unit staff, nutrition assessment of patients at moderate nutrition risk to dietetics technicians, and survival skills nutrition education of inpatients to dietetics technicians. Opportunities to streamline may also be identified—for example, the decision to use a standard template for nutrition assessment documentation. At times, evaluation of productivity may reveal a disproportion in time use, as, for example, the use of the majority of RD time for initial patient assessment and care planning to meet established time standards. As a result, inadequate time may be spent on follow-up monitoring and reassessment. Evaluation of weekend coverage may reveal inadequate staffing to meet needs or, conversely, lower productivity than on weekdays. In facilities with computerized medical records, many opportunities are available for achieving efficiencies while also improving communication with team members about patients' nutrition care. At the author's facility, Vanderbilt University Medical Center (VUMC), members of the clinical staff save their inpatient notes in both the permanent medical record and draft form. They are able to use the previous draft version of a note as a template for their next note, saving much documentation time. On-line documentation is also readily accessible when patients transition to other care settings, as from inpatient to outpatient settings, ensuring that outpatient dietetics staff are aware of discharge goals and nutrition care plans.

- Orientation and training: Time spent orienting staff to new positions, whether the result of hiring new employees or internal transfers, is time well spent. Adequate orientation and training promote improved patient safety and compliance with regulatory standards for performance competency. They also contribute to enhanced job satisfaction.

- Staff retention and turnover: In general, facilities seek to retain good employees and to minimize turnover. Although some turnover is unavoidable—owing to transfer of family members, family-related responsibilities, and the desire to obtain additional education or explore new professional opportunities—much of it is avoidable. Turnover is costly in terms of the time and energy required to recruit and train new staff and the emotional cost to existing staff of actual or perceived overwork during periods of vacancy. Many facilities are implementing formal recognition programs to be proactive in communicating to staff their value to the organization. Managers at these facilities hope that this will translate into increased staff retention.

- Joint Commission on Accreditation of Healthcare Organizations (JCAHO) activities: With the advent of periodic performance reviews and unannounced JCAHO surveys have come increased requirements for performance monitoring to support the levels of compliance that are reported to JCAHO. This may lead to increased use of staff time for data collection and review, depending on existing procedures.

OPPORTUNITIES FOR COST SAVINGS

Systems that lead to early identification of patients at nutrition risk, such as nutrition screening programs, promote rapid assessment of nutrition problems and initiation of interventions that address these problems and contribute to reduced lengths of hospital stay.[46,47] Follow-up monitoring and reassessment ensure that patient tolerance of nutrition interventions, including nutrition supplements and tube feeding products, is evaluated and that changes are made when needed. As an example, avoidance of overfeeding of nutrition support reduces the likelihood of hyperglycemia and its associated risk of infection. Tracking the outcomes of nutrition care provided in the inpatient setting is important to demonstrate the value of nutrition care and the clinical dietetics practitioners who provide this care.

Members of the clinical dietetics staff need to be alert for ways to improve quality and reduce costs. These two examples from the author's facility illustrate ways that this can be done.

CASE EXAMPLE: DEVELOPMENT OF A SUPPLEMENT AND ENTERAL PRODUCTS FORMULARY OPPORTUNITY

Clinical dietitians used a large number of nutrition supplements and enteral products, including similar types of products from different vendors. Storeroom staff found it hard to maintain adequate supplies of products, and as a result, formulas frequently had to be shipped via overnight express, resulting in increased costs. The decision was made to develop and implement a supplement and enteral nutrition formulary that would meet patients' needs yet provide limits on the number of products used.

STRATEGIES

The process for developing a formulary included these steps:

1. Assemble a formulary committee. Include representatives from nursing units with high enteral feeding use, physicians who regularly order enteral nutrition, and dietetics professionals who were managers or supervisors involved with purchasing supplements and enteral products, in addition to members of the clinical dietetics staff.
2. Review the role of the committee and the process that will be used to select formulary products. Explain limits on product selection due to buying contracts and be clear about the decision-making process and the level of involvement the committee will have in this process.
3. Define patient needs and list categories of supplements and enteral products that meet these needs; for example, standard, standard with fiber, concentrated, and elemental tube feedings.
4. Define each category in specific terms, listing calorie concentrations and protein ranges that are acceptable for each category and any limitations that must be met—for example, whether an elemental category includes only products composed of amino acids or whether products with both amino acids and short-chain peptides are acceptable.
5. Define indications for using products in each category and indications for discontinuing their use.
6. Review the list of product categories, definitions, and indications carefully and reach agreement on these within the committee. Defining indications for use of high-cost products helps to limit inappropriate use and unnecessary expense. Product names are omitted until step 7 in the process.
7. Put each product that meets established criteria and is available on the facility's buying contract into the appropriate formulary category. In the interest of time, this step can be done by one member of the committee and shared with the entire committee for review and approval.
8. For oral supplements only, share feedback on patient acceptance from past experience with the use of such products. The committee may want to complete a blind taste test of products in each category; however, committee members should be aware that their taste preferences might differ significantly from those of patients. Another option is to include patients in the taste-testing process. Omit any products that do not meet acceptability criteria.
9. At this point in the process, all products listed in each category should be acceptable for use on the formulary. List cost per unit or per serving for products in each

category; compare products based on cost; and select the least expensive product in each category. This step may be done by a subgroup of the committee and selections reported to the entire committee.

10. Approve the formulary, submit to any facility committees for final approval, and communicate to appropriate staff and dietetics department managers. Determine a schedule for implementation, allowing adequate time for transition. This can include:

    a. Notifying vendors and distributors of product changes.
    b. Obtaining codes for computer order entry systems and internal charges.
    c. Ordering new products to have on hand on the date of implementation.
    d. Depleting existing stores of products that are being discontinued.
    e. Determining a strategy for patients on tube feedings that are being discontinued on the implementation date so as to ensure continuity in tolerance. Existing inventories of these products may be sufficient to meet needs for the remainder of the patients' hospital stay.

The formulary committee developed policies and procedures to support the use of the formulary. One issue addressed was how to meet the needs of patients who are admitted on nonformulary tube feedings. Refer to Table 4-2 for solutions to this issue. Another issue considered was how to transition tube-fed patients to nonformulary tube feedings for discharge in cases where nursing homes and home care agencies responsible for patients' postdischarge nutrition care have their own formularies of products that are not on the VUMC formulary. On the one hand, staff understand that other facilities and agencies have their own financial limits and must operate within contractual arrangements. On the other hand, they do not want patient care to be compromised because comparable products are not available. To avoid inappropriate substitutions, emphasis has been given to documentation of discharge nutrition goals and interventions in the medical record, provision of a copy of this documentation to postdischarge care providers, and communication with staff in the postdischarge setting directly or through case managers. In addition, clinical dietitians developed an enteral feeding discharge order set that specified tube-feeding orders, allowed substitutions, and provided for postdischarge monitoring of orders and protocols. Generally, product substitutions are allowed with prior notification of the inpatient clinical dietitian.

Careful consideration was also given to the issue of providing supplies of tube feeding products for postdischarge use. Providing more than a minimal amount of product, such as more than the remainder of the feeding for the day of discharge, results in substantial unreimbursed costs to the facility. This is because charges for products to be used after the day of discharge cannot be added to patients' hospital bills. A system for patients to purchase tube feedings through the hospital cashier has been implemented, with product prices that are comparable to retail prices. Exceptions are made in special circumstances—for example, for infants being discharged to home on formulas requiring special recipe ingredients. In these cases, one can or bottle of each product used in the recipe is provided by the hospital at no charge.

Economic Impact

Use of a formulary has allowed high-quality nutrition care to be provided and budget targets to be met. Inclusion of the clinical dietetics staff in the process enhanced their understanding of the economic issues involved.

TABLE 4-2	Enteral Nutrition Formulary Issues
ISSUE	**SOLUTION**
• Patients admitted to the hospital on tube feedings that are not on the approved formulary	• Most adult patients can be changed to formulary products without difficulty.
	• Physicians and parents may not want to change tube-feeding products of children on tube feedings when tolerance is well established. A small supply of nonformulary products is kept in the storeroom for use in these situations.
• Patients discharged to facilities or home-care programs with their own formularies that include alternate products	• Determine when a "no substitution" policy is clinically necessary. Document rationale for tube-feeding product in medical record. Communicate postdischarge tube-feeding orders in writing and through case managers.

EVIDENCE-BASED PRACTICE

The process of formulary development provides an excellent opportunity to incorporate evidence-based principles into the practice of dietetics. This can be done by relying on national practice guidelines, such as the clinical guidelines published by the American Society of Parenteral and Enteral Nutrition and the Canadian Clinical Guidelines, to define indications for use of products that make claims for specific diagnoses or conditions.[48,49] Committee members may decide to do their own analysis of the professional literature. If so, use of a systematic process, such as the one used by the ADA to develop its Medical Nutrition Therapy Evidence-Based Guides for Practice, is recommended.[50] Use of an evidence-based approach enhances the quality of the formulary that is developed, although it also adds time to the process.

CASE EXAMPLE: DEVELOPMENT OF A TUBE-FEEDING CARE-MANAGEMENT PROGRAM OPPORTUNITY

Numerous staff provided education of patients discharged on tube feedings and patients whose tube feedings were initiated in the outpatient setting. As a result, education was inconsistent in content and thoroughness. Feedback from patients indicated that they often had questions about tube-feeding orders and administration after discharge, which led to a failure to meet their nutrition goals.

STRATEGIES

A team of two RDs (tube-feeding program RDs) worked with the clinical dietetics manager (the author) to develop a program that included:

- Education of patients and their caregivers on patients' tube feedings prior to hospital discharge by unit RDs and prior to or immediately after tube placement in the outpatient setting by a tube-feeding program RD.
  - Written educational materials were developed for four different methods of tube-feeding administration.
  - Inpatient RDs were trained on core content to ensure their competency in teaching patients and their caregivers.

- A teaching checklist was developed for use during patient and caregiver education to ensure consistency. The checklist is also used for documentation.
- A tube-feeding discharge order set was developed and implemented to communicate postdischarge orders and monitoring protocols to home care providers. The order set contains a referral to the outpatient nutrition clinic to alert program RDs to patients' discharge.
- Monitoring via phone and in-person follow-up that is focused on the first 3 months after discharge or tube feeding initiation that includes:
  - Phone follow-up by a program RD within 72 hours of discharge or initiation of tube feeding to reinforce content of tube-feeding teaching, answer questions, and evaluate adequacy of feeding and fluid infusion.
  - Two follow-up appointments, scheduled at times of regular physician visits, at approximately 2 weeks and 2 months postdischarge or tube-feeding initiation and three additional phone follow-up calls during the 3-month interval.
  - Use of a short standard assessment tool to collect relevant data on weight, amount of tube feeding and fluids infused, occurrence of side effects, and unplanned calls or visits to primary care providers or specialists related to tube feeding.
  - Ongoing follow-up after the initial 3-month interval when warranted.

ECONOMIC IMPACT

Although data have not been aggregated at the time of writing, it will be possible to compare outcome indicators such as weight, percent of goals met, frequency of complications, and frequency of unplanned provider calls and visits between program patients and tube-feeding patients who are not enrolled in the program. Potential opportunities for cost savings include reducing the frequency of tube-feeding complications, unplanned provider calls and visits, emergency room visits, and hospital readmissions.

SUMMARY

In summary, the delivery of nutrition care affects the cost of healthcare directly through the costs of resources used in care provision, such as staff time, products, equipment, and supplies, and the cost savings achieved through careful monitoring of nutrition interventions. Nutrition care can also affect healthcare costs indirectly by contributing to reduced inpatient lengths of stay, unplanned care, and hospital readmissions. Clinical dietetics professionals need to understand the economic implications of their care or, in some instances, the lack of their care. They also need to design and implement programs and services to maximize efficiencies and achieve appropriate cost reductions. Doing so allows them to be proactive in demonstrating their economic value to patients, healthcare administrators, providers, and payers. In this way, they can position themselves as essential members of the healthcare teams of today and tomorrow.

SECTION 3   Performance and Value
                of the Dietetics Profession
                Sylvia Escott-Stump

Professional service is not free. Nutrition assessment, diagnosis, interventions, evaluation, and monitoring are essential to the maintenance of health or the return to it. Therefore, the budget of every healthcare facility or program should include sufficient compensation for the necessary human "collateral" required to provide excellence in nutrition services. This section describes how dietetics professionals can demonstrate leadership in any facility, how they can market their services, and how they can negotiate for compensation in a more appropriate manner than in the past.

At the beginning of the decade, the ADA's representative body, the House of Delegates, found that the number-one issue for members was the concern that salaries did not always meet expectations relative to the required training and education in sciences and management. Other issues were fear of competition or encroachment from other professionals, limited public recognition of the dietetics professional as "the" food and nutrition expert, and a perspective that the demands of professional competency and expectations for continuing education exceeded member interest levels.[51]

Data on employment and salaries of ADA members registered as dietitians (RDs) and dietetics technicians (DTRs) are reported regularly in the professional *Journal of the American Dietetic Association*. Employment levels reported by member RDs and DTRs were consistent and high throughout the 1990s and, overall, salaries for RDs and DTRs in all areas of practice have risen. According to the 2002 Dietetics Compensation and Benefits Survey,[52] a number of factors can be identified that affect the perceived value of the profession by its members and by the public. Table 4-3 delineates a demographic profile of the profession and potentially relevant concerns related to these factors.

This study of the perception and image of dietetics professionals by the public is not new. Over the years, greater visibility has enhanced public perception of the ADA,[53] but the individual dietetics professional must continue to focus on his or her own performance. Knowing the trends (the external environment) and conducting regular self-assessments (the internal, personal environment) helps the dietetics practitioner to achieve a higher level of success than if either set of factors remains unclear. For a review of trends and implications, refer to Chapters 1 and 5.

PUBLIC PERCEPTION AND PROFESSIONAL COMPETENCY

The Nutrition Trends Survey published by the ADA in 2002 reported that primary sources for nutrition information among Americans are television (48%) and magazines (47%); registered dietitians and nutritionists (90%) and doctors (92%) are the most valued sources of nutrition information.[54] According to this same survey, most

TABLE 4-3	Practitioner Profile: A Snapshot of the Dietetics Profession (DP) in 2001–2002	
PROFILE FACTOR	**FINDINGS**	**RELEVANT CONCERNS**
Sex	97% female	May reflect tendency to be less competitive in the job marketplace; viewed as less assertive profession? Some dietitians take time off from employment to raise a family; this may delay their rise on the "career ladder."
Age	Median age 43; 11% are 55 or older; 27% are under 35	Generational synergy is needed to meet different expectations.
Racial demographics	92% Caucasian; 3% Hispanic; 5% African American or other	Diverse viewpoints may be limited.
Education	Minimum BS degree plus supervised practice for RD; 45% hold master's degree and 3% doctoral degrees. 26% of DTRs hold a BS degree or higher.	Entry-level competencies may require more than 4 years; salary not competitive with other careers where a bachelor's degree is sufficient.
Specialty training	16% of RDs and 6% of DTRs hold one or more specialty certifications (CSR, CSP).	No specialty certifications offered in nonclinical roles, even though the profession supports preparation for practice in other areas.
Employers	40% work for a nonprofit firm; 19% work for the government; 30% work for a for-profit firm; 10% of dietitians are self-employed.	Nonprofit perspective may not require a competitive stance by dietitians. Those who work in business or private practice will understand the need for marketing and staying competitive.
Clinical positions	Clinical nutrition, acute care (28% RDs, 41% DTRs) Clinical nutrition, ambulatory care (14% RDs, 1% DTRs) Clinical nutrition, long-term care (12% RDs, 20% DTRs)	54% of RDs and 62% of DTRs employed in positions recognized as "clinical"; concern that salaries are not competitive with other allied health practitioners, and facilities often do not retain excellent practitioners.
Community and education/research positions	Community nutrition (11% RDs, 10% DTRs) Education and research (6% RDs, 1% DTRs)	17% of RDs and 11% of DTRs are in positions related to community or education and research in the field.
Management and consultation or business positions	Food and nutrition management (13% RDs, 20% DTRs) Consultation and business (11% RDs, 2% DTRs)	24% of RDs and 22% of DTRs work in positions that require regular inclusion of skills such as negotiation, marketing, conflict resolution, business planning, and evaluation. These skills may be minimally addressed at entry level.
Full-time employment	68% of respondents worked full time (35 or more hours a week).	Part-time employment may not reflect total cash compensation, especially for consultants. Part-time employment may limit compensation packages for RDs and DTRs who are not self-employed or who do not supervise others.
Compensation	Highest-paying nonacademic RD positions: Executive-level professional Sales representative Research and development Director of nutrition Public relations or marketing Director of food and nutrition School/child care nutritionist Communications consultant Clinical nutrition manager	Years of experience, level of supervisory and budgetary responsibility, and area of practice contribute the most to better-paying positions. Many dietetics professionals do not understand the career ladder and how to achieve desired goals or positions.

Data reflect responses from 13,694 respondents to the American Dietetic *Association's 2002 Dietetics Compensation and Benefits Survey.* Chicago: American Dietetic Association, 2003. Relevant concerns were added by the author of this section.

Americans (90%) have heard of registered dietitians, yet only 32% know that an RD is certified or has a degree or license. Now that a majority of states have some form of licensure or certification, public perception of competency may gradually improve for the dietetics professional as awareness of licensure and credentialing for the profession becomes more widely recognized by the public.

Competency-based practice is a common buzzword for professionals. Understanding the skill base of staff members and improving those skills with training is the responsibility of management. Each professional should realize as well that competency assessment and continuing development will be needed to maintain a high level of job success and satisfaction. Competency-based evaluations allow the manager to explain areas needed for improvement during reviews and to describe how an employee can acquire needed skills for other positions or for promotions in the organization.

To assist dietetics professionals in reaching their goals of recognition for competency, position descriptions must include a complete list of preset, job-specific standards. The level of expected performance must be carefully aligned with strategic goals and objectives in the organization. Specific clinical or technical, management, and interpersonal skills must be delineated to assure that the job is assigned a suitable scale for compensation. The ADA has published sample job descriptions that can be used to establish consistency across geographic areas and from one facility to another.[55]

Behavioral performance standards that lead to job success should be available to the employee. Individuals should be encouraged to perform regular self-assessments, manager-directed assessments, customer assessments, and assessments by staff members who report to them. Applying competency-based standards and performance reviews may help reduce turnover because expectations are clear for both employer and staff member. Concrete examples of skill sets should be presented to minimize ambiguity.

Dietetics professionals have to meet not only the internal expectations of their employers but also the external expectations from outside agencies. According to the Joint Commission on Accreditation of Healthcare Organizations (JCAHO), staff members in all health professions need to be able to address the need and expectations of population groups that differ from one another.[56] Competency implies current knowledge and capability for conducting the work assignments of a position. Overall, management teams are responsible for selecting, hiring, and training employees who are competent and *remain* competent over time. Organizations will continue to strive to improve their human capital through training and development programs, workforce planning, and performance management. Knowledge and skills are constantly evolving. If a practitioner does not acquire these content updates or enhance his or her skill sets as the field changes, members of the public will not receive the best level of care. Table 4-4 provides a sample format for staff competency development related to the skill of nutrition counseling. Table 4-5 provides a competency-based assessment tool for evaluating skills such as communication, teamwork, and collaboration.

In addition to job duty competency, dietetics professionals must be able to demonstrate cultural competence, which is the integration and transformation of knowledge about individuals and groups of people into specific standards, policies, practices, and attitudes to increase the quality of services and outcomes.[57] Addressing cross-cultural perspectives has become increasingly important in

TABLE 4-4	Staff Competency Development Plan for Nutrition Counseling Skills

Name: John Doe, new RD   Date:

Competence Area: Ambulatory care unit

Competency: Nutrition counseling skills

Goal: Employs appropriate counseling techniques in helping clients meet needs or goals

OBJECTIVES	ACTIONS	TARGET DATES
John will observe seasoned RD practitioners and receive coaching.	Coaching—receiving feedback while practicing	3–6 months after hire
John will receive computer-aided instruction from a designated counseling module.	Computer-assisted instruction and distance learning	1–6 months after hire
John will participate in clinical case reviews.	Clinical case reviews and participation	6–9 months after hire
John will attend relevant seminars or conferences related to counseling skills.	Attend counseling seminars and conferences, poster sessions	6–12 months after hire
John will practice simulated counseling skills with an assigned mentor.	Participate in a designated "experiential lab" on site or on field trip assignment	9–12 months after hire

Anticipated obstacles: Financial constraints if activities are too distant from home facility

Sources for help: Clinical nutrition manager; designated websites; journal club; available externships

Adapted from Inman-Felton A, Rops MS. Ensuring Staff Competence. Chicago: American Dietetic Association, 1998.

healthcare and business sites. Cultural knowledge involves being familiar with cultural characteristics, history, values, belief systems, and behaviors of the members of another ethnic group.[58] Cultural awareness is one of the important trends that affect the future of the dietetics profession.

CAREER LADDERING AND OPPORTUNITY

Various healthcare systems offer career ladders and options for dietetics professionals. For example, the Veterans Administration offers career laddering to encourage promotions and professional growth. Administrative dietitians in the Veterans Administration are responsible for applying effective resources management, cost containment, planning, and utilizing current foodservice systems; applying and analyzing automated information; managing quality improvement programs; offering staff education; coordinating activities with clinical programs; and implementing applied research.[59] Clinical dietitians in these same systems may choose specialty areas of geriatrics, preventive health, nutrition support, spinal cord injury, renal disease, psychiatric care, and hospital-based home care as well as educational positions, clinical nutrition management, or research.[59] Other facilities offer career ladders to dietetics professionals where the individual begins at an entry level, moving to a level of greater responsibility and higher salaries over time.

When individuals find themselves limited in their positions because of perceived or real financial constraints, they should choose behaviors that are more likely to achieve improved results. To get motivated to change, a road map will be needed to identify strengths, close any gaps, and make aspirations a reality.[60] "People change

TABLE 4-5	Competency-Based Assessment Tool for Evaluating Communications, Teamwork, and Collaboration			
		RANKING		
SKILL	EXPECTED STANDARD	MEETS	EXCEEDS	DOES NOT MEET
Instructing	Expanding knowledge or skills enhancement of others, formally or informally			
Interviewing	Conducting interviews directed toward specific goal or objective			
Public speaking	Making formal presentations before internal or external audiences			
Writing	Writing and editing concise, clear chart notes, letters, reports, articles, e-mails			
Negotiating	Successfully reaches an agreement or solution to build consensus in negotiations			
Persuading	Influencing others toward some action or point of view			
Listening	Actively engaging in conversations in order to clearly understand others' message and intent			
Establishing rapport	Establishing and maintaining good rapport and cooperative working relationship with others			
Taking initiative	Showing flexibility in joining unit teams and taking on extra responsibilities when required or beneficial to the facility			
Choosing communication methods	Effectively selecting the appropriate communication method to fit the situation			
Involving others	Involving coworkers and direct reports by sharing information through reports, meetings, or presentations			
Soliciting input	Asking for input from others through reports, meetings, or presentations			
Influencing	Using relationships to influence others to take risks for the good of the overall organization			
Respecting others	Treating others with respect, regardless of position or function			
Facilitating brainstorming	Initiating brainstorming sessions when required to ensure that team members are invested in team activities and decisions			

Source: Adapted with permission from Gravett and Associates, 2004. Available at: http://www.e-hresources.com. Accessed March1, 2006.

when they are emotionally engaged and committed."[60] Table 4-6 lists some ideas that may be useful in making a more successful dietetics career.

To address the need for equitable career growth for dietitians, a formal career ladder may be developed by a facility. Table 4-7 provides a sample of one such career ladder. In this ladder, the first level (RD-I) demonstrates novice through competent levels of practice during the early years of practice. The second level (RD-II) demonstrates proficiency through demonstration of a depth of knowledge about subtle needs and changes needed in caring for patient. The third level (RD-III) recognizes expert levels of practice, demonstrated through an intuitive grasp of situations without considering unproductive alternatives, a talent for leadership, and recognition by peers and managers. Each level provides a separate range of

TABLE 4-6	Ideas for Moving Ahead in a Dietetics Career
Changing perceptions	Change how the public views the profession; enhance perception through "professionalism." Maintain high visibility. Take opportunities to showcase your talents. Become involved in local, national, departmental, or organizational initiatives that keep you in the spotlight. Share success stories of how your work has had an impact. Customer satisfaction keeps patients coming back and keeps revenue high.
Achieving salary equity	Investigate the salary structure of other allied health professionals; identify similar functions, skill sets, and responsibilities. Review and revise your job description to clearly outline the position and the complex scope of services you manage or provide. Use the results of outcomes research to reinforce and validate your perceived value and income potential. Know your employer's or customer's goals and how you can be of help in achieving those goals. Keep a running list of your achievements and share them monthly with your employer or customer. Report financial achievements monthly to administrators.
Reducing encroachment by competitors	Offer services that are mutually beneficial to the customer and you. "Be different" and offer more than the average practitioner. Go beyond the expected in customer service; "exceed" rather than "meet" expectations. Keep tabs on the competition. What are they doing that you are not? Be competitive with what customers want. Find out what your customers want and then be sure to deliver. Develop other skill sets, as in publishing, financial management, organizational leadership.
Breaking out of a limited career track	Be positive; take advantage of opportunities that present themselves. Be creative with your current position; you may be able to redesign certain elements to benefit you. Seize opportunities—do not sit back and wait for someone else to do it for you. Accept challenges that are nontraditional, especially those that are creative and require problem solving. Be flexible and open to new ideas. Be able to relocate from one geographic area to another.
Enhancing job satisfaction and growth	Develop mutually beneficial relationships. Add dimension and skills to your resume. Network extensively; network with people from other professions and those in power positions. Accept mentoring from a revered colleague. Work in a positive work environment. Provide constructive feedback to administration regarding your needs. Have fun!

Sources: Tips offered as per author telephone interviews with Veronica McLymont, MS, RD; Janet McKee, MS, RD; and Becky Dorner, RD. June and July 2003.

compensation. Dietitians may apply by submitting a portfolio for the new ladder step after a designated period of practice. More information about creating a career portfolio is available from multiple resources, such as one that includes a CD-ROM for simplified use.[61]

LEADERSHIP TRAITS

Many dietitians have indicated that greater career success has evolved from the demonstration of effective leadership skills. Indeed, the career ladder described above indicates that leadership is one factor for advancement. Having a clear personal mission and then creating a vision to achieve that mission are important initial

TABLE 4-7	Dietetics Career Ladder (Dietitian)		
LEVEL	**EDUCATION**	**CLINICAL EXPERIENCE**	**OTHER REQUIREMENTS**
Entry level—level I compensation	RD-eligible; licensure-eligible	Experience in acute care preferred	Able to instruct students in basic skills
Level II starting $/week/1–2 years of experience $/week/ 2–3 years $/week/ 3–4 years $/week/ 4–5 years $/week/5–6 years 1% for each additional years experience ($1,000 more if master's in nutrition or field directly applicable)	RD and licensed	Experience in acute care preferred	Instructs students actively
Level III starting $/week/2–3 years $/ week/3–4 years $/week/ 4–5 years $/week/5–6 years 1.5% for each additional years exp ($1,000 more if master's in nutrition or field directly applicable or if CNSD) IF 5 or more years of experience and supervisory responsibilities $5,000 more	RD/license required plus one specialty certification	Two years of experience in teaching hospital	Instructs students and peers actively
Level IV educator level starting $/week/ 5–6 years 1.5% for each additional years of experience ($4,000 more if CNSD/ $5,000 more if management responsibilities)	RD/license required plus one specialty certification and master's degree	Five years of experience in teaching hospital	Active membership contributions to DPG; presents at professional presentations or poster sessions; instructs students and peers actively, author of at least one professional document: newsletter, diet manual sections, texts, educational materials, or journal articles/research grants; trains staff

Reprinted with permission from Cincinnati Children's Hospital Medical Center, 2004.

steps. Flexibility, a good sense of humor, keeping perspective, removing obstacles to success, engaging customers effectively, and maintaining high standards are also essential qualities for a personal leadership strategy.

According to Kovner and Channing,[62] the skill sets for being a successful leader include (1) motivating others, (2) scanning the environment, (3) negotiating the political terrain, and (4) generating and allocating resources. For motivating others, key roles include serving as "figurehead, liaison, or leader"; for scanning the environment, one accepts the roles of "monitor and disseminator"; for negotiating office politics, one must be a "spokesperson, negotiator and disturbance handler"; and to handle resources successfully, one must be an "entrepreneur and a resource allocator."[63]

The work of Goleman and colleagues in *Primal Leadership*[60] indicates that intelligence quotient (IQ) is just a small part of career and personal success. The real story involves the sensitive use of emotional intelligence (EI) to enhance the personality and environmental influences among relationships in the workplace. Social skills—communicating with and motivating others—are paramount to success in the workplace.[64] In fact, the word "resonance" is used to evaluate how effective a leader is in establishing a positive climate, so that work can be accomplished at the highest possible level.[60] According to Goleman and colleagues,[60] climate can determine 20 to 30% of business performance (p. 18) and "gifted leadership occurs where heart and head—feeling and thought—meet" (p. 26).

A self-assessment tool to identify current and desired leadership attributes can be found in Table 4-8. It is useful to know one's current abilities and limitations in designing a self-improvement plan to achieve career success. For the purposes of this section, negotiation skills, conflict resolution, and marketing tips are offered, since these are business skills that dietetics professionals often identify as weaknesses in their preparation for practice.[59]

NEGOTIATION SKILLS THAT WORK

According to Veronica McLymont (personal telephone interview, Memorial Sloan-Kettering Hospital, New York, July 2, 2003), it is important to research the issues extensively before proposing a change in strategy, financial plan, or relationship, and, where possible, to obtain benchmarking data for comparison. Successful individuals recognize that others in the organization may have more information and experience and may have valuable input from outside the department or organization.

It can be helpful to enroll in electronic (e-mail) discussion groups where professional questions can be easily answered by others who have undertaken a similar challenge. Effective participation allows one to find out what works and what does not!

Timing is also a key factor for negotiations. By listening and being attuned to what is going on in the organization, it is possible to maintain one's composure and wait for the right time. It makes good sense to stay in touch with the strategic plan of the unit and the organization.

One can also stay ahead of the curve by offering useful suggestions to administration; effective upward communication is critical. Having regular buy-in from people across the organization will help to sell a good idea and to market a plan. Use of colorful charts and graphs helps busy administrators key into a summary or business plan more readily. Because many administrators do not fully understand the field of dietetics, it may be necessary to educate them regularly, but in a pleasing manner! For example, it never hurts to offer a food or snack item at a business meeting.

MARKETING TO YOUR CUSTOMERS

Juran has pointed out that there are two types of customers: the "useful many" and the "vital few."[65] While the useful many affect numerous decisions because they represent a larger number, the vital few must also be considered because they make important referrals or contacts that have a potentially larger outreach.[65,66] In the field of dietetics, practitioners must clearly identify their target markets,

TABLE 4-8	Self-Assessment of Leadership Attributes

LEADERSHIP ATTRIBUTE	RANKING				
	1 LOW	2 EVOLVING	3 COMPETENT	4 PROFICIENT	5 EXPERT OR MASTER
Dedicated to quality and improved outcomes, systemwide					
Driven by nutrition ideals in personal life and in professional activities					
Visionary; creates a shared vision of the future and fosters consensus					
Concerned for the public/community; promotes access to food and nutrition					
Effective with marketing and promotion; broadly applies marketing techniques					
Uses a global approach; considers bigger consequences for events and decisions					
Functions effectively as a change agent in a proactive manner; uses anticipatory skills to see the need for change and new approaches					
Enhances customer relations through relationships, partnerships and use of high standards					
Ethical; decision making follows the law, the standards and guidelines of the profession					
Cost-effective, holistic resource utilization					
Uses scientific perspective to translate research into practice					
Maximizes multicultural knowledge and receptivity					
Enhances human potential; brings out the best in others					
Ensures empowerment of others with collective sense of responsibility					
Lifelong learner; curious and open; committed to learning continuously					
Integrative systems thinker; big picture comprehension					
Professional development through coaching, counseling, and mentoring others					
Effective communicator; influences others positively and listens actively with open mind					
Creative; fosters innovation					
Negotiator; influences and builds consensus and collaboration					
Political; influences policy and decisions; networks effectively to gain support for desired outcomes					
Information seeker; seeks new sources for improving practice; uses databases and expert systems					
Process improvement supporter; continually evaluates processes and uses creative problem-solving methods					
Uses electronic media and computers effectively to mobilize collaboration					
Respectful team builder; encourages group decisions with collaboration and participation					
Positive and optimistic; inspirational to others; finds opportunities in problems					
Research mindset; seeks applications for practice					
Scans for strategic technology and new ideas; scans ahead					

Source: Adapted with permission from Schiller RS. Shifting sands: leading in times of transition. In: Biesmeier C, Marino L, Schofield MK, eds. Connective Leadership: Linking Vision with Action. Chicago: American Dietetic Association, 2000:32–33.

including those who are customers (the useful many) and the gatekeepers who may make important referrals (the vital few). Customers may include patients or clients (the many) and the referring agencies or physicians or industry partners (the vital few).

Being aware of both internal and external markets is also essential. Internal customers include those individuals within the healthcare or food industry systems who indirectly or directly receive or refer to the products and services that are provided by the practitioner; external customers would include the patients, family, and payers who actually purchase the products and services.[65,66] If one forgets the internal customer (the person "along the way"), business can be lost by a drop in referrals, an increase in complaints, or damage to a good reputation.

To stay in touch with both types of customers, practitioners will want to focus with "laser-beam clarity" on customer wants and demands.[67] To keep a grasp on external as well as internal perspectives, it is important to attend other meetings or forums besides those in dietetics. The Disney Institute, for example, offers training on the best ways to meet customer expectations. Thinking "outside of the box" by offering the unexpected, the exciting, and the "nice to know" lends itself well to enhanced marketing outcomes.

A successful marketing plan should include target market evaluation, public relations strategies, advertising and promotions, publications and presentations, use of the Internet, and other creative ideas. Being clever and being different lend themselves to being memorable.

SUPPORT FROM THE AMERICAN DIETETIC ASSOCIATION AND OTHER ORGANIZATIONS

Reading about how others manage to achieve career success can be useful. Self-assessment and regular introspective activities may also be enlightening. Often, clarifying one's beliefs, values, and attitudes is in order. Life stages affect perspectives, and what was important at age 20 may not be relevant to the practitioner at age 50.

TABLE 4-9	Getting Prepared for Job Success
STEP	**DESCRIPTION**
Take calculated risks.	Sometimes a new challenge requires moving beyond your usual comfort zone.
Tailor your resume or curriculum vitae.	Include more than just clinical context; include business and management tasks in which you were successful.
Learn as much as possible.	Learn all that you can; expand your horizons when possible. Do a little bit of everything in your worksite.
Everything worth waiting for takes time.	Build your credentials and expertise for the job that you want.

Source: Adapted with permission from Brown D. Considering opportunities in high level management. J Am Diet Assoc 2003;103:819.

Executive newsletters and organizations are helpful in acquiring valid perspectives on world issues. Media-related magazines are useful for identifying new ways to market services and products. Management and consultant dietetics practice groups provide tips in their newsletters and articles, and one can often benefit from following advice from a network of friends and mentors.

Becoming active in a professional organization can bring rewards, not only from leadership roles but also from the natural networking liaisons that develop from sharing common interests and values. The ADA, sister organizations, and business organizations are member driven. Understanding the business side of organizations can help give dietetics professionals the edge they are seeking to enhance personal and professional achievement.[64] Table 4-9 provides a final list of suggestions for career success, economically and personally. Figure 4-1 provides a thought-provoking summary of how the adoption of a positive outlook can lead to

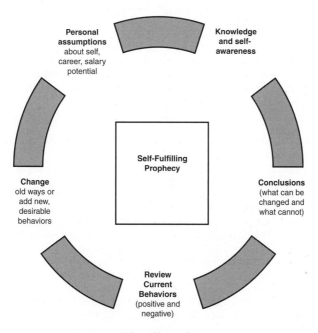

FIGURE 4-1 *The self-actualizing career.*

an optimal self-fulfilling prophecy: the self-actualizing career that provides both personal satisfaction and economic success. Anything is possible!

REFERENCES

1. Massachusetts Dietetic Association. Nutrition Services Improve Health and Save Money: Evidence from Massachusetts. Boston: Massachusetts Dietetic Association, January 1993.
2. Ohio Dietetic Association. Cost Savings Through Medical Nutrition Therapy in Ohio.
3. Wisconsin Dietetic Association. Nutrition Services Health Effective: Cost Effective Evidence from Wisconsin. Madison: Wisconsin Dietetic Association, 1994.
4. Derelian D. ADA urges congress to expand Medicare coverage for medical nutrition therapy. J Am Diet Assoc 1995;95:997.
5. Kaye GL. Outcomes Management: Linking Research to Practice. Columbus, OH: Ross Products Division, Abbott Laboratories, 1996.
6. Splett P. Cost Outcomes of Nutrition Intervention: A Three Part Monograph. Evansville, IN: Mead Johnson & Company, 1996.
7. Gallagher-Alred C, Voss AC, Gussler JD. Nutrition Intervention and Patient Outcomes: A Self-Study Manual. Columbus, OH: Ross Products Division, Abbott Laboratories, 1995.
8. Franz MJ, Monk A, Barry B, et al. Effectiveness of medical nutrition therapy provided by dietitians in the management of non–insulin-dependent diabetes mellitus: a randomized, controlled clinical trial. J Am Diet Assoc 1995;95:1009–1017.
9. Sheils JF, Rubin R, Stapleton DC. The estimated costs and savings of medical nutrition therapy: the Medicare population. J Am Diet Assoc 1999;99:428–435.
10. Johnson EQ, Valera, S. Medical nutrition therapy in non–insulin dependent diabetes mellitus improves clinical outcome. J Am Diet Assoc 1995;95:700–701.
11. McGehee MM, Johnson EQ, Rasmussen HM, et al. Benefits and costs of medical nutrition therapy by registered
dietitians for patients with hypercholesterolemia. J Am Diet Assoc 1995;95:1041–1043.
12. Sikand G, Kashyap ML, Yang I. Medical nutrition therapy lowers serum cholesterol and saves medication costs in men with hypercholesterolemia. J Am Diet Assoc 1998;98:889–894.
13. Sikand G, Kashyap ML, Wong ND, Hsu JC. Dietitian intervention improves lipid values and saves medication costs in men with combined hyperlipidemia and a history of niacin noncompliance. J Am Diet Assoc 2000;100:218–224.
14. Pastors JG, Warshaw H, Daly A, Franz M, Kulkarni K. The evidence for the effectiveness of medical nutrition therapy in diabetes management. Diabetes Care 2002;25(3):608–613.
15. Institute of Medicine. The Role of Nutrition in Maintaining Health in the Nation's Elderly: Evaluating Coverage of Nutrition Services for the Medicare Population, Committee on Nutrition Services for Medicare Beneficiaries. Washington, DC: National Academy Press, 2000.
16. US Department of Health and Human Services. Report to Congress on Medical Nutrition Therapy. Washington, DC: US Department of Health and Human Services, 2004.
17. Institute of Medicine. To Err Is Human: Building a Safer Health System. Committee on Quality of Health Care in America. Washington, DC: National Academy Press, 2000.
18. Institute of Medicine. Crossing the Quality Chasm: A New Health System for the 21st Century. Washington, DC: National Academy Press, 2001.
19. Medical Nutrition Therapy Across the Continuum of Care: Patient Protocols, vol. 1. Chicago: American Dietetic Association, 1996.
20. Medical Nutrition Therapy Across the Continuum of Care: Patient Protocols, Supplement. Chicago: American Dietetic Association, 1997.
21. Medical Nutrition Therapy Across the Continuum of Care: Patient Protocols, Chicago: American Dietetic Association, 1998.
22. Medical Nutrition Therapy Evidence-Based Guides for Practice. Hyperlipidemia Medical Nutrition Therapy Protocol [CD-ROM]. Chicago: American Dietetic Association, 2002.
23. Medical Nutrition Therapy Evidence-Based Guides for Practice. Nutrition Practice Guidelines for Type 1 and 2 Diabetes Mellitus [CD-ROM]. Chicago: American Dietetic Association, 2002.
24. Medical Nutrition Therapy Evidence-Based Guides for Practice. Nutrition Practice Guidelines for Gestational Diabetes Mellitus [CD-ROM]. Chicago: American Dietetic Association, 2002.
25. Medical Nutrition Therapy Evidence-Based Guides for Practice. Chronic Kidney Disease (non-dialysis) Medical Nutrition Therapy Protocol [CD-ROM]. Chicago: American Dietetic Association, 2002.

26. Disorders of Lipid Metabolism Evidence Based Nutrition Practice Guideline. Chicago: American Dietetic Association, 2005. Available at: http://www.ebg.adaevidencelibrary.com/topic.cfm?cat=2651. Accessed February 20, 2006.

27. Rollins G. Guidelines outline effectiveness of medical nutrition therapy in managing and preventing diabetes. Rep Med Guide Outcomes Res 2002;25:13:5–7.

28. Lacey K, Pritchett E. Nutrition care process and model: ADA adopts road map to quality care and outcomes management. J Am Diet Assoc 2003;103:1031–1072.

29. American Dietetic Association. Position of the American Dietetic Association: integration of medical nutrition therapy and pharmacotherapy. J Am Diet Assoc 2003;103:1363–1370

30. Wolf A , Hazen K , Conaway M, Crowther J, Nadler J, Bovbjerg V. Improving Control with Activity Nutrition (ICAN): impact of lifestyle intervention on glucose control medication use. (abstr). Diabetes 52 (suppl 1):A558, 2003.

31. Baranoski CLN, King, SL. Insurance companies are reimbursing for medical nutrition therapy. J Am Diet Assoc 2000;100:1530–1532.

32. Chima CS, Pollack HA. Position of the American Dietetic Association: nutrition services in managed care. J Am Diet Assoc 2002;102:1471–1478.

33. Aetna US HealthCare web page. Available at: http://www.aetna.com/cpb/data/CPBA0049.html. Accessed February 20, 2006.

34. Blue Cross/Blue Shield Massachusetts web page. Available at: http://www.bcbsma.com. Accessed August 25, 2003.

35. Larson E. MNT: an innovative employee-friendly benefit that saves. Empl Benefits J. 2000;25:33–36.

36. Israel DA. McCabe M. Using disease-state management as the key to promoting employer sponsorship of medical nutrition therapy. J Am Diet Assoc 1999;99:583–588.

37. Final MNT Regulations. CMS-1169-FC. Federal Register, November 1, 2001. US Department of Health and Human Services. 42 CFR Parts: 405, 410, 411, 414, and 415. Available at: http://cms.hhs.gov/physicians/pfs/cms1169fc.asp. Accessed June 27, 2003.

38. Medicare Coverage Policy Decision: Duration and Frequency of the Medical Nutrition Therapy (MNT) Benefit (No. CAG-00097N). Available at: http://cms.hhs.gov/ncdr/memo.asp?id=53. Accessed June 2, 2003.

39. Medicare MNT Payment Schedule 2003 by State/City. Available at: http://www.eatright.org/Member/Files/MNT_payment_schedule_-3.28DM.xls. Accessed June 9, 2003.

40. Impasse with APASS soon to be resolved. The Medicare MNT provider. J Am Diet Assoc 2003;2:1–3.

41. Bodenheimer T, Wagner EH, Grumbach K. Improving primary care for patients with chronic illness, part 1. JAMA 2002;288:1775–1779.

42. Bodenheimer T, Wagner EH, Grumbach K. Improving primary care for patients with chronic illness. The chronic care model, part 2. JAMA 2002;288:1909–1914.

43. Robert Wood Johnson Foundation. Improving chronic illness care. Available at: http://www.improvingchroniccare.org/. Accessed August 30, 2003.

44. Institute for Healthcare Improvement. Pursuing perfection. Available at: http://www.ihi.org/pursuingperfection/background/index.asp. Accessed August 30, 2003.

45. Biesemeier CK. Achieving Excellence: Clinical Staffing for Today and Tomorrow. Chicago: American Dietetic Association, 2004.

46. American Dietetic Association. Position of the American Dietetic Association: nutrition services in managed care. J Am Diet Assoc 2002;102:1471–1478.

47. American Dietetic Association. Position of the American Dietetic Association: cost-effectiveness of medical nutrition therapy. J Am Diet Assoc 1995;95:88–91.

48. American Society for Parenteral and Enteral Nutrition Board of Directors and the Clinical Guidelines Task Force. Guidelines for use of parenteral and enteral nutrition in adult and pediatric patients. J Parenter Enter Nutr 2002(suppl);26:1SA–138SA.

49. Heyland DK, Rupinder D, Drover JW, Gramlich L, Dodek P, Canadian Critical Care Clinical Practice Guidelines Committee. Canadian clinical practice guidelines for nutrition support in mechanically ventilated, critically ill adult patients. J Parenter Enter Nutr 2003;27:355–373.

50. The American Dietetic Association Scientific Affairs and Research. ADA Evidence Analysis Guide. 2nd Ed. Chicago: American Dietetic Association, 2003.

51. Balch GI. Employers' perceptions of the role of dietetics practitioners: challenges to survive and opportunities to thrive. J Am Diet Assoc 1996;96:1301.

52. American Dietetic Association. 2002 Dietetics Compensation and Benefits Survey. Chicago: American Dietetic Association, 2003.

53. Winterfeldt EA, Bogle ML, Ebro LL. Dietetics: Practice and Future Trends. Gaithersburg, MD: Aspen Publishers, 1998.

54. Stahl P. Status report on nutrition in the news. J Am Diet Assoc 2002;100:1298.

55. Hornick B. Job Descriptions: Models for the Dietetic Profession. Chicago: American Dietetic Association, 2003.
56. Inman-Felton A, Rops MS. Ensuring Staff Competence. Chicago: American Dietetic Association, 1998.
57. Davis K. Exploring the Intersection Between Cultural Competency and Managed Behavioral Health Care Policy: Implications for State and County Mental Health Agencies. Alexandria, VA: National Technical Assistance Center for State Mental Health Planning, 1997.
58. Adams DL, ed. Health Issues for Women of Color: A Cultural Diversity Perspective. Thousand Oaks, CA: Sage Publications, 1995.
59. American Dietetic Association. Performance, proficiency and value of the dietetics professional. J Am Diet Assoc 2002;102:1304.
60. Goleman D, Boyatsis R, McKee A. Primal Leadership: Realizing the Power of Emotional Intelligence. Boston: Harvard Business School Press, 2002.
61. Williams AG, Hall KJ, Shadix K, Stokes M. Creating Your Career Portfolio: At-a-Glance Guide for Dietitians. Upper Saddle River, NJ: Prentice-Hall, 2005.
62. Kovner AR, Channing AH. Really Trying: A Career Guide for the Health Services Manager. 2nd Ed. Chicago: Health Administration Press, 1994.
63. Mintzberg H. The Nature of Managerial Work. Englewood Cliffs, NJ: Prentice-Hall, 1980.
64. Brown D. Considering opportunities in high-level management. J Am Diet Assoc 2003;103:819.
65. Juran JM. Juran on Leadership for Quality: An Executive Handbook. New York: Free Press, 1989.
66. Jackson R. Nutrition and Food Services for Integrated Health Care: A Handbook for Leaders. Gaithersburg, MD: Aspen Publishers, 1997.
67. Marino L. Succeeding in a market-driven environment. In: Biesemeier C, Marino L, Schofield MK, eds. Connective Leadership: Linking Vision with Action. Chicago: American Dietetic Association, 2000, pp. 14–15.

DEVELOPMENT OF THE DIETETICS PROFESSIONAL'S ROLE AS A MEMBER OF A HEALTHCARE TEAM

Beth Leonberg

Dietetics is a young and dynamic profession that continues to evolve. The role of the dietetics professional within the healthcare team has expanded dramatically. Professionals have opportunities to affect care in significant ways by assuming many and varied roles within the team. Learning to work with other team members to provide seamless care adds tremendous value to patient outcomes. Evolving practice roles provide great rewards for the professional who seizes the opportunities available.

VISIBILITY ON THE TEAM

The clinical dietetics professional has gained increasing visibility as a key member of the healthcare team. Following the publication of landmark articles, such as Butterworth's "Skeleton in the Hospital Closet" in 1974, it became common practice to screen patients for malnutrition on admission.[1] Typically, the screen, performed by the dietetics department, included evaluation of risk based on parameters such as diagnosis, diet order, and laboratory values. Yet as recently as the 1980s, dietitians in clinical practice were in a reactive role; in most settings, they assessed patients and provided recommendations solely in response to physician consult. Physicians were informed of the dietitian's nutrition risk assessment, often only by notes in the medical record. Dietitians were generally required to receive a consult before providing a full assessment and recommendations on patients identified at risk.

The development of nutrition support teams was a significant step forward in giving dietitians a more proactive role in nutrition care and provided the first hospital-based model for the widespread participation of dietitians on a formal multidisciplinary team. Nutrition support teams were fostered largely through the activities of the American Society for Parenteral and Enteral Nutrition (ASPEN), which conducted symposia and developed standards to guide their function. Typically made up of a dietitian, nurse, pharmacist, and physician, nutrition support teams allowed the unique knowledge and skills of dietitians to become much more visible. Nutrition support dietitians performed assessments, determined nutrition goals, and provided the daily data-collection activities. The effectiveness of dietitians in the care of these patients was especially evident during the transition from parenteral and/or enteral nutrition to oral diets. Nutrition support teams have continued to evolve, with many facilities that previously had a formal team now reverting to a less formal structure. But regardless of the team's formality, dietitians gained both visibility and critical skills through their work on nutrition support teams.

Although past practice may have dictated that nutrition care be provided to patients on a consult-only basis, current practice dictates that all patients be screened for nutrition risk on admission using an interdisciplinary assessment tool. The American Dietetic Association (ADA) and ASPEN were instrumental in convincing the Joint Commission on Accreditation of Healthcare Organizations (JCAHO) to include nutrition risk screening, assessment, and development of the nutrition care plan as a core aspect of care for every patient. The current JCAHO guidelines have moved nutrition care from something done exclusively and separately by the dietetics department to an aspect of care for which all members of the team are to a degree responsible. The role of the registered dietitian in the development of an interdisciplinary nutrition therapy plan is clearly outlined in the intent of the JCAHO standards.[2] JCAHO has also been instrumental in moving the concept of team care from multidisciplinary, in which disciplines operate in parallel, to interdisciplinary, in which disciplines operate interdependently. JCAHO has further influenced the visibility of dietitians through its strong focus on interdisciplinary care and treatment plans, ongoing performance improvement activities, and staffing standards. Dietitians now regularly sit on committees throughout the facility, well beyond the traditional pharmacy and therapeutic standards committees. Patient education, documentation, and ethics committees all now frequently include dietitian members, due to the increased focus on interdisciplinary care. In addition, staffing standards that promote coverage 7 day per week have raised the awareness of facility administration about the need for adequate dietitian coverage. As a result of these expectations, dietetics professionals have achieved greater prominence on the team.

Professional organizations such as ASPEN and the Cystic Fibrosis Foundation have developed standards that promote the key role of the dietetics professional on the healthcare team. The ASPEN standards for the treatment of patients on specialized nutrition support clearly delineate the specific role the registered dietitian plays in performing the formal nutrition assessment of patients and residents while reinforcing the importance of developing an interdisciplinary nutrition care plan.[3–6] The Cystic Fibrosis Foundation has developed minimum criteria for cystic fibrosis (CF) center accreditation.[7] These include the requirement that a dietitian/nutritionist (RD) must regularly attend outpatient clinics and team conferences and be available for inpatient consultation or coordination of care with inpatient staff. Reinforcing this requirement, the foundation's recent consensus report on nutrition for pediatric patients with CF states, "A registered dietitian must be part of the team to provide the discipline-specific expertise needed for optimal nutritional management."[8] In this way, professional associations have helped to increase visibility of dietetics professionals.

Specialty and advanced-level credentials have also played a role in increasing the visibility of dietetics professionals. The Certified Nutrition Support Dietitian (CNSD) credential and the Certified Diabetes Educator (CDE) credential have become expected for practice in those areas of care in many facilities. Schwartz reported on the development and success of the CNSD credentialing program, which had 2,000 active credentialed practitioners in 2003.[9] These credentials help to position dietitians with their healthcare peers as well as to demonstrate their competence to patients. In addition, the Commission on Dietetic Registration's board certifications in pediatric nutrition and renal nutrition have provided an opportunity to demonstrate competence in these areas of practice, increasing visibility of these practitioners within their practice settings.[10]

Federal regulations have also played a role in increasing dietitian visibility. In the late 1970s, the regulations governing care in outpatient dialysis units stipulated the patient care plan be developed by a professional team that included a "qualified dietitian."[11] The regulations defined a qualified dietitian as a person either eligible for registration by the Commission on Dietetic Registration or holding a bachelor's or advanced degree in food and nutrition or dietetics, with a minimum of 1 year of clinical nutrition experience.[12] A decade later, the U.S. Congress enacted the Omnibus Budget Reconciliation Act of 1987, which established the Resident Assessment Instrument (RAI), developed by the Health Care Financing Administration (HCFA), to be used in all nursing homes certified to participate in Medicare or Medicaid. Today the RAI, composed of the Minimum Data Set (MDS) and Resident Assessment Protocols (RAPs), includes an extensive section on oral/nutritional status, which has placed registered dietitians and dietetics technicians as core members of the healthcare team in long-term-care facilities.[13]

The visibility of registered dietitians and nutrition professionals changed dramatically when the Centers for Medicare and Medicaid (CMS) designated RDs as the only authorized providers of medical nutrition therapy (MNT) in 2001. The passage of this act placed dietetics professionals in an entirely new relationship with insurers and healthcare providers by recognizing them and providing reimbursement for services that have been demonstrated to be cost effective in improving patient outcomes. Although limited in scope to outpatient diabetes and nondialysis kidney disease in its first few years, Medicare MNT should be expanded in scope to include other chronic illnesses. Early indications are that commercial insurers will follow the lead of Medicare in making reimbursement of nutrition services for selected chronic illnesses universally reimbursed.[14] In addition, Medicare has authorized the development of disease management insurance plans to include MNT. This new role for the clinical dietetics professional offers great opportunities to broaden the impact beyond the walls of the facility and into the community, expanding visibility to community physicians and public health providers as well as patients.

Visibility within the healthcare team has been achieved by a combination of initiatives moving in the direction to support the key role dietitians play on the team. This visibility has given dietetics professionals the opportunity to significantly affect patient outcomes. Dietetics professionals are encouraged to seize this opportunity to make a difference for the profession, their careers, and the outcomes of their patients.

IMPACT ON PATIENT CARE

The increased visibility of dietetics professionals within the healthcare team is due in no small part to the tremendous effect they have had on patient care. Early nutrition risk screening and effective intervention have led to improved patient outcomes in a variety of patient populations. For example, in a 3-year intervention study of adult heart failure patients, the impact of the registered dietitian as a member of the multidisciplinary team was evaluated.[15] Nutrition intervention focused on decreasing sodium and fluid intake, following a protocol that used both educational and counseling techniques. In a group of 79 patients followed over three visits, highly significant decreases in sodium intake (0.5 g) and fluid intake (15 oz at 2 to 3 months and 12 oz at 6 to 9 months) were documented. Out of a total of 83 hospital readmissions for this patient group in 3 years, only 6 were attributed to excessive sodium intake. As a result of these patient outcomes, permanent funding was provided for the registered dietitian in the heart failure center.

A similar study evaluated the impact of the registered dietitian as a member of the multidisciplinary care team on the growth of very-low-birth-weight (VLBW) infants in the first year.[16] Catch-up growth as demonstrated by length and head circumference was compared for two groups of similar VLBW infants at 8- and 12-month growth-corrected age. Although the input of the registered dietitian and other ancillary members of the healthcare team was available to both groups of infants, the group cared for routinely by the multidisciplinary team approach, which included a registered dietitian, demonstrated significantly better catch-up growth in length and head circumference at both 8 and 12 months. The impact of this improved growth in the first year on the long-term outcomes of these children cannot be overestimated.

Studies like these demonstrate the positive effect of nutrition intervention and the impact of the dietitian's role as part of the team on improved nutrition status and overall health of patients with chronic illnesses. The ADA's Quality Management Team has published *Medical Nutrition Therapy Evidence-Based Guides for Practice* based on careful review of the documented evidence supporting nutrition intervention for several key populations. To date these include type 1, type 2, and gestational diabetes; chronic kidney disease (nondialysis); and hyperlipidemia.[17-20] It is continuing to review the available research and is working to develop similar evidence-based guidelines for other diseases. Kulkarni and colleagues demonstrated the efficacy of ADA's diabetes protocols in improving patient outcomes.[21] In a comparison of 24 patients seen by dietitians using practice guidelines with 30 seen by dietitians providing usual care, improvements in hemoglobin A_{1C} (HbA_{1C}) levels were seen in 21 (88%) versus 16 (53%) of the patients respectively. Among the patients in the protocol group, these improvements were found to be significantly greater, and the group demonstrated sustained differences from baseline at 3 months.

Positive patient outcomes translate into healthcare cost savings. The economic impact of poor nutrition status on the healthcare costs of hospitalized patients has been documented since the 1980s.[22] The documentation of healthcare cost savings as a result of nutrition intervention, however, has occurred more recently. The ADA's position statement on the cost-effectiveness of medical nutrition therapy outlines economic benefits in settings across the continuum of care.[23] More recently, using diabetics as an example, a 10-year case-control study of patients who had access to comprehensive diabetes care, including diabetes education on nutrition therapy, demonstrated significant improvements in HbA_{1C}, a decrease in the annual ratio of emergency room visits (diabetic versus nondiabetic patients) from 2.5 to 1.8 visits per patient and a decrease in the ratio of acute-care patient days (diabetic versus nondiabetic patients) from 3.6 to 2.5 per year.[24] Similarly, a report of 2,394 diabetic adults over 4 years indicated a direct correlation between HbA_{1C} levels and hospital days.[25] While patients with HbA_{1C} levels less than 8% averaged 13 inpatient treatment days per 100 patients, those with HbA_{1C} levels between 8 and 10% averaged 16 days per 100 patients, and those with HbA_{1C} greater than 10%

averaged 31 days per 100 patients. When translated to charges, the patients with poor glycemic control averaged $3,040, compared to only $970 for those with good glycemic control. Among patients with long-term diabetic complications and poor glycemic control, these charges averaged $8,320. Clearly, medical nutrition therapy aimed at improved glycemic control can result in substantial cost savings to patients, facilities, and the healthcare delivery system as a whole.

The overall patient experience can also be positively affected by the role of the dietetics professional. Customer satisfaction is a major emphasis in an increasingly competitive healthcare environment. Millions of dollars are spent annually nationwide on consultants and external survey instruments that provide feedback to facilities on their patients' experience with the facility. Nutrition services, both clinical and patient foodservice, play a critical role in influencing a patient's perception of the facility. Newer patient foodservice delivery methods, including spoken menus and room service, have greatly improved patient satisfaction.[26] In a long-term study of dietary satisfaction among renal patients, those whose protein intake was usual (typical U.S. diet) but focused on heart-healthy food choices had higher satisfaction ratings than those on low-protein or very low protein diets.[27] The authors report that higher dietary satisfaction was associated with improved adherence to the diet and suggest that the measurement of dietary satisfaction may be a way to help identify patients requiring more intensive intervention. Similarly, more liberal diets for short-stay and long-term-care patients promote better dietary intake and may improve patient satisfaction.[28–30]

The dietetics professional is uniquely positioned to provide continuity of care from inpatient to outpatient settings, a critical aspect sometimes missed by other disciplines. As inpatient length of stay continues to shorten, more care is being provided in the outpatient setting. In recent years we have come to appreciate that nutrition education of patients promotes acquisition of knowledge, but nutrition therapy promotes behavior change. The "nutrition therapist" has been described as a dietitian who practices long-term, client-centered nutrition counseling, often as part of a multidisciplinary team.[31] Since nutrition therapy is most effective when a care relationship is established between patient and provider, the short length of stay common for most acute-care admissions makes effective therapy in the inpatient setting limited. However, providing patients and caregivers with survival skills as inpatients and establishing follow-up plans for more extensive intervention in the outpatient setting may be effective in producing lasting diet and lifestyle changes and positive disease outcomes. Looking ahead at the future of dietetics in 2017, Julie O'Sullivan Maillet, past president of the ADA, commented "The RD's counseling focuses on the needs of the individual based on age, genetics, body composition, health status, and lifestyle. Most nutrition care is done within the community or online, at home."[32] As we move towards this future, staffing models for dietetics professionals that promote a combination of inpatient and outpatient responsibilities, as well as those that allow specialization, should be encouraged to provide optimal patient care and allow dietitians to develop into experts.

Dietetics professionals also significantly influence patient care when they participate in data collection for clinical research. The Diabetes Control and Complications Trial (DCCT) provides an excellent example of how this can occur.[33] In this large multicenter trial, the input of the dietetics professionals during the planning phase was limited to providing input on macronutrient composition of the diet and dietary history techniques. During the feasibility phase of the trial, their role expanded to include participant screening, research diet histories, nutrition education, team meetings, appointment of a dietitian coordinator for the study, and an annual meeting of dietitians. As the full-scale trial took place, the role of the dietitian expanded further to include recruitment; eligibility and screening; data collection; diabetes care and management; attaining normoglycemia; weight control; more active team participation; expanded dietitian annual meeting; nutrition counseling and team-boosting workshops; adherence promotion; site visits; ancillary studies; and newsletters/publications. The dietitian's role was central to the success of this important national trial, which has subsequently had such a significant impact on the treatment of diabetes.

Dietetics professionals have demonstrated their ability to affect patient care in varied and critical ways. Demonstration of outcomes is a critical aspect of today's healthcare environment, and the collection and reporting of outcomes must be a core aspect of the clinical professionals' job. Dietetics professionals need to be conscious of their potential to contribute to care and take responsibility for continuing to seek out new ways to improve nutrition health.

AUTHORITY WITHIN THE TEAM

Dietetics professionals assume varying degrees of authority within healthcare teams, dependent largely on their demonstration of competence, the scope of practice, and the unique knowledge, skills, and preferences of the team members. Authority may be formally delegated by way of position descriptions, job competencies, and facility bylaws, or informally as an outgrowth of team personalities, time constraints, and the natural growth of the team or patient population. Authority is seldom an absolute; it is extended for certain aspects of a patient's care or team function, but not others, and changes in delegation of authority are necessary over time. There appears to be a greater likelihood of a more flexible and informal designation of authority in outpatient settings than in inpatient settings.

Typically, clinical dietetics professionals are granted authority to assess nutrition status, recommend and/or implement a nutrition care plan, and educate and counsel patients on necessary diet and lifestyle modifications. Over the years, gaps between physicians' and dietetics professionals' perceptions of the dietitian's role have been revealed.[34–36] Most recently, Boyhtari and Cardinal surveyed 410 physicians and clinical dietitians in Michigan and found significant differences in role perception in 10 of 15 clinical dietitian responsibilities.[37] The greatest differences were seen in responsibilities related to patient foodservice activities, such as menu distribution and the selection and checking of meal trays, with physicians agreeing more strongly than dietitians that this was part of the dietitian's responsibility. Although there was good agreement between the two groups in response to assessing nutrition needs, making a dietary regimen, and planning nutrition support, physicians were significantly less likely to agree with dietitians contributing to discussion during medical rounds and with managing or controlling diseases and medical complications with therapeutic diets or nutrition support. In fact, when asked to respond to the question of who should be responsible for making a diet order change, 34% of physicians responded the physician alone, and none responded that a dietitian alone should change the order. Conversely, 2% of the dietitians responded that the physician alone should change the order, and 17% responded the dietitian alone should change the order. Of interest is the significant relationship between specialization and responses to this question, with highly specialized professionals believing that interaction should occur between physicians and dietitians when changing a diet order rather than either professional making the change alone. The authors postulate that this difference from generalists may be the result of the specialists being more experienced with and placing a higher value on a team approach to patient care.

Similarly, Hart and coworkers surveyed internal medicine physicians and nephrologists about their expectations of renal dietitians and general clinical dietitians.[38] There was general agreement between the groups on the types of activities dietitians should perform, with more than 50% of both groups agreeing that either generalist or renal dietitians should conduct nutrition assessments, determine patient's energy needs, evaluate medication-nutrient interactions, recommend diet and tube-feeding orders, instruct patients on physician-ordered diets, and teach nutrition concepts to hospital interns. Although few physicians agreed dietitians should order diets, tube feedings, or diet instructions, 23% of nephrologists responded that a renal dietitian should "prescribe diet (dietitian writes order)" and 14% that a renal dietitian should "prescribe a tube-feeding order (dietitian writes order)," versus 16 and 12%, respectively, of internal medicine physicians. These findings reinforce that physicians who work more closely with dietitians in team settings may be more likely to agree with giving them greater authority.

CARE MODELS

Formal care models for healthcare team functioning, based largely in nursing, have been described in the literature and may be used to guide team development in some healthcare facilities.[39–41] As healthcare organizations have responded to the demand to integrate care and bring all disciplines to the table, both benefits and challenges have been identified. While early attempts at interdisciplinary care were relatively unstructured, there has been an increasing focus in the last few years on the need to more clearly identify roles and practice accountability for the disciplines.

Each profession's scope of practice, standards of performance, and code of ethics serve as the basis for establishing the interdisciplinary care model, whether formally or informally. The ADA's Code of Ethics and Standards of Professional Performance provide dietetics professionals with a framework for their professional interactions.[42,43] The ADA House of Delegates and board of directors recently developed a model scope of practice for the dietetics profession that broadly outlines the key knowledge and skills dietitians bring to healthcare.[44] ADA dietetics practice groups (DPGs) have also published both scopes of practice and standards of professional practice specific to their area of practice. The Diabetes Care and Education DPG has developed a scope of practice specific to dietitians who work in caring for diabetic patients.[45]

Similarly, the Gerontological DPG has published standards of professional practice for dietetics practitioners working with older adults.[46] These documents help to guide practitioners in establishing their role within the practice team.

ROLES OF DIETETICS PROFESSIONALS ON TEAMS

Along with traditional responsibilities attributed to dietetics professionals, clinical dietetics professionals assume a variety of roles that impact greatly on patient care, team function, and job satisfaction (Table 5-1). A focus group study of dietitian roles on healthcare teams was conducted with 49 dietitians practicing medical nutrition therapy in an acute care setting who attended the 1997 ADA Annual Meeting and Exhibition.[47] The group discussions were guided by the following questions: "What do you perceive as the dietitian's current role on the interdisciplinary team?"; "Is the dietitian's current role on the interdisciplinary team as it should be?"; and "What measures must dietitians take to remain a vital component of future healthcare teams?" Participants generally identified with formal team participation and saw their role as clinically focused, primarily as educators and subject-matter experts. They did not view staff dietitians as being participants on an interdisciplinary team. Although the participants indicated they would like the opportunity for more responsibilities, they were generally comfortable with their current roles, and some participants expressed discomfort with change, especially related to assuming more direct patient care or hands-on skills. In response to the third question, participants believed dietitians need to engage in outcomes research, become more proactive, take on new skills and acquire new knowledge, increase efforts to market their services, take risks, and struggle to overcome traditional stereotypes.

Some of the roles or functions that dietitians frequently assume within teams include consultant, patient caregiver, nutrition therapist, case manager/lifestyle coach, patient advocate, administrator, educator, and researcher. Most clinical nutrition positions require dietitians to assume multiple roles, depending on the number of team members and the scope of services they offer. Thompson has written about the role of the neonatal nutritionist in *Nutritional Care of High-Risk Newborns*.[48] She describes the primary functions as patient care and physician consultation rounds, education and research, and administration and other aspects. In this highly specialized area of dietetics, the role of consultant to physicians and other members of the healthcare team are emphasized. Neonatal nutritionists are sought out within the unit to provide input and recommendations on specific patient's treatment as well as information on specialized nutrition products and regimens. They routinely educate other team members about aspects of neonatal nutrition, both formally and informally, on rounds and patient care conferences. They contribute to or initiate research to increase the understanding of the needs of neonates. Administratively, they assume responsibility for development of policies and

TABLE 5-1	Roles of Dietetic Professionals on Teams
Consultant to patient care	
Patient caregiver	
Nutrition therapist	
Case manager/lifestyle coach	
Patient advocate	
Administrator/director of services	
Educator	
Researcher	

procedures, participate in quality improvement projects, and interface with or supervise the preparation and delivery of infant formulas.

CONSULTANT TO PATIENT CARE

As a consultant, a dietitian provides recommendations for nutrition-related care that others will carry out. In this role, the dietitian uses assessment skills to determine the patient's nutrition status and develops a recommended nutrition-care plan. By effectively working with the other members of the team, the dietitian ensures that the nutrition aspects of care are included in the patient's care and treatment as provided by nurses, physicians, and other direct caregivers. As the role of dietitians on teams has evolved, this role remains at the heart of clinical care; improving the nutrition status of individual patients is still the primary objective.

PATIENT CAREGIVER

In some settings, the role of consultant has expanded to involve more direct patient-care activities. These may include skills that were more traditionally employed by other members of the team, such as physical assessment skills used by nurses and physicians. Taking blood pressure, drawing blood, teaching, and performing blood glucose monitoring, body composition analysis, and measurement of resting energy expenditure are now more commonly being performed by dietitians in monitoring nutrition status and providing care. The 2000 Commission on Dietetic Registration Dietetic Practice Audit included 63% of beyond-entry-level RDs who reported practicing in clinical nutrition.[49] Of the total beyond-entry-level RDs responding to the audit, the following reported performing these tasks: performing blood-glucose monitoring, 15%; measuring blood pressure, 10%; conducting cholesterol screening, 8%; conducting fitness testing, 7%; drawing blood, 4%; performing swallowing evaluation, 4%; checking placement of nasogastric feeding tubes, 2%; and inserting nasogastric feeding tubes, 1%. In all cases, a greater proportion anticipate performing these tasks in the future, with more than one-third anticipating that they will perform blood glucose monitoring and approximately one-fourth anticipating that they will measure blood pressure, conduct cholesterol screening, and conduct fitness testing.

Specialization and advanced skill development has allowed some dietetics professionals to provide direct care related to feeding tubes, including passing tubes and monitoring tube placement. Cresci has described her experience as a nutrition support dietitian who has expanded her skills to include bedside placement of small bowel feeding tubes.[50] After appropriate training and certification, she reports her experience with placing 135 small bowel feeding tubes in surgical and medical patients, both in the intensive care unit and on the ward. Ninety-five percent of the tubes were successfully placed postpylorically, with an average time of 28 minutes for tube placement, and 92% of placed tubes were confirmed radiographically with only one radiograph. No acute complications were associated with tube placement. Cresci believes that nutrition support dietitians should function in this role as a means to both facilitating earlier enteral feeding by obtaining access more quickly and to improve the utilization of scarce hospital resources.

Opportunities exist for expanding clinical privileges to allow dietitians to have a more direct role in patient care by way of writing orders and diagnosing problems involving nutrition. In 1996, Mueller and colleagues surveyed nutrition support practitioners to evaluate the practice of dietitians writing parenteral nutrition orders and reported that 37% sometimes or usually wrote parenteral nutrition orders.[51] In spite of this relatively high reported participation almost 10 years ago, expansion of privileges for dietitians has moved slowly. In 2002, Moreland and associates described the successful development of a program that grants clinical privileges to dietitians to write orders for nutrition care in a long-term acute-care hospital.[52] With approval of the medical staff, dietitians are granted privileges after a minimum 6 months of employment by demonstrating initial competence using multiple measures, completing a 3-month probationary period during which orders written are tracked and reviewed, and gaining final approval by the medical director. The authors report that expedited order implementation, improved patient nutrition response, and increased RD responsibility have all been seen as benefits of the program.

Simultaneously, Myers and coworkers provided a comprehensive discussion of the issue of clinical privileges for dietitians, laying out the related considerations and encouraging an ongoing dialogue on the subject.[53] Their article included consideration of the impact on the dietitian's role within the practice team when clinical privileges are expanded. Silver and Wellman further advocated for both the value to practitioners and the quality for clients that can be achieved with expansion of privileges for both order writing and nutrition diagnosing.[54]

NUTRITION THERAPIST

Private practice dietitian and entrepreneur Lisa Licavoli, RD, advocated for the role of nutrition therapist when she wrote, "We must discard the role of 'food cop,' replacing it with a counseling style attuned to the needs and life issues of our clients."[31] As compared to traditional nutrition education, she described nutrition therapy with the following characteristics: more time, fosters choice among options, dietitian and client develop a relationship, gives motivation and praise, is open-ended, explores personal issues, can evaluate adherence and make adjustments, dietitian and client are partners, promotes client's independence, and a team approach is emphasized. She strongly urged dietetics professionals to refine their counseling skills through additional training but also acknowledged the importance of recognizing the limits of their scope of practice and making appropriate referrals to other disciplines when indicated.

Role of the Dietetics Professional: Nutrition Therapist

Molly Kellogg, RD, LCSW, is a successful nutrition therapist in private practice in Philadelphia. She says that she became a nutrition therapist after years of work with patients who suffered from disordered eating and had weight concerns, which led her to seek additional training so as to improve the effectiveness of her interventions (personal communication, M. Kellogg, October 21, 2004). Although she obtained a master's degree in social work and is a licensed clinical social worker, she continues to see patients for nutrition therapy, separating her role in the realm of dietetics from the treatment for broader psychosocial issues. Sharing her expertise with other dietitians, she publishes a free e-mail bulletin series entitled *Counseling Tips for Nutrition Therapists*.[55] Recent topics speak to the development of skills needed to be an effective nutrition therapist, including asking "how?" and "what?" instead of "why?"; unpacking meaning; making use of time boundaries in sessions and triangulation; defining the role of the nutrition therapist; and getting clients to return after the first visit.

Israel and McCabe described a model for providing nutrition therapy to 80,000 subscribers of Texas Instruments health plan through a preferred nutrition therapist network of registered dietitians.[56] The services entitled each subscriber with a nutritionally related diagnosis to receive four visits with a dietetics professional per year. Using disease-specific protocols as the guide, nutrition therapists provided personalized services based on individual needs while also monitoring disease-specific clinical and behavioral measures and patient satisfaction. To prepare for this role, dietetics professionals received training in evaluating readiness for change. The authors attribute the success of this approach to being a health partner along with the company's occupational health nurses, a toll-free nurse counseling service, the employee assistance program, the clinical and health plan networks, and fitness services. This illustrates a clear model for the nutrition therapist in an integrated but dispersed healthcare team.

CASE MANAGER/LIFESTYLE COACH

The role of the dietitian as lifestyle coach and case manager was described in the Diabetes Prevention Program (DPP).[57] In this study of 3,234 individuals with impaired glucose tolerance at high-risk for the development of diabetes, dietitians at 27 centers participated as lifestyle coaches. This intensive intervention was compared to traditional treatment with medications and demonstrated significantly greater reductions in the risk of developing diabetes. As lifestyle coaches, dietitians followed a 16-module core curriculum as the basis of their intervention. They also employed counseling skills, flexible scheduling, and toolbox strategies to overcome barriers while tailoring courses or developing additional modules and moving from a structured educational approach to a skill-building, motivational approach over time. Case management functions included scheduling, reporting adverse events, reviewing progress with the care team weekly, and making referrals to other team members when indicated.

Similarly, Saffel-Shrier and Athas advocated for the role of the dietitian as nutrition case manager for the elderly in response to the Nutrition Screening Initiative of the early 1990s.[58] They saw a role for the dietitian in coordinating support for dietitians implementing screening and intervention programs; communicating nutrition status to other members of the healthcare team; educating outreach workers, discharge planners, and third-party payers; and orchestrating nutrition information to policymakers, the public, the elderly, and their families and caregivers. It is not clear to what degree dietetics practitioners have embraced this role, though they are uniquely positioned to do so.

PATIENT ADVOCATE

The role of patient advocate is one that dietetics professionals often perform informally. As value-driven individuals, dietetics professionals exhibit a strong association with and concern for their patients. This often plays out in the individualized attention dietetics professionals offer their patients in developing or modifying diet or enteral nutrition regimens, writing letters to insurance providers to obtain coverage for specialized nutrition therapies, and actively participating in patient support groups. As a means to ensure food security for their patients outside the facility, dietitian advocates often work to address hunger in the community and volunteer at local food banks.

Role of the Dietetics Professional: Patient Advocate

Elaine Hagen, RD, CD, of Elkhart General Hospital in Elkhart, Indiana, had a unique opportunity to participate in her facility's Health Advocacy Program for employees (personal communication, E. Hagen, December 18, 2003). Following the precept that 20% of the employees are using 80% of the facilities' resources spent on healthcare, the hospital identifies and invites employees to be part of the program based on their healthcare needs. After agreeing to participate, clients are assessed for their individual needs by a nurse, physician, and behavioralist. Elaine becomes involved by referral when nutrition is identified as an issue. Once involved, she is given broad authority to set up and provide services as she deems necessary, including individual counseling sessions, home visits, and supermarket tours. She reports being given a lot of latitude and the freedom to think outside the box to meet the clients' needs.

As a part of the team, Elaine is expected to be fully committed to the values of the program and the interdisciplinary team. Although she does not routinely attend regular team meetings, she reports that developing a rapport with the other team members, demonstrating trust, communicating regularly, having a broad view of the patient's needs, and referring needs back to the team have been key to being part of the team. Elaine says that being a good listener, being able to show compassion, being willing to go the extra mile, fostering a familylike atmosphere, and being mentally prepared for what she will encounter are skills she has developed in this role that help her to be successful. She has high job satisfaction in this role because she sees the results of her work and is making a difference in her clients' lives.

An important advocacy role for dietetics professionals is in the ethical deliberation of care options. In situations in which the ethics of patient feeding are in question, dietitians have a role in ensuring that patients and their caregivers understand their options and the anticipated outcomes.[59] In this manner, they contribute to patients providing informed consent for care, an aspect of critical importance to patient autonomy.

ADMINISTRATOR/DIRECTOR OF SERVICES

Dietetics professionals have a role on interdisciplinary teams as administrators of programs related to nutrition. In this role, clinical dietitians develop and implement policies and procedures to support the most effective patient care and positive patient outcomes. Screening and intervention policies, diet-ordering procedures, enteral formularies, and the preparation and delivery of diets and enteral formulas are just some of the administrative aspects of care in which dietetics professionals are involved. In recent years, the consolidation of management positions has allowed some dietitians to take on administrative responsibility for multiple departments, using skills that are common to management across healthcare functions.

Role of the Dietetics Professional: Administrator/Director of Services

As neonatal nutritionist at INOVA Fairfax Hospital in Fairfax, Virginia, Sandy Robbins, RD, CSP, is an integral member of the interdisciplinary team in the neonatal intensive care unit (personal communication, S. Robbins, December 18, 2003). She sees her primary role on the team as developing protocols—designing and implementing a plan and then monitoring its effectiveness. She focuses on assessing the global needs of the patients in the unit versus only the needs of the individual patients and collaborates with the team to achieve the best possible outcomes. Examples are seen in Sandy's oversight of the infant formula room that prepares and delivers all formulas not available in ready-to-feed form. Her involvement in this function of the unit ensures that the appropriate products are in the formulary, that the ordering systems promote selection of the most appropriate product, and that the products are prepared and handled correctly to minimize error and maximize safety. All of these aspects contribute substantially to positive patient outcomes.

Sandy reports she balances this role with her patient-care responsibilities and other activities, such as teaching and research. Her credibility within the interdisciplinary team has been earned by a willingness to look at the big picture, be flexible with her time and commitments, and continuously develop her communication and management skills. She believes in developing relationships with team members by always being a couple of favors ahead and by extending herself to her teammates when they ask, whether or not the request is technically part of her job. It is this involvement with the team that she believes is responsible for the development of advanced-level practice skills and the job satisfaction that is achieved over an extended career.

EDUCATOR

Dahlke and coworkers have described the role of educator of other health professionals as one dietetics professionals are comfortable with.[47] This role takes various forms, depending on the setting. The training of dietetics interns is a commitment to the profession that many dietitians participate in. Dietitians provide inservices and participate in new-hire orientation for nurses in most hospitals. In teaching facilities, dietitians may be called on to have a more active role in the training of other healthcare providers.

Role of the Dietetics Professional: Educator

Dorene Balmer, MA, RD, neonatal nutritionist at the University of Pennsylvania Medical Center and The Children's Hospital of Philadelphia, identifies her primary role as educator of pediatric medical residents (personal communication, D. Balmer, December 13, 2003). She recognizes that her time with each individual patient is limited, and she can maximize her impact on both current and future patients by educating residents. Her teaching focuses not only on the nutrition concepts and knowledge that residents need to care for patients but also on the role of the dietitian in caring for these patients. As this role has developed on the interdisciplinary team, the team has come to expect it in addition to her role as consultant on nutrition therapies for individual patients. Dorene says that respect for others has been the key to her success on the interdisciplinary team. Her respect for the knowledge of other professionals, as well as developing their trust, has helped her to develop the role of nutrition educator.

As the expectation for all healthcare providers to be competent in nutrition increases, the opportunity for dietetics professionals to be educators of other health professionals also increases. Touger-Decker and colleagues reported on a survey of dental schools, physician assistant, nurse practitioner, and certified nurse midwifery programs to assess their perceived need for nutrition education.[60] The respondents agreed that their graduates need some discipline-specific competence in nutrition and reported that the most frequent provider of nutrition education (47%) was an RD. The study concluded that significant opportunities exist for dietitians as educators of other healthcare disciplines.

RESEARCHER

As discussed earlier, clinical dietitians have a unique opportunity to contribute to and build a role in research. They also play an important role in conducting or contributing to translational research, which is required to apply findings of basic science research to clinical practice. The dietitian role in the DCCT demonstrates how central dietitians can be to establishing the outcomes of the study. Although this role was developed in the context of a large multisite study, dietetics professionals also have significant opportunities to conduct research in independent facilities.

Role of the Dietetics Professional: Researcher

Leila Beker, PhD, RD, formerly the pediatric nutritionist on the cystic fibrosis (CF) team at Children's National Medical Center in Washington, D.C., identifies her primary role there as researcher (personal communication, L. Beker, December 17, 2003). She reports that the physician she worked with had strong research interests and approached patient care from this perspective. Her research involvement started out by doing a chart review of all the patients enrolled at the CF center to establish a baseline of their nutrition status. Data were compared to those published by the CF Foundation and used as the basis of both assessing their population and prioritizing patients for nutrition intervention. This initial project led to multiple other funded and unfunded research opportunities over successive years.

Leila's role as researcher was balanced with her other roles as consultant, caregiver, educator, and case manager. She emphasizes the importance of dietitians acting as part of a team, even if there is no formal team organization, and sees bonding with nurses as an important activity. She reports that dietitians may have a tendency to be too adversarial and need to see the big picture, use more finesse in communicating, and develop the buy-in of other team members to be more successful in their roles.

CREATING SEAMLESS CARE

The goal of multidisciplinary or interdisciplinary team care is to bring the combined expertise and skills of multiple professionals to the table to promote positive patient outcomes. This occurs best when the team functions effectively, bringing out the strengths in each member of the team while compensating for weak areas. The advantages to the patient and to the healthcare system are that resources, including both time and money, are used effectively to the benefit of the patient. Collaboration and communication are two key aspects to creating seamless care. In the outpatient setting, patients are typically triaged to receive the care of the professional(s) indicated at the time, rather than each patient being seen by all members of the team at every visit. This requires a coordinated effort by the team to make sure that the most pressing issues are uncovered and addressed. Although the scope of practice of each of the team members is a consideration, dietitians experienced in working on teams report that established teams function less on the basis of scope of practice and more on the basis of trust and respect. To be an effective team member, dietitians must know their own scope of practice and readily refer care beyond their scope to other members of the team and/or to dietetics specialists as indicated. The dietitian is responsible for understanding how the team functions, what formal roles are expected of each team member, and developing personal skills that contribute not only to patient care but also to team function.

Beth Winthrop, MS, RD, CNSD, Clinical Nutrition Manager at Southcoast Health System in Massachusetts, described a successful model for the nurse/dietitian team on the inpatient unit in an acute care setting, when the dietitian is not functioning as part of a formal interdisciplinary team.[61] Her team developed a three-question nutrition screening/referral system completed by nursing, which led to a twofold increase in patients receiving diet teaching and a threefold increase in nutrition reassessments over an 18-month period. Although the screening questions do not differ from those used at other facilities, the implementation of the program and the attitude of the dietitians appear to produce different outcomes. Winthrop emphasizes the importance of building relationships with nursing leadership and has developed a guide for dietitians entitled *Clinical Dietitian's Guide to a Win-Win Relationship with Nursing*. Winthrop holds that when dietetics professionals work in a collegial, collaborative, and coordinated manner with nursing, the result is better patient care, better communication with physicians, and a better work life for dietetics professionals. The main recommendations are listed in Table 5-2.

ACQUIRING SKILLS

Employers responding to the 2000 Dietetics Practice Audit identified a movement towards multidisciplinary care over the late 1990s.[49] They reported that the most valued team members were those with more global views and more competencies. Technical competencies were seen as important and expected, but employers emphasized the importance of dietitians developing business competencies, specifically persuasive communication, negotiation skills, supervisory abilities, and financial knowledge. Professional characteristics identified as important include flexibility, creativity, initiative, a problem-solving mindset, and a heightened focus on the patient or customer.

The concept of emotional intelligence (EI) has gained attention in the last decade as being a significant contributor to healthcare workplace performance.[62] Although intelligence (IQ) had long been acknowledged as a contributor to individual success, the contribution of an individual's EI had previously not been recognized. Goleman is credited with bringing the concept into prominence in the late 1990s.[63] In *Primal Leadership: Realizing the Power of Emotional Intelligence*, he offers a modified and streamlined model.[64] Goleman defines EI as the ability to be aware of emotions and able to regulate them, both inwardly and outwardly. He identifies four domains of EI—self-awareness, self-motivation, social awareness, and relationship management—and 18 competencies that can be developed to strengthen each domain. An important tenet of Goleman's work is that these competencies are not innate talents but rather learned abilities.

Healthcare educators have begun to include EI in their training programs for entry-level practitioners.[65] Sylvia Escott-Stump, MA, RD, LDN, Dietetic Program Director at East Carolina University in Greenville, North Carolina, describes using several standardized measures to evaluate EI, with the goal of helping her interns to develop skills to make them "leadership ready" (personal communication, S. Escott-Stump, December 18, 2003). She reports seeing a reduction in interpersonal problems between interns and their preceptors since introducing EI and believes that her interns are better prepared to be successful in the job market.

TABLE 5-2	Clinical Dietitians' Guide to a "Win-Win" Relationship with Nursing Staff

1. Nursing has well-developed systems; work within them.

- Use the data on the nursing assessment to avoid asking patients the same questions repeatedly. Ask "I notice you told your nurse you avoid salt at home; do you restrict any other foods?" Patients feel confident when they feel that caregivers communicate well.

- Know the nurse manager on your unit. Request an invitation to "unit council" meetings, and ask to be on the unit's e-mail distribution list. Be "in the loop."

- Understand and use the ways in which nurses communicate with one another (shift-to-shift report; nursing kardex, interdisciplinary patient care plan).

- Work with nursing professional development to include nutrition messages in nursing orientation, on-line training, "skills days," and nurse's aid training. If you develop educational content for nurses, apply for nursing CEUs.

- Use nursing awards and recognition systems to document your appreciation for the nurses that you find to be outstanding to work with.

2. The delivery of nursing care in a hospital setting is stressful. Nurses appreciate colleagues who save them time, help them avoid errors, and put user-friendly resources into their hands.

- Be aware of top priorities and "hot issues" for nursing staff. Be supportive of projects on medication errors, restraints, pain, and length of stay. Evaluate the role of nutrition in nursing initiatives.

- Provide simple nutrition education materials for nurses to use off shift.

- Inpatient nurses tend to focus on the inpatient world. Raise awareness of the advantages of outpatient nutrition counseling.

- Provide quick and helpful guides for nurses, such as formula substitution charts.

- Coordinate efforts with other disciplines, such as speech-language pathology and clinical pharmacy, to give nurses and doctors one consistent recommendation.

- Get to know nursing "off shifts." Get up to your units and do rounds at supper at least once a week. It's a great opportunity to see and teach family members.

3. Involve nurses in the nutrition care plan as a team member. Be aware of nursing practice standards and regulations.

- Never work with a doctor to change the patient's plan and then leave the nurses in the dark. They are responsible for coordinating the patient's care; keep them informed.

- Introduce yourself to unfamiliar nurses and clarify your role on the unit, so that they know it is appropriate to share protected health information with you.

- Do not ask nurses to transcribe a verbal order given to you by a physician.

4. Be sensitive to work flows, time demands, and space issues on the unit.

- Do not monopolize the charts or take over someone's "designated" workspace.

- To minimize the risk of medication errors, do not interrupt the nurse who is passing medications unless it is absolutely necessary.

- Know and respect time-critical periods of the day. "Listen in" on shift-to-shift reports if you can, but realize that this is not a good time for a nurse to respond to questions or discuss clinical cases.

5. Work to reduce meal-service issues for your nursing staff.

- When your schedule permits, be visible on the floors at mealtimes so as to identify problems while they are manageable.

- Teach unit secretaries how to order complex diets. Show nurses (in a nondefensive way) when order-entry mistakes result in problems with patients' meals.

- Include nurses in tray assessments so that they know what the meals taste like (even purees). They will be better able to encourage patient intake if they know the meals are tasty.

- Empower diet office staff to solve minor meal-service issues to prevent a call light.

- Encourage foodservice managers and production staff to do meal rounds with you on your unit and get firsthand interaction with patients and nurses.

6. Use your global knowledge of the patient and unit procedures to develop an appropriate nutrition care plan.

- Never chart on a patient whom you have not gone in to see. Even if you just need to "crunch the numbers" on a tube feeding, get face-to-face with the patient and talk to the nurse. You will access information that is not in the chart.

- Know what nurses do to hang tube feedings and TPN. Know how to check in a TPN bag against the physician's order. It is their job, not yours, but you need to know the process.

TABLE 5-2	Clinical Dietitians' Guide to a "Win-Win" Relationship with Nursing Staff *(cont)*

- Make sure you know what is really happening so that your recommendations will be sound. Consider the fluid in IV meds and the water used to give meds via PEG before you recommend additional water flushes. Remember to check for suction/drain losses.
- Once you are trained, feel free to help nurses with "boosts" and bed scales. Do not be afraid to touch patients.

7. Be a part of the unit.
- Answer the phone if you're sitting at the desk. Answer the patients' call lights. You can do it! Just go into the room and say "I'm Beth, your dietitian. Do you need your nurse, or is there something I can take care of for you?"
- Ask if the patient needs anything else before you leave the room. Check that the patient can reach his or her phone and call light and train your staff to check as well.
- Be aware of the timing on the unit. When are labs drawn? Breathing treatments scheduled? Insulin administered? Does this make sense with mealtimes?

8. Welcome opportunities to demonstrate that you are the nutrition expert.
- Make sure that nutrition counseling is a covered service in the hospital employees' health plan. Provide expert services when nurses are personally in need; they will remember your help and be more likely to refer patients for counseling.
- Help answer personal nutrition questions for your colleagues in nursing. Help them deal with their picky toddler or their frail mother.
- Work with public relations on nutrition communication in the media. Media exposure enhances your department's reputation and confirms you as the nutrition expert.

9. Keep an open mind even if you "agree to disagree."
- Pick your battles regarding controversial nutrition issues. Recognize that in many cases the data are not all in. Offer information/advice if requested or if you are aware that a colleague is doing something potentially dangerous (i.e., suggesting or using ephedra for weight loss).
- Learn a little more about complementary and alternative approaches in the world of nursing. Knowing a bit more about Reiki, aromatherapy, and massage will help you talk to your patients about what they are doing. Try not to be judgmental.

Source: Adapted with permission from Winthrop B. Dietitian Orientation Handbook. New Bedford, MA: Southcoast Health System, 2003.

Goleman and others have described the importance of EI to successful team function. Two professors of organizational behavior and management, Urch Druskat and Wolff, have described in the *Harvard Business Review* the significance of EI to teams.[66] They contend that three conditions are critical to a team's success: trust among members, a sense of group identity, and a sense of group efficacy. The most effective teams are those that build group norms to support these three conditions. They outline norms that create awareness of emotions, working progressively from the individual to the group to cross-boundary communication, including interpersonal understanding, perspective taking, team self-evaluation, the seeking of feedback, and organizational understanding. In addition, they outline a group of norms that help regulate emotions, including confronting, caring, creating resources for working with emotion, creating an affirmative environment, solving problems proactively, and building external relationships. Their research indicates that norms can be introduced by formal team leaders, informal team leaders, courageous followers, through training, or from the larger organizational culture. Finally, the authors conclude the most effective teams are emotionally intelligent ones and that any team can become emotionally intelligent. These findings reinforce the power that individual team members have to influence the effectiveness of the team, not only by their technical knowledge and skills but also by their own EI.

TELEHEALTHCARE

As medical care moves forward in the next 10 years, electronic technology and the Internet will no doubt play a significant role in shaping it. Dietetics professionals have an opportunity to evaluate their roles and make sure that they will have a place at the table as care models employing new technologies are developed. The ADA's 2002 Environmental Scan includes information technology as becoming an integral part of health and medical care and recommends that dietitians embrace the Internet for client communications, learning, and promotion.[67]

Dietetics professionals are using new technology in their practice in a variety of ways.[68] As practice develops, unique issues related to technology use have been recognized. Rodriguez summarized her experience and learning as a result of posting articles and responding to questions about nutrition on a Spanish-language website.[69] She identified 10 major legal, ethical, and professional issues that need to be considered when practicing nutrition through this medium, including the global nature of cyberspace; cultural variations in food and nutrition or models; differences in scope and standards of practice; presentation of the self and one's credentials, area(s) of knowledge, and scope of practice; source or nature of the inquirers information and knowledge; nature of the cyberspace client-practitioner relationship; protection of the self, the client, and the public; need for a response model or process; and the need for a professional electronic communication policy.

Telehealthcare allows patients at remote locations to receive timely services at a fraction of the cost it would take for them or the provider to travel to meet in person. Cline and Wong reported on the successful use of videoconferencing to provide nutrition counseling from Oahu, Hawaii, to patients on the Kwajalein Atoll on the Marshall Islands in the South Pacific.[70] Telehealthcare's efficacy has also been reported in less distant, medically underserved, rural areas of the United States. In rural central New York, dietitians at Bassett Healthcare reported using interactive videoconferencing (IATV) to counsel patients referred from regional health centers.[71] They saw improvements in participation rates from 74 to 79% and high satisfaction ratings, with 85% of clients indicating the visit led to better understanding of the treatment, and 98% indicating they benefited from the visit and would advise family members to receive care from this consultant.

Ethical issues around the practice of telemedicine have been addressed by a number of organizations. A panel of international experts convened in January 2000, by the Internet Health Organization, sponsored by the World Health Organization/Pan-American Health Organization. The group developed an e-Health Code of Ethics with guiding principles organized under the headings of candor, honesty, quality, informed consent, privacy, professionalism in online healthcare, responsible partnering, and, accountability.[72] "Telemedicine: Legal, Ethical and Liability Considerations" by Ashley identifies dietetics issues.[73]

Clearly, the evolution of technology will change the way in which healthcare is delivered. Forkner-Dunn describes Internet-based patient self-care as the next generation of healthcare delivery.[74] Others have described use of the Internet to implement standardized clinical practice guidelines across multiple sites.[75] In January 2004, the American Medical Association released a temporary Current Procedural Terminology (CPT) code, 0074T, for online consultations, describing the service as a type of Evaluation and Management (E&M) service provided by a physician or qualified health care professional, to a patient using Internet resources, in response to the patient's online inquiry. Reportable services involve the physician's personal timely response to the patient's inquiry and must involve permanent storage (electronic or hard copy) of the encounter. This service should not be reported for patient contacts (e.g., telephone calls) considered to be preservice or postservice work for other E&M or non-E&M services. A reportable service would encompass the sum of communication (e.g., related telephone calls, prescription provision, laboratory orders) pertaining to the online patient encounter or problem(s).[76]

It is reasonable to expect that insurance providers will begin to reimburse services of dietetics professionals in a similar fashion in the future.

As telehealthcare evolves, the complexities of dealing in an electronic medium will be sorted out. Dietetics professionals are encouraged to seek out current resources and familiarize themselves with legislation before entering into this arena.

Issues to Ponder

- What additional outcome studies should be done to demonstrate the effect on patients of nutrition intervention?
- What additional studies should be done on the impact of the dietitian's role as part of the team on improved nutrition status and overall health of patients with chronic illnesses?
- What are the effects of more liberal diets on patient intake and satisfaction?
- Why do MD specialists tend to give more autonomy to dietitian decision making than the generalist MDs?
- What are the similarities and differences among the diversity of roles for dietetics professionals: consultant, patient caregiver, nutrition therapist, case manager/lifestyle coach, patient advocate, administrator, educator, and researcher?
- Should the goal be that all dietitians have the privilege to write orders and diagnose problems involving nutrition or should these be restricted to specialty or advanced practitioners?
- How can dietetics professionals' role on the team support development of advanced level practice skills and job satisfaction?
- All healthcare providers need to understand and support the role of nutrition in health and disease. How can the RD promote this increased knowledge?
- What are the composite of skill sets necessary to an effective team member?
- What legal, ethical, and liability issues need to be explored in telehealthcare?

SUMMARY

The practice of dietetics in clinical settings has developed to make the role of the dietetics professional integral to the comprehensive treatment of patients. The increasing value placed on this role is evident in a number of ways: practice standards and federal regulations specifying the role of dietetics professionals; authorization by the Centers for Medicare and Medicaid of dietetics professionals as sole providers of medical nutrition therapy; and documentation of positive patient outcomes resulting from the intervention of dietetics professionals. The impact of dietitians' central role in the healthcare team can be seen in better continuity of care from inpatient to outpatient settings, cost savings, and increased opportunities for collecting data to contribute to clinical research.

Inherent in this increased recognition of value is an increased responsibility of the dietetics professional to move beyond traditional roles and assume new and expanded roles within the healthcare team. This requires the development of new skills and attitudes. As medical care continues to evolve to outpatient settings and telehealthcare, dietetics professionals have an opportunity to position themselves as central players. Dietetics professionals who embrace this opportunity and take a leadership role, both personally and professionally, can create rewarding career opportunities for themselves and their peers.

REFERENCES

1. Butterworth CE. The skeleton in the hospital closet. Nutr Today 1974;9:4–8.
2. JCAHO: The Joint Commission on Accreditation of Healthcare Organizations. 2006 Comprehensive Accreditation Manual for Hospitals: The Official Handbook. Oakbrook Terrace, IL: JCAHO, 2005.
3. ASPEN Board of Directors and the Standards for Hospitalized Patients Task Force. Standards for specialized nutrition support: adult hospitalized patients. Nutr Clin Pract 2002;17:384–391.
4. ASPEN Board of Directors. Standards for nutrition support for adult residents of long-term care facilities. Nutr Clin Pract 1997;12:284–293.
5. ASPEN Board of Directors and Task Force on the Standards for Specialized Nutrition Support for Hospitalized Pediatric Patients. Standards for specialized nutrition support: hospitalized pediatric patients. Nutr Clin Pract 2005;20:103–116.
6. ASPEN Board of Directors. Standards of practice for nutrition support dietitians. Nutr Clin Pract 2000;15:53–59.
7. Cystic Fibrosis Foundation. Clinical Practice Guidelines for Cystic Fibrosis. Bethesda, MD: Cystic Fibrosis Foundation, 1997.
8. Drucy B, Baker RD, Stallings V. Consensus report on nutrition for pediatric patients with cystic fibrosis. J Pediatr GI Nutr 2002;35:246–259.
9. Schwartz DB. History and evolution of a successful certification program in nutrition support; CNSD experience. J Am Diet Assoc 2003;103:736–741.
10. Leonberg B, Stivers Rops M. The current state of specialty practice in pediatric nutrition and renal nutrition. J Am Diet Assoc 1998;98:1339–1352.
11. Fed. Reg. October 19, 1978;43:203.
12. Fed. Reg. June 3, 1976;41:108.
13. CMS's RAI Version 2.0 Manual, Section K. Available at: http://www.cms.hhs.gov/quality/mds20/raich3.pdf. Accessed November 16, 2004.
14. Fitzner K, Myers EF, Caputo N, Michael P. Are health plans changing their views on nutrition service coverage? J Am Diet Assoc 2003;103:157–161.
15. Kuehneman T, Salsbury D, Splett P, Chapman, DB. Demonstrating the impact of nutrition intervention in a heart failure program. J Am Diet Assoc 2002;102:1790–1794.
16. Bryson SR, Theriot L, Ryan NJ, Pope J, Tolman N, Rhoades P. Primary follow-up care in a multidisciplinary setting enhances catch-up growth of very-low-birth-weight infants. J Am Diet Assoc 1997;97:386–390.
17. Medical Nutrition Therapy Evidence-Based Guides for Practice. Nutrition Practice Guidelines for Type 1 and 2 Diabetes Mellitus [CD-ROM]. Chicago: American Dietetic Association, 2002.
18. Medical Nutrition Therapy Evidence-Based Guides for Practice. Nutrition Practice Guidelines for Gestational Diabetes Mellitus [CD-ROM]. Chicago: American Dietetic Association, 2002.
19. Medical Nutrition Therapy Evidence-Based Guides for Practice. Chronic Kidney Disease (non-dialysis) Medical Nutrition Therapy Protocol [CD-ROM]. Chicago: American Dietetic Association, 2002.
20. Medical Nutrition Therapy Evidence-Based Guides for Practice. Hyperlipidemia Medical Nutrition Therapy Protocol [CD-ROM]. Chicago: American Dietetic Association, 2002.
21. Kulkarni K, Castle G, Gregory R, et al. Nutrition practice guidelines for Type 1 diabetes mellitus positively affect dietitian practices and patient outcomes. J Am Diet Assoc 1998;98:62–70.
22. Reilly JJ, Hull SF, Albert N, Waller A, Bringardener S. Economic impact of malnutrition: a model system for hospitalized patients. J Parenter Enteral Nutr 1988;12:371–376.
23. Position of the American Dietetic Association: cost-effectiveness of medical nutrition therapy. J Am Diet Assoc 1995;95:88–91.

24. Menzin J, Langley-Hawthorne C, Friedman M, Boulanger L, Cavanaugh R. Potential short-term economic benefits of improved glycemic control: a managed care perspective. Diabetes Care 2001;24:51–55.

25. Betz Brown J, Nichols GA. Case-control study of 10 years of comprehensive diabetes care. West Med J 2000;172:85–90.

26. Sheehan-Smith LM. Hotel-style room service in hospitals: the new paradigm of meal delivery for achieving patient satisfaction of food service. J Am Diet Assoc 2004;104:A43.

27. Coyne T, Olson M, Bradham K, Garcon M, Gregory P, Scherch L. Dietary satisfaction correlated with adherence in the modification of diet in renal disease study. J Am Diet Assoc 1995;95:1301–1306.

28. Position of the American Dietetics Association: liberalized diets for older adults in long-term care. J Am Diet Assoc 2002;102:1316–1323.

29. Chima C. To the editors. J Am Diet Assoc 1998;98:1400–1401.

30. Miller MA, Schiller MR. To the editors. J Am Diet Assoc 1998;98:1401.

31. O'Sullivan Maillet J. Dietetics in 2017: what does the future hold? J Am Diet Assoc 2002;102:1404–1406.

32. Licavoli L. Dietetics goes into therapy: nutrition therapists replace rules with understanding. J Am Diet Assoc 1995;95:751–752.

33. The DCCT Research Group. Expanded role of the dietitian in the Diabetes Control and Complications Trial: implications for clinical practice. J Am Diet Assoc 1993;93:758–764,767.

34. Schiller MR, Vivian VM. Role of the clinical dietitian. I. Ideal role perceived by dietitians and physicians. J Am Diet Assoc 1974;65:284–287.

35. Gaare J, Maillet JO, King D, Gilbride JA. Perceptions of clinical decision making by dietitians and physicians. J Am Diet Assoc 1990;90:54–58.

36. Rosen O, Downes NJ, Sucher KP, Shifflett B. Physicians' perceptions of the role of clinical dietitians are changing. J Am Diet Assoc 1991;91:1074–1077.

37. Boyhtari ME, Cardinal BJ. The role of clinical dietitians as perceived by dietitians and physicians. J Am Diet Assoc 1997;97:851–855.

38. Hart JJ, Hurley RS, Garrison MEB, Stombaugh I. Nephrologists' and internal medicine physician's expectations of renal dietitians and general clinical dietitians. J Am Diet Assoc 1997;97:1389–1393.

39. Davis B, Heath O, Reddick P. A Multi-disciplinary professional practice model: supporting autonomy and accountability in program-based structure. Can J Nurs Leader 2002;15:21–25.

40. Grigsby K, Westmoreland D, Shiparski L. Capacity building of leaders in healthcare organizations: monitoring organization-wide implementation of the clinical practice model. J Nurs Adm 2002;32:398–404.

41. O'Rourke MW. Rebuilding a professional practice model: the return of role-based practice accountability. Nurs Admin Q 2003;27:95–105.

42. American Dietetic Association. The American Dietetic Association standards of professional practice for dietetics professionals. J Am Diet Assoc 1998;98:83–87.

43. American Dietetic Association. Code of ethics for the profession of dietetics. J Am Diet Assoc 1999;99:109–113.

44. O'Sullivan Maillet J, Skates J, Pritchett E. American Dietetic Association: scope of dietetics practice framework. J Am Diet Assoc 2005;105:634–640.

45. Kulkarni K, Boucher JL, Daly A, et al. American Dietetic Association: standards of practice and standards of professional performance for registered dietitians (generalist, specialty, and advanced) in diabetes care. J Am Diet Assoc 2005;105:819–824.

46. Shoaf LR, Bishirjian KO, Schlenker ED. The geronotological nutritionists standards of professional practice for dietetics professionals working with older adults. J Am Diet Assoc 1999;99:863–867.

47. Dahlke R, Wolf KN, Wilson SL, Brodnik M. Focus groups as predictors of dietitian's roles on interdisciplinary teams. J Am Diet Assoc 2000;100:455–457.

48. Thompson M. Perspectives on the neonatal nutritionist's role. In: Groh-Wargo S, Thompson M, Cox JH, eds. Nutritional Care for High-Risk Newborns. Chicago: Precept Press, 2000.

49. Rogers D, Leonberg BL, Broadhurst CA. 2000 Commission on Dietetic Registration dietetics practice audit. J Am Diet Assoc 2002;102:270–292.

50. Cresci G, Martindale R. Bedside placement of small bowel feeding tubes in hospitalized patients. Nutrition 2003;19:843–846.

51. Mueller CM, Colaizzo-Anas T, Shronts EP, Gaines JA. Order writing for parenteral nutrition by registered dietitians. J Am Diet Assoc 1996;96:764–768.

52. Moreland K, Gotfried M, Vaughan L. Development and implementation of the clinical privileges for dietitian order writing program at a long-term acute-care hospital. J Am Diet Assoc 2002;102:72–74, 79–81.

53. Myers EF, Barnhill G, Bryk J. Clinical privileges: missing piece of the puzzle for clinical standards that elevate responsibilities and salaries for registered dietitians? J Am Diet Assoc 2002;102:123–132.

54. Silver HJ, Wellman NS. Nutrition diagnosing and order writing: value for practitioners, quality for clients. J Am Diet Assoc 2003;103:1470–1472.

55. Counseling Tips for Nutrition Therapists. Available at: http://www.mollykellogg.com/archive2004.htm. Accessed November 29, 2004.

56. Alexander Israel D, McCabe M. Using disease-state management as the key to promoting employer sponsorship of medical nutrition therapy. J Am Diet Assoc 1999;99:583–588.

57. Wylie-Rosett J, Delahanty L. An integral role of the dietitian: implications of the diabetes prevention program. J Am Diet Assoc 2002;102:1065–1068.

58. Saffel-Shrier A, Athas BM. Effective provision of comprehensive nutrition case management for the elderly. J Am Diet Assoc 1993;93:439–444.

59. Position of the American Dietetic Association: ethical and legal issues in nutrition, hydration and feeding. J Am Diet Assoc 2002;102:716–726.

60. Touger-Decker R, Benedict Barracato JM, O'Sullivan-Maillet J. Nutrition education in health profession programs: a survey of dental, physician assistant, nurse practitioner, and nurse midwifery programs. J Am Diet Assoc 2001;101:63–69.

61. Winthrop B. The nurse/dietitian team. Future Dimensions 2003;22:1–5.

62. Segal J. Good leaders use "emotional intelligence." Health Prog 2002;83:44–46, 66.

63. Goleman D. Emotional Intelligence: Why It Can Matter More Than IQ. New York: Bantam Books, 1997.

64. Goleman D, Boyatzis R, McKee A. Primal Leadership: Realizing the Power of Emotional Intelligence. Boston: Harvard Business School Press, 2002.

65. Evans D, Allen H. Emotional intelligence: its role in training. Nurs Time 2002;98:27, 41–42.

66. Urch Druskat V, Wolff SB. Building the emotional intelligence of groups. Harvard Business Rev 2001;79:80–90, 164.

67. Jarratt J, Mahaffie JB. Key trends affecting the dietetics profession and the American Dietetic Association. J Am Diet Assoc 2002;102:1821–1839.

68. Palumbo C. Using new technology for nutrition counseling. J Am Diet Assoc 1999;99:1363–1364.

69. Rodriguez JC. Legal, ethical, and professional issues to consider when communicating via the Internet: a suggested response model and policy. J Am Diet Assoc 1999;99:1428–1432.

70. Cline AD, Wong M. New frontiers in using telemedicine for nutrition intervention. J Am Diet Assoc 1999;99:1442–1443.

71. Johnson A, Gorman M, Lewis C, Baker F, Coulehan N, Rader J. Interactive videoconferencing improves nutrition intervention in a rural population. J Am Diet Assoc 2001;101:173–174.

72. e-Health Ethics Initiative. E-Health code of ethics. J Med Internet Res 2000;2:e9.

73. Ashley RC. Telemedicine: legal, ethical and liability considerations. J Am Diet Assoc 2002;102:267–269.

74. Forkner-Dunn J. Internet-based patient self-care: the next generation of health care delivery. J Med Internet Res 2003;5:e8.

75. Jeannot JG, Scherer F, Pittet V, Burnand B, Vader JP. Use of the World Wide Web to implement clinical practice guidelines: a feasibility study. J Med Internet Res 2003;5:e12.

76. Category III CPT Codes. American Medical Association, 2004. Available at: http://www.ama-assn.org/ama/pub/article/3885-4897.html. Accessed January 13, 2004.

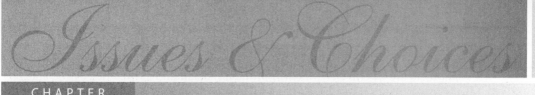

CHAPTER

6

IS THE DIETETICS PROFESSIONAL AN EQUAL
PLAYER ON THE HEALTHCARE TEAM?

*Robert F. Kushner, Cecelia Echevarria, Jane V. White,
and Laura Heald Watson*

SECTION 1   A Physician's Perspective

Robert F. Kushner

A major healthcare challenge for the 21st century will be caring for the increasing number of Americans with chronic illnesses, including diabetes, hypertension, heart disease, respiratory diseases, and obesity, among others. Unfortunately, today's healthcare system is designed to deal with acute, episodic care and has not kept pace with the changing demands of medical practice. In the current traditional medical model, physicians spend their time principally addressing acute symptoms, ordering and reviewing laboratory and other diagnostic tests, providing advice, and prescribing medications. Management of chronic illnesses, which requires empowering patients to effectively manage their own health through the acquisition of self-care skills, is less optimally addressed. The Institute of Medicine (IOM) report, *Crossing the Quality Chasm: A New Health System for the 21st Century*, highlights this discrepancy (the "chasm") between the medical care made possible by advances in clinical and behavioral therapies and the care received by the majority of Americans.[1] The report concludes that making incremental improvements in current systems of care will not suffice and instead focuses more broadly on how the healthcare system can be reinvented to foster innovation and improve the delivery of care. Among the 10 rules suggested to redesign the healthcare system is that "Cooperation among clinicians is a priority—clinicians and institutions should actively collaborate and communicate to ensure an appropriate exchange of information and coordination of care." It is within this principle of collaboration and communication that the registered dietitian (RD) should become an equal valued player on the healthcare team.

HISTORICAL PERSPECTIVE OF TEAM-BASED MEDICINE

According to Wagner, a patient care team is "a group of diverse clinicians who communicate with each other regularly about the care of a defined group of patients and participates in that care."[2] In a general sense, patient care teams currently exist in the hospital if we use a broad definition of the term. A hospitalized patient is cared for by his or her physician, the physician in training (resident, intern, medical student), registered nurse, dietitian, social worker, satellite pharmacist, and members of other disciplines as needed. The cumulative effort of each professional contributes to the care of the patient. In this "medical model," written and/or ver-

109

bal orders are usually generated from the physician and carried out by the ancillary staff. Successful outcomes of this "team effort" are typically cure or control of the event that prompted hospitalization, limited length of hospital stay, and avoidance of iatrogenic complications.

The first adaptation of a more structured team approach was naturally born out of the hospital environment. Nutrition support teams were formed in the late 1970s shortly after the introduction of new technology for the invasive administration of specialized parenteral and enteral nutrition care. Composed of an attending physician, pharmacist, RD, and registered nurse, these teams were established to provide safe delivery of optimal nutrition support while minimizing complications. The teams functioned as a unit, crossing departmental and divisional boundaries. Each of the four disciplines possessed skills and training that were unique to its own field and applied to a common purpose: care of the malnourished patient. Communication among team members was direct, via team meetings, conferences, and patient-care rounds. The effectiveness of team-managed nutrition support has been documented by a decrease in the complications in patients receiving parenteral and enteral nutrition support and more judicious and cost-effective use of specialized nutrition care.[3,4] The American Society for Parenteral and Enteral Nutrition (ASPEN)—an organization formed in 1975 to foster and support an interdisciplinary approach to nutrition care, education, and research—stands as one of the few societies that emphasizes the value of a team approach to patient care.

The team-oriented, multidisciplinary approach to patient care has been more recently affirmed in the concept of disease management (DM), broadly defined as a process of organizing care for a special high-cost and/or high volume diagnosis in a coordinated way, using teams and information systems to improve health status and quality of life and, when possible, lowering overall costs.[5] The DM approach, utilizing a multidisciplinary collaborative team of clinicians, has been applied to the care of patients with hyperlipidemia,[6] diabetes,[7] renal failure,[8] and obesity.[9] In contrast to the conception of the hospitalized nutrition support teams, this model was developed to function in the outpatient setting to aid patients in the management of their chronic disease. The model presents a multidimensional, multidisciplinary solution to a complex chronic problem. The American Heart Association Lipid Disorders Training Program was designed to enable physicians to diagnose and manage patients with complex lipid abnormalities. One of the course objectives was to promote a collaborative interdisciplinary approach to long-term management of patients with lipid abnormalities.[10] Other lipid clinics were formed using a similar collaborative approach.[6] To meet the needs of this population, the healthcare team often consists of a nurse practitioner, RD, and clinical psychologist. The model of care has been shown to increase the achievement of targeted lipid levels, improve office efficiency, and increase patient satisfaction.

The importance of a team approach has also been exemplified in two landmark diabetes studies: the Diabetes Control and Complications Trial (DCCT)[11] and the Diabetes Prevention Program.[12] In both studies, dietitians, nurse educators, and mental health professionals worked alongside diabetologists as equal participants in patients' care, strengthening key treatment recommendations of the other team members. The long-term goals of the diabetes treatment in the DCCT were summarized as follows[13]: "These intensive interventions involve training by a multidisciplinary staff to provide participants with skills in self-care, regimen self-correction, problem solving, and self-motivation. The goal is to prepare patients to leave the program able to participate more actively in their own self-care."

The DCCT showed that patients were able to achieve improved adherence to treatment, as reflected by lowering of blood glucose concentrations and glycosylated hemoglobin values and delaying the onset and slowing the progression of diabetic retinopathy, nephropathy, and neuropathy. The DPP showed that patients with impaired glucose tolerance can significantly delay the onset of type 2 diabetes with lifestyle management. The importance of a team approach is reflected in the American Diabetes Association (ADA) Education Recognition for institutions; it requires an instructional team that includes at least an RD and a registered nurse who have continuing education and experience in both diabetes and behavioral teaching/counseling skills.[14] This model of care is perhaps most pertinent to the treatment of patients with obesity since approximately 80% of patients with type 2 diabetes are also obese. A series of articles recommending a multidisciplinary approach to obesity care was previously published as a supplement to the *Journal of the American Dietetic Association*.[15]

DEVELOPING A NEW CHRONIC CARE MODEL

Effective management of patients with chronic illnesses requires a team-based approach in which a division of labor allows nonphysician personnel to take a greater responsibility in patient care.[16] According to Bodenheimer et al., "the chronic model envisions an informed, activated patient interacting with a prepared, proactive practice team, resulting in high-quality, satisfying encounters and improved outcomes." Since a substantial component of the treatment for chronic diseases includes dietary counseling, RDs would function in a complementary role, that is, one in which the physician often has neither the skills nor the time to do well, such as counseling on diet and behavior change.[2] Physicians do not have the training, time, or confidence to provide optimal nutrition care.[17] This "MD-RD" partnership is fundamental to successful implementation of a new chronic care paradigm. A recent article addressing this collaboration described several MD-RD healthcare models in which professionals either work "hand-in-hand," the MD employs or retains an RD for referrals, or the MD serves as medical director with an RD to design and implement nutrition management programs[18] (Figure 6-1).

The Wellness Institute of Northwestern Memorial Hospital in Chicago provides an example of the third MD-RD healthcare model. The Wellness Institute is an innovative team-based lifestyle medicine program where physicians, dietitians, health psychologists, and exercise specialists work side-by-side to provide care for patients with chronic illness. In this academic center, outpatient consultative program, patients with chronic disease conditions such as obesity, diabetes, hypertension, heart disease, and cancer are provided with interventions that emphasize the skills and strategies to enhance self-management. Patients are typically referred by their primary care physician for services and programs that include nutrition and physical activity counseling, behavioral and psychological care, or specialized medical/surgical management of obesity. Collaborative integration also exists with specialty hospital programs such as cardiovascular surgery and solid organ transplantation. The team utilizes clinical policies, protocols, and standards of care based on evidence-based

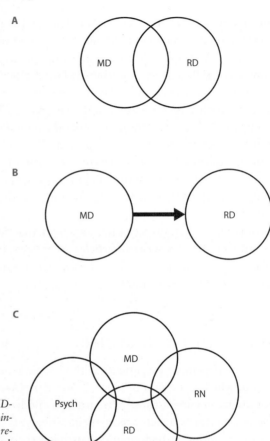

FIGURE 6-1 *Three models of an MD-RD partnership.* **A.** *Upper panel, hand-in-hand.* **B.** *Middle panel, MD employs or retains an RD for referrals.* **C.** *Lower panel, MD serves as medical director of a health-care team.*

medicine and best practices.[19] Weekly case-based discussions, monthly research updates, a journal club, and administrative meetings ensure that all team members regularly communicate with each other and function as a coordinated unit. Integration with the medical center is maintained by offering clinical rotations to residents, medical students, and dietetics interns; sending consultative letters to referring physicians; and participating in collaborative clinical research.

RDs will become equal players on the healthcare team in the care of patients with chronic illness. The challenge will not be in defining their unique role but rather in redesigning the healthcare system that will support a team-based process of care. Two initiatives, Put Prevention Into Practice (PPIP), a national campaign of the Agency for Health Care Policy and Research (AHCPR), and Improving Chronic Illness Care (ICIC), a national program of The Robert Wood Johnson Foundation, are designed to facilitate the transition from delivering acute care to providing chronic care.[20,21] The essential elements for improving the care of people with chronic illness include

Issues to Ponder

- How will the MD role in disease management evolve and how will this impact the RD and other team members?
- What changes in the healthcare system need to occur to support a team-based process of care?

the need for assisting with self-management, decision support based on guidelines, development of clinical information systems, using well-designed delivery systems that meet the needs of patients, adapting a unified organizational philosophy of healthcare, and involvement of community resources. These programs are excellent resources for redesigning the healthcare system. It is important for thought leaders and policy makers in the medical and dietetics profession to promulgate this new paradigm. One way is by example, as we have demonstrated in the integrated, team-based Wellness Institute at Northwestern Memorial Hospital.

A Nurse's Perspective
Cecelia Echevarria

Interactions among healthcare professionals, which had been historically author-itarian and dominated by physicians, were altered in the 1980s with the intro-duction of primary nursing and the nursing process.[22,23] As financial issues and evidence-based practice affected service delivery, the concept of total patient care in the 1990s shifted the emphasis to interdisciplinary teamwork, which became the central focus for specialist service delivery.[24] Medicine, nursing, and dietetics pro-fessionals are required to provide integrated care in an interprofessional context that supports specialization and avoids duplication.[25] Hospitals remain the single largest employer for dietetics professionals, and "a place at the table" is ensured for dietitians by standards and regulations of the Joint Commission on Accreditation of Healthcare Organizations and the Centers for Medicare and Medicaid Services.[26] The trend in healthcare to value clinicians for what they do in performing procedures and treatments versus what they know in advising on content is of some concern to dietetics professionals, who are more familiar with dietetics as being advisory.[27]

COLLABORATION AND PROFESSIONAL IDENTITY

A critical aspect of professional competence is managing to get results collabora-tively.[28] Collaboration becomes even more essential as the complexity of patient care increases.[29] An effectively functioning team integrates complementary competence and skills to achieve identified goals and outcomes.[30] Success requires a high level of negotiation and cooperation between team members.[29] A concern of all disciplines that contributes to poor collaboration is encroachment, the gradual assumption of elements of practice of one profession into areas of traditional service of another profession.[31] Individuals can sabotage interprofessional interactions if they are pro-tecting personal reputations.[32]

Collaborative interactions in general are little researched.[33] Studies on teamwork and team building in healthcare rarely mention perceptions, hierarchy, and conflicts that develop among different personalities and professions. One hypothesis states that allegiance to the team and acknowledgment of conflict may impinge on one's role on the team.[34] It may also be threatening when professional issues or personal identity are at stake, particularly in confronting those higher up the hierarchical ladder. Such con-frontations are often dealt with by avoidance tactics designed to maintain the status quo and minimize the potential threat of change.[35] All groups are not teams, and too many teams are simply groups.[30] Current concepts of teams and teamwork must move beyond the rhetoric of cooperation and toward a more authentic depiction of skills and strategies required to function in the competitive setting of the healthcare team.[28] Many reports indicate how to set up teams and manage them, although research ex-plaining how interdisciplinary team members manage their concerns and work to-gether in everyday practice is minimal.[36]

Anecdotes in a study using the critical incident technique describing interactions among dietitians with nurses reveal much about the practice of clinical dietitians.[37] Dietitians associated positive incidents with patient, family, physician, and nurse interactions as well as the impact of dietetics intervention on quality of life and health. The negative incidents were linked to role conflicts, complaints, and lack of communication. Dietitians were noted to associate twice as many negative incidents with nurses as positive.

Sample anecdotes reported in this 2002 study were:

- The surgeon installed a feeding tube following the dietitian's recommendation, although the nurses did not agree.
- A dietitian read that a cardiologist had written in the patient's medical file: "To receive, from the nurse, instructions for a liquid diet."
- . . . After a few weeks, the patient was feeling better and a nurse said that she would never interfere with a dietitian's recommendations again.
- A training session for diabetic educators was limited to nurses.
- Although nurses disagreed with the dietitian's intervention, her contribution to the patient's well-being was acknowledged.
- A nurse interrupted a dietitian while she was providing clinical services to inform her that the food was not appetizing and that the patient preferred fast-food meals.
- A nurse told the physician that the dietitian was fussy and that her request to have the patient weighed and measured was not important.
- Nurses receiving a course from a dietitian complained because they wanted to learn how to take charge of the nutrition plans of patients with diabetes.

Communication profoundly affects teamwork. A study of the perceptions of nurses regarding collaboration and quality of care identified an association with three communication styles: dominant, contentious, and attentive.[38] A "dominant style" communicates by speaking frequently, strongly, in a dominating and take-charge manner. A "contentious style" communicates in an argumentative, quick-to-challenge manner in which one insists upon very precise definitions, asks for documentation of what the other is arguing, and has a hard time stopping the conversation. An "attentive style" communicates in a very careful and empathetic manner, deliberately showing that one is listening and is always able to repeat back to others what was said. Promoting an attentive style and avoiding contentious and dominant styles does not necessitate teaching new skills. Introspection and reflection allows practitioners to see where their styles may interfere with collaboration and reinforce the value of communication styles that promote collaborative behaviors.

Dialogue is the key to success, as it facilitates discussion of the team philosophy, values, and a shared approach to quality.[39] Value systems and professional identity affect teamwork, and successful teamwork revolves around a common worldview.[40] Values are usually viewed to be the norm, conservative, and often unspoken, or as aspirational, sought after, and often written in mission statements.[41] Values attributed to nurses include individualism, caring, autonomy, holism, and patient well-being, while social workers internalize collectivity, liberty, equality, and justice.[39] A physician's professional identity is shaped by personal beliefs, cultural values, gender, professional expectations, and societal influences. Dietitians also possess a professional identity that can alter the course of their interactions with others through the discourse associated with being "the nutrition expert" (Gingras J, Dietitians' experience of their education: the identity and socialization of "nutrition experts." Unpublished doctoral dissertation, University of British Columbia, 2005). Although an explicit set of values is a key feature of a profession, it is often an incomplete indication of how members of a profession actually carry out their day-to-day work.[39]

Research on dietetics professional socialization indicates a dominant reliance on technical rationale and scientific processes that consider theoretical knowledge as objective and value-free.[42] Technical thinking is required at lower levels of practice and often stressed by academic programs. Technical rationale contradicts a more empowering professionalism of reflective practitioners and inhibits moral action. Aptitudes identified as essential to communications and business are conceptual skills, and these integrative thinking skills are important at higher levels of practice.[43] Human and conceptual skills are also more highly compensated in the marketplace.[44] A standardized and validated scoring instrument administered to clinical dietitians reflected a dichotomy of two dominant modes of thinking and behavior, self-actualized and dependent. The "self-actualized" style identified persons who believe in their ability, strive to continue self-growth, and show independence. The "dependent" style identified characteristics of persons with self-doubt, who tend to be submissive and influenced by others. The data documented an emergence of self-actualized leaders but indicated the existence of many dietitians who seek security rather than satisfaction with people or tasks. Only when dietetics professionals are cognizant of their professional self-concept can they set goals to strengthen positive traits and minimize limiting attributes.[45]

Attitudes are not fixed but develop and evolve amid reflections and interactions in environments that are neutral yet dynamic.[46] New ways of thinking are important, as one health professional can no longer meet all client needs.[47] Many writers have concluded that separate disciplinary education does not foster interprofessional practice.[48] Separatism denies students the opportunity to develop the collaborative relationships essential for cross-fertilization between disciplines, yet few health professionals are taught teamwork skills.[36,49] Problems associated with disciplinary diversity fade once the team focuses on patient outcomes.[39] What is important is what teams do, how they do it, whether it improves patient outcomes, and whether it benefits the organization and the service funder.[48] Fundamental to the team approach to healthcare is that each team member have a clear understanding of the role of the other members.[29]

NUTRITION, NURSING, AND THE DIETETICS PROFESSIONAL

It is the position of the American Dietetic Association that nutrition education is an essential curricular component for the majority of healthcare professionals. Curricula should include nutrition principles and identification of nutrition risk factors to ensure appropriate and timely referral to a qualified dietetics professional for comprehensive nutrition services.[50] Topics included in general nutrition courses—such as food fads, processing, additives, nutrition history, economics, or world problems—are not relevant for preparing acute-care practitioners.[51] Topics considered important for application in acute-care settings are quite basic: nutrient digestion and metabolism, nutrition throughout the life cycle, and nutrition disorders of various body systems. Nutrition education is included in all nursing curricula as the RN National Council Licensing Examination, which includes a nutrition component and is taken for the registered nurse credential.[52] A survey of baccalaureate nursing programs revealed that 71% of the nutrition faculty were RDs.[53]

Nursing care is allocated depending on the education, licensure, and credentialing of student nurses, certified nursing assistants, licensed practical nurses, diploma, nurse associates-degree and baccalaureate-prepared registered nurses, master's level clinical nurse specialists, registered nurse practitioners, certified registered nurse anesthetists, certified nurse midwives, and doctors of nursing science and practice. An increased level of nursing education has been determined to be significant for greater perception of multidisciplinary collaboration.[54] The nurse is a valuable conduit for the dietitian for both the patient and the healthcare team. The primary responsibility of entry-level nurses is direct patient care, which is mirrored in frequently performed functions including patient assessment, preparing patients for procedures, monitoring patients' conditions or reactions, administering medications and treatments, and assisting with the provision of nourishment to patients. Two of the most frequent nutrition nursing functions, recording fluid intake and output and monitoring hydration status, reinforce an important topic in nursing curriculum: fluids, electrolytes, and acid-base balance. Other frequently performed nutrition nursing functions involve patients receiving nothing by mouth, enteral and parenteral nutrition, and postsurgical diet progression.[51] Nutrition issues are common topics in the nursing literature.[55–58] Nurses play an important role in the provision of general dietary advice. Referral to a dietitian most often occurs when nutrition needs are complex or the patient is anxious about a dietary prescription.[31]

The traditional clinical role of the dietetics professional is screening for nutrition risk, assessment of nutrition status, implementation and evaluation of nutrition care plans, and nutrition education. There are indications that expectations are higher for the dietetics professional's participation on the healthcare team than is currently accepted. The traditional role was found to meet expectations and perceptions of hospital administrators and directors of medicine and nursing, yet these activities were negatively associated with the level of education, professional development, and research capabilities of dietitians.[59] A survey conducted among maternity-care nurses to gather data on the state of breast-feeding in Utah hospitals indicated that of dietitians, physicians, and nurses, those perceived by nurses to be the least likely to provide breast-feeding assistance and information were dietitians.[60] Medical directors, dietitians, and nurses from New York State end-stage renal disease facilities were surveyed regarding opinions of legal responsibility in a dietitian providing a lethal amount of dietary potassium for an anephric patient. Nurses saw the dietitian as being legally accountable, as consistent with the standard-of-care expectations of prudent healthcare professionals defined by professional malpractice jurisprudence.[61] A narrower scope of practice and responsibility for greater numbers of patients than comprised by the work of other team members has limited the dietetics professional's participation on the healthcare team.[62] Dietitians are often viewed as consultants to the team rather than as active team members.[63,64]

Within the dietetics profession itself, performance, proficiency, and value of the dietetics professional is a controversial issue.[27] Focus groups were conducted as predictors of dietitians' roles on healthcare teams. These dietitians reported limited respect from other healthcare professionals and lower salaries, which were attributed to lack of appreciation for dietitians' knowledge and education. The strong emphasis placed on the dietitian's knowledge and how to convey that knowledge to team members—rather than collaboration with team members to determine the best course of treatment—was determined to be problematic for dietetics professionals. New tasks suggested for dietitians—such as taking blood pressures, drawing blood, or inserting feeding tubes—were reported to be both surprising and disturbing by the focus group dietitians and revealed that they may not wish to assume nontraditional roles.[65] The present acute-care environment is not anticipated to support the need for dietitians without new skills.[27]

EXPANDING THE ROLE OF THE DIETETICS PROFESSIONAL IN NUTRITION CARE

Strategic partnerships and networking must be utilized to identify and share best practices of dietetics professionals. Recommendations to upskill and cross-train have been plagued by professional liability and malpractice coverage issues as well as state licensure affecting the boundaries of practice.[26] Poorly defined advanced-practice skills hinder recognition and compensation efforts for dietetics professionals. Conversely, the nursing profession offers specialized and advanced practice through clearly structured pathways that support professional development and career advancement. Current career pathways in nursing are products of years of evolution, negotiation, opportunity, and litigation. Dietetics is rapidly moving toward an intervention-oriented, outcome-focused discipline. Specialty practice credentials are available to dietitians in nutrition support; diabetes education and management; weight management for adults, children, or adolescents; and pediatric and renal specialties. Dietetics professionals need to identify skills of value to patients and healthcare organizations and become proficient in performing these skills.[27] Recommendations for dietetics professionals to create an environment for respect and appreciation through the manner in which they practice include[66]:

- Understand the view from the other side: Discern areas of mutual agreement and begin there.
- Establish credibility through evidence-based practice.
- Be there: Adjust work schedule to allow attendance at unit rounds and be present when team members are present.
- Build relationships: Establish connections and take advantage of meetings and conversations to generate dialogue or collaboration.
- Meet team needs: Organize communications and documentation to focus on need-to-know information.
- Take the initiative: Contact team members to ensure recommendations are received and discuss plans.
- Seek to expand your role.
- Be courteous: Discuss concerns directly with team members.
- Do not burn bridges: Always leave the door open to future collaboration.
- Appreciate incremental success: Build on small accomplishments for long-term success.

To improve the RD-RN team as well as provide the best nutrition care, the dietetics professional should nurture collaboration with nurses at the bedside. The student nurse or certified nursing assistant responsible for feeding the patient on calorie count may not be mindful of nutrient density, the licensed practical nurse may not accurately thicken for honey consistency in the patient at risk for aspiration, and the novice registered nurse may not remember that medications are administered via the gastric port of a percutanous gastrostomy– jejunostomy tube. Understanding the need for an accurate weight for nutrition assessment on a cachectic patient may not be the priority for a nurse with another patient experiencing chest pain.

Issues to Ponder

- What suggestions do you have to improve the RN–RD team?
- How should education change to foster interprofessional practice?

The current nursing shortage affects the nutrition care of patients throughout the healthcare system and dietetics professionals are encouraged to support legislation to improve nursing staffing ratios.[67] A negative impact on nutrition care of the most vulnerable populations is now evident. In July 2000, a federal report addressed the fact that understaffing contributes to increased incidence of severe bed sores, malnutrition, and abnormal weight loss among nursing home residents.[68] Nurse-to-patient ratios were determined to be associated with frequency of bloodstream infections of hospitalized patients receiving total parenteral nutrition.[69] Many team members work in conjunction with nurses providing bedside care: speech pathologists perform swallow evaluations, occupational therapists treat and dress burn wounds, and respiratory therapists administer treatments and maintain endotracheal and tracheostomy tubes. Could, should, or would the dietetics professional participate in nutrition care to weigh and feed patients, maintain patent enteral feeding tubes, or assist in wound care to monitor healing?

Many areas of complementary competence and skills exist between nutrition nursing functions and the role of the dietetics professional. These shared components of nutrition care offer opportunities to improve collaboration as well as potential to expand the role of the dietetics professional. Enhancement of pertinent knowledge and skills in clinical practice and group process is important to the performance, proficiency, and value of the dietetics professional to enable effective and equal partnership as a member and a leader on the healthcare team.

SECTION 3   A Dietitian's Perspective

Jane V. White

Opportunities to become equal players on the healthcare team are available to dietetics professionals as never before. The global call for provision of clinical nutrition services to the public in numerous clinical guidelines published by preventive and therapeutic committees and task forces is unprecedented.[70–78] Widespread recognition of obesity as a preventable risk factor with morbidity, mortality, and costs approaching a health impact of the magnitude of cigarette smoking positions our profession to become global players in assuring the health and well-being of Americans and the people of the world.[79–82] Q7 Recognition that small changes in lifestyle can yield big health benefits continues to accrue.[83]

Although the American public consistently cites the media as its primary source of general nutrition information, the 2002 American Dietetic Association (ADA) Nutrition Trends Survey[84] found that 90% of Americans surveyed were aware of RDs and viewed them as credible sources of nutrition information.

The Institute of Medicine (IOM) published guidelines related to the provision of high quality healthcare[1] and health professions education.[85] These reports encourage providers to significantly increase their focus on prevention of disease and disability and maintenance of functional status throughout life.[1] This calls for all healthcare professionals to deliver patient-centered care as members of interdisciplinary teams that rely on evidence-based practice, continuous quality improvement, and informatics.[85] It encourages physicians to develop expertise in working in a collaborative fashion, which necessitates shared decision making regarding patient care.

Thus, the dietetics profession is in a better position than at any time previously regarding equal status on healthcare teams. Whether the individual dietitian/dietetics technician capitalizes on the opportunities available in his or her practice environment and how "equality," and thus "success," is defined by dietetics professionals is less evident.

VALUES AND PROCESSES NECESSARY TO TEAM FORMATION AND MAINTENANCE

Team building and teamwork are complex processes that require continual reevaluation and modification in order to succeed. For the most part, the quality of care provided is a function of the effectiveness of communication among team members.[86] Essential elements of team building include the development of a culture that fosters trust, healthy conflict resolution, commitment, accountability, and a focus on outcomes.[87] These elements must be in place if team members are to feel comfortable in communicating frustrations, talking out differences, and benefiting from lessons learned from past mistakes. When these elements are present, team members can more easily offer and accept apologies, give or receive feedback, admit knowledge or skills deficits, and accept help. The ability to thoroughly and frankly discuss problems and reach mutual decisions regarding their resolution allows team members to act in unison and to accept responsibility for care plans implemented. Identifying and sharing outcomes and revising the approach used based on routinely identified best practices can improve patient care and job satisfaction.[87] As the U.S. population becomes more diverse and increased numbers of care delivery systems move to the virtual realm, development of the fundamental elements required for team-building assume increased importance. Dietetics practitioners must develop the cultural sensitivity and communications technology skills to enable them to prosper in the 21st century.

Barriers to team cohesion and effective functioning include petty jealousies, ignorance, and perceived losses of autonomy or threats to professional status.[88] Individuals new to professional practice or those that are firmly entrenched in scope of practice distinctions tend to simplify and distort other professions' roles and motivations, particularly when team communications are tense.[89]

DIETETICS PROFESSIONALS' PERCEPTIONS REGARDING TEAM STATUS

Dahlke and colleagues[65] reported that dietitians in interdisciplinary team settings had the lowest sense of personal accomplishment and greatest sense of depersonalization of the health professionals assessed (physicians, nurses, social workers, and dietitians). They suggested that dietitians' self-perception of their professional role and value may need to be addressed. Most dietitians appear to view their primary role on interdisciplinary teams as the provision of optimal nutrition education and treatment to the patient. Yet many seem to fail to recognize their larger and more significant role in the determination of the best course of treatment for the patient, irrespective of the degree to which medical nutrition therapy is employed.

When clinical dietitians were asked about assuming additional or alternative functions in interdisciplinary settings, they tended to believe that there would be resistance from other team members or voiced discomfort in the performance of tasks outside the traditional realm of dietetics practice.[65] Dietitians voiced similar concerns in focus groups regarding ADA's Physician Nutrition Education Project[90] relative to their willingness to educate physicians in the course of daily practice. The physicians' focus group response to a similar query was to express delight that dietitians would be willing to assume this role. Held back by such misperceptions and the tendency to resist movement into unfamiliar or uncomfortable practice settings, dietitians tend to serve as "consultants" to healthcare teams versus active members. They do not attain the level of respect that more active and innovative team participants enjoy, and they receive lower salaries.[65]

Fuhrman[91] identified similar issues in her survey of members of the dietitians in the ADA Nutrition Support (DNS) Dietetic Practice Group. She emphasized the necessity for dietetics professionals to maintain competence and skills in one's chosen area of practice. She gave equal importance, however, to the need for DNS members to understand how nutrition fits into the larger healthcare plan for each patient and to be prepared to expand professional alliances to optimize nutrition services delivery. She encouraged members to share information and expertise with other professionals directly, to be confident in making recommendations, and to be open to new learning opportunities and practice paradigms.

Dietetics professionals must be prepared to justify nutrition recommendations to members of the healthcare team with evidence-based guidelines and peer-reviewed literature.[10,91] Rather than viewing the need to provide documentation for recommendations as an insult or taking a refusal to accept a recommendation personally, dietetics professionals should view such instances as sincere requests by professionals of other disciplines to understand the "science" behind a nutrition-care approach. Such requests, regardless of how they are stated, offer an opportunity to provide peer education and mentoring. They also offer dietetics professionals the opportunity to ask why a particular nonnutrition intervention was provided and to learn more about the provision of nonnutrition aspects of healthcare. Direct, collegial communication with physicians and other team members offers the opportunity to demonstrate a willingness to acquire knowledge and skills beyond dietetics traditional scope of practice and to become a more fully engaged participant in the healthcare team's treatment decisions.

The 2002 published dietetics practice audit[92] states that multidisciplinary-care teams appear to have become the modus operandi in institutional settings. It further states that employers value team members who demonstrate flexibility in patient care and who pitch in to do whatever tasks needs to be accomplished. Those who are most valued are those with more global views of healthcare and more competencies. Institutions are increasingly configuring teams using fewer members, using team members more synergistically, and diverting care provision to lower-cost practitioners.

CONCLUSIONS AND RECOMMENDATIONS

Dietetics professionals want the demand for dietetics services to increase.[26] Yet they frequently fail to recognize and capitalize upon the very real opportunities that our daily participation in the healthcare team process provides. Many of them tend to equate recognition and status with the unquestioned acceptance of dietetics recommendations as infallible and resent being asked to document their perspective and provide their evidence base.[10,91,93] Dietetics professionals want equality in the healthcare team environment but are often reluctant to commit to the development of skills and performance of tasks beyond the more traditional realms of nutrition screening, assessment, and intervention.

Issues to Ponder

- How will the focus on prevention of disease impact the role of the dietitian as a team member?
- What traits contribute to and deter team development?
- How can the dietitian shift from being viewed as a "consultant" to the healthcare team to being an active member?

As a group, clinical dietetics professionals tend to be detail oriented and territorial; they often have difficulty in determining the roles of dietitians and dietetics technicians in the delivery of nutrition care in addition to that of other nonnutrition professionals.[92] The focus is usually narrowly directed toward nutrition concerns, and dietitians often feel slighted, although insult is usually unintended, when the rest of the team pursues a more global approach with nutrition considerations viewed as important but perhaps not the number-one issue to be pursued. Dietetics professionals want higher salaries, but as individuals they tend to be reluctant to build an outcomes portfolio and enter into negotiations to improve their personal compensation rate (personal communication with ADA members on electronic forums, 1999–2003).

A number of dietetics professionals have attained equality and key leadership in the healthcare team environment. If all are to become full and equal partners in the healthcare team environment, dietetics practitioners must do the following:

- Attain comfort with defined and potential roles and responsibilities of dietitians and dietetics technicians; work in partnership with other team members.
- Develop expertise in the principles of healthcare team formation, building, and maintenance.
- Demonstrate competence and confidence in the recommendations made regarding a patient's nutrition care but be open to objective discussion of alternatives.
- Demonstrate interest and contribute fully to the global plan of care while serving as the nutrition ombudsman on the healthcare team.
- Diversify knowledge and skills sets as team needs indicate; do not hesitate to volunteer to develop unique expertise in needed areas others may be reluctant to pursue (communications technology, cultural sensitivity, alternative/complimentary care, drug-nutrient interactions, health risk appraisal, motivational counseling, case management, physical fitness, etc.).
- Document outcomes and provide evidence of the effectiveness and cost-efficiency of medical nutrition therapy.
- Track team participation and document contribution of dietetics input to seamless team functioning and improved quality of care.
- Leverage patient outcomes and administrative data in salary negotiations.

Highly functional healthcare teams require time to establish cohesion and shared values. Every dietetics professional has the opportunity to become an equal if not superior member of his or her healthcare team as the team-building process proceeds. To accomplish this goal, dietetics practitioners must become active participants in the process and be prepared to demonstrate cost-effectiveness, efficiency, a willing spirit, and the ability to provide optimal and relevant patient care.

Dietetics professionals often question whether they are considered by administrators to be valued members of the healthcare team. To persuade administrators—those in the organization who can make decisions and remove barriers—that dietetics professionals have a unique and valuable contribution to make, the story must be told regularly in a convincing and credible manner. Personal and team skills discussed in this section can be learned and improved with training. Personal development, with or without a mentor, depends on knowing one's particular strengths and weaknesses, knowing the needs and values of the organization, and developing skills sets to match those needs.

The apparent value of the clinical dietitian on a team is as the technical expert on nutrition care of patients. The administrator's perceived value of this contribution is limited. The greater value of nutrition care to the business of healthcare is demonstrated through more efficient use of resources, creating new business, growing existing business, or demonstrating improved outcomes. Even though the clinical nutrition budget may be a small percentage of the total hospital budget, it is not insignificant from an administrator's perspective. Everyone in an organization is a potential player, but the magnitude of an individual's success depends on effective team skills, leadership development, and business acumen.

EFFECTIVE TEAM SKILLS

It is all too common, in hospitals, that policies affecting the delivery of nutrition care to patients are implemented without including input from dietetics professionals. This may create barriers to the provision of medical nutrition therapy. Altering a policy after the fact is often a difficult and uphill battle. It would have been so much eas-

Jane's Story, Part 1

Jane has been a clinical dietitian at General Hospital for 8 years. She is an excellent clinician and valued team member on her assigned patient care units. Jane is passionate about facilitating behavior change to improve the health and well-being of her patients. She is a certified diabetes educator and serves as a resource for the healthcare team. She has conducted a limited study to demonstrate improved patient outcomes through improved management of her patients' diabetes. She presented her findings at a recent meeting within the hospital. The chief financial officer and chief nursing officer were impressed with Jane's business approach and presentation. They have asked her to facilitate a team's process of exploring the feasibility of establishing an American Diabetes Association (ADA)-certified diabetes program. How did Jane gain this level of confidence and trust to facilitate such an important team?

ier to be invited to the table at the beginning of the process. The RD is frequently overlooked when teams are developed. Nurses and physicians are the first to be invited as team members, leaders, and facilitators. Dietitians are often not seen for the unique and valuable perspective they can offer. Only an RD can effectively tell the clinical nutrition story and strategically position the role of medical nutrition therapy in patient care.

The work of an organization is accomplished through teams. For individuals to reach their potential or accomplish their goals, they must participate in teams that make critical decisions.[93] A team is a group of people who are passionate about a cause and who come together to work toward a mutually shared purpose. They are motivated to work together because of their shared vision. Individuals begin to learn team skills by participating on teams within their immediate sphere of influence (e.g., clinical nutrition teams or interdisciplinary teams on patient care units). A myopic focus on one team member's goal alone can prevent overall improvement. Seeking opportunities to interact with the multidisciplinary team will broaden the group's perspective and allow clinical nutrition to be accepted as an integral part of decisions and protocols.

Other disciplines frequently tell their story in an effort to maintain or increase their numbers within the organization. Clinical dietitians have not been as effective in getting their message across. Looking at the multitude of books, articles, and websites on communication, it is not hard to come to the conclusion that effective communication skills are among the most important personal skills that determine success or failure. The Commission on Dietetic Registration identified verbal and written communication skills as two of the top three professional skill-learning needs of the RD.[94] Acquiring and maintaining effective communication skill requires lifelong learning. In today's age of technology, communication continuously assumes new faces and dimensions. It is as crucial to use effective skills in written and electronic communications as in face-to-face communication.

First and foremost, an excellent communicator is a good listener. Identify the audience and listen carefully and critically to learn what the administrator or organization wants and needs. To be effective requires knowing the audience and matching communication to their needs and values.[95-97] Listening also makes it possible to identify the perceptions and biases of the audience, so that the message can be appropriately modified.

Good communication is clear, concise, and specific. It is helpful to identify three or four key messages and then stay focused by developing those points. The use of stories, analogies, metaphors, and "compare and contrast" creates a visual image for the listener and makes the presentation more powerful.[96] The message should be positioned in a positive perspective whenever possible. People with a positive outlook attract a greater following than those who have a multitude of reasons why something will not work. One needs to develop one's own communication style while remaining flexible and versatile to adapt to different situations.

Credibility is critical to effective communication. Evidence-based studies offer the real outcomes information that is critical in making healthcare decisions. Be sure that the message is supported by data. Know the source of the data. It is better to offer to get back with an answer rather than to risk providing less than accurate information.

Jane's Story, Part 2

As a new dietitian, Jane was thrilled that physicians asked for her input in the care of their patients. She was careful to use evidence-based data for medical nutrition therapy and in recommendations to the physicians. She noticed that a new clinical initiative for her organization was to improve care of patients with decubitus ulcers. Jane had recently attended a seminar where a team approach had been presented. She knew that nutrition was an essential component of the care process. She approached the nurse who had been designated to lead the project. Because the nurse had observed Jane's effectiveness in working with physicians and other health team members, she asked Jane to join the team in developing protocols for patient care. Jane has an opportunity to prove her value as an RD but, more importantly, through her efforts, nutrition will be included as part of the total approach to patient care.

Seek the support of others in the organization to tell your story frequently. The food and nutrition department should have a common message. Tell the story with enough data so that those in leadership positions in the department can promote clinical nutrition and dietetics professionals to those higher in the organization. Network with peer leaders within and outside of dietetics practice. One of those individuals may become a mentor.

Being invited to participate on the team is only the first step to demonstrating value and guaranteeing success. Being effective on that team is dependent on additional skills. Spend time preparing for the topic of discussion. One of the biggest time-wasters for a team is lack of preparation by team members. Talk with dietetics peers to obtain their perspectives within the area of practice. Review the literature to have the most current research at hand. Doing homework creates confidence to speak up and contribute to discussion at meetings. Challenge the status quo when it is appropriate.

Listening carefully and critically enables individuals to understand others on the team, particularly those with differing views. Diversity of views can result in more thorough discussion, unique solutions, and more effective outcomes. Everyone on the team should have the opportunity to express his or her views. Observe those on the team whose excellent communication and team skills help bring the team to consensus. Consensus-building skills are critical in effective team work.[97]

Invest time and energy in the team. Participate every time the team meets. Trust and loyalty are essential to building consensus and implementing the plan. When the group makes a decision, every team member should support the decision. Following through with assignments after the meeting is as important as planning prior to meetings. Deliver what is promised for the team.

SELF-ASSESSMENT

Individuals can develop personal and team skills through practice as well as through formal training. Self-awareness opens the doors to personal growth.[95–97] Spend time developing strengths.[98] No one person is strong in every area. Individuals have a greater capacity to grow by building on strengths first. It takes more time and energy to develop skills in areas of weakness.

Self-reflection can be a good starting place for identifying strengths and levels of effectiveness. Self-assessments, however, often do not reflect the views of others. Frank conversation with a trusted leader within the organization can be helpful. This can be an immediate supervisor, a mentor, or other peer leaders. Both formal and informal assessments have value. Informal, frequent feedback from colleagues may be less threatening than formal assessment and can take place more often. Formal assessment includes such tools as periodic performance reviews, personality inventories, or 360-degree feedback.

A 360-degree feedback tool gathers information about performance and effectiveness from multiple people—peers, subordinates, supervisors, customers, and oneself.[99–101] This type of evaluation is more reliable and objective than an evaluation from a single source. No one person generally sees every aspect of an individual's job performance. Input from multiple sources allows each rater to evaluate those dimensions of performance of which he or she has knowledge. For example, a supervisor and a customer assign ratings on the basis of their very different expectations of competence. This type of survey more accurately reflects the differences in the way individuals normally relate to different types of people. Although individuals may select the participants in their 360-degree survey, the responses are anonymous, making the results less biased or skewed. A 360-degree survey can be especially helpful in identifying opportunities for personal development.

Numerous tools are available that attempt to describe our natural tendencies to act and react to people and situations. Two commonly used tools are the Myers-Briggs Type Indicator and the Johari Window. The premise for these types of assessments is that people are different from each other and that the more individuals understand about themselves and others, the more effective the relationships. The Johari Window is a tool that identifies an individual's preferred method for giving and receiving feedback.[102,103] Communication provides information on how behaviors affect others' feelings and perceptions. The assessment provides a window through which one can give information about oneself to others and receive information about oneself from them.

The Myers-Briggs identifies and describes natural behavioral preferences.[104,105] There is a natural preference for using the right hand or the left hand. Using the preferred hand occurs naturally, as a matter of habit. Individuals can learn to write with the other hand, but it would not feel as natural or effective. In the same way, individuals have natural behavior preferences. Understanding preferences gives insight into an individual's reactions to other people and situations.

Self-knowledge is the first step to self-development. Better understanding allows greater opportunity to adapt one's style to be more effective. Reassessment should be ongoing to ensure that development efforts are having the intended outcome. Individuals encounter many different personalities as they become more involved in the organization. Learning to adapt to different styles enhances value.

WHAT IS THE VALUE OF THE DIETETICS PROFESSIONAL?

Do administrators value the dietetics professional as an equal player on the team? The answer depends on you. Developing effective communication and team skills are the core competencies required for multidisciplinary team participation. Individuals gain trust and respect as they demonstrate leadership capabilities across the organization.

Issues to Ponder

- With healthcare being a big business, what value can nutrition bring to the business of healthcare?
- What can dietitians do to become more involved in the decision/policy making in their institutions?
- Why is the team such an important concept in healthcare?
- What methods are available to understand one's strengths and weaknesses and set a self-development plan?

Methods to increase management and leadership skills include using professional networks outside the organization, networking with peers in professional organizations to foster sharing of resources, benchmarking to strengthen practice, and communicating that information with superiors so that they see professional growth.

Development of business acumen enables clinical dietitians to speak the language of administrators. Learn how to read financial reports and, more importantly, what drives the numbers. Use technology effectively. Measure and document outcomes to demonstrate the value of practice. Be familiar with regulatory requirements and how they impact dietetics practice. Get involved in the legislative process as it impacts the profession and the organization. Being vital and valued requires lifelong learning.

The 2002 Compensation and Benefits Survey conducted by the American Dietetic Association found a positive correlation with RD compensation and years of experience, level of supervisory responsibility, and budget responsibility.[106,107] These are factors that demonstrate value to those in administration and justify higher compensation. The value that RDs add to the organization through commitment to professional growth and lifelong learning can yield rewards through recognition as the head of a team or task force, a promotion, and/or increased compensation.

REFERENCES

1. Institute of Medicine. Crossing the Quality Chasm: A New Health System for the 21st Century. Washington, DC: National Academy Press, 2001.
2. Wagner EH. The role of patient care teams in chronic disease management. BMJ 2000;320:569–572.
3. Brown RO, Carlson SD, Cowan GSM Jr, Powers DA, Luther RW. Enteral nutritional support management in a university teaching hospital: team vs nonteam. J Parenter Enteral Nutr 1987;11:52–56.
4. Faubion WC, Wesley JR, Khalidi N, Silva J. Total parenteral nutrition catheter sepsis: impact of the team approach. J Parenter Enteral Nutr 1986;10:642–645.
5. Kibbe DC. Disease management: who's caring for your patients? Fam Pract Mgt 1998;5(9). Available at: http://www.aafp.org/fpm/981100fm/disease.html. Accessed September 26, 2005.
6. Shaffer J, Wexler LF. Reducing low-density lipoprotein cholesterol levels in an ambulatory care system. Results of a multidisciplinary collaborative practice lipid clinic compared with traditional physician-based care. Arch Intern Med 1995;155:2330–2335.
7. Messing C, Boucher J, Cypress M, et al. National standards for diabetes self-management education. Diabetes Care 2003;26(Suppl 1):S149–S156.
8. Callahan MB, Bender K, McNeely M. The role of the health care team in the implementation of the National Kidney Foundation–Dialysis Outcomes Quality Initiative: a case study. Adv Renal Replace Ther 1999;6:42–51.
9. Kushner R, Pendarvis L. An integrated approach to obesity care. Nutr Clin Care 1999;2:285–291.
10. Czerwinski BS, Hymann DJ, Jones EV, Scott LW, Jones PH. Physician education in hyperlipidemia management: the impact on collaboration. South Med J 1979;90:685–690.
11. Diabetes and Control Complications Trial Research Group. The effect of intense treatment of diabetes on the development and progression of long-term complications in insulin-dependent diabetes mellitus. N Engl J Med 1993;329:977–986.

12. Diabetes Prevention Program Research Group. Reduction in the incidence of type 2 diabetes with lifestyle intervention or metformin. N Engl J Med 2002;346:393–403.

13. Rubin RR, Peyrot M. Implications of the DCCT. Looking beyond tight control. Diabetes Care 1994;17:235–236.

14. American Diabetes Association (ADA) Education Recognition Program. Available at: http://diabetes.org/for-health-professionals-and scientists/recognition/edrecognition.jsp. Accessed September 26, 2005.

15. Rippe JM. The obesity epidemic: a mandate for a multidisciplinary approach. J Am Diet Assoc 1998;98(suppl 2): S16–S54.

16. Bodenheimer T, Wagner EH, Grumbach K. Improving primary care for patients with chronic illness. JAMA 2002;288:1775–1779.

17. Kushner RF. Barriers to providing nutrition counseling by physicians: a survey of primary care practitioners. Prev Med 1995;24:546–552.

18. Mathews A, Heimburger DC, Myers EF. Collaboratively enhancing nutrition care: RD and physician nutrition specialist. Nutrition & the MD 2004;30:1–4.

19. Gibbs J, Kattapong K, St. John J, Kushner RF. Assessing hospital-based wellness services using an outcome measurement system. Health Prom Pract 2002;2:60–75.

20. 10 Steps: Implementation Guide. Put Prevention into Practice. Adapted from The Clinicians' Handbook of Preventive Services. 2nd Ed. Publication No. 98-0025, 1998. Rockville, MD: Agency for Healthcare Research and Quality, 1998.Available at: http://www.ahrq.gov/ppip/impsteps.htm. Accessed September 26, 2005.

21. Improving chronic illness care. Available at: http://improvingchroniccare.org/. Accessed September 26, 2005.

22. Fagin CM. Collaboration between nurses and physicians: no longer a choice. Acad Med 1992;67(5):295–303.

23. Lyon JC. Models of nursing care delivery and case management: clarification of terms. Nurs Econ 1993;11(3);163–169.

24. Stein LI, Watts DT, Howell T. The doctor-nurse game revisited. N Engl J Med 1990:322;546–549.

25. Leathard A, ed. Going Interprofessional: Working Together for Health and Welfare. London: Routledge, 1994.

26. Summo EO, Schofield M, Cochran N, et al. Performance, proficiency, and value of the dietetics professional. J Am Diet Assoc 2002;102(9);1304–1307.

27. Skipper A. The history and development of advanced practice nursing: lessons for dietetics. J Am Diet Assoc 2004;104(6):1007–1012.

28. Lingard L, Espin S, Evans C, Hawryluck L. The rules of the game: interprofessional collaboration on the intensive care unit team. Crit Care 2004;8(6):R403–408.

29. Baggs JG, Ryan SA, Phelps CE, Richeson JF, Johnson, JE. The association between interdisciplinary collaboration and patient outcomes in a medical intensive care unit. Heart Lung 1992;21:18–24.

30. Kezsbom DS, Schilling DL, Edward KA. Dynamic Project Management: A Practical Guide for Managers and Engineers. New York: Wiley, 1989.

31. White JV, Bielk KM, Rogers ES, Lennon ES. Professional partnerships: key to dietetics practice success. Top Clin Nutr 2003;18(4):22–228.

32. Chapman T, Hugman R, Williams A. Effectiveness of interprofessional relationships: a case illustration of joint working. In: Soothill K, Mackay L, Web C, eds. Interprofessional Relations in Health Care. London: Edward Arnold, 1995.

33. Jones RAP. Multidisciplinary collaboration: conceptual development as a foundation for patient-focused care. Holistic Nurs Pract 1997;11:8–16.

34. Long S. Primary health care team workshop: team members' perspectives. J Adv Nurs 1996;23:935–941.

35. Wall VS, Nolan LL. Perceptions of inequity, satisfaction, and conflict in task oriented groups. Hum Rel 39:1033–1051.

36. Larson EL. New rules for the game: interdisciplinary education for health professionals. Nurs Outlook 1995;43:180–185.

37. Marquis M, Gayraud H. Exploring clinical dietitians'day to day practice through the critical incident technique. J Am Diet Assoc 2002;102:1461–1465.

38. Coeling HVE, Cukr PL. Communication styles that promote perceptions of collaboration, quality, and nurse satisfaction. J Nurs Care Qual 2000;14:63–74.

39. Wilmot S. Professional values and interprofessional dialogue. J Interprofess Care 1995;9:257–266.

40. Waugman WR. Professionalism and socialization in interprofessional collaboration. In: Casto RM, Julia M, eds. Interprofessional Care and Collaborative Practice: Commission on Interprofessional Education and Practice. Pacific Grove, CA: Brooks/Cole, 1994.

41. Pattison S, Roisin P. Values in professional practice: lessons for health, social care and other professionals. Oxford, UK: Radcliffe Medical Press, 2004.
42. Liquori T. Food matters: changing dimensions of science and practice in the nutrition profession. J Nutr Ed Behav 2001;33:234–236.
43. Moore KK. Criteria for acceptance to preprofessional dietetics programs vs desired qualities of professionals: an analysis. J Am Diet Assoc 1995;195:77–81.
44. Rinke J, Finn SC. Winning strategies to excel in dietetics. J. Am Diet. Assoc 1990;90:935–938.
45. Schiller MR, Foltz MB, Campbell SM. Dietitians' self-perceptions: implications for leadership. J Am Diet Assoc 1993;93:868–876.
46. Clark PG. Values in health care professional socialization: implications for geriatric education in interdisciplinary teamwork. Gerontologist 1997:37:441–451.
47. Harbough GL. Assumptions of interprofessional collaboration: interrelatedness and wholeness. In: Casto RM, Julia MC, eds. Interprofessional Care and Collaborative Practice: Commission on Interprofessional Education and Practice. Pacific Grove, CA: Brooks/Cole, 1994.
48. McCallin A. Interdisciplinary practice—a matter of teamwork: an integrated literature review. J Clin Nurs 2001;10:419–428.
49. Hilton RW, Morris DJ, Wright AM. Learning to work in the health care team. J Interprofess Care 1995;9:267–274.
50. Position of the American Dietetic Association: nutrition education for health care professionals. J Am Diet Assoc 1998;98:343–346.
51. Weigley ES. Nutrition in nursing education and beginning practice. J Am Diet Assoc 1994;94:654–655.
52. Matassarin-Jacobs E. The nursing licensure process and the NCLEX-RN. Nurse Ed 1989;14:32–35.
53. Cutler L. Nutrition education in baccalaureate degree nursing schools: 1983 survey results. J Am Diet Assoc 1986;86:933–937.
54. Mansourimoaied M, Boman K, Causle, T. Nurses' perceptions of interdisciplinary collaboration. Nurs Connect 2000;13:21–31.
55. Dudek S. Malnutrition in hospitals: who's assessing what patients eat? Am J Nurs 2000;100:36–43.
56. Kowanko I, Simon, S, Wood, J. Nutritional care of the patient: nurses' knowledge and attitudes in an acute care setting. J Clin Nurs 1999;8:217–224.
57. Cortis JD. Nutrition and the hospitalized patient: implications for nurses. Br J Nurs 1997;6:666–667, 670–674.
58. Perry L. Nutrition: A hard nut to crack. An exploration of the knowledge, attitudes, and activities of qualified nurses in relation to nutritional nursing care. J Clin Nurs 1997;6:315–324.
59. Schwartz NE. A study of the clinical role of the dietitian as viewed by allied health professionals. J Allied Health 1984;13:288–298.
60. Helm A, Windham CT, Wyse B. Dietitians in breastfeeding management: an untapped resource in the hospital. J Hum Lact 1997;13(3):221–225.
61. King D. Interdisciplinary perceptions of the dietitian's legal responsibility for lethal dietary prescription errors for patients with end-stage renal disease. J Am Diet Assoc 1993;93:1269–1273.
62. Schmitt MH, Heineman GD, Farell M. Discipline differences in attitudes toward interdisciplinary teams, perceptions of the process of teamwork, and stress levels in geriatric health care teams. Interdisciplinary Health Care Teams: Proceedings of the Sixteenth Annual Conference, 1994;92–105.
63. Schiller, MR. Role of the clinical dietitian. J Am Diet Assoc 1974;65:284–285.
64. Ryan FS, Folt MB, Finn SC. The role of the clinical dietitian: staffing patterns and job functions. J Am Diet Assoc 1988;88:659–683.
65. Dahlke R, Wolf KN, Wilson SL, Brodnik M. Focus Groups as predictors of dietitians' role on interdisciplinary teams. J Am Diet Assoc 2000;100:455–456.
66. Peregrin R. A place at the table: marketing dietetics professionals' expertise to other health care providers in a clinical setting. J Am Diet Assoc 2004;104;1781–1782.
67. American Dietetic Association. Liberalized diets for older adults in long term care. Available at: http://www.eatright.org/cps/rde/xchg/ada/hs.xsl/advocacy_3772_ENU_HTML.htm. Accessed February 20, 2006.
68. US Senate: Special Committee on Aging. Nursing Home Residents: Short-changed by Staff Shortages, Part II. 106th Congress, July 27, 2000. Available at: http://grassley.senate.gov/index.cfm. Accessed February 20, 2006.
69. Fridkin SK, Pear SM, Williamson TH, Galgianai JN, Jarvis, WR. The role of understaffing in central venous catheter associated bloodstream infections. Infect Control Hosp Epidemiol 1996;17:150–158.
70. US Department of Health and Human Services. Healthy People 2010: Understanding and Improving Health. 2nd Ed. Washington, DC: US Government Printing Office, November 2000. Available at: http://www.healthypeople.gov. Accessed August 11, 2003.

71. US Preventive Services Task Force. Behavioral counseling in primary care to promote a healthy diet. Am J Prev Med 2003; 24:93–100. Available at: http://www.ahcpr.gov/clinic/uspstfix.htm. Accessed August 11, 2003

72. Chobanian AV, Bakris GL, Black HR, et al. Seventh report of the Joint National Committee on Prevention, Detection, Evaluation and Treatment of High Blood Pressure: the JNC 7 report. JAMA 2002; 289:2560–2572. Epub 2003 May 14.

73. American Diabetes Association. Clinical practice recommendations 2003. Diabetes Care 2003;26(suppl 1):S51–S61, S70–S72.

74. Thomas DR, Ashmen W, Morley JE, et al. Nutritional management in long-term care: development of a clinical guideline. J Gerontol Med Sci 2000;55A(12):M725–M734.

75. Nutrition Screening Initiative. Physician's Guide to Nutrition in Chronic Disease Management in Older Adults. Washington, DC: American Academy of Family Physicians and American Dietetic Association, 2002.

76. National Cholesterol Education Program. Third Report of the Expert Panel on Detection, Evaluation and Treatment of High Blood Cholesterol in Adults (Adult Treatment Panel III). Final Report. Bethesda, MD: National Institutes of Health, 2002. Available at: http://www.nhlbi.nih.gov/guidelines/cholesterol/atp3_rpt.htm. Accessed August 11, 2003.

77. Institute of Medicine. The Role of Nutrition in Maintaining Health in the Nation's Elderly: Evaluating Coverage of Nutrition Services for the Medicare Population. Washington, DC: National Academy Press, 2000. Available at: http://books.nap.edu/catalog/9741.html. Accessed

78. D'Alto M, Pacileo G, Calabro R. Nonpharmacologic care of heart failure: patient, family and hospital organization. Am J Cardiol 2003;91(suppl):51F–54F.

79. Calle EE, Rodriguez C, Walker-Thurmond K, Thun MJ. Overweight, obesity, and mortality from a prospective studied cohort of US adults. N Engl J Med. 2003:348:1625–1638.

80. Banegas JR, Lopez-Garcia E, Gutierrez-Fisac JL, Guallar-Castillon P, Rodriguez-Artalejo F. A simple estimate of mortality attributable to excess weight in the European Union. Eur J Clin Nutr. 2003;57:201–208.

81. Wolf AM, Colditz GA. Current estimates of the economic cost of obesity in the United States. Obes Res 1998;6:97–106.

82. Chopra M, Galbraith S, Darnton-Hill I. A global response to a global problem: the epidemic of overnutrition. Bull WHO 2002;80:952–958.

83. Knowler WC, Barrett-Connor E, Fowler SE, et al. Reduction in the incidence of type 2 diabetes with lifestyle intervention or metformin. N Engl J Med 2002;346:393–403.

84. American Dietetic Association. Nutrition and You: Trends Survey. Chicago: American Dietetic Association, 2002.

85. Committee on Health Professions Education Summit. Board on Health Care Services. In: Greiner AC, Knebel E, eds. Health Professions Education: A Bridge to Quality. Washington, DC: Institute of Medicine, National Academy Press, 2003. Available at: http://www.nap.edu. Accessed August 31, 2003.

86. Burd A, Cheung KW, Ho WS, et al. Before the paradigm shift: concepts and communication between doctors and nurses in a burns team. Burns 2002;28:691–695.

87. Cox S. Building dream teams. Nurs Mgt 2003;34(3):58.

88. Gibbon B, Watkins C, Barer D, et al. Can staff attitudes to team working in stroke care be improved? J Adv Nurs 2002;40:105–111.

89. Lingard L, Reznick R, DeVito I, Espin S. Forming professional identities on the health care team: discursive constructions of the "other" in the operating room. Med Ed 2002;36:728–734.

90. Goldstein /Krall Marketing Resources, Inc. Focus Groups Conducted to Guide the Development of the ADA Physician Nutrition Education Program. Stamford, CT: 1993.

91. Furhman MP. Issues facing dietetics professionals: challenges and opportunities. J Am Diet Assoc 2002;1021618–1620.

92. Rogers D, Leonberg BL, Broadhurst CB. 2000 Commission on Dietetics Registration practice audit. J Am Diet Assoc 2002;102:270–292.

93. Maxwell, JC. The 17 Indisputable Laws of Teamwork. Nashville, TN: Thomas Nelson, 2001.

94. Keim, KS, Johnson, CA, Gates, GE. Learning needs and continuing professional education activities of professional development portfolio participants. J Am Diet Assoc 2001;6:697–702.

95. Covey, SR. The Seven Habits of Highly Effective People. New York: Simon & Schuster, 1989.

96. Kouzes JM, Posner BZ. The Leadership Challenge. 3rd Ed. San Francisco: Jossey-Bass, 2002.

97. Patterson K, Grenny J, McMillan R, Switzler A. Crucial Conversations. New York: McGraw-Hill, 2002.

98. Buckingham, M, Clifton, DO. Now, Discover Your Strengths. New York: The Free Press, 2001.

99. Edwards, MR, Ewen, AJ. 360 Feedback: The Powerful New Model for Employee Assessment & Performance Improvement. New York: AMACOM, 1996.

100. Congruence of job-performance ratings: a study of 360° feedback examining self, manager, peers, and consultant ratings. Hum Rel 1998;4:517–530.

101. Tornow, W, London, M. Maximizing the Value of 360-Degree Feedback. San Francisco: Jossey-Bass, 1998.

102. The 1973 Annual Handbook for Group Facilitators. In: Jones, JE, Pfeiffer, JW, eds. San Diego, CA: Pfeiffer & Company, 1974.

103. Boje, DM. Johari Window and psychodynamics of leadership and influence in intergroup life. Available at: http://cbae.nmsu.edu/dboje/503/johari_window.htm. Accessed March 1, 2006.

104. Kirby, LK, Myers, KD. Introduction to Type: A Guide to Understanding Your Results on the Myers-Briggs Type Indicator. Palo Alto, CA: Consulting Psychologists Press, 1998.

105. Keirsey, D, Bates, M. Please Understand Me. 5th Ed. Del Mar, CA: Prometheus Nemesis Book Co, 1984.

106. ADA Reports: performance, proficiency and value of the dietetics professional. J Am Diet Assoc 2002:9:1304–1315.

107. 2002 Dietetics Compensation and Benefits Survey. Chicago: American Dietetic Association, 2003.

108. Jarratt J, Mahaffie JB. Key trends affecting the dietetics profession and the American Dietetic Association. J Am Diet Assoc 2002;102:S18221–S1839.

109. ADA. Strategic Plan. Chicago: American Dietetic Association, 2003. Available at: http://www.eatright.org. Accessed February 20, 2006.

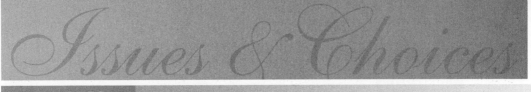

GLOBAL DIETETICS ISSUES

Patricia S. Anthony

A dietetics professional is defined by the American Dietetic Association (ADA) as a highly trained food and nutrition expert who has met minimum academic and professional requirements.[1] The European Federation of the Associations of Dietitians (EFAD) and the International Confederation of Dietetic Associations (ICDA) define a dietitian as a person with a legally recognized qualification (in nutrition and dietetics) who applies the science of nutrition to the feeding and education of groups of people and individuals in health and disease.[2,3] Do these definitions travel internationally? Is the dietitian legally recognized in all countries? Are the educational and professional requirements of dietitians similar across the world? Are dietitians recognized as nutrition experts? Does the dietitian practice similarly across the globe? What are the challenges of dietetics professionals across the world? With over 220,000 dietitians across the world, there are amazing similarities in the practices, goals, and challenges of dietitians. This is true despite vast differences in economic, political, cultural, and religious practices. With the leadership of organizations such as ICDA, EFAD, the Asian Federation of Dietetic Associations (AFDA), the Latin American Confederation of Nutritionists and Dietitians (CONFELANYD), and the Caribbean Association of Nutritionists and Dietitians (CANDI) (Table 7-1), dietetics organizations are working together regionally and globally to improve the communication between dietitians, enhance the image of the profession, and increase awareness of the standards of education, training, and practice of dietetics.

DIETETICS ORGANIZATIONS

The ADA is the world's leading dietetics organization and serves as a model for many others.[4] The British Dietetic Association, Dietitians of Canada, and the Dietetic Association of Australia are also looked to by many countries as models of organization and practice.

In Europe, 24 national dietetics associations are members of EFAD. EFAD has the following goals:

- To improve the nutrition of the population of its member states.
- To develop dietetics on a scientific and professional level.
- To promote the development of the dietetics profession.
- To improve the teaching of dietetics.
- To equate the criteria for the qualification within dietetics.[5]

A major goal of EFAD is to unify the dietetics profession across the European Union (EU), ultimately enabling dietitians trained in any EU country to practice in any

133

TABLE 7-1	Organizations of Dietetics Associations		
ORGANIZATION	**ABBREVIATION**	**NO. OF ASSOCIATION MEMBERS**	**GEOGRAPHIC DISTRIBUTION**
International Confederation of Dietetic Associations	ICDA	34	Global
European Federation of the Associations of Dietitians	EFAD	22	Europe
Caribbean Association of Nutritionists and Dietitians	CANDI	11	Caribbean islands
Latin American Confederation of Nutritionists and Dietitians	CONFELANYD	12	South America
Asian Federation of Dietetic Associations	AFDA	9	Asia

other EU country (Table 7-2). This goal is consistent with the Bologna Declaration from the European Ministers of Education (1999),[6] which states a common goal: to create a European Area for Higher Education. It also pledges to reform the European Union higher education structures in a convergent way. Owing to significant variation in education and recognition of the role of the dietitian, a dietitian in one EU country today cannot practice as a dietitian in another EU country. Currently, however, cross-border recognition exists within the EU of physicians and pharmacists.

EFAD has done several studies looking at dietetics in Europe and concluded that the education and work of dietitians in Europe is complex and multifaceted.[2] The different cultures in each country give rise to different expectations from professionals, politicians, and the public. This, in turn, affects the education process, the qualifications gained, and the work undertaken.[2] In June 2005, EFAD published the European Academic and Practitioner Standards for Dietetics, which has been accepted by all EFAD members as the European Benchmark Statement for Dietetics.[7] This benchmark establishes the minimum standard required for qualification as

TABLE 7-2	Members of the European Federation of the Associations of Dietitians
Austria	Italy
Belgium	Luxembourg
Cyprus	Netherlands
Denmark[a]	Norway[b]
Finland	Poland
France	Slovenia
Germany	Spain
Greece	Sweden[a]
Hungary	Switzerland[b]
Iceland[b]	Turkey[b]
Ireland	United Kingdom

[a]Denmark and Sweden each have two dietetic association memberships, one for clinical dietitians and one for dietitians.
[b]Not a member of the European Union.

a dietitian in any of the member countries of EFAD. It also includes additional statements that supplement the minimum core statements and are the threshold level for the areas of specialization within dietetics in Europe. This document is an advisory document; it outlines the standard that must be achieved by dietitians on qualification and maintained through continuing professional development. EFAD will continue to work toward the convergence of dietetics education across Europe, so that dietitians will be able to work and move freely among European nations.

In Africa, only a few dietetics organizations exist, with the Association for Dietetics in South Africa being the most formally organized and developed. Organizations are present as well in Sudan and Nigeria. Countries where dietitians have been known to work are Morocco, Egypt, Gambia, Sierra Leone, Ghana, the Democratic Republic of Congo, Tanzania, Mozambique, Zimbabwe, the Republic of South Africa, Malawi, Lesotho, Swaziland, Namibia, Botswana, and the island of Mauritius.[8] Reports in 1985 and 1991 by the East, Central, and Southern Africa Food and Nutrition (ECSAFAN) Cooperation looking at dietitian and nutrition positions for food and nutrition programs leave one with the impression that the role of the dietitian is not understood in Africa and that possibly the dietitian and the nutritionist are regarded as being the same.[8]

In the Middle East, there are five organized dietetics associations—in Turkey, Cyprus, Lebanon, Saudi Arabia, and Israel. Dietitians are also known to be practicing in Jordan, the United Arab Emirates (UAE), Bahrain, Iran, Iraq, Oman, and Qatar (personal communication, E. Edwards, February 2004).

Asia's rapid economic development over the past few decades has brought with it concomitant nutrition and lifestyle-related problems similar to those experienced in western societies. With this has come an increased awareness of nutrition and health among the general public, and the dietetics profession has undergone transformation to meet the demand.[9] Dietetics organizations in Asia are working closely with their governments as well as healthcare and education systems to increase the visibility and level of practice of the dietitian. They are working aggressively to move the dietitian from the traditional foodservice role to that of a food and nutrition expert and professional. They feel a significant pressure to make this transition very quickly, stating that "we do not have 20 years to move the profession forward, it needs to happen now" (personal communication, S. Taechangam, April 2004). Nine dietetics associations in Asia belong to the AFDA, including those of Malaysia, Hong Kong, Taiwan, Singapore, the Philippines, Indonesia, Thailand, Korea, and Japan. AFDA, formed in 1990, has conducted several surveys looking at workforce needs, training, and the role of dietitians in their member countries. AFDA has also hosted an educational conference every 4 years.[10]

Both Australia and New Zealand have well-established dietetics organizations, with over 2,800 dietitians in the two countries. Although not formal members of AFDA, Australia and New Zealand work closely with AFDA, participating in surveys and conferences. As in Europe, significant variation is present in the education, practice, and recognition of dietitians within Asia and the Pacific.

Dietetics associations are well-established in Central and South America and the Caribbean. A 1995 survey of dietitians in the Americas (North, Central, and South America as well as the Caribbean) showed that 80% of Canadian and South American nutritionists belong to professional organizations. Only four countries participating in the survey (Bolivia, Honduras, Nicaragua, and Paraguay) did not have a professional organization.[11] Mexico, Venezuela, Chile, and several other countries have professional organizations administered through universities. In South America, 12 nutrition and dietetics organizations participate in CONFE-LANYD, which conducts a symposium every 3 years. CANDI, a well-established consortium of dietetics professionals on 11 Caribbean islands, conducts meetings of the island associations and focuses on upgrading the leadership and management skills of its members and strengthening research.[11]

There appear to be no dietetics organizations in the Middle East and Africa. What makes these parts of the world different, that we see this void? Does the role of women in the Arab world impact the role of the dietetics professional in these countries? Does the severe poverty and political unrest in Africa play a role in slowing the progression of the profession? Does the similarity between a dietitian and a nutritionist in Africa underestimate the true number of "nutrition professionals" if one is looking at only dietetics organizations and dietitians?

WHAT IS A DIETITIAN? IS THE DIETITIAN LEGALLY RECOGNIZED?

Throughout the world, the official definition of dietitian usually includes a reference to the necessary educational requirements and to the role of the dietitian in providing nutrition information to groups of people with relation to health and disease. Dietitians are portrayed as working within the medical community and the general public with a goal of improving overall general nutrition well-being. Common terms used to describe dietitians include "expert," "specialist," "consultant," "practitioner," and "professional." Dietitians:

- Translate and apply the science of food, nutrition, dietetics, and alimentation into practice.
- Educate, advise, and counsel people and groups of people.
- Promote good health through optimal nutrition.
- Are in charge of meal management and nutrition services to prevent diseases and improve the health of individuals, groups, and communities.
- Play an important role in the medical management of disease with nutrition.
- Play an important role in the education of the population on the role of food and nutrition with health and lifestyle.
- Play an important role in the delivery of safe food to the population.

In most developed countries there is mention of the dietitian as a member of a multidisciplinary team, although the recognition by the members of the multidisciplinary team of the dietitian as the nutrition expert is often a goal and not yet reality.

EFAD has three official specialty definitions of the dietitian, which were felt to be necessary due to the different types of work done by dietitians. The *administrative* dietitian has an education focused on foodservice management, with responsibility for feeding groups of people in health and disease in an institution or community. The *clinical* dietitian has an education focused on clinical nutrition and dietetics, with responsibility for dietary prevention and treatment of individuals in an institution or community. A *general* dietitian has an education in clinical nutrition, dietetics, and foodservice management, with overall responsibilities for both aspects in an institution or community. Some members of EFAD have all three categories of dietitians and some only two, but the majority qualify in only one category. Within the three categories, it appears that dietitians do more or less the same type of work.[2]

About half of the dietetics associations surveyed by the author indicated that dietitians are legally recognized by the country in which they find themselves. In some countries, an official legal definition of dietitian is noted in an official government regulation; in others, this definition may apply to the dietitian/nutritionist. Often, the official definition has been formulated in cooperation between the national dietetics association and the Ministry of Health, the outcome being the recognition of a formal definition by the Ministry of Health. In some countries (e.g., Mexico), there is a legal definition, but it is not enforced; in other countries (e.g., India), there is a dietetics examination, but it is not mandatory and not observed by most dietitians. In some countries, the recognition of the dietitian is not on the national level but on the state or regional level. In Canada, the terms "registered dietitian," "professional dietitian," and "dietitian" are protected by provincial legislation. In the United States, the registered dietitian is certified by the Commission on Dietetic Registration (CDR), and completion of a specific educational program is required, as well as successful completion of an examination and ongoing continuing education; the actual recognition of the dietitian credential, however, is on the state level. Over the last 20 years, there has been a significant effort for dietitians to become licensed in each state; as of mid-2005, 46 states regulated dietitians or nutritionists through licensure, statutory certification, or registration.[12] In Switzerland, the Swiss Red Cross has regulated dietitians' training since 1984, in accordance with a mandate from the cantonal (provincial) board of directors of medical affairs. As of July 1999, the title "registered dietitian" is government protected there.[13]

There appears to be a link between the level of dietetics practice, an official definition, and whether the term dietitian is legally protected in a country. In India, the dietitian is anyone who has studied nutrition and works in a hospital clinic or freelance and who defines herself as such (personal communication, N. Jesudason, March 2004). In Pakistan, a dietitian is a professional who works in a hospital or runs an outpatient department advising nutrition and diet therapy in different disease conditions. In neither of these countries is the term "dietitian" legally protected, but the local association is working to obtain legal protection and recognition of the term by the government. In both India and Pakistan, and in many other countries, the term dietitian may not be legally protected, but there is a government definition that is used for the hiring of dietitians for government jobs (i.e., hospitals, public health, education, etc.). Numerous countries within Asia, the Middle East, and Africa either do not offer training for dietitians or the level of training for dietitians is low, and/or a high percentage of dietitians practicing in the country were trained outside the country. Many of these countries do officially recognize the title of dietitian, but often that definition is dependent on a person meeting the education and dietitian qualification criteria of another country. Singapore and Hong Kong are excellent examples of this. Today, there is no training program for dietitians in Singapore. Singaporean dietitians are usually trained in Malaysia, Australia, New Zealand, Canada, the United Kingdom, or the United States. There is no registration or licensure requirement to practice dietetics in Singapore, but you must show that you meet the criteria for credentialing in the country where you obtained your education.[14] Until recently, Hong Kong was similar, but in the last 5 years a dietetics education program has been started. Most dietitians in Hong Kong have been trained in the United States, the United Kingdom, Canada, or Australia, and most continue to be trained outside the country. The title of dietitian is not protected in Hong Kong, but you must have graduated from either the approved Hong Kong program or one of the four overseas "equivalent" programs to work for either of the two major dietetics employers in Hong Kong, the Department of Health or the Hospital Authority.[15] In the United Arab Emirates, the Ministry of Health description for clinical dietitian includes a bachelor of science degree plus an internship. To practice as a clinical dietitian in the United Arab Emirates, one must be eligible for registration as a clinical dietitian in the same country as the internship was done and have a minimum of 2 years of clinical experience. The Ministry of Health does administer an examination for the dietitian specialty, which is evaluated as a qualified dietetics technician. For dietitians trained abroad, there is a diploma attestation process, but there is no requirement to take an examination (personal communication, E. Edwards, February 2004).

DIETITIAN VERSUS NUTRITIONIST— HOW DO THEY DIFFER?

According to the American Heritage Dictionary, a dietitian is a person specializing in dietetics, while a nutritionist is a person specializing in the study of nutrition.[16] According to the U.S. Bureau of Labor Statistics, dietitians and nutritionists plan food and nutrition programs and supervise the preparation and serving of meals. They help to prevent and treat illnesses by promoting healthy eating habits and recommending dietary modifications. Dietitians manage foodservice systems for institutions, promote sound eating habits through education, and conduct research. Dietitians and nutritionists need at least a bachelor's degree in dietetics, food and nutrition, foodservice systems management, or a related area.[17]

As mentioned before, ADA defines a dietitian as a highly trained food and nutrition expert who has met minimum academic and professional requirements.[1] The American College of Nutrition defines a nutritionist as a health specialist who devotes his or her professional activity exclusively to food/nutrition science, preventive nutrition, diseases related to nutrient deficiencies, and the use of nutrient manipulation to enhance the clinical response to human diseases. The American College of Nutrition offers a certification for a certified nutrition specialist, which is open to dietitians with a master's degree as well as other nutritionists meeting the criteria specified and passing a certification examination. The criteria to take the examination include between 1,000 and 4,000 hours of practical experience, depending upon the type of experience.[18] Thus, the differentiating factor between a dietitian and a nutritionist in the United States is the specific education process of a dietitian, the successful mastering of the registration examination, and maintenance of ongoing continuing education.

Can a nutritionist be a dietitian and a dietitian a nutritionist? In the United States, the answer is yes, but it depends on the specific state licensing, certification, and registration laws in addition to the education and training of the person. This leads to the question: Why would a dietitian want to be both a nutritionist and a dietitian? What are the benefits? Which title is more respected by the public and by other healthcare professionals? Do the public and other healthcare professionals understand the distinction between dietitians and nutritionists? Over the last few years, ADA has worked aggressively to increase the awareness of the training and expertise of the registered dietitian and has made significant inroads, especially with the passing of the Medical Nutrition Therapy legislation.

In Canada, the term "nutritionist" is not protected by law in all provinces, thus people with different levels of training and education can call themselves nutritionists. In some Canadian provinces, the title "nutritionist" is protected for dietitians, and dietitians do use the title nutritionist. So it depends on where one lives in Canada whether a dietitian and a nutritionist are the same.[19]

The distinction between dietitian and nutritionist becomes even more confusing outside North America. Many of the dietetics associations referenced earlier are professional organizations of dietitians and nutritionists. In many countries the title "nutritionist" actually refers to someone with a higher level of education than that of a dietitian (i.e., holding an advanced degree.) In Jamaica, all professionals with specific core training in nutrition are called nutritionists. In Brazil, a nutritionist has an advanced degree. In Germany, both the titles "dietitian" and "nutritionist" are authorized and recognized by the government. In Hungary, a dietitian has a medical and nutrition education, whereas a nutritionist is a food industry engineer. In Hong Kong, there has been a recent effort to separate the dietetics and nutrition professional organizations with the formation of the Hong Kong Dietitians Association. The association differentiates dietitians and nutritionists by the fact that nutritionists do not study dietetics nor have a clinical practicum. In many countries the terms "dietitian" and "nutritionist" are synonymous. Sometimes the term "nutritionist" is perceived to indicate a higher level of expertise than the term "dietitian," with the dietitian relegated to the kitchen. As mentioned before, in most of Africa there is no distinction between the two terms.

Thus, in trying to understand the professions of dietetics and nutrition across the globe, it is first necessary to determine who practices nutrition and dietetics in a given country and what title they use to identify themselves. If you speak with Germans about dietitians, you get a very different perspective than if you ask them about nutritionists. In this example, many nutritionists are actually medical physicians, scientists, researchers, and/or dietitians. The German Nutrition Society is an agency comprising dietitians and nutrition scientists that develops nutrition policies, provide scientific and educational materials, and host conferences. Members of this agency are considered to be the leading authorities on nutrition in Germany, and every 4 years the society publishes a scientific document on the nutrition status of the German population. This document also contains reviews of important aspects of the current science of nutrition, such as breast-feeding and infant nutrition, geriatric nutrition, toxicological aspects of nutrition, technological aspects of food processing, etc.[20] The society works closely with the government to coordinate the assurance of quality nutrition education and to promote and maintain the health and fitness of the population. This organization may actually have the most similarity with the ADA, even though there is a German Dietetic Association, which is a member of ICDA. In trying to understand the field of nutrition and dietetics in Germany, it is essential to be aware of the German Nutrition Society, the German Dietetic Association, and the German Diet Technician Association. Germany is an excellent example of the interchangeability of the terms dietitian and nutritionist. To understand the dietetics profession globally, one must also explore the practice of nutritionists. In short, one is definitely not exclusive of the other.

WHERE DO DIETITIANS PRACTICE?

Across the world, the most common employment for dietitians is in a hospital setting, as evidenced by 33% of U.S. dietitians,[21] greater than 50% of European dietitians,[2] and some 70% of dietitians in Argentina practicing in such settings. Of those countries surveyed by the author, all listed hospitals as a primary setting of employment for dietitians. In Brazil as of 1996, some 50% of nutrition professionals were practicing in food service.[11] Other sites of employment are nursing homes, rehabilitation centers, or extended-care facilities; community nutrition and public health; the food and pharmaceutical industries; educational institutions; the catering industry; quality management; private practice; the government; environmental health; health clubs; the health insurance industry (i.e., managed care companies); nongovernmental organizations; and home economics (Table 7-3). In these practice settings, dietetics/nutrition professionals counsel, advise, and educate; develop and implement policy; do marketing and product development; work in food development, production, and service; act as supervisors, managers, or administrators; conduct research; communicate on issues of disease prevention and health promotion; and more. Fifty-four percent of U.S. dietitians still practice in the field of clinical nutrition, with the remainder practicing in the areas of community nutrition, food and nutrition management, consultation and business, and education and research.[22] In Pakistan, 1 of 6 dietitians works in health education/public health (personal communication, N. Safdar, March 2004); in Mexico, 35% work in the community setting.[11] The work settings of dietitians across the world are very similar. The actual tasks and responsibilities of the dietetics/nutrition professional in the various job settings vary

TABLE 7-3	Sites of Dietetic Employment Globally	
Hospitals[a]	Quality management
Nursing homes	Private practice
Rehabilitation centers	Government
Extended-care centers	Environmental health
Community nutrition	Health clubs
Public health	Health insurance industry
Food and pharmaceutical industries	Nongovernmental organizations
Educational institutions	Home economics
Catering industry	Media

[a]Primary site of employment in most countries.

greatly depending on the country, the general recognition and acceptance of the dietetics/nutrition professional, and the individual performing the job.

EDUCATION OF DIETITIANS

As noted previously, the specific educational requirements of dietitians are often what differentiate them from nutritionists; this difference has led to formal recognition by authorities. But what specifically are the educational requirements for dietitians? Are these requirements universal? These questions were asked prior to the XIIth International Congress of Dietetics in Manila in 1996, where a report was given on the education and training of dietitians in the different regions of the world. This work has been followed up by EFAD, which has looked extensively at the education and training of dietitians in Europe.

Dietetics is a combined science, an interdisciplinary science that brings together basic science, applied science, and social science. It involves the application of knowledge gained through science toward the ultimate goal of improving human well-being.[23] Dietetics education should thus be a combination of theoretical science and practice, each part being of equal importance. Globally there appears to be a similar emphasis on basic and biological sciences, clinical nutrition, and dietetics in academic-based programs[23] despite the fact that not all programs are university based. EFAD has found that, as of 2002, a total of 14 of its 22 member states have educational programs leading to the equivalent of a bachelor of science degree. Six member states have programs that do not equate to a bachelor of science degree, instead awarding a diploma or the equivalent. Two countries do not have education programs to train dietitians (Luxembourg and Cyprus). Within Europe, the amount of time a dietitian spends in training does not necessarily equate to the completion of a bachelor of science degree. Training time in Belgium, Hungary, Lithuania, Sweden, and the United Kingdom ranges between 4,000 and 6,000 hours, with a bachelor of science degree being granted upon completion. In Germany and Switzerland, 4,000 to 6,000 hours are spent in training, leading to the awarding of a diploma. In the majority of the EFAD countries, most of the training time is spent on food and nutrition science followed by basic science. All EFAD countries have practical programs, which make up between 15 and 30% of the total education in countries granting a bachelor of science degree and 35 to 50% of the training time in countries granting a diploma or its equivalent.[2] In the Americas (the United States, Canada, Brazil, the Caribbean, and Mexico), basic dietetics training is university based. In the 1990s, university training programs for dietitians were created in Jamaica and Trinidad, but there continues to be a void of training programs on the other nine Caribbean islands represented by CANDI. Dietitians on these islands are usually trained in the United Kingdom, the United States, or Canada. A wide variety exists between the credit hours required for completion of the degree, but all programs contain courses in the following areas: basic sciences, food and nutrition sciences, foodservice administration, nutrition education, and community nutrition. With the exception of Brazil, all the countries studied by the author indicated a requirement for a postgraduate internship, which ranges from 30 weeks to 1 year.[24]

In Asia and Africa, there appears to be no uniformity of academic require-ments. In many countries no dietetics training exists, but nutrition and/or home economics training may be available. The availability of training is not necessarily related to the economic prosperity of the country, as in the example of Singapore, which is a progressive nation both economically and in health care but does not have a dietetics training program. This situation may be to some degree reflective of the small size of the country (as with Luxembourg), but does it also reflect the perceived importance of the profession? Trostler noted in 1996 that in many parts of the world, clinical dietetics is still thought of as a luxury, like advanced medical treatment or a very specific medication. In the survey done by Trostler in 1996, of 18 countries in Africa and the Middle East surveyed, only four (Greece, Israel, South Africa, and Nigeria) had dietetics programs leading to a bachelor of science degree.[25] In Asia and the Pacific, Australia, New Zealand, the Philippines, Hong Kong, and Malaysia require a university degree to practice as a dietitian. In both Japan and Korea, one can become a dietitian by completing anything from a 2-year program to a full university degree. In Japan, one must complete work experience, which is between 1 and 3 years, depending upon education. An examination must be successfully completed in both countries prior to being recognized as a dietitian (personal communication, S. Tomomi, October 2003).[26]

It is clear that dietetics education varies greatly across the globe, but dietetics associations appear to be working toward the requirement of a bachelor of science degree, including the basic science, food, and nutrition science components in addi-tion to practical experience. This focus has likely been stimulated by the efforts of ICDA with its member organizations in working toward increasing the awareness of standards of education, training, and practice of dietetics. The topic of dietetics education across the world was presented at the ICDA congresses in Manila (1996), Edinburgh (2000), and Chicago (2004). The ICDA delegates (representatives from each country) voted that the bachelor of science degree should be the international minimal education level.

COMMON GLOBAL DIETETICS CHALLENGES

As one speaks with dietitians around the world, it is amazing that despite variations in education, practice levels, and cultures, many similar themes emerge as challenges to dietitians as individuals and as a profession. Common challenges include:

- Professional recognition
- Compensation
- Job security

In spring 2001, the ADA identified that the number-one issue of its member-ship was the concern that salaries do not always meet expectations when compared with the required scientific background for dietetics professionals. This salary con-cern was also related to the competition and encroachment of the marketplace, the promotion of the profession as the food and nutrition experts, and the need for competencies, training, and continuing education. The question discussed by the

ADA House of Delegates (HOD) was "How do we reduce the gap between the level of performance and proficiency and the value of the dietetics professional? What is the responsibility of the individual dietitian and what is the responsibility of ADA?"[27] This issue, although it may at first glance appears to focus on compensation, actually touches on the three common challenges of dietitians globally and indicates that all three issues are deeply intertwined. Out of this issue came recognition that the profession of dietetics is moving forward quickly but possibly not at the same speed as other healthcare professions, thus leaving dietitians at a disadvantage. A need to expand the role of the dietetics professional was also recognized. The responsibility for addressing these issues was seen as a joint responsibility between the ADA and the individual dietitian.[28] This issue demonstrated that dietetics professionals need to develop the skills to help create greater value of the dietitian in the workforce, which should ultimately have an effect on professional recognition, compensation, and job security. Dwyer stated in 2000 that "Dietitians with the unique combination of a strong scientific base coupled with practical skills in therapy, education and management are proving to be equal to the challenges of the 21st century."[29] The ADA HOD work clearly demonstrated a need for dietetics professionals to become better negotiators and more adept at business; they also need to develop better marketing skills and to improve their ability to convey to others the value of their professional work. The ADA HOD work reinforced the need for further development of the skills identified by Dwyer as being essential for success in the 21st century. Trostler and Myers further highlighted this theme in their discussion of the need for dietitians to perform outcomes research showing the impact of dietetics practice. They reinforced the need for dietetics education including research skills, computer proficiency, marketing, entrepreneurship, and management, as without these skills dietitians will have less than optimal professional interaction with other healthcare professionals and acceptance into the healthcare team.[23]

Issues to Ponder

- Is a dietitian a nutritionist or vice versa? How does this translate globally?
- Does the cultural role of women have an impact upon the recognition of the dietetics practice?
- How does the perceived value of dietetics professionals relate to financial compensation?
- What are the similarities and differences among dietetics practitioners across the globe?
- What are roles of professional associations across the globe?

In 2000, EFAD concluded from its work that "the profession must analyze and be aware of new trends in the community related to new technologies, demographic changes, increased demands for cost-effectiveness, and increased expectations from well-informed clients." Most of the European Dietetic Association felt that dietitians in the future will be in higher positions, and that the dietetics organizations need to plan to meet their members' needs. EFAD also stressed that dietitians would need skills outside the traditional dietitian skills; that they must become adept at strategic thinking, lobbying, and marketing of the profession instead of just being experts in dietetics.[30]

REFERENCES

1. American Dietetic Association website. Available at: http://www.eatright.org/cps/rde/xchg/ada/hs.xsl/career_748_ENU_HTML.htm. Accessed February 20, 2006.
2. Middleton C, Lawson M, Hadell K, Soerensen MA. Education programmes and work of dietitians in the member states of EFAD (summary report). Available at: http://www.efad.org/Reports/Education% 20ProGrammes.htm. Accessed October 14, 2003.
3. About ICDA. Available at: http://www.internationaldietetics.org/abouticda.asp. Accessed February 29, 2004.
4. Smith Edge M. Dietetics on a global scale. J Am Diet Assoc 2004;104:15.
5. European Federation of the Associations of Dietitians. The history of EFAD. Available at: http://www.efad.org/reports/. Accessed February 20, 2006.
6. The Bologna Declaration of 19 June 1999. Available at: http://www.bologna-berlin2003.de/pdf/bologna_declaration.pdf. Accessed October 15, 2005.
7. European Academic and Practitioner Standards for Dietetics. Available at: http://www.efad.org/Reports/ EFAD_BenchmarkJune2005_UK.pdf. Accessed October 15, 2005.
8. Kennedy RD. Trends in the work of dietitians in Africa and the Middle East. In: Proceedings of Two Minisymposia. Trends in the Work of Dietitians Around the World and Trends in the Education and Training of Dietitians Around the World. Twelfth International Confederation of Dietetics Associations, 1998:20–24.
9. Chwang LC. New perspectives of dietitians in Asia. In: Thirteenth International Congress of Dietetics Invited Speaker Abstracts, 2000:S55.
10. Chwang LC. Trends in the work of dietitians in Asia and the Pacific. In: Proceedings of Two Minisymposia. Trends in the Work of Dietitians Around the World and Trends in the Education and Training of Dietitians Around the World. Twelfth International Confederation of Dietetics Associations, 1998:13–19.
11. Derelian D. Trends in the work of dietitians in the Americas. In: Proceedings of Two Minisymposia. Trends in the Work of Dietitians Around the World and Trends in the Education and Training of Dietitians Around the World. Twelfth International Confederation of Dietetics Associations, 1998:9–12.
12. CDR certification and state licensure. Available at: http://www.cdrnet.org/certifications/index.htm. Accessed October 12, 2005.
13. Oliveira SV. Professional certification in Switzerland. ICDA newsletter. 1999;6:5.
14. http://www.snda.org.sg. Accessed January 3, 2004.
15. Hong Kong Dietitians Association Limited. Dietetic education and career in HK. Available at: http://www.hkda.com.hk/education&career.html. Accessed February 2, 2004.
16. The American Heritage Dictionary. 2nd College Ed. Boston: Houghton Mifflin, 1982:395,853.
17. US Department of Labor, Bureau of Labor Statistics. Dietitians and Nutritionists Occupational Handbook. Available at: http://www.bls.gov/oco/content/ocos077.stm. Accessed March 21, 2004.
18. American College of Nutrition. Certification board for nutrition specialists. Available at: http://www.cert-nutrition.org. Accessed April 4, 2004.
19. What is the difference between a dietitian and a nutritionist? A career in nutrition. Available at: http://www.dietitians.ca/career/i1.htm. Accessed March 21, 2004.
20. German Nutrition Society. Nutrition reports. Available at: http://www.dge.de/Pageslnavigation/english_version1nutrition revorts.htm. Accessed March 14, 2004.
21. Rogers D. Salary survey work group. Report on the ADA 2002 Dietetics Compensation and Benefits Survey. J Am Diet Assoc 2003;103:244–245.
22. Rogers D. Salary survey work group. Report on the ADA 2002 Dietetics Compensation and Benefits Survey. J Am Diet Assoc 2003;103:245.
23. Trostler N, Myers EF. Mainstreaming international outcomes research in dietetics. J Am Diet Assoc 2004;104:279.
24. Corby L. Education and training of dietitians in Canada, Ceara (Brazil), the Caribbean, Mexico, and the United States. Trends in the work of dietitians in the Americas. In: Proceedings of Two Minisymposia. Trends in the Work of Dietitians Around the World and Trends in the Education and Training of Dietitians Around the World. Twelfth International Confederation of Dietetics Associations, 1998:34–35.
25. Trostler N. Education and training of dietitians in the Middle East and Africa. In: Proceedings of Two Minisymposia. Trends in the Work of Dietitians Around the World and Trends in the Education and Training of Dietitians Around the World. Twelfth International Confederation of Dietetics Associations. 1998:40.

26. Brochure of the Korean Dietetic Association, 2002. Available at: http://www.dietitian.or.kr. Accessed February 20, 2006.
27. The Performance, Proficiency and Value Tactical Workgroup of the ADA House of Delegates. Performance, proficiency and value of the dietetics professional. J Am Diet Assoc 2002;102:1304–1315.
28. Thorpe M. Performance, proficiency and value of the dietetics professional: an update. J Am Diet Assoc2003;103:1376–1379.
29. Dwyer JT. Six revolutions that challenge us and move dietetic practice forward. In: Thirteenth International Congress of Dietetics Invited Speaker Abstracts, 2000: S53.
30. Sorensen MA, Hadell K. Profile of the European dietitian and challenges for the future. In: Thirteenth International Congress of Dietetics Invited Speaker Abstracts. 2000:S57.

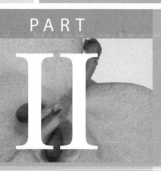

CLINICAL PRACTICE ISSUES: AN EVIDENCE-BASED PERSPECTIVE

Editor: Marion F. Winkler

CHAPTER

8

NUTRITION SCREENING IN ACUTE CARE
Pam Charney

Malnutrition is a known risk factor for increased morbidity and mortality, but there is no commonly agreed upon method for determining nutrition status of individuals. Various regulatory agencies have mandated that nutrition risk screening be completed on admission to acute care. There are many screening tools utilized in clinical settings, but few have been validated. Most screening tools are very complicated and more closely resemble nutrition assessment protocols, thus leading to confusion regarding definitions of screening and assessment. Nutrition risk screening should provide a mechanism to rapidly determine which patients require more comprehensive assessment and medical nutrition therapy. The screening process should be rapid and cost-effective while also maintaining sufficient sensitivity and specificity. This chapter reviews some of the parameters and tools in use and provides recommendations for rapid nutrition screening in acute care as well as a brief overview of the nutrition risk screening process in other settings.

NUTRITION RISK SCREENING

Nutrition risk screening has been defined as "the process of identifying characteristics known to be associated with nutrition problems. Its purpose is to pinpoint individuals who are nutritionally at risk for malnutrition or are malnourished." Those individuals who are identified to be at risk should be referred for nutrition assessment, or "a comprehensive evaluation to define nutrition status, including medical history, dietary history, physical examination, anthropometric measurements, and laboratory data."[1,2] A screening protocol should be designed to be a quick, easy, and cost-effective approach to detect risk for developing nutrition-related complications during hospitalization or admission to a healthcare institution or setting. If it is determined that risk is present, then the nutrition assessment protocol should provide a mechanism to determine the presence and extent of deficiencies and the care plan needed.

In the United States, regulatory agencies including the Joint Commission on Accreditation of Healthcare Organizations (JCAHO) and many state agencies require that patients admitted to an acute-care facility be screened for nutrition risk early during their admission. The screening process should be interdisciplinary, and it is mandated that the screen be completed within 24 hours of admission. Although the requirement for rapid screening may affect workload and staffing, given the shorter length of hospitalization today, it only makes sense to rapidly identify those patients requiring intervention. In spite of this, it is not known if completion of nutrition risk screening within 24 hours of admission is the most appropriate time frame or whether doing so will influence the outcome. Quick determination of risk/no risk does allow for better utilization of resources by concentrating care on those patients identified as nutritionally at risk upon admission.

Patients found to be at nutrition risk through the screening process are referred for comprehensive assessment of nutrition status. Most facilities have a process in place that allows for the "rescreening" of those patients who were initially not at risk but who have a length of stay that is beyond some predetermined cutoff, depending on the population. Healthcare professionals have developed screening and assessment tools for use in a variety of settings. Many of these tools have not been validated, and some appear to be more suited for nutrition assessment (see Chapter 9).

WHY IS NUTRITION RISK SCREENING SO IMPORTANT?

Since the publication of the landmark "Skeleton in the Hospital Closet,"[3] it has been noted that a significant proportion of patients admitted to an acute-care setting have nutrition deficits.[4] Malnutrition has been associated with increased morbidity and mortality in acutely ill patients. In spite of the growing awareness of the interactions between nutrition status and recovery from illness, there is evidence that nutrition status deteriorates over the course of hospitalization. Weinsier and coworkers assessed nutrition status at admission and 14 days after admission for patients who were still hospitalized.[5] Parameters utilized for this assessment included eight different anthropometric and biochemical measures (folate, vitamin C, albumin, absolute lymphocyte count, hematocrit, triceps skinfold, height, and weight). When available, preexisting cutoff values for each parameter were used. When standards for hospitalized patients did not exist, arbitrary levels were used, depending on the investigator's clinical experience. Using these criteria, it was found that 48% of patients had a high likelihood of malnutrition on admission, which increased to 69% when subjects still hospitalized after 14 days were reevaluated. Poor nutrition status correlated with increased length of stay and poor outcomes.[5] A follow-up study was completed 12 years later in the same setting using the same criteria.[6] A similar likelihood of malnutrition at admission (38% versus 48%, $p = .09$) was detected. Likelihood of malnutrition increased by 8% after 2 weeks in the follow-up study, compared to a 14% increase in the original study. These results indicate that while nutrition status does not deteriorate to the same degree during hospitalization, a significant number of patients admitted to an acute-care setting are malnourished on admission.[6] It should be noted that these studies utilized multiple parameters to identify patients who may be malnourished. It is unknown if a similar percentage would be identified if fewer parameters were used or if those parameters without objective criteria for evaluation were omitted.

More recently in the United Kingdom, it was found that approximately 20% of patients newly admitted to four hospitals could be identified as malnourished, using anthropometrics, "commonsense" evaluation, and advice of the hospital staff.[7] These authors evaluated 850 of 1,611 eligible patients within 48 hours of admission. Intensive-care unit (ICU) and bedbound patients were excluded. Malnutrition was defined by suboptimal body mass index (BMI), triceps skinfold, midarm muscle circumference, or weight. Dietetics professionals at each study site used severity of illness criteria, "common sense," and anthropometric measurements to assess patients and grade malnutrition as mild, moderate, or severe. True prevalence of malnutrition in this study was probably underestimated because of the exclusion of ICU and bedbound patients.

NUTRITION STATUS AND OUTCOME

The important relationship between nutrition status and outcome cannot be overlooked. In 1936, Studley noted that there was a significant relationship between preoperative weight loss and risk for death following surgery for peptic ulcer disease.[8] A similar relationship between weight loss at time of a cancer diagnosis and outcome has been noted. Patients with certain tumor types and as little as 5% weight loss had shorter survival time from diagnosis than patients who had not lost weight.[9] Others have found that malnourished patients with bladder cancer had higher postoperative morbidity and mortality than did well-nourished patients.[10] More recently, malnourished elderly patients diagnosed by the Subjective Global Assessment (SGA) had significantly increased mortality at 90 days and 1 year following admission.[11] Similarly, increased risk for mortality up to 4.5 years following discharge from acute care was found in a group of malnourished elderly patients.[12] Because of the association between nutrition status and outcome, it is important to identify those individuals who may either be malnourished or at risk for becoming malnourished during the course of hospitalization. This is challenging for dietetics practitioners because there is no universally agreed-upon marker of nutrition status. Misdiagnosis of malnutrition may occur with some frequency depending on the setting or the parameter used. As a result, to increase diagnostic accuracy, a combination of parameters should be used for nutrition screening.[13]

Issues to Ponder

- What is the screening protocol designed to detect? What are the desired outcomes?
- Define the term "nutrition risk." Be specific concerning the risk to be lessened by screening and early intervention.
- Propose an outcomes study to demonstrate the benefits of screening for a desired condition or end result.

NUTRITION SCREENING PARAMETERS

The parameters that follow are thought to be readily available or easy to obtain, have shown a link to nutrition status, and could feasibly be completed within 24 hours of admission.

DIET

Malnutrition results from inadequate nutrient intake, malabsorption of nutrients, or altered metabolism. Because of the identified link between nutrition status and outcome, it is important to identify potential causes of nutrition deficiencies as rapidly as possible so that appropriate therapy can be initiated. There is little research investigating diet intake prior to or during hospitalization and the effect of intake on outcome. Incalzi and colleagues studied 286 patients admitted to medicine or geriatrics wards in a university hospital.[14] Nutrition assessment was completed using percent of ideal body weight, BMI, skinfold measurements, albumin, total lymphocyte count, and hemoglobin. They found that 27% of patients were malnourished on admission and that most of the patients consumed less than 70% of their actual needs,[14] with a relationship between the percent of needs met and degree of malnutrition. In another study, approximately 20% of 497 elderly patients admitted to a Veterans Affairs hospital were found to have an average daily intake of less than 50% of calculated needs during hospitalization.[15] Study patients received a comprehensive nutrition assessment consisting of a clinical history, review of records for all primary and secondary diagnoses, laboratory values, functional status assessment, and neuropsychological examination. Evaluation of nutrient intake was completed by direct observation for the first 3 days of hospitalization and every other day thereafter until discharge. Patients were divided into two groups for analysis: those who consumed more than 50% of calculated requirements and those who consumed less. Admission weight, albumin, and prealbumin levels did not differ between the low- and high-intake groups. The low-intake group had a higher rate of in-hospital mortality as well as a higher rate of mortality within 90 days of admission. Additionally, they were more likely to be functionally dependent at discharge than the group with higher intake.[15] These findings indicate that patients who are malnourished have poor intake prior to and during hospitalization, that poor intake is associated with adverse outcomes, and that traditional markers of poor nutrition status do not accurately identify those patients who will eat poorly during hospitalization.

Clinical studies investigating dietary intake suffer from lack of an objective measurement of intake. The gold standard for determining nutrient intake is the analysis of weighed aliquots taken from foods eaten along with weights of foods before and after meals. Such measurements are obviously time-consuming and expensive and are not often done in a clinical setting. Although indirect calorimetry is the gold standard for determining energy requirements, it is still not known what level of intake results in increased risk. It is possible to determine energy requirements with a high amount of certainty, but it is not feasible in most clinical settings to determine how well those requirements are met. The presence of observers, researchers, or assistants during meals may also threaten validity from interaction with the researcher in studies investigating food intake. Intake may therefore differ in a nonresearch setting.

These studies indicate the need for a rapid, nonintrusive method to identify those patients who are at risk for inadequate intake during hospitalization to better determine the impact of nutrient intake on outcomes prior to and during hospitalization. Many clinicians are familiar with the "calorie count" or "nutrient intake analysis" (see Chapter 10). These methods attempt to quantify intake by monitoring meal and snack consumption during hospitalization. Most methods used to estimate in-hospital food and beverage consumption are fraught with error and may significantly over- or underestimate actual intake. Additionally, given the short length of hospitalization, delaying nutrition therapy until the results of a 3-day calorie count are determined may not allow sufficient time for development and implementation of appropriate plans for nutrition care. Calorie-count methods are also not appropriate for determination of intake prior to hospitalization.

Alternate methods of estimating nutrient intake may be more useful than calorie counts or diet records in acute-care settings. If a rough estimate of adequacy of intake is needed, it may be best to simply monitor the percent of meals consumed, given knowledge of meals delivered. Room service is becoming popular for meal delivery in hospitals but may compromise the ability to determine what was eaten. Consumption of 50% of a meal of tea and toast is obviously suboptimal compared to 50% of a meal of meat, potatoes, and vegetable. Patients or family members may be able to provide a 24-hour recall of foods consumed. This method will not provide information on habitual diet prior to admission but can give a good estimate of adequacy of current intake. A simple food-frequency questionnaire can also be utilized in an inpatient setting (see Chapter 10).

Weight Loss

Weight loss can be an important indicator of the presence of malnutrition and is used as a prognostic indicator in many settings. Unintentional weight loss was a predictor of future neoplastic diagnosis in a group of patients admitted to an internal medicine service.[16] Examination of the National Health and Nutrition Examination Survey (NHANES) data for 4,710 subjects aged 55 to 74 years showed an increased risk for mortality (relative risk 1.3 to 1.6) among those with low BMI (<22 kg/m^2).[17] A large national survey found that individuals with unintentional weight loss had poorer outcomes than those with intentional weight loss.[18] Weight loss was compared to other parameters thought to reflect nutrition status, including serum albumin, total lymphocyte count, and total iron-binding capacity in 398 patients undergoing surgery for gastrointestinal (GI) cancer. Multiple logistic regression analysis using these parameters showed that weight loss had the best ability to predict surgery-related infections ($p = .02$), with 10% weight loss shown to be the minimum value associated with risk.[18] The addition of serum albumin less than 3.5 g/dL to the predictive equation did not improve the ability of weight loss alone to predict postoperative complications in this group.[19]

Weight loss alone may not reflect functional capacity for healing and rehabilitation. Windsor and Hill completed a preoperative assessment including evaluation of weight changes and an assessment of functional status on 102 patients admitted for elective GI surgery.[20] History and physical examination data were used to determine functional status by focusing on clinically relevant factors. Physiologic impairment was defined as a change in activity level at home or work along with symptoms of tiredness, malaise, depression, and apathy. Muscle function was assessed by asking patients to squeeze the examiner's hand. A single clinician who had no knowledge of the objective data then categorized patients as having weight loss <10% with no impairment, weight loss >10% with no impairment, and weight loss >10% with impairment. These subjective measurements were then compared to objective anthropometric measures of body composition and muscle function. Patients were followed until discharge. Results showed a correlation between clinical assessment and objective measures such as serum albumin and weight loss. Patients with both weight loss and functional impairment had significantly more complications, septic complications, pneumonia, and increased length of stay compared to the other groups.[20]

Although weight loss appears to be an important indicator of outcome, there is no agreement on interpretation of weight changes in acute-care settings. Most dietetics professionals compare current weight to "ideal" weight, as determined from life insurance tables. However, tables of ideal body weight (IBW) developed using actuarial data from healthy middle-class populations do not apply to hospitalized adults. BMI also suffers from the same problems, as it was not developed for use in acutely ill adults. Dietetics professionals also compare current weight to usual weight. This may be more applicable for the individual patient but still lacks accuracy, as usual weight is often obtained by patient recall. Although 10% weight loss is often cited as being significant,[21] there is no agreement on the amount or percentage of weight loss that accurately identifies increased risk for nutrition-related complications. Beck and Ovesen suggest that risk for nutrition-related complications in elderly patients increases with 5% loss of usual weight.[22] Additionally, no objective methods are available for evaluation of functional status for clinical use that can be rapidly applied across all inpatient populations.

Issues to Ponder

- How much time is required to conduct a screening?
- What is the cost of conducting a nutrition screen?
- What is the cost/benefit ratio of the screening protocol?
- How much does it cost to identify one patient with the condition in question?

HEPATIC TRANSPORT PROTEINS*

Serum levels of albumin and prealbumin are often used as markers of nutrition risk and status in the clinical setting as they appear to respond to nutrient, specifically protein, intake. Albumin levels are thought to reflect long-term intake, while prealbumin, owing to its shorter half-life and smaller body pool, appears to be reflective of short-term intake. It is often forgotten, however, that both of these hepatic proteins act as negative acute-phase proteins and may reflect underlying disease or injury severity more than nutrition status. During acute illness, hepatic protein synthesis is shifted away from transport proteins as acute-phase proteins are produced in response to release of cytokines and other metabolic mediators. There is also capillary leak of serum proteins, with the result that levels of albumin and prealbumin are decreased irrespective of prior nutrition status.[23] Proteins that show an increase in plasma levels during stress, such as fibrinogen and ceruloplasmin, are considered to be positive acute-phase proteins.

There is agreement in the nutrition community that albumin levels are a poor reflection of short-term nutritional status, but such levels may be useful as a measure of overall long-term intake and status. While albumin levels may reflect nutrition status in healthy populations, interpretation of serum albumin levels in acute-care settings is difficult because albumin concentrations change rapidly during the first

*See Chapter 9 for more information on this topic.

few hours of admission to the ICU.[24] McMillan and associates provide further evidence of lack of specificity of albumin in acute care.[25] Albumin levels were measured in 40 male patients with cancer (12 esophageal, 7 stomach, 3 pancreas, 7 colon, and 11 non–small-cell lung cancer) and compared to body cell mass (BCM) as estimated by total body potassium and C-reactive protein (CRP) levels. A small but significant correlation was found between albumin and BCM, while a stronger, negative correlation was found between albumin and CRP, indicating that albumin may better reflect inflammatory changes due to the disease process.[25] This study is flawed by lack of information concerning weight changes, as weight loss was estimated based on an initial reported weight and the nonequivalent study sample as evidenced by the variety of cancer types studied.

Potter and Luxton investigated the use of prealbumin levels as a screening parameter in an acute-care setting.[26] Prealbumin and albumin levels were determined on a cohort of 147 consecutive admissions from the emergency department in a tertiary care facility. Protein-calorie malnutrition (PCM) was diagnosed if prealbumin was less than 16 mg/dL or albumin was less than 3.5 g/dL. The investigators compared length of stay, in-hospital mortality, and cost of care between those who were identified as having PCM and those who were well nourished. Results indicated that 24% of the patients had at least mild PCM as determined by prealbumin levels, that prealbumin was associated with a significantly longer length of stay and higher mortality rate, and that prealbumin screening on admission led to a cost savings of $414 for each patient.[26] Although these results appear impressive on the surface, the study raises several questions. The authors assume that prealbumin is the gold standard for determination of nutrition status. There was no assessment of weight, diagnosis, nutrient intake, or injury severity. It is known that prealbumin acts as a negative acute-phase protein, such that prealbumin levels in these patients could have simply reflected degree of illness. Sicker patients would have longer lengths of stay and higher mortality. With no other marker for comparison, it is difficult to ascribe prealbumin levels simply to nutrition.

Others have suggested that prealbumin may be a useful screening parameter.[27,28] Brugler and coworkers investigated the use of prealbumin levels in nutrition risk screening.[29] Eligible patients were randomly assigned to have results of prealbumin testing reported to the medical record or hidden from practitioners. On closer review of the study methods, it appears that the usefulness of prealbumin was determined at some point following the initial screen, as patients included in the study were classified as "risk level 3 or 4." Therefore the study does not really evaluate the usefulness of prealbumin as a nutrition risk screen. Additionally, 76% of eligible patients were not enrolled and another 47 dropped out during the study period. It is difficult to analyze these results because of differences in the groups.[29] Use of hepatic transport values alone as a nutrition risk screen would lead to false-negative results in screening patients with chronic malnutrition, as serum protein levels are often maintained at or near normal levels until fairly late in starvation.

There has recently been some interest in the use of CRP as a tool to assist with evaluation of prealbumin or albumin levels. CRP, named for its ability to precipitate C-polysaccharide particles from *Streptococcus pneumoniae*, is felt to be a sensitive marker of inflammation.[30] CRP concentrations are very low in normal, healthy individuals and rise quickly in response to inflammation and activation of the acute-phase response. Because CRP responds to a general inflammatory stimulus, it cannot be used as a diagnostic tool for a specific disorder. CRP is useful in determining the presence and extent of the inflammatory response.[31,32] There have been no clinical studies determining relationships between hepatic transport proteins and CRP in the assessment of nutrition status. It can be expected that in an ICU setting, low levels of prealbumin and albumin are most likely related to the acute-phase response and that these patients would also have an elevated CRP. Before recommendations for the use of CRP and prealbumin in nutrition risk screening can be made, it is necessary to evaluate the cost of the tests in comparison to their usefulness in clinical decision making.

NUTRITION RISK SCREENING PROTOCOLS

No agreed-upon mechanism exists for completing nutrition risk screening in an inpatient setting. Available screening tools may be too cumbersome for use in rapid screening or may include laboratory parameters that are not readily accessible within the 24-hour framework required by JCAHO. Screening programs have been developed for use in community and clinic settings and include the Mini Nutrition Assessment and the Nutrition Screening Initiative questionnaires.[33,34] Both of these tools are too time-consuming to be utilized in an inpatient setting. The Mini Nutritional Assessment–Short Form (MNA–SF) was developed from the Mini Nutrition Assessment to rapidly identify elderly patients who may need in-depth assessment (Figure 8-1). Although not yet validated for use in an inpatient population, the MNA–SF may be more useful, as it can be completed rapidly using information that should be readily available on admission.[35]

Many tools developed for use in inpatient settings cannot be used rapidly because of complex scoring systems to determine risk. Kovacevich and colleagues designed a nutrition risk screening tool to be administered by nurses.[36] This tool uses diagnosis, intake and GI symptoms, IBW standards, and weight history. It is not clear how certain diagnoses were chosen to indicate nutrition risk. The tool was validated using prealbumin levels as the gold standard, which may not be appropriate for certain inpatient populations.[36] Brugler and coworkers developed a screening tool that utilizes a scoring system consisting of 10 history factors and 8 laboratory parameters.[37] Completion of the screen requires two steps: nurses complete questions about medical history and dietitians enter laboratory data and assign risk level.[37] Neither the Kovacevich nor the Brugler screen allows rapid determination of nutrition risk because of the inclusion of laboratory data in the scoring of results. There should be some concern about compliance with completion of these complicated screening tools by busy nurses.

Rapid screens have been used for a number of medical conditions including cardiovascular disease, diabetes, and cancer.[38] The goal of a screening test in any setting is to separate those individuals who might be at risk for a disease or disorder from those who are not. An appropriate screening process should not attempt to define levels of care or be time-consuming or expensive. The American Dietetic Association has suggested that the nutrition screen be tailored to the population served (inpatient versus outpatient) and that the dietetics professional be involved in monitoring the effectiveness of the screening process.[39] Any screening tool chosen

NESTLÉ NUTRITION SERVICES

Mini Nutritional Assessment
MNA®

Last name:	First name:	Sex:	Date:
Age:	Weight, kg:	Height, cm:	I.D. Number:

Complete the screen by filling in the boxes with the appropriate numbers.
Add the numbers for the screen. If score is 11 or less, continue with the assessment to gain a Malnutrition Indicator Score.

Screening

A Has food intake declined over the past 3 months
due to loss of appetite, digestive problems,
chewing or swallowing difficulties?
0 = severe loss of appetite
1 = moderate loss of appetite
2 = no loss of appetite   ☐

B Weight loss during last months
0 = weight loss greater than 3 kg (6.6 lbs)
1 = does not know
2 = weight loss between 1 and 3 kg (2.2 and 6.6 lbs)
3 = no weight loss   ☐

C Mobility
0 = bed or chair bound
1 = able to get out of bed/chair but does not go out
2 = goes out   ☐

D Has suffered psychological stress or acute
disease in the past 3 months
0 = yes   2 = no   ☐

E Neuropsychological problems
0 = severe dementia or depression
1 = mild dementia
2 = no psychological problems   ☐

F Body Mass Index (BMI) (weight in kg) / (height in m)²
0 = BMI less than 19
1 = BMI 19 to less than 21
2 = BMI 21 to less than 23
3 = BMI 23 or greater   ☐

Screening score (subtotal max. 14 points)   ☐ ☐

12 points or greater   Normal – not at risk –
no need to complete assessment

11 points or below   Possible malnutrition – continue assessment

Assessment

G Lives independently (not in a nursing home or hospital)
0 = no   1 = yes   ☐

H Takes more than 3 prescription drugs per day
0 = yes   1 = no   ☐

I Pressure sores or skin ulcers
0 = yes   1 = no   ☐

J How many full meals does the patient eat daily?
0 = 1 meal
1 = 2 meals
2 = 3 meals   ☐

K Selected consumption markers for protein intake
• At least one serving of dairy products
(milk, cheese, yogurt) per day?   yes ☐ no ☐
• Two or more serving of legumes
or eggs per week?   yes ☐ no ☐
• Meat, fish or poultry every day   yes ☐ no ☐
0.0 = if 0 or 1 yes
0.5 = if 2 yes
1.0 = if 3 yes   ☐ . ☐

L Consumes two or more servings
of fruits or vegetables per day?
0 = no   1 = yes   ☐

M How much fluid (water, juice, coffee, tea, milk…)
is consumed per day?
0.0 = less than 3 cups
0.5 = 3 to 5 cups
1.0 = more than 5 cups   ☐ . ☐

N Mode of feeding
0 = unable to eat without assistance
1 = self-fed with some difficulty
2 = self-fed without any problem   ☐

O Self view of nutritional status
0 = views self as being malnourished
1 = is uncertain of nutritional state
2 = views self as having no nutritional problem   ☐

P In comparison with other people of the same age,
how do they consider their health status?
0.0 = not as good
0.5 = does not know
1.0 = as good
2.0 = better   ☐ . ☐

Q Mid-arm circumference (MAC) in cm
0.0 = MAC less than 21
0.5 = MAC 21 to 22
1.0 = MAC 22 or greater   ☐ . ☐

R Calf circumference (CC) in cm
0 = CC less than 31   1 = CC 31 or greater   ☐

Assessment (max. 16 points)   ☐ ☐ . ☐
Screening score   ☐ ☐
Total Assessment (max. 30 points)   ☐ ☐ . ☐

Malnutrition Indicator Score

| 17 to 23.5 points | at risk of malnutrition | ☐ |
| Less than 17 points | malnourished | ☐ |

FIGURE 8-1 *Mini Nutritional Assessment.* ® *Société des Produits Nestlé S.A., Vevey, Switzerland, trademark owners. Used with permission. Ref.: Guigoz Y, Vellas B, and Garry PJ. 1994. Mini Nutritional Assessment: a practical assessment tool for grading the nutritional state of elderly patients. Facts and Research in Gerontology. Supplement #2:15–59.*

for use in acute care must be designed to rapidly identify those who may need more in-depth intervention and also have sensitivity and specificity to detect nutrition risk or malnutrition that preclude high numbers of false-positive or false-negative results (Table 8-1).

TABLE 8-1	Hallmarks of an Effective Screening Test	
FEATURE	**ALTERNATE NAME**	**DEFINITION**
Sensitivity	True-positive rate	How good is this test at picking up people who have the condition?
Specificity	True-negative rate	How good is this test at correctly excluding people without the condition?
Positive predictive value	Posttest probability of a positive test	If a person tests positive, what is the probability that he or she has the condition?

Source: Adapted with permission from Greenhalgh T. Papers that report diagnostic or screening tests. In: Greenhalgh T, ed. How to Read a Paper: The Basics of Evidence Based Medicine. London: British Medical Journal Books, 2001:105.

Ferguson and colleagues developed and validated a simple nutrition risk screening tool.[40] Following review of the literature, a set of screening questions was identified. The nonrandom sample consisted of 408 patients who were admitted to an acute-care facility. Within 2 days of admission, the patients were assessed by the SGA.[40] SGA is a nutrition assessment tool that was developed as a method to incorporate clinical judgment in the assessment process. It relies heavily on results of the medical history and a nutrition-focused physical examination to assist in determining nutrition status.[40–42] Scores on the screening questions were compared with SGA results. Three questions demonstrated ability to predict the SGA score and were used to develop the screening tool (Table 8-2).[43] Validity of the simple screen was not determined outside of the originating institution. Outcome studies using this tool are needed to determine if increased morbidity and mortality can be predicted.

A complicated screening tool using actual height and weight measurements, calculation of BMI, and knowledge of surgical history has been validated for use in patients with chronic obstructive pulmonary disease.[44] The tool was compared to results of a complete nutrition assessment. A point system was used to determine risk. When a cutoff of 4 points on the screen was utilized, there was good agreement with the complete assessment.[45] A simpler tool using only BMI and percent weight loss over time was also shown to have good agreement with a comprehensive assessment, but it may be limited in practice by the requirement to obtain actual weight measurement needed to calculate BMI.[46] These tools also presume that measurements taken upon admission will be accurate.[46]

Further research is needed to develop and validate screening tools for use in acute-care settings. Although virtually all healthcare facilities have a screening mechanism in place, few are collecting data or publishing outcomes. A review of 44 screening tools showed that none of the published tools were sufficiently tested or validated to allow for replication.[47]

Issues to Ponder

- Discuss reasons why weight loss and poor intake are markers of poor outcome.
- Discuss why screening tools that focus on nutrient intake may be useful to identify risk for poor outcome in acute care (for example, increased infections, poor wound healing, increased length of stay).
- Discuss how nutrition risk screening leads to an entry point to the nutrition care process (see Chapter 9).

TABLE 8-2	Malnutrition Screening Tool[a]
PARAMETER	**POINT VALUE**
Have you lost weight recently without trying?	
No	0
Unsure	2
If yes, how much weight (kilograms) have you lost?	
1–5	1
6–10	2
11–15	3
>15	4
Unsure	2
Have you been eating poorly because of a decreased appetite?	
No	0
Yes	1
Total points	

[a]Score of 2 or more indicates patient at risk of malnutrition.
Source: Reprinted with permission from Ferguson M, Capra S, Bauer J, Banks M. Development of a valid and reliable malnutrition screening tool for adult acute hospital patients. Nutrition 1999;15:458–464.

SCREENING IN ALTERNATE HEALTHCARE SETTINGS

Dietetics professionals responsible for provision of medical nutrition therapy in outpatient settings should be aware of the connections between diet, nutrition status, and outcomes in patients/clients with a variety of conditions. Screening protocols that are appropriate for an inpatient setting may not identify the issues relevant to an outpatient population or vice versa. For example, a nutrition risk screening protocol for an outpatient lipid clinic might be designed to identify diets that are high in saturated fat and calories associated with a sedentary lifestyle and the presence of overweight.

CONCLUSIONS AND RECOMMENDATIONS FOR PRACTICE

There is currently no agreed-upon method to rapidly identify those patients who may be at risk for nutrition-related complications during hospitalization. Although most agree that diet, weight loss, and hepatic transport proteins should be evaluated, there is no agreement on the best way to accomplish this. Complicating the dilemma is the added requirement that nutrition risk screening be completed as soon as possible following admission, preferably within the first 24 hours of admission. It is most reasonable to include the screening process as part of the initial assessment completed

Issues to Ponder

- Why is one definition of risk not sufficient in outpatient settings?
- Consider the differences in screening for cardiovascular risk and screening for risk of nutrition-related complications.
- How should nutrition screening protocols be adapted for different healthcare settings, life cycle, and primary disease states?

by nursing personnel at the time of admission. In many settings it is currently difficult or impossible to have results from laboratory testing, particularly prealbumin levels, available at admission. Technological advances in electronic medical records and data management systems may positively influence the screening process. Dietetic professionals should collaborate with nurses and information technology experts to design these systems.

It makes sense to identify parameters that are readily available at admission that can be used as indicators of nutrition status. Those responsible for developing nutrition risk screening protocols should also consider the cost of the screen in terms of personnel and resource utilization. Although the cost of an individual laboratory test may be low, in the current climate of limited inpatient reimbursement, use of laboratory testing should be minimized until the benefits of laboratory testing for nutrition risk screening are proven. Given the desire to create an interdisciplinary approach to screening, it would also be important to include items in the nutrition risk screen that are easily obtainable and understood by other healthcare practitioners. It has been suggested that nutrition screening tools designed to be completed by nurses be easy to use, cost-effective, provide for an action plan, and have proven validity and reliability.[48]

Weight change and nutrient intake should be utilized to conduct nutrition screening, as this information can be gathered quickly and noninvasively. Assessment of weight change and dietary intake can be taught to other healthcare professionals, thus increasing compliance with timely completion of nutrition risk screening. Given the known difficulty in obtaining actual height and weight measurements in acute-care settings, a proxy measure of weight status, such as change in clothing size, can be utilized if actual weights are not available. Use of such proxy measures has not been validated at this time. Stated weight is known to be associated with inaccuracy.[49] A rough estimate of change in intake can be obtained by determining quartiles of usual intake. There is some evidence that measures of weight and intake reflect nutrition status and the need for further intervention.

Further development and testing of methods to gather information used in nutrition risk screening is necessary, as some methods currently in use may not be valid in hospital settings. The complex relationship between serum levels of hepatic transport proteins, nutrient intake, and illness must be better understood. Dietetics professionals should investigate the best way to determine weight status given inaccurate or absent weights on admission. There is also a need to determine at which level of weight loss nutrition risk increases, and if this level is different for different age groups and diagnoses. Finally, research should be conducted to determine at what level of usual intake nutrition risk increases, so that sensitive and specific screening tools can be developed to identify those patients needing a comprehensive nutrition assessment.

REFERENCES

1. ASPEN Board of Directors. Definition of terms used in ASPEN guidelines and standards. Nutr Clin Pract 1995;10:1–3.
2. JCAHO (Joint Commission on Accreditation of Healthcare Organizations). Comprehensive Accreditation Manual for Hospitals. Oakbrook Terrace, IL: JCAHO, 2002.
3. Butterworth CE. The skeleton in the hospital closet. Nutr Today 1974;9:4–8.

4. Bistrian BR, Blackburn GL, Vitale J, Cochran D, Naylor J. Prevalence of malnutrition in general medical patients. JAMA 1976;235:1567–1570.

5. Weinsier RL, Hunker EM, Krumdieck CL, Butterworth CE Jr. Hospital malnutrition: a prospective evaluation of general medical patients during the course of hospitalization. Am J Clin Nutr 1979;32:418–426.

6. Coats KG, Morgan SL, Bartolucci AA, Weinsier RL. Hospital-associated malnutrition: a reevaluation 12 years later. J Am Diet Assoc 1993;93:27–33.

7. Edington J, Boorman J, Durrant ER, et al. Prevalence of malnutrition on admission to four hospitals in England. The Malnutrition Prevalence Group. Clin Nutr 2000;19:191–195.

8. Studley HO. Percentage of weight loss: a basic indicator of surgical risk in patients with chronic peptic ulcer. JAMA 1936;106:458–460.

9. Dewys WD, Begg C, Lavin PT, et al. Prognostic effect of weight loss prior to chemotherapy in cancer patients. Am J Med 1980;69:491–497.

10. Mohler JL, Flanigan RC. The effect of nutritional status and support on morbidity and mortality of bladder cancer patients treated by radical cystectomy. J Urol 1987;137:404–407.

11. Covinsky KE, Martin GE, Beyth RJ, Justice AC, Sehgal AR, Landefeld CS. The relationship between clinical assessments of nutritional status and adverse outcomes in older hospitalized medical patients. J Am Geriatr Soc 1999;47:532–538.

12. Sullivan DH, Walls RC. Protein-energy undernutrition and the risk of mortality within six years of hospital discharge. J Am Coll Nutr 1998;17:571–578.

13. Neithercut WD, Smith AD, McAllister J, La Ferla G. Nutritional survey of patients in a general surgical ward: Is there an effective predictor of malnutrition? J Clin Pathol 1987;40:803–807.

14. Incalzi RA, Gemma A, Capparella O, Cipriani L, Landi F, Carbonin P. Energy intake and in-hospital starvation. A clinically relevant relationship. Arch Intern Med 1996;156:425–429.

15. Sullivan DH, Sun S, Walls RC. Protein-energy undernutrition among elderly hospitalized patients: a prospective study. JAMA 1999;281:2013–2019.

16. Rabinovitz M, Pitlik SD, Leifer M, Garty M, Rosenfeld JB. Unintentional weight loss: a retrospective analysis of 154 cases. Arch Intern Med 1986;146:186–187.

17. Tayback M, Kumanyika S, Chee E. Body weight as a risk factor in the elderly. Arch Intern Med 1990;150:1065–1072.

18. Meltzer AA, Everhart JE. Unintentional weight loss in the United States. Am J Epidemiol 1995;142:1039–1046.

19. Gianotti L, Braga M, Radaelli G, Mariani L, Vignali A, Di Carlo V. Lack of improvement of prognostic performance of weight loss when combined with other parameters. Nutrition 1995;11:12–16.

20. Windsor JA, Hill GL. Weight loss with physiologic impairment: a basic indicator of surgical risk. Ann Surg 1988;207:290–296.

21. DeSanti L. Involuntary weight loss and the nonhealing wound. Adv Skin Wound Care 2000;13(suppl 1):11–20.

22. Beck AM, Ovesen L. At which body mass index and degree of weight loss should hospitalized elderly patients be considered at nutritional risk? Clin Nutr 1998;17:195–198.

23. Gabay C, Kushner I. Acute phase proteins and other systemic responses to inflammation. N Engl J Med 1999;340:448–454.

24. McCluskey A, Thomas AN, Bowles BJ, Kishen R. The prognostic value of serial measurements of serum albumin concentration in patients admitted to an intensive care unit. Anaesthesia 1996;51:724–727.

25. McMillan DC, Watson WS, O'Gorman P, Preston T, Scott HR, McArdle CS. Albumin concentrations are primarily determined by the body cell mass and the systemic inflammatory response in cancer patients with weight loss. Nutr Cancer 2001;39:210–213.

26. Potter MA, Luxton G. Prealbumin measurement as a screening tool for protein calorie malnutrition in emergency hospital admissions: a pilot study. Clin Invest Med 1999;22:44–52.

27. Bernstein LH, Leukhardt-Fairfield CJ, Pleban W, Rudolph R. Usefulness of data on albumin and prealbumin concentrations in determining effectiveness of nutritional support. Clin Chem 1989;35:271–274.

28. Bernstein L, Pleban W. Prealbumin in nutrition evaluation. Nutrition 1996;12:255–259.

29. Brugler L, Stankovic A, Bernstein L, Scott F, O'Sullivan-Maillet J. The role of visceral protein markers in protein calorie malnutrition. Clin Chem Lab Med 2002;40:1360–1369.

30. Pepys MB, Hirschfield GM. C-reactive protein: a critical update. J Clin Invest 2003;111:1805–1812.

31. Povoa P. C-reactive protein: a valuable marker of sepsis. Intens Care Med 2002;28:235–243.

32. Matson A, Soni N, Sheldon J. C-reactive protein as a diagnostic test of sepsis in the critically ill. Anaesth Intens Care 1991;19:182–186.

33. Posner BM, Jette AM, Smith KW, Miller DR. Nutrition and health risks in the elderly: the Nutrition Screening Initiative. Am J Public Health 1993;83:972–978.

34. Garry PJ, Vellas BJ. Practical and validated use of the Mini Nutritional Assessment in geriatric evaluation. Nutr Clin Care 1999;2:146–154.

35. Cohendy R, Rubenstein LZ, Eledjam JJ. The Mini Nutritional Assessment-Short Form for preoperative nutritional evaluation of elderly patients. Aging Clin Exp Res 2001;13:293–297.

36. Kovacevich DS, Boney AR, Braunschweig CL, Perez A, Stevens M. Nutrition risk classification: a reproducible and valid tool for nurses. Nutr Clin Pract 1997;12:20–25.

37. Brugler L, DiPrinzio MJ, Bernstein L. The five-year evolution of a malnutrition treatment program in a community hospital. Joint Commission J Qual Impr 1999;25:191–206.

38. Grimes DA. Schultz KF. Uses and abuses of screening tests. The Lancet 2002;359:881–884.

39. Lacey K, Pritchett E. Nutrition Care Process and Model: ADA adopts road map to quality care and outcomes management. J Am Diet Assoc 2003;103:1061–1072.

40. Detsky AS, McLaughlin JR, Baker JP, et al. What is subjective global assessment of nutritional status? J Parenter Enteral Nutr 1987;11:8–13.

41. Baker JP, Detsky AS, Wesson DE, et al. Nutritional assessment: a comparison of clinical judgment and objective measurements. N Engl J Med 1982;306:969–972.

42. Detsky AS, Baker JP, O'Rourke K, et al. Predicting nutrition-associated complications for patients undergoing gastrointestinal surgery. J Parenter Enteral Nutr 1987;11: 440–446.

43. Ferguson M, Capra S, Bauer J, Banks M. Development of a valid and reliable malnutrition screening tool for adult acute hospital patients. Nutrition 1999;15:458–464.

44. Thorsdottir I, Eriksen B, Eysteinsdottir S. Nutritional status at submission for dietetic services and screening for malnutrition at admission to hospital. Clin Nutr 1999;18:15–21.

45. Thorsdottir I., Gunnarsdottir I, Eriksen B. Screening method evaluated by nutritional status measurements can be used to detect malnourishment in chronic obstructive pulmonary disease. J Am Diet Assoc 2001;101:648–654.

46. Laporte M, Villalon L, Payette H. Simple nutrition screening tools for healthcare facilities: development and validity assessment. Can J Diet Pract Res 2001;62:26–34.

47. Jones JM. The methodology of nutritional screening and assessment tools. J Hum Nutr Diet 2002;15:59–71; quiz 73–75.

48. Arrowsmith H. A critical evaluation of the use of nutrition screening tools by nurses. Br J Nurs 1999;8:1483–1490.

49. Kuczmarski MF, Kuczmarski RJ, Najjar M. Effects of age on validity of self-reported height, weight, and body mass index: findings from the Third National Health and Nutrition Examination Survey, 1988–1994. J Am Diet Assoc 2001;101:28–34, quiz 35–36.

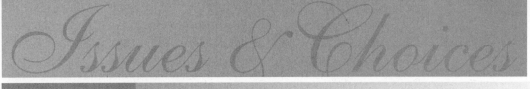

NUTRITION ASSESSMENT
Marion F. Winkler and Riva Touger-Decker

Nutrition assessment is defined as a "systematic process of obtaining, verifying, and interpreting data in order to make decisions about the nature and cause of nutrition-related problems."[1] Implicit in this definition is the recognition that nutrition assessment results from critical thinking by the dietetics professional and the evaluation of data from multiple sources. In other words, assessment is based on clinical judgment using both subjective and objective information. Nutrition assessment is an ongoing, dynamic process that involves not only initial data collection but also continual reassessment and analysis of patient/client/group needs. The specific types of data gathered in the assessment will vary depending on practice settings, individual or groups' present health status, how data are related to outcomes to be measured, recommended guidelines, and whether the assessment is an initial one or a reassessment. Nutrition assessment requires clinical judgment and making comparisons between the information obtained and reliable standards (ideal goals). Its purpose is to obtain adequate information to identify nutrition-related problems and establish the nutrition care plan. Nutrition assessment is initiated by referral and/or screening of individuals or groups for nutrition risk factors.

Dietetics professionals have spent decades trying to design an assessment tool that encompasses the categories of diet history, anthropometric measurements, laboratory markers, subjective data, and physical examination findings, yet debate continues to focus on the reliability and validity of the instrument and how best to differentiate effects of the underlying disease or clinical condition from energy and/or nutrient inadequacy or deficiency. It is generally well accepted that no gold standard exists for determining nutrition status; this is in part due to the lack of a universally accepted definition of malnutrition.[2] Practical difficulties also arise with individual measurement components and their interpretation across the life span and within different care settings.[3,4] Even the 2002 clinical guidelines from the American Society for Parenteral and Enteral Nutrition suggest "in the absence of an outcomes validated approach to nutrition assessment, a combination of history, physical exam, and biochemical parameters should be used to assess the presence of malnutrition."[5] (Updates of these guidelines, when available, may be found at http://www.clinnutr.org.) Realization that nutrition assessment is a systematic process, which requires judgment on the part of the dietetics professional to review, analyze, and synthesize data from multiple sources, moves us closer to defining a nutrition problem and establishing a nutrition diagnosis. It also underscores the need to think of nutrition assessment on a continuum, with requisite monitoring and periodic reassessment at designated intervals and whenever there is a change in the clinical course. Heymsfield stated that nutrition assessment is a

Issues to Ponder

- Why do we assess nutrition status?
- How is the 21st-century patient different from the patient 10 years ago?
- What is the value of nutrition assessment to the dietetics professional and the rest of the healthcare team?
- Are we assessing nutrition diagnoses, the impact of medical or surgical status on nutrition, or both?
- What are the outcomes of the nutrition assessment component of the nutrition care process?

scientific frontier and that "scientific revolutionaries tend to be divergent thinkers who conceive of multiple solutions to a problem . . . outside of the accepted paradigm . . . systematically evaluating their novel and non-mainstream hypotheses."[6]

The focus of nutrition assessment has shifted in the last half century. In the 1950s, the focus was on identifying nutrient deficiencies. From the 1950s through the 1970s, emphasis was placed on recognizing and diagnosing malnutrition. In the 1980s, the process of nutrition risk screening was introduced and comprehensive assessment following screening was the standard of practice. Since the 1990s, the focus of nutrition assessment has expanded to include disease prevention, cost reduction and control, and quality of life, while the process expanded to include physical assessment. In 1996, a *New England Journal of Medicine* article highlighted this new focus, suggesting that what we eat today would be a major factor shaping clinical problems that will be evident in 20 to 30 years.[7] Health promotion, disease prevention, individualized patient/client assessment, and treatment comprise the current focus of nutrition assessment. Dietetics professionals must also consider nutrient/food excesses; uniqueness of age, gender, and ethnicity; and genetic profile in conducting the nutrition assessment. The 21st-century patient/client may be cared for in many different settings, such as the hospital, home, long-term care facility, rehabilitation unit, community health center, or school. The hospitalized patient today is typically older, heavier, more likely to be overweight or obese, a user of more medications (both prescription and over-the-counter agents, including dietary supplements and herbal remedies), and sicker.

TERMINOLOGY

In practice, the terminology that is used to define nutrition assessment has been confusing. Dietetics professionals often interchange the terms "nutrition screening" and "nutrition assessment," when in fact they represent two distinct processes. Nutrition screening (see Chapter 8) is the process of identifying characteristics known to be associated with dietary or nutrition problems to differentiate individuals who are at high risk of nutrition problems or have altered nutrition status, with the goal of categorizing patients according to need for further assessment and intervention.[8,9] Nutrition assessment allows us to gain a measure of actual nutrition status in clinically meaningful terms, with dietary or nutrition-related indicators.[8,9] The reasons to perform nutrition assessment may vary according to the underlying clinical condition or the healthcare or research setting. Nutrition assessment may be conducted to:

- Assess and define the nutrition status of a patient.
- Identify the risk of malnutrition.

- Evaluate the risk of nutrition-related complications that could affect outcome.
- Diagnose a state of malnutrition.
- Measure intake and absorption of food.
- Determine requirements and the type and amount of nutrition support needed.
- Establish a baseline to monitor changes in response to nutrition therapy.

Nutrition assessment measures changes in body composition and associated functional changes that positively or adversely affect clinical outcome.[3] The evaluation of nutrition status includes an examination of alterations caused by over- or undernutrition and a metabolic assessment that focuses on organ system function and the effect of altered metabolism on body composition.[5] This can be illustrated by a practical example, whereby depletion of lean body mass results in a decline of performance status and diminished cardiopulmonary function because it affects breathing and the workload of the heart owing to impaired respiratory muscle strength and altered ventilatory drive.

Issues to Ponder

- In what setting is nutrition assessment being performed?
- Who is paying for services?
- Who is performing the assessment?
- What is the rationale or purpose of the assessment and intervention?
- What instrument or methodological approach should be used?
- How can technology assist in nutrition assessment?
- What outcomes should be measured to determine success?
- What diagnostic nutrition codes should be used?

RELIABILITY AND VALIDITY OF NUTRITION ASSESSMENT TOOLS

The process of nutrition assessment has suffered from a number of methodological issues. First is the confusion among terms, including "nutrition status," "nutrition screening," "malnutrition," and "nutrition assessment," as previously described. Second, nutrition assessment outcomes are reported in different ways. For example, depending on the instrument or technique used, patients may be classified on the basis of normal versus abnormal criteria (well versus malnourished), graded by severity of risk (low, moderate, high), or degree of malnutrition (mild, moderate, severe), or they may receive a nutrition score based on predefined criteria or questions. Third, the procedures used to develop nutrition assessment tools are not uniform and many do not have appropriate evaluation of reliability or validity.[10] Fourth, much of the data used to derive predictive equations utilized in nutrition assessment and body composition estimations were derived in populations that may not be comparable to the setting where they are applied.[11] Furthermore, appropriate reference data for lean body mass and fatness are not yet available for all populations.[12] Waitzberg and Correia added an additional concern as to how accurately staff members document the information necessary to identify nutrition risk in different populations.[11] They cited examples of inaccurate measurements of height and weight and under- or over-estimations of intake.

Lyne and Prowse, in their review of the literature of nutrition assessment, summarized three types of validation studies that have been conducted.[9] Some studies compared results obtained with a nutrition assessment instrument to expert clinical judgment. They suggest that interprofessional issues may present difficulties in comparing studies because the application of nutrition concepts between professions (e.g., nursing and dietetics) may be different. Results of nutrition assessments conducted with a particular instrument or technique have also been compared to physiological or anthropometric measures. Validation using this approach has been fraught with problems owing to the lack of association between nutrition assessment results and indicators such as body weight or serum proteins, which are affected by the underlying disease or clinical condition. Finally, a limited number of nutrition risk assessment tools have been validated concurrently against other instruments (see Table 9-1). These studies are usually limited to specific patient populations and may not be applicable in all settings or to all individuals.

Jones critically appraised 44 published reports of nutrition screening or assessment tools on the basis of scientific merit and by applying principles of sound design and analysis.[10] Of the studies reviewed by Jones, only two-thirds assessed validity, 45% reliability, and 39% both reliability and validity. Only two reports selected factors to be included in the nutrition assessment instrument based on multivariate techniques. Jones suggested that a nutrition assessment tool should be of

TABLE 9-1   Comparison of Nutrition Risk Screening Tool for Dental Professionals to Other Nutrition Risk Screening Tools

TOOL	CRITERIA FOR NUTRITION RISK	SENSITIVITY	SPECIFICITY	PPV	NPV
Nutrition Risk Screening Tool for Dental Professionals[16]	Expert clinical opinion by two registered dietitians	95.19%	46.30%	85.99%	73.53%
Mini Nutritional Assessment[50]	Nutrition assessment by physician trained in nutrition	96%	98%	Not reported	Not reported
Nutrition Risk Classification in Hospitalized Patients[51]	Prealbumin level	84.6%	62.7%	40.7%	93.1%
Nutrition Screening Tool for Healthcare Facilities[52]	Nutrition assessment by dietitian	82%	80%	Not reported	Not reported
Nutrition Screening Tool for use in hospital in UK[53]	Having one or more of four markers of malnutrition (BMI, mid-upper-arm circumference, % weight loss, energy intake)	78%	52%	74%	57%
Adult Nutrition Screening Tool for Community Hospital[54]	Nutrition assessment by dietitian	72%	84%	66%	87%
Nutrition Screening Initiative Checklist[55]	Intake of ≥3 nutrients below 75% RDA				
	Four-point cutoff	60.9%	62.7%	24.9%	Not reported
	Six-point cutoff	36.2%	84.9%	37.9%	Not reported
	Eight-point cutoff	23.2%	94.8%	53.3%	Not reported
Screening Tool for Risk of Undernutrition in the Community[56]	Nutrition assessment by dietitian	Not reported	Not reported	94.6%	81.1%

PPV = positive predictive value, NPV = negative predictive value, RDA = recommended dietary allowance.
Source: Is oral disadvantage predictive of nutrition risk? Doctoral dissertation. Newark, NJ: University of Medicine and Dentistry of New Jersey, 2004. Reprinted with the permission of Diane Rigassio Radler.

benefit to the users, relevant, acceptable, have value, and be reliable and valid.[10] Nutrition assessment instruments should be:

- Published with sufficient information to allow correct usage.
- Based on information known to be associated with malnutrition.
- Pretested to identify and rectify problems with content and format.
- Reliable based on the measure of agreement between the results of a tool when more than one user or rater applies the tool to the same subject.
- Valid based on the agreement between a patient's "true" nutrition status and that indicated by the tool.
- 100% (or close to 100%) sensitive and specific; that is, should correctly classify those with nutrition deficits and those without.

In subsequent publications, Jones offered detailed methodology for development of a nutrition screening or assessment tool using multivariate techniques and for demonstrating reliability and validity.[13–15] Radler and colleagues[16] explored those factors predictive of oral health nutrition risk in an ambulatory clinic population. They found few nutrition risk screening tools in the literature with acceptable sensitivity and specificity. Jones reviewed the nutrition screening literature and found that the majority of nutrition risk screening tools have not been tested for sensitivity or specificity in large populations, thereby significantly limiting their generalizability.[10]

NUTRITION ASSESSMENT: DOES ONE APPROACH FIT ALL?

Nutrition assessment should be patient-specific but may also need to be age-, disease-, and setting-specific. Although all evaluations should include a detailed medical and nutrition history and body composition analysis, there may need to be focused physical examination, selected pertinent laboratory markers, and other objective parameters depending on the impact on health risk.

A thorough nutrition assessment should identify the mechanisms for nutrition deficiency, either a primary deficiency due to inadequate intake or a secondary deficiency due to increased nutrient requirements, altered nutrient utilization, or increased nutrient losses. An assessment should also consider whether the progression of the deficiency has led to an adaptive state (reduced requirements with normal or diminished function) or a malnourished state (depletion of stores with altered nutrient dependent function and clinical symptoms). Nutrition assessment may identify nutrient excess or toxicity. In the case of overweight and obesity, the assessment should focus not only on nutrition status but also on associated health risks. When nutrition assessment confirms a well-nourished healthy individual, it may be important to review family history and environmental exposures in an effort to focus on health promotion, fitness, and well-being.

In the community setting (clinics, home care, physicians' offices, long-term care), the nutrition assessment should focus on factors that may be associated with reduced intake and increased risk of malnutrition as well as health promotion. Components of the evaluation should include[4]:

- Depression
- Disease
- Disease risk based on family history

- Economic resources
- Functional impairment
- Need for assistance with self-care
- Polypharmacy, alcohol, or substance abuse
- Poor dentition
- Recency of hospitalization
- Social isolation
- Swallowing ability
- Weight status

Measurements, if conducted, should ideally be performed with calibrated instruments. Dietetics professionals should also consider how to address patients with edema, fluid overload, heart failure, and dehydration.[4] For patients at risk of nutrition-associated diseases, more focused questions should be incorporated into the medical and diet history. For example, assessment of protein and calcium intake and frequency and intensity of exercise would be pertinent for those at risk of osteoporosis. Similarly, for patients with dyslipidemia, coronary heart disease, or risk of coronary heart disease, assessment should focus on family history, dietary composition and adequacy, weight history, body fat, and physical activity. Pediatric nutrition assessment should incorporate evaluation of feeding behaviors, developmental milestones, and growth (normal growth velocity; catch-up growth).[17] Because of the prevalence of obesity in children, particular attention should be given to the assessment of dietary adequacy, physical activity, and BMI.[18]

Dietetics professionals conducting nutrition assessment of hospitalized patients should examine the characteristics that are likely to preclude adequate oral intake. Patients who are ill or injured usually do not eat because of:

- Effects of pain
- Altered level of cognition
- Dependence on others
- Food delivery issues
- Immobility
- Imposed dietary restrictions
- Lack of desire
- Medications
- Physical constraints
- Treatment limitations
- Withholding of meals for diagnostic tests and procedures

Issues to Ponder

- What is the feasibility of conducting nutrition assessment in the intensive care unit?
- What are the advantages and limitations of measuring biochemical tests?
- What are the limitations of obtaining anthropometrics?
- What methods are available to measure body composition in the acute-care setting?

The ability to predict the clinical course and the resumption of adequate oral food intake is a key component of nutrition assessment in the acute-care setting.[19] Since it has long been known that malnutrition is strongly associated with increased morbidity and mortality among critically ill patients, it is extremely important that risk of development or presence of the condition be documented.[20] Critically ill patients will always be identified at high nutrition risk or assessed as malnourished regardless of the technique employed.[5] Nutrition assessment not only identifies a state induced by nutrient deficiency but also reflects the severity of the metabolic derangement caused by the underlying illness, disease, or injury.

Whatever the setting, assessment parameters should be sensitive, accurate, and reproducible by different dietetics professionals in different populations; broadly applicable; and cost effective. According to Carney and coworkers, "the ultimate clinical utility of any method of nutrition assessment lies in its ability to assess risk of morbidity and mortality related to malnutrition, and to predicate that the patient will benefit."[21]

THE NUTRITION CARE PROCESS

As a first step in addressing these inconsistencies, the American Dietetic Association (ADA) in 2002 introduced the Nutrition Care Process (NCP).[1] The NCP "gives dietetics professionals a consistent and systematic structure and method by which to think critically and make decisions,"[1] "Nutrition assessment" is the first step of the NCP. Assessment provides the foundation for the nutrition diagnosis at the next step of the NCP. The NCP (Figure 9-1) clearly defines where screening and referral initiate the need for assessment.

"Nutrition diagnosis" is the second step of the NCP; it refers to the identification and labeling that describes an actual occurrence, risk of, or potential for developing a nutrition problem that dietetics professionals are responsible for treating independently. The ADA has developed nutrition diagnostic codes for use by practitioners (see Figure 9-2). At the end of the assessment step, data are grouped, analyzed, and synthesized. This helps to identify a nutrition diagnostic code from which a specific nutrition diagnostic statement can be made. Nutrition diagnosis is not synonymous with medical diagnosis. A nutrition diagnosis changes as the patient/client's condition changes. A medical diagnosis remains the same provided the disease or condition exists. A patient/client/group may have the medical diagnosis of "Type 2 diabetes mellitus"; however, after performing a nutrition assessment, dietetics professionals may diagnose, for example, "undesirable overweight status" or "excessive carbohydrate intake." The analysis of assessment data and determination of the nutrition diagnosis provide links to setting realistic and measurable expected outcomes, selecting appropriate interventions, and tracking progress in attaining those expected outcomes.

The third step in the model is "intervention." This step involves planning and implementation of appropriate care for individuals or groups. In the NCP, this step is conceived of as "client-driven." The fourth and final step (although the process is circular, so one would go back to the first step) is monitoring and evaluation. Monitoring specifies the measurement and review of outcomes based on the diagnoses and planned interventions and outcomes. Evaluation is the comparison of findings on monitoring with initial or previous measures.

As the model is implemented, one needs to keep in mind that screening and referral systems are important to "activate" the nutrition care process. The NCP is dependent on accurate and valid screening and referral mechanisms that may be

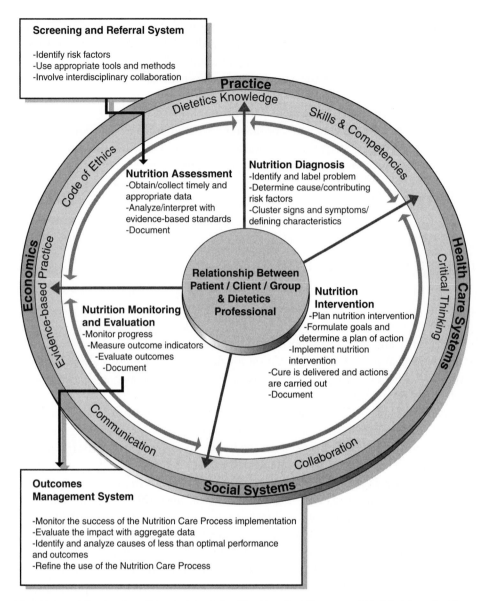

FIGURE 9-1 *The American Dietetic Association Nutrition Care Process and Model. Adapted with permission from Lacey K, Pritchett, E. Nutrition Care Process and Model: ADA adopts road map to quality care and outcomes management. J Am Diet Assoc 2003;103:1061-1072.*

initiated by dietetics or other health professionals. The NCP "provides dietetics professionals with the updated road map to follow the best path for high quality patient/client/group-centered nutrition care."[1] It provides a 21st-century infrastructure from which professionals or institutions can build their nutrition care process.

ROLE OF SERUM PROTEINS IN NUTRITION ASSESSMENT

There is an ongoing clinical discussion with respect to the role of serum proteins in nutrition assessment. Albumin has long been associated with assessment of nutrition

NUTRITION DIAGNOSTIC TERMINOLOGY

INTAKE   NI

Defined as "actual problems related to intake of energy, nutrients, fluids, bioactive substances through oral diet or nutrition support"

Caloric Energy Balance (1)
Defined as "actual or estimated changes in energy (kcal)"

- Hypermetabolism   NI-1.1
  (Increased energy needs)
- Hypometabolism   NI-1.2
  (Decreased energy needs)
- Inadequate energy intake   NI-1.3
- Excessive energy intake   NI-1.4

Oral or Nutrition Support Intake (2)
Defined as "actual or estimated food and beverage intake from oral diet or nutrition support compared with patient goal"

- Inadequate oral food/   NI-2.1
  beverage intake
- Excessive oral food/   NI-2.2
  beverage intake
- Inadequate intake from   NI-2.3
  enteral/parenteral nutrition
  infusion
- Excessive intake from   NI-2.4
  enteral/parenteral nutrition
- Inappropriate infusion of   NI-2.5
  enteral/parenteral nutrition

Fluid Intake (3)
Defined as "actual or estimated fluid intake compared against patient goal"

- Inadequate fluid intake   NI-3.1
- Excessive fluid intake   NI-3.2

Bioactive Substances (4)
Defined as "actual or observed intake of bioactive substances, including single or multiple functional food components, ingredients, dietary supplements, alcohol"

- Inadequate bioactive   NI-4.1
  substance intake
- Excessive bioactive   NI-4.2
  substance intake
- Excessive alcohol intake   NI-4.3

Nutrient (5)
Defined as "actual or estimated intake of specific nutrient groups or single nutrients as compared with desired levels"

- Increased nutrient needs   NI-5.1
  (specify)_____
- Evident protein-energy   NI-5.2
  malnutrition
- Inadequate protein-   NI-5.3
  energy intake
- Decreased nutrient needs   NI-5.4
  (specify)_____
- Imbalance of nutrients   NI-5.2

Fat and Cholesterol (51)
- Inadequate fat intake   NI-51.1
- Excessive fat intake   NI-51.2
- Inappropriate intake   NI-51.3
  of food fats
  (specify)_____

Protein (52)
- Inadequate protein intake   NI-52.1
- Excessive protein intake   NI-52.2
- Inappropriate intake   NI-52.3
  of amino acids
  (specify)_____

Carbohydrate and Fiber Intake (53)
- Inadequate carbohydrate   NI-53.1
  intake
- Excessive carbohydrate   NI-53.2
  intake
- Inappropriate intake of   NI-53.3
  types of carbohydrate
  (specify)_____
- Inconsistent   NI-53.4
  carbohydrate intake
- Inadequate fiber intake   NI-53.5
- Excessive fiber intake   NI-53.6

Vitamin Intake (54)
- Inadequate vitamin   NI-54.1
  intake *(specify)_____*
- Excessive vitamin   NI-54.2
  intake *(specify)_____*

A	C
Thiamin	D
Riboflavin	E
Niacin	K
Folate	Other_____

Mineral Intake (55)
Inadequate mineral intake   NI-55.1
Excessive mineral intake   NI-55.2

Calcium	Iron
Potassium	Zinc
Other	

FIGURE 9-2 *Nutrition diagnostic terminology sheet. Adapted with permission from Nutrition Diagnosis: A Critical Step in the Nutrition Care Process. Chicago: American Dietetic Association, 2006.*

(Continued next page)

NUTRITION DIAGNOSTIC TERMINOLOGY

CLINICAL   **NC**

Defined as "nutritional findings/problems identified as related to medical or physical conditions"

Functional (1)
Defined as "change in physical or mechanical functioning that interferes with or prevents desired nutritional consequences"

- ☐ Swallowing difficulty   NC-1.1
- ☐ Chewing   NC-1.2
  (masticatory) difficulty
- ☐ Breastfeeding difficulty   NC-1.3
- ☐ Altered GI function   NC-1.4

Biochemical (2)
Defined as "change in capacity to metabolize nutrients as a result of medications, surgery, or as indicated by altered lab values"

- ☐ Impaired nutrient utilization NC-2.1
- ☐ Altered nutrition-related   NC-2.2
  laboratory values
- ☐ Food medication interaction   NC-2.3

Weight (3)
Defined as "chronic weight or changed weight status when compared with usual or desired body weight"

- ☐ Underweight   NC-3.1
- ☐ Involuntary weight loss   NC-3.2
- ☐ Overweight/obesity   NC-3.3
- ☐ Involuntary weight gain   NC-3.4

BEHAVIORAL-
ENVIRONMENTAL   **NB**

Defined as "nutritional findings/problems identified as related to knowledge, attitudes/beliefs, physical environment, or food supply and safety"

Knowledge and Beliefs (1)
Defined as "actual knowledge and beliefs as observed or documented"

- ☐ Food and nutrition-related   NB-1.1
  knowledge deficit
- ☐ Harmful beliefs/attitudes   NB-1.2
  about food or nutrition-
  related topics
- ☐ Not ready for diet/   NB-1.3
  lifestyle change
- ☐ Self-monitoring deficit   NB-1.4
- ☐ Disordered eating pattern   NB-1.5
- ☐ Low adherence to nutrition-   NB-1.6
  related recommendations
- ☐ Undesirable food choices   NB-1.7

Physical Activity
and Function (2)
Defined as "actual physical activity, self-care, and quality of life problems as reported, observed or documented"

- ☐ Physical inactivity   NB-2.1
- ☐ Excessive physical activity   NB-2.2
- ☐ Inability to manage self care NB-2.3
- ☐ Impaired ability to   NB-2.4
  prepare foods/meals
- ☐ Poor nutrition quality of life NB-2.5
- ☐ Self-feeding difficulty   NB-2.6

Food Safety and Access (3)
Defined as "actual problems with food access or food safety"

- ☐ Intake of unsafe food   NB-3.1
- ☐ Limited access to food   NB-3.2

Date Identified	Date Resolved

#1 Problem_____

   Etiology_____

   Signs/Symptoms_____

#2 Problem_____

   Etiology_____

   Signs/Symptoms_____

#3 Problem_____

   Etiology_____

   Signs/Symptoms_____

FIGURE 9-2 *Nutrition diagnostic terminology sheet (cont).*

status, and some practitioners still define degree of malnutrition by the serum albumin level.[22] This interpretation is thought to be inaccurate in the acute-care setting. Selberg and Sel's review of the literature over the past 20 years reveals numerous studies in which serum albumin concentration is associated with increased morbidity and mortality in conditions such as old age, critical illness, renal disease, lymphoma, HIV infection, carcinoma, stroke, pneumonia, presence of a gastrostomy tube, and gastrointestinal surgery.[23] Dietetics professionals also associate these same conditions with increased nutrition risk.

Serum albumin has been shown to be a reliable prognostic indicator of morbidity and mortality, but its role as a diagnostic indicator for the state of malnutrition has not been confirmed. In an evaluation of 87,000 noncardiac surgeries as part of the National Veterans Affairs Surgical Risk study, reduced preoperative serum albumin was the strongest predictor of postoperative 30-day mortality.[24] In a subsequent report of 54,215 noncardiac surgery patients, it was demonstrated that a continuous increase in morbidity and mortality occurred as serum albumin progressively decreased.[25]

In multivariable analyses adjusting for potential confounders, patients with a serum albumin level below 3.5 g/dL had a significantly increased risk of renal failure, postoperative atrial fibrillation, and increased length of stay.[26] Patients with a serum albumin level below 2.5 g/dL also had an increased risk of death, low cardiac output, and reexploration for bleeding.[26] In a study of 44 patients admitted to a respiratory intensive care unit (ICU) for nontraumatic medical conditions compounded by respiratory failure, reduced serum albumin concentrations were associated with increased severity of illness and high severity scores; furthermore, albumin levels below 2.8 g/dL predicted mortality.[27]

Delgado-Rodrigues and colleagues, in a prospective cohort study of 2,989 hospitalized patients, demonstrated an adjusted odds ratio of 19 for serum albumin levels and showed an inverse and highly significant relationship with nosocomial infection, an odds ratio of 58 with in-hospital death, and independent, significant, and inverse relationships with length of stay.[28] In a large meta-analysis of cohort studies and controlled clinical trials, hypoalbuminemia was found to be a potent, dose-dependent, independent predictor of poor outcome.[29] Results from this review concluded that each decline of 1.0 g/dL in serum albumin concentration significantly raised the odds of mortality by 137%, morbidity by 89%, prolonged ICU stay by 28%, and length of hospitalization by 71%.[29] The unfavorable sequelae associated with serum albumin in these studies were evident in hospitalized patients overall, in populations undergoing cardiac or noncardiac surgery, and in those suffering from renal dysfunction. These authors also noted a significant association between hypoalbuminemia and poor outcome that persisted after adjustment for BMI and other measures of nutrition status as well as markers of inflammation.[29]

Albumin, prealbumin, retinol-binding protein, transferrin, fibronectin, and insulin-like growth factor make up a group of proteins classified as having a negative acute-phase response, Negative acute-phase proteins decrease during inflammation by at least 25%.[30] Mueller provides an extensive review of this topic, in which he reports that there is overwhelming evidence to suggest that severity of illness and inflammation are the dominant factors determining the direction of acute-phase protein metabolism and serum concentrations.[31] He concludes that the "findings argue against using serum hepatic proteins as indicators of nutritional status although they can indicate severity of illness which is a predictor of future malnutrition." Clochesy and associates suggest that albumin level may be useful for adjusting the risk associated with severity of illness when health outcomes are monitored rather than being used as a unique nutrition assessment variable.[32]

INTERPRETING ABNORMAL LEVELS

The dietetics professional needs to consider what is being assessed and the underlying mechanism contributing to an abnormal laboratory value. It is not sufficient to say, on the basis of a low albumin level, that protein stores are depleted. All proteins in the body are functional; they may be enzymes, muscle, transport carriers, etc. Proteins do not serve as a storage depot for energy. Loss of lean body mass and diminished circulating proteins affect function or performance status. This concept needs to be recognized in conducting nutrition assessment and interpreting the findings. Low albumin levels have prognostic value, but whether the decreased levels are caused by inflammation, disease, or poor nutrient intake cannot be determined simply by looking at the laboratory value. The entire clinical picture must be appreciated.

APPLICATIONS TO PRACTICE

Traditionally, dietetics professionals performing nutrition assessment have taken diet histories, obtained anthropometric measurements, reviewed medical and clinical data, observed patients for signs and symptoms of nutrient deficiency or excess, and calculated nutrient requirements.[33] Today, dietetics professionals obtain vital signs, perform nutrition-focused physical examinations (including head, neck, and oral assessment), assess cranial nerve function, screen for dysphagia, palpate and auscultate the abdomen, evaluate range of motion, and assess functional and performance status.[34] Dietetics professionals also perform indirect calorimetry and bioelectrical impedance studies to better assess energy requirements and evaluate body composition. Mackle and colleagues reported that dietitians who have received training in physical assessment competencies most frequently assessed presence of peripheral edema, evaluated the skin, and performed dysphagia screening.[34] Fewer dietetics professionals conducted an assessment of the head, neck, oral cavity, cranial nerves, and abdomen or listened to breath, heart, or bowel sounds, but these techniques are being taught and applied. The 1995 practice audit conducted by the Commission on Dietetic Registration included "conduct physical assessment" and "perform swallowing evaluation" in the list of skills and tasks.[35] More dietetics professionals were conducting basic physical assessment and evaluating body composition in the 2000 practice audit than that reported in 1995.[36] From 1995 to 2000, the number of dietitians reporting integration of basic physical assessment into their nutrition care increased 28%. The 2000 practice audit of registered dietitian members of ADA indicated that 60% of dietetics professionals integrated basic physical assessment into their nutrition care.[36] Similarly, the role delineation study for certified nutrition support dietitians found nutrition support specialists performed physical examinations among the tasks and skills audited.[37]

Despite its methodological limitations, nutrition assessment is an essential component of the care and management of patients in the acute-, long-term-, and home-care setting and for health promotion and disease prevention programs in the community. Advances in technology allow better assessment of body composition, and these data can nicely complement the history and physical examination. Pichard and colleagues recently analyzed fat-free mass and fat mass in patients using bioelectrical impedance and compared this to classifications on the basis of a subjective global assessment (SGA) and BMI.[38] They found that the fat-free mass index was significantly associated with an increased length of stay and was a more sensitive determinant than using percent weight loss or BMI alone. A study by Barbosa-Silva and colleagues also compared bioelectrical impedance analyses in the diagnosis of malnutrition with the SGA score.[39] Their results suggested that some alterations in tissue electrical properties with malnutrition can be detected by bioelectrical impedance and that this technique is a complementary method in nutrition assessment. Bioelectrical impedance has also been used to assess muscle and adipose tissue at single sites, including skinfold thickness. Air-displacement plethysmography is a technique used to measure body composition on the basis of the same whole-body measurement principle as hydrostatic weight but using air-displacement technology instead of water. It is now considered to be more precise than hydrodensitometry, making it a potentially useful tool both in the clinical setting and in fieldwork.[40]

FUTURE PERSPECTIVES

Metabolic assessment is taking on new meaning as we increase our understanding of cellular abnormalities associated with disease and the impact of nutrition therapies. Knowledge of skeletal muscle catabolism and the resultant loss of both structural and functional proteins, impaired muscle function, and alterations in body composition have grown from skeletal muscle energetics.[41] Technological advances are providing new insights in our understanding of structure and function. For example, the use of body cell mass and fat-free mass as markers of metabolically active tissue—estimated by underwater weighing, neutron activation, dual-photon absorptiometry, and multicomponent methods—has added to our knowledge of body composition at the organ and tissue level and to resting metabolic rate.[42] More is known about the regulation of lipolysis and glucose metabolism at the tissue level thanks to minimally invasive sampling tools such as microdialysis.[43] Noninvasive technology, such as miniaturization of assays, is also contributing to more acceptable diagnostic tests of nutrition status for field studies and community-based nutrition research.[44] In addition, nutrition biomarkers are being used in large-scale population surveys and epidemiologic studies to provide measures of nutrition status and may someday be applicable to the clinical setting.[45]

Personal metabolomics may be the next-generation nutrition assessment.[46] Metabolomics is the analysis of small molecules and metabolites and metabolic flux in biological fluids, cells, and tissues using mass spectrometry, nuclear magnetic resonance, and chromatographic techniques.[47,48] This approach may be useful for identifying the metabolic status of an individual or the effects of diet and individual metabolism on nutrition status.[48] Metabolic profiling, a term often used to describe these analyses, is helping researchers learn more about glucose, amino acid, and fatty acid metabolism. Metabolite profiles will provide biomarkers for diagnostic and therapeutic monitoring.[47] This technology should lead to the quantification of entire classes of metabolites. "The role of nutritionists will be to build the knowledge that explains the variations in metabolism among individuals ultimately linking functional genomics, proteomics, metabolite concentrations, metabolic regulation, and accurate phenotypic information."[49] It will be necessary to build an integrated knowledge base of all metabolites and their responsiveness to nutrition.[48]

REFERENCES

1. Lacey K, Pritchett E. Nutrition Care Process and Model: ADA adopts road map to quality care and outcomes management. J Am Diet Assoc 2003;103:1061–1072.
2. Klein S, Kinney J, Jeejeebhoy K, et al. Nutrition support in clinical practice: review of published data and recommendations for future research directions. National Institutes of Health, American Society for Parenteral and Enteral Nutrition, and American Society Clinical Nutrition. J Parenter Enteral Nutr 1997;21:133–156.
3. Baxter JP. Problems of nutritional assessment in the acute setting. Proc Nutr Soc 1999;58:39–46.
4. Edington J. Problems of nutrition assessment in the community. Proc Nutr Soc 1999;58:47–51.
5. ASPEN Board of Directors and the Clinical Guidelines Task Force. Guidelines for the use of parenteral and enteral nutrition in adult and pediatric patients. J Parenter Enteral Nutr 2002;26(suppl):11SA.
6. Heymsfield SB. Nutrition support at the scientific frontier. J Parenter Enteral Nutr 1997;21:252–258.
7. Kumanyika S. Improving our diet—still a long way to go. N Eng J Med 1996;335:738–740.
8. Barrocas A, Belcher D, Champagne C, Jastram C. Nutrition assessment practical approaches. Clin Geriatr Med 1995;11:675–713.
9. Lyne PA, Prowse MA. Methodological issues in the development and use of instruments to assess patient nutritional status on the level of risk of nutritional compromise. J Adv Nurs 1999;30:835–842.
10. Jones JM. The methodology of nutritional screening and assessment tools. J Hum Nutr Diet 2002;15:59–71, quiz 73–75.
11. Waitzberg DL, Correia MI. Nutritional assessment in the hospitalized patient. Curr Opin Clin Nutr Metab Care 2003;6:531–538.
12. Davidson J, Getz M. Nutrition screening and assessment of anthropometry and bioelectrical impedance in the frail elderly: a clinical appraisal of methodology in a clinical setting. J Nutr Elder 2004;23:47–63.
13. Jones JM. Development of a nutritional screening or assessment tool using a multivariate technique. Nutrition 2004;20:298–306.
14. Jones JM. Reliability of nutritional screening and assessment tools. Nutrition 2004;20:307–311.
15. Jones JM. Validity of nutritional screening and assessment tools. Nutrition 2004;20:312–317.
16. Radler DR. Is oral disadvantage predictive of nutrition risk? Doctoral dissertation. Newark, NJ: University of Medicine and Dentistry of New Jersey, 2004.
17. Mascarenhas MR, Zemel B, Stallings VA. Nutritional assessment in pediatrics. Nutrition 1998;14:105–115.
18. Barlow SE, Dietz WH. Obesity evaluation and treatment: expert committee recommendations. The Maternal and Child Health Bureau, Health Resources and Services Administration and the US Department of Health and Human Services. Pediatrics 1998;102:E29.
19. Pomp A, Bates B, Albina JE. Specialized nutritional support in surgical patients. Prob Gen Surg 1988;5:271–295.
20. Dempsey DT, Mullen JL, Buzby GP. The link between nutritional status and clinical outcome: can nutritional intervention modify it? Am J Clin Nutr 1988;47(suppl 2):352–256.
21. Carney DE, Meguid MM. Current concepts in nutritional assessment. Arch Surg 2002;137:42–45.
22. Fuhrman MP. The albumin-nutrition connection: separating myth from fact. Nutrition 2002;18:199–200.
23. Selberg O, Sel S. The adjunctive value of routine biochemistry in nutritional assessment of hospitalized patients. Clin Nutr 2001;20:477–485.
24. Khuri SF, Daley J, Henderson W, et al. Risk adjustment of the postoperative mortality rate for the comparative assessment of the quality of surgical care: results of the National Veterans Affairs Surgical Risk Study. J Am Coll Surg 1997;185:315–327.
25. Gibbs J, Cull W, Henderson W, Daley J, Hur K, Khuri SF. Preoperative serum albumin level as a predictor of operative mortality and morbidity: results from the National VA Surgical Risk Study. Arch Surg 1999;134:36–42.
26. Engelman DT, Adams DH, Byrne JG, et al. Impact of body mass index and albumin on morbidity and mortality after cardiac surgery. J Thorac Cardiovasc Surg 1999;118:866–873.

27. Ravasco P, Camilo ME, Gouveia-Oliveira A, Adam S, Brum G. A critical approach to nutritional assessment in critically ill patients. Clin Nutr 2002;21:73–77.

28. Delgado-Rodriguez M, Medina-Cuadros M, Gomez-Ortega A, et al. Cholesterol and serum albumin levels as predictors of cross infection, death, and length of hospital stay. Arch Surg 2002;137:805–812.

29. Vincent JL, Dubois MJ, Navickis RJ, Wilkes MM. Hypoalbuminemia in acute illness: is there a rationale for intervention? A meta-analysis of cohort studies and controlled trials. Ann Surg 2003;237:319–334.

30. Gabay C, Kushner I. Acute-phase proteins and other systemic responses to inflammation. N Eng J Med 1999;340:448–454.

31. Mueller C. True or false: serum hepatic protein concentrations measure nutritional status. Support Line 2004;26:8–16.

32. Clochesy JM, Davidson LJ, Piper-Caulkins E, Carno MA, Bauldoff GS. Use of serum albumin level in studying clinical outcomes. Outcomes Mgt Nurs Pract 1999;3:61–66.

33. Winkler MF. Change: challenge and opportunity for nutrition support dietitians. Nutrition 1999;15:805–808.

34. Mackle TJ, Touger-Decker R, O'Sullivan Maillet J, Holland BK. Registered dietitians' use of physical assessment parameters in professional practice. J Am Diet Assoc 2003;103:1632–1638.

35. Kane MT, Cohen AS, Smith ER, Lewis C, Reidy C. 1995 Commission on Dietetic Registration Dietetics Practice Audit. J Am Diet Assoc 1996;96:1292–1301.

36. Rogers D, Leonberg BL, Broadhurst CB. 2000 Commission on Dietetic Registration Dietetics Practice Audit. J Am Diet Assoc 2002;102:270–292.

37. Nutrition Support Dietitians Role Delineation Survey. Silver Spring, MD: National Board of Nutrition Support Certification, 1997.

38. Pichard C, Kyle UG, Morabia A, Perrier A, Vermeulen B, Unger P. Nutritional assessment: lean body mass depletion at hospital admission is associated with an increased length of stay. Am J Clin Nutr 2004;79:613–618.

39. Barbosa-Silva MC, Barros AJ, Post CL, Waitzberg DL, Heymsfield SB. Can bioelectrical impedance analysis identify malnutrition in preoperative nutrition assessment? Nutrition 2003;19:422–426.

40. Elia M, Ward LC. New techniques in nutritional assessment: body composition methods. Proc Nutr Soc 1999;58:33–38.

41. Jacobs DO, Wong M. Metabolic assessment. World J Surg 2000;24:1460–1467.

42. Guigoz Y, Lauque S, Vellas BJ. Identifying the elderly at risk for malnutrition. The Mini Nutritional Assessment. Clin Geriatr Med 2002;18:737–757.

43. Binnert C, Tappy L. Microdialysis in the intensive care unit: a novel tool for clinical investigation or monitoring? Curr Opin Clin Nutr Metab Care 2002;5:185–188.

44. Solomons NW. Methods for the measurement of nutrition impact and adaptation of laboratory methods into field settings to enhance and support community-based nutrition research. Nutr Rev 2002;60:S126–S131.

45. Potischman N. Biologic and methodologic issues for nutritional biomarkers. J Nutr 2003;133:875S–880S.

46. German JB, Roberts MA, Watkins SM. Personal metabolomics as a next generation nutritional assessment. J Nutr 2003;133:4260–4266.

47. Schmidt C. Metabolomics takes its place as latest up-and-coming "omic" science. J Natl Cancer Inst 2004;96:732–734.

48. Watkins SM, German JB. Toward the implementation of metabolomic assessments of human health and nutrition. Curr Opin Biotechnol 2002;13:512–516.

49. German JB, Roberts MA, Fay L, Watkins SM. Metabolomics and individual metabolic assessment: the next great challenge for nutrition. J Nutr 2002;132:2486–2487.

50. Guigoz Y, Vellas B, Garry PJ. Assessing the nutritional status of the elderly: the Mini Nutritional Assessment as part of the geriatric evaluation. Nutr Rev 1996;54:S59–S65.

51. Kovacevich DS, Boney AR, Braunschweig CL, Perez A, Stevens M. Nutrition risk classification: a reproducible and valid tool for nurses. Nutr Clin Pract 1997;12:20–25.

52. Laporte M, Villalon L, Payette H. Simple nutrition screening tools for healthcare facilities: development and validity assessment. Can J Diet Pract Res 2001;62:26–34.

53. Burden ST, Bodey S, Bradburn YJ, et al. Validation of a nutrition screening tool: testing the reliability and validity. J Hum Nutr Diet 2001;14:269–275.

54. Elmore MF, Wagner DR, Knoll DM, et al. Developing an effective adult nutrition screening tool for a community hospital. J Am Diet Assoc 1994;94:1113–1118, 1121; quiz 119–120.

55. Posner BM, Jette AM, Smith KW, Miller DR. Nutrition and health risks in the elderly: The Nutrition Screening Initiative. Am J Public Health 1993;83:972–978.

56. Ward J, Close J, Little J, et al. Development of a screening tool for assessing risk of undernutrition in patients in the community. J Hum Nutr Diet 1998;11:323–330.

CHAPTER

10

MEASURING NUTRIENT INTAKE: ARE THE TOOLS VALID FOR CLINICAL PRACTICE AND/OR RESEARCH?

Phyllis J. Stumbo

Diet is an important but sometimes overlooked factor in medical practice. Diet may affect the absorption and action of medication; it plays a prominent role in disease prevention; and it is a central part of health promotion. It may even constitute the primary treatment of a disease. Thus the measurement of dietary intake plays a major role in clinical and research dietetics.

This chapter contrasts dietary methods used for research and those common in the clinical setting. Both sectors make important contributions to the practice of dietary assessment. Many research questions grow from experience in the clinical area. More has been written about research methods, so this factor may seem to be overemphasized here. A major role of the dietetics professional is to translate research findings into clinical practice; therefore, emphasis on research findings serves to improve clinical practice. More needs to be known about nutrition assessment from the dietetics practitioner's perspective, however, as a way to better inform the research process. Dietetics professionals possess a rich store of knowledge that is more difficult to tap, because publication is not rewarded in the clinical setting and fewer outlets are available for disseminating clinical knowledge than are available for research findings. Clinical knowledge is becoming better known since the Internet has provided a structure, in the form of list serves, for dietetics practitioners to share information among themselves and with scholars, who hopefully will translate this dialogue into published reports of practice knowledge.

Dietetics practitioners typically have a dietary assessment objective that differs from typical research objectives. The clinical goal is usually to assess current intake to help develop and guide a nutrition care plan. Although long-term intake is of considerable interest, it is usually not the dominant goal. In the clinical setting diet is seldom used to determine cause of disease or serve as a baseline from which to assess effectiveness of treatment. The nutritional epidemiologist, on the other hand, relies on dietary assessment to capture a subject's habitual intake, which forms the basis for a study hypothesis. The hypothesis that food intake leads to specific health outcomes often rests on the knowledge of an individual's lifetime (or at least long-term) intake. Thus, the ability of the data collection method to reflect habitual food intake is critical for the epidemiologist but of limited concern for the busy practitioner. Methods that are suitable for most clinical purposes may be of limited benefit to the epidemiologist.

Despite the differences in purpose, accuracy in assessment of intake is a goal for both dietetics practitioners and researchers. The dietetics practitioner is mindful of treatment effectiveness, and each new client becomes a case study used to formulate and refine ideas about the effectiveness of dietary strategies.

The line between research and clinical practice is often blurred, with professionals from both being interested in the most accurate method that their time and budget can afford.

DIETARY ASSESSMENT METHODS

Dietary assessment methods have been classified into five groups for the purpose of describing the varied characteristics of tools in common use. These groups are unstructured interview, food records, dietary recalls, food frequency questionnaires, and brief dietary screeners. The division of tools into five categories suggests that they are distinctly different instruments. Actually the instruments have many commonalties. For example, an unstructured interview may involve a review of food intake from a list of food groups, thus mimicking the food frequency questionnaire. A food record may involve probing to elicit forgotten foods as one would in reviewing a dietary recall. A food frequency questionnaire and screener differ primarily in length, especially in number of foods listed and number of nutrients reported.

The apparent simplicity of recording intake as it is consumed is deceptive. Careful diet studies have found that approximately 80% of adults who record or recall their food consumption underestimate their true intake by an average of 700 calories.[1] The presumed reasons for reporting error are varied, including inaccurate estimates of portion size or description of foods eaten, forgetting to record part or all of some snacks or meals, and the tendency to eat less when food intake is being recorded. Knowing a person's habitual intake would be helpful for planning an intervention, but reporting error and the tremendous variability in amounts consumed from day to day makes estimating "usual" or "typical" intake a challenge.[2–10]

Various groups of dietetics practitioners and researchers have favorite ways to gather information about intake and different notions about accuracy of the methods they use. Researchers in England and the rest of Europe consider a 7-day weighed food record as the gold standard for intake,[11] whereas researchers in the United States typically rely on a 3- to 4-day record or recall covering 1 weekend and 2 to 3 weekdays.[12] Selecting a method for research requires tradeoffs, either selecting methods that minimize subject burden to facilitate capturing data from many individuals or seeking highly motivated subjects who are willing to provide more detailed data. Each strategy has its place; the real problem is in knowing when the burden caused by detailed data collection is justified and when less rigorously collected information is sufficient.

In an effort to simplify dietary assessment, researchers have pioneered the use of short food lists to assess intake of key foods that provide most of the nutrient(s) of current interest. A list-based questionnaire is an economical way to survey the food intake of large groups of subjects. These lists may be extensive, designed to capture intake of a wide range of nutrients, or composed of fewer foods, designed to capture a single or limited group of nutrients. Comprehensive lists and their accompanying response forms are called food frequency questionnaires (FFQs) and more abbreviated instruments are often called "dietary screeners." The following section gives a brief overview of methods commonly used to collect dietary intake data and some information about the accuracy of each method.

UNSTRUCTURED INTERVIEW

The unstructured interview is probably the most common clinical assessment tool, beginning with the question, "Tell me what you usually eat." The aim is to gather enough information about number and type of meals usually eaten, the resources for obtaining food, facilities for preparing and eating food, difficulties encountered in obtaining food, and the types of food usually eaten. The information is recorded as a brief or detailed clinical note and processed mentally as the dietetics practitioner formulates a judgment about the nutritional quality of the intake. Data from the interview are used as a framework for developing a therapeutic plan.

Assessment of the unstructured interview is done by classifying the foods reported into groups based on their nutritional composition; these groups are then used to devise a dietary treatment plan. Numerous grouping schemes are used by dietetics practitioners to achieve clinical objectives. When general nutrition is the focus, the food guide pyramid may provide the basis for analysis. This tool divides foods into six groups (see Table 10-1).

The dietetics practitioner usually has an ideal pattern of intake in mind and will compare the subject's responses to this ideal pattern. Recommendations will often center on over- or underrepresented food groups.

When the clinical objective is control of either calories or macronutrients, a slightly different food grouping system is used where foods are classified into groups with similar macronutrient and energy values. An exchange system developed cooperatively by the American Dietetic and American Diabetes Associations serves a variety of clinical purposes. The exchange system (Table 10-2) also has six groups but is based not on overall nutrition but on carbohydrate, protein, fat, and total energy content of the foods. Treatments for other diseases require clinicians to use other food grouping systems, such as foods high and low in potassium and sodium for diets used in treatment of renal disease or protein control in the treatment of liver disease.

No studies have evaluated the validity of the unstructured interview, largely because its structure and content depends on the practitioner's experience and interview style. The assumption is that the method is a useful clinical tool but not precise enough to determine habitual nutrient intake for research purposes. A form such as the one shown in Figure 10-1 may be used to guide and facilitate evaluating the unstructured interview.

TABLE 10-1	Nutrient Contribution of the 2005 Pyramid Servings for Use in Assessing Diets[a]		
		RECOMMENDED SERVINGS OR AMOUNTS	
GROUP	**IMPORTANT FEATURE**	**1,600 CALORIES**	**2,600 CALORIES**
Sugar and fats	To be limited in use	5 tsp oil; 130 calories	8 tsp oil; 410 calories
Dairy	Calcium, potassium, and vitamin D	3 cups	3 cups
Meat and alternates	Protein, iron, zinc, magnesium, B vitamins	5 oz	6.5 oz
Vegetables	Vitamins A, C, E; folate, fiber, potassium	2 cups	3.5 cups
Fruit	Vitamins C, A; folate, fiber, potassium	1.5 cups	2 cups
Grains	Carbohydrate, fiber, B vitamins, folate, iron; include whole grains	5 oz	9 oz

[a]Available at: http://www.mypyramid.gov/pyramid/index.html. Accessed February 26, 2006.

CALORIE COUNTS

The diabetic exchange list (Table 10-2) is equally useful in nutrition planning and assessment. As a planning tool it is used to develop diet patterns for energy and carbohydrate control. Its use in assessment is often referred to as a "calorie count," because the primary interest is often to monitor the energy value of the diet. For a person well versed in food composition, the exchange system is extremely simple and efficient for calculating intake of energy and the energy nutrients. The outpatient dietetics practitioner can quickly assess the energy value of reported intake, comment on which foods or meals are typically the most energy dense, and recommend alternative foods from an assessment based solely on a calculation system committed to memory. The hospital-based dietetics practitioner uses this system to monitor intake of extremely ill patients who are unable to take in enough food to cover their energy needs and whose health status is at risk of deteriorating rather than improving unless adequate nourishment is provided. The calorie count system is a convenient tool to monitor intake in the acute setting.

In the hospital setting, the calorie count system relies on the cooperation of nursing and dietetics staff, with nursing carefully recording the amount of food eaten and the dietetics professional later determining the calorie intake and, if requested, the carbohydrate, protein, and/or fat intake based on the diabetic exchange system. The nursing staff that record intakes may not be certain of the amount of food served to the patient but rather must record intake based on what remains on the tray. Dietetics staff usually develop the rules for recording intake that are followed by the nursing staff. Communicating between services is sometimes delayed, which can contribute to tension between services. Many dietetics professionals try to avoid this source of stress and campaign to keep the use of calorie counts to a minimum so as to avoid unnecessary tension when the information is not critical to patient care or is not used by the physician in making medical decisions. Calorie counts are most valuable in pediatrics, burn units, and surgical intensive care, where energy needs are great for healing and growth, and anywhere else in the clinical setting where personnel rotations may jeopardize continuity of care.

TABLE 10-2	Food Exchange Lists for Carbohydrate and Calorie Control			
GROUP	**CALORIES**	**CARBOHYDRATE**	**PROTEIN**	**FAT**
Starch, 1 serving	80	15	3	0
Fruit, 1 serving	60	15	0	0
Milk, skim, 1 cup	80	12	8	0–3
Milk, 2% fat, 1 cup	120	12	8	5
Milk, whole, 1 cup	150	12	8	8
Vegetables, 1 serving	25	5	2	0
Meat, lean, 1 oz	50	0	7	1–3
Meat, medium fat, 1 oz	75	0	7	5
Meat, high fat, 1 oz	100	0	7	8
Fat, 1 tsp or serving	45	0	0	5

Source: The American Dietetic Association and the American Diabetes Association, Exchange Lists for Meal Planning. Chicago: American Dietetic Association, 1995.

Name	Usual Intake/24 Hour Recall
Address	
Telephone:	
Diet Concerns:	

Height:	cm	Weight:	kg
Age		Birthdate	
BEE:		TEE:	
Bee Women = 655 + (9.46*ht) + (1.86*wt)-(4.68*age)			
Bee Men = 66.47 + (13.75*ht) + (5*wt)-(6.76*age)			
TEE= BEE * Activity Factor (1.2 sedentary, 1.5 active)			

Usual Physical Activity	Supplement Intake (years taken):

Diet Modifications/Concerns

		Lab Data					
Date	Weight	Notes:	Date Lab				

FIGURE 10-1   *Form to guide unstructured interview.*

FOOD DIARY

Outside the hospital setting, the patient or client is the source of information. One of the many ways to assess intake in a free-living population is by asking clients to record what they eat, either as a food log or diary. A food diary is written by the client and consists of a carefully recorded list of everything eaten and drunk for a day or more. Dietetics practitioners and researchers typically ask for at least a 3-day diary because of the normal variability expected in food intake from day to day. The specific days recorded are also important, with both weekdays and weekends included, because eating habits often change when the weekday routine is broken, and the weekend offers a wider variety of eating places and opportunities.[13] Although 3 days is commonly chosen as a reasonable sample of intake, careful stud-

Food Probes:

Protein Foods:

Snack Foods & Sweets:

Fruits and Vegetables:

Type of Fat:

Calcium Sources:

Fiber-rich Foods:

Problem List:

Appetite:

Constipation:

Diarrhea:

Nausea:

Heartburn:

Vomiting:

Teeth:

Hair, skin, vitality:

BMI Guide

Underweight	<18.5
Normal	18.5-24.9
Overweight	25.0-29.9
Obesity I	30-34.9
Obesity II	35-39.9
Obesity III	$\geq$40

Waist Circumference
Normal:
Men $\leq$102 cm ($\leq$40 in)
Women $\leq$88 cm ($\leq$35 in)

BMI	19	20	21	22	23	24	25	26	27	28	29	30	31	32	33	34	35
Height (inches)	Body Weight (pounds)																
58	91	96	100	105	110	115	119	124	129	134	138	143	148	153	158	162	167
59	94	99	104	109	114	119	124	128	133	138	143	148	153	158	163	168	173
60	97	102	107	112	118	123	128	133	138	143	148	153	158	163	168	174	179
61	100	106	111	116	122	127	132	137	143	148	153	158	164	169	174	180	185
62	104	109	115	120	126	131	136	142	147	153	158	164	169	175	180	186	191
63	107	113	118	124	130	135	141	146	152	158	163	169	175	180	186	191	197
64	110	116	122	128	134	140	145	151	157	163	169	174	180	186	192	197	204
65	114	120	126	132	138	144	150	156	162	168	174	180	186	192	198	204	210
66	118	124	130	136	142	148	155	161	167	173	179	186	192	198	204	210	216
67	121	127	134	140	146	153	159	166	172	178	185	191	198	204	211	217	223
68	125	131	138	144	151	158	164	171	177	184	190	197	203	210	216	223	230
69	128	135	142	149	155	162	169	176	182	189	196	203	209	216	223	230	236
70	132	139	146	153	160	167	174	181	188	195	202	209	216	222	229	236	243
71	136	143	150	157	165	172	179	186	193	200	208	215	222	229	236	243	250
72	140	147	154	162	169	177	184	191	199	206	213	221	228	235	242	250	258
73	144	151	159	166	174	182	189	197	204	212	219	227	235	242	250	257	265
74	148	155	163	171	179	186	194	202	210	218	225	233	241	249	256	264	272
75	152	160	168	176	184	192	200	208	216	224	232	240	248	256	264	272	279
76	156	164	172	180	189	197	205	213	221	230	238	246	254	263	271	279	287

FIGURE 10-1   *Form to guide unstructured interview (cont).*

DIETARY INTERVENTION STUDY IN CHILDREN

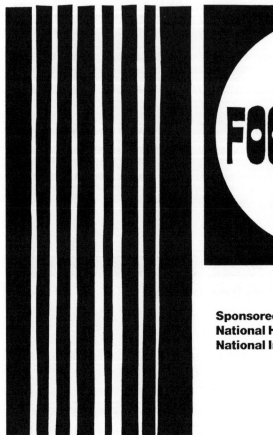
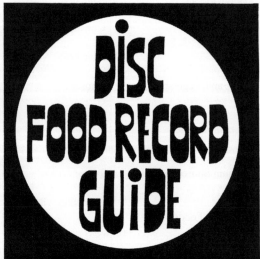

**Sponsored by the
National Heart, Lung, and Blood Institute
National Institutes of Health**

FIGURE 10-2   *DISC Food Record Guide. Shown are selected pages from a 35-page booklet used in the Dietary Intervention Study in Children for training and as a visual aid for estimating intake among children. Reprinted with permission from Van Horn et al.* [23]

ies show that longer periods are required to assess intake of nutrients with a high day-to-day variation, such as typical intakes of vitamin A and iron.[14]

Diaries kept by untrained clients often do not include enough detail about each food to make accurate assessment possible. Subjects need to be trained in how to record food and beverage intake, and diaries should be reviewed with the client to add essential details about ingredients, preparation methods, brands, and other descriptive details that materially influence nutritive values of the food. The dietetics practitioner who plans to collect multiple food records over an extended treatment period may simplify training initially and rely on repeated follow-up visits to fill in missing details, expecting the client to gain skill in record keeping with continued practice. The researcher who will use data obtained from every single diary recorded, however, requires a detailed training process to ensure that each diary from first to last has adequate details to enable locating the appropriate food on a food composition database. Training may involve watching a video training tape,[15] practicing with three-dimensional food models,[16,17] using two-dimensional sheets and booklets,[18,19] and/or practicing with real food. Figure 10-2 shows selected

Squares and Rectangles

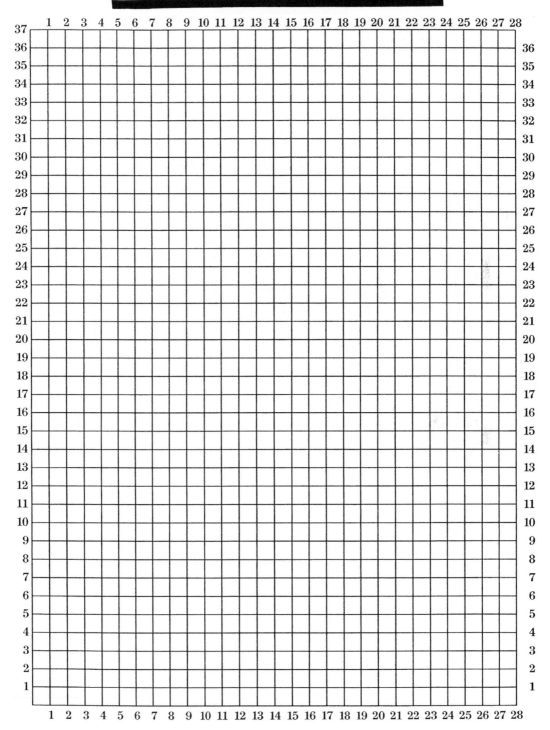

FIGURE 10-2   *DISC Food Record Guide (cont).*
Note: Not to scale.

Circles

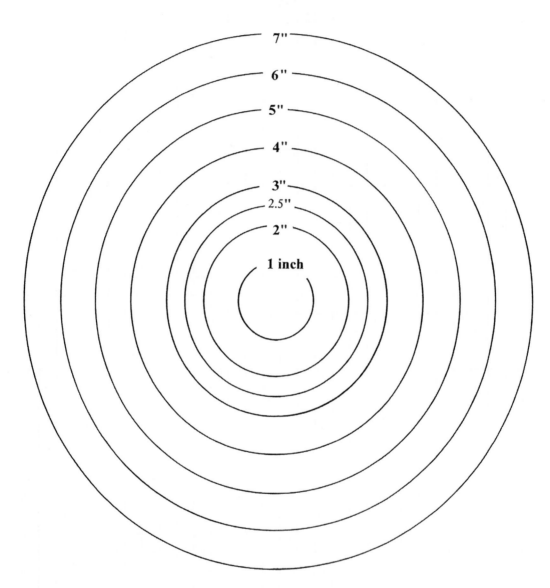

FIGURE 10-2   *DISC Food Record Guide (cont).*
Note: not to scale.

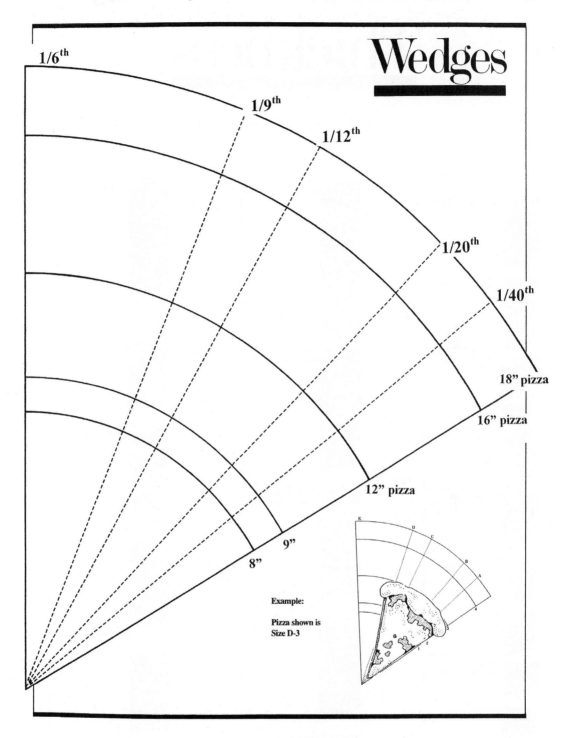

FIGURE 10-2   *DISC Food Record Guide (cont).*
Note: not to scale.

Thickness

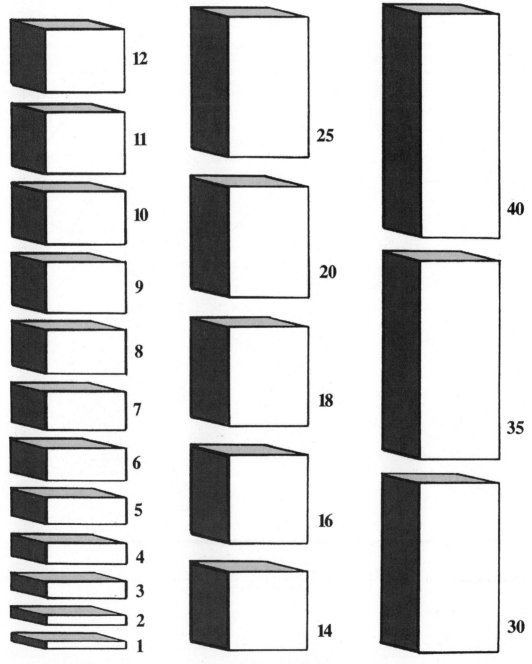

FIGURE 10-2   *DISC Food Record Guide (cont).*
Note: not to scale.

pages form a booklet used for training in the Dietary Intervention Study in Children (DISC).[20] Research subjects and clients need to be instructed in good record-keeping procedures and reminded to describe everything consumed. A carefully designed food diary is helpful in prompting clients to record important details about their intake. Diary forms take many shapes; Figure 10-3 (A and B) shows two styles, the first is a one-page trifold that fits easily in a pocket or bag; the second consists of several pages, giving ample room to carefully record details about foods consumed. The smaller version is more likely to be carried for use away from home, but the larger form facilitates recording greater detail.

Recording the size of portions eaten can be difficult in some circumstances. Recording packaged foods is convenient, since the weight of the portion is often printed on the label, and in fast-food and chain restaurants, the portion is standardized. In independent restaurants and at home, however, portion sizes can vary widely. Dietetics practitioners have suggested comparing portion sizes to common objects that might be found around the house or even parts of the body, such as the thumb for a chunk of cheese or the palm of the hand for a hamburger. Ellen Schuster, of the Oregon Extension Service, compiled a list of several familiar objects that can be referred to in describing food portions (Figure 10-4). The U.S. Department of Agriculture (USDA) Food Survey Research Group developed a food model booklet for use with the 1994–1996 Continuing Survey of Food Intake of Individuals (CSFII) containing life-size photographs and drawings of food portion sizes (see sample pages in Figure 10-5). Nutritionists developing this tool thought it was important that the food models were life-size. The booklet measured 11 by 12 inches and is of a general nature but is not available for purchase. Nutritionists at the General Clinical Research Center used a digital camera to develop their own food models, as shown in Figure 10-6. These models are available at http://www.medicine.uiowa.edu/gcrc/who/nutrientintakeassessment.htm (scroll down to "Portion Size Estimation"). Two-dimensional portion models often form part of the assessment package given to subjects to use at home in recording food intake (see Figures 10-2, 10-5, and 10-6). The National Health and Nutrition Survey (NHANES) conducted by the U.S. Department of Health and Human Services uses the CSFII food models for telephone interviews and a set of three-dimensional portion-size aids (Figure 10-7) to facilitate accurate portion-size estimates in face-to-face interviews.[18]

The most accurate way to report size of food portions eaten is to weigh the food before it is eaten. Numerous researchers use this method for documenting portion size.[12] The quality of the scale determines in large part how easy it will be to keep a weighed diary. A wide variety of scales are available, but small postal scales are not satisfactory for food work. The most useful scales have a capacity of 1,000 grams or more and have a mechanism to allow for taring the scale to zero after the empty food plate is placed on the scale. With this functionality, the food can then be placed on the plate and the weight of the food recorded. Then the plate with the food can be taken to the table. When the empty plate along with leftovers is placed back on the scale after eating, the exact weight of the portion eaten can be determined. A high-quality scale that makes this process easy is relatively costly, and keeping track of the scales and retrieving them for the next client or subject requires bookkeeping and sometimes repeated attempts to retrieve the equipment, so that using this method is usually restricted to very serious endeavors. Also, the weighing of food requires a highly motivated subject who will use the scale on a regular basis.

Guidelines for recording foods in your food diary:

1) Record day and date.
2) Record all foods and beverages consumed for each day.
3) Describe each food and beverage item.
   Examples: chocolate milk, 2% milk, fried chicken leg, scrambled eggs.
4) Give brand names when possible.
   Examples: Snickers® candy bar, Wheaties®, Gatorade®.
5) Estimate foods eaten in common measurements:
   Cup = c.
   Tablespoon = Tbsp.
   Teaspoon = tsp.
   Examples: ½ c. apple juice, 1 Tbsp. butter, 1 c. tuna casserole, 1 tsp. sugar.
6) Record amount of extras.
   Examples: 1 slice of toast with 1 tsp. butter and 1 tsp. of jelly; ½ c. oatmeal with 2 tsp. sugar and ½ c. 2 % milk; ¼ c. mashed potatoes with 2 Tbsp. gravy.
7) When completed mail this form back to your dietitian. Be sure to include your name and return address.

The University of Iowa Hospitals and Clinics
Food and Nutrition Services, W146 GH
200 Hawkins Drive
Iowa City, IA 52242-1051

RD

3 Day Food Diary

Name: _____	Address: _____	
Day of Week: ____ Date: ____	Day of Week: ____ Date: ____	Day of Week: ____ Date: ____
Time	Food/Beverage & Amount	Time	Food/Beverage & Amount	Time	Food/Beverage & Amount

MEAL / SNACK

MEAL / SNACK

MEAL / SNACK

FIGURE 10-3   *A. 3-day diary form. © 2005 Food and Nutrition Services, University of Iowa Hospitals and Clinics, Iowa City, IA. Reprinted with permission.*

Nutrition Study

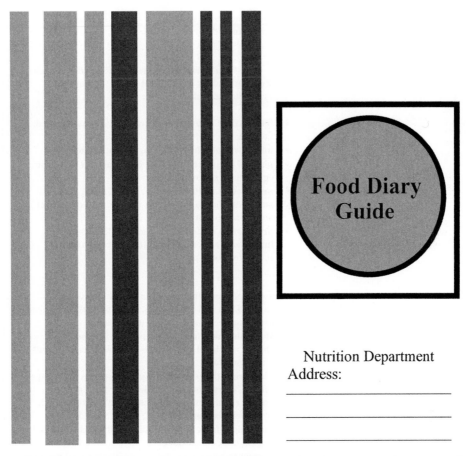

Food Diary Guide

Nutrition Department
Address:

_____

_____

_____

FIGURE 10-3   B. *Food diary guide. Reprinted with permission form the University of Iowa Hospitals and Clinics.*

Therefore these scales are most useful when most meals are eaten at home, and they are most likely to be used in a roomy, well-organized kitchen or dining room where the scale can be conveniently and more or less permanently located. U.S. Department of Agriculture (USDA) researchers have developed a food scale connected to a computer that gives the user instant information not only about the portion weight but also the nutrient content.[21] This scale (Figure 10-8) was developed for use in a research setting but could be adapted for consumer use.[22]

Problems with food diaries are many. Subjects may neglect the task and fail to record intake as promised; food diaries may not be complete when presented several days after they are recorded, too late for clients to reliably recall forgotten details; and the mere act of recording intake may alter what is eaten. These problems are often so severe that other methods for collecting dietary data have been developed.

Food Record Directions

Time:	**The Time indicates how often you eat**
Food or beverage name	**Please name and describe your foods as completely as possible. Include brand names.**
Type and/or preparation	**Give details that identify unique characteristics of each food (include labels for unusual foods). Record the following features of your food:** • **form (salted or unsalted, sweetened or unsweetened, fat-free, low cholesterol)** • **how it was purchased (fresh, frozen, canned)** • **place of preparation: home or restaurant (list name, eg., Wendy's, Bonanza)** • **preparation method (boiled, baked, fried, creamed) and added fat, salt, coatings or marinades; were fat and skin eaten or removed?** • **preparation directions: from mix (list brand and ingredients added) or "scratch" (record unusual recipes on form provided)**
Amount	**Please record only the amount actually eaten. For example, if you serve ½ cup peas but only half are eaten, record ¼ cup peas in the "Amount" column.** • **If possible, weigh on a scale: meat, fish, poultry, cheese, and hard to measure foods such as pizza and baked potatoes.** • **Measure with measuring cups and spoons: beverages, cereals, margarine, vegetables. For fluid ounce measurements, please label as "fl oz" to distinguish from weighed ounces.** • **List weight from label of individually packaged food (e.g., 1.75 oz candy bar)** • **Record common units for food with standard portions (e.g., 1 slice bread, 1 large egg, 1 large banana)**

FIGURE 10-3   B. *Food diary guide (cont).*

FOOD RECALL

The food recall is one way to overcome some of the problems encountered with diaries. The most common food recall is a 24-hour recall, where the foods eaten during the previous 24 hours are recalled upon prompting by an interviewer. The time period for data collection varies; sometimes the previous day's intake is requested, and sometimes the past 24 hours, starting from the time the interview was conducted and going back in time for 24 hours. This time period is often preferred if the interview occurs late in the day. The advantage of this time period is the recall of the most recent eating events. This time period might be preferred in collecting data from schoolchildren who are available to be interviewed only after school and/or in the evening. The disadvantage is that major eating occasions may be completely missed if the time period is strictly followed. For example, if the interview

Food Record

(include one page for each day)

Name:_____   Day:_____   Date:_____

[Record 2 weekdays and 1 weekend day]

Vitamin/Mineral Supplements:	Was your food intake for this day:
_____	1. Typical?
_____	2. **More** than usual?
_____	3. **Less** than usual?

Time	Foods and Beverages	Type and/or Preparation	Amount

FIGURE 10-3   B. *Food diary guide (cont).*

occurs at 6 PM and on the previous day the child had supper at 5 PM, but today supper will be at 7 PM, then data would be collected during a 24-hour period without including the major meal of the day. In this case, common sense should be exercised to select a representative 24-hour period.

Advantages of the recall are many. You collect data about meals that have already been eaten, so the recording process does not alter what is eaten and the subject or client cannot forget to provide the data because he or she is contacted directly when the data are needed. Disadvantages are that the time at which data are

Making Sense of Portion sizes

Finding it hard to show others what a serving or portion size is? Below are some ways you can help others picture a serving or portion size using everyday objects. Using these everyday examples can help show others that they may actually be eating more servings from the Food Guide Pyramid than they think! (Note: hands and finger sizes vary from person to person! These are GUIDES only).

The Bread, Cereal, Rice, and Pasta Group

1 cup of potatoes, rice, pasta	is a tennis ball, ice cream scoop
1 pancake	is a compact disc (CD)
1/2 cup cooked rice	is a cupcake wrapper full
1 piece of cornbread	is a bar of soap
1 slice of bread	is an audiocassette tape
1 cup of pasta, spaghetti, cereal	is a fist
2 cups cooked pasta	is a full outstretched hand

The Vegetable Group

1 cup green salad	is a baseball or fist
1 baked potato	is a fist
3/4 cup tomato juice	is a small styrofoam cup
1/2 cup cooked broccoli	is a scoop of ice cream or a light bulb
1/2 cup serving	is 6 asparagus spears; 7 or 8 baby carrots or carrot sticks or 1 ear of corn on the cob

The Fruit Group

1/2 cup of grapes (15 grapes)	is a light bulb
1/2 cup of fresh fruit	is 7 cotton balls
1 medium size fruit	is a tennis ball or fist
1 cup of cut-up fruit	is a fist
1/4 cup raisins	large egg

The Milk, Yogurt, and Cheese Group

1 1/2 ounces cheese	is a 9-volt battery, 3 dominoes or your index and middle fingers
1 ounce of cheese	is a pair of dice or your thumb
1 cup of ice cream	is a large scoop the size of a baseball

The Meat, Poultry, Fish, Dry Beans, Eggs, and Nuts Group

2 tablespoons peanut butter	is a ping-pong ball
1 teaspoon peanut butter	is a fingertip
1 tablespoon peanut butter	is a thumb tip
3 ounces cooked meat, fish, poultry	is a palm, a deck of cards or a cassette tape
3 ounces grilled/baked fish	is a checkbook
3 ounces cooked chicken	is a chicken leg and thigh or breast

Fats, Oils, and Sweets

1 teaspoon butter, margarine	is the size of a stamp the thickness of your finger or a thumb tip
2 tablespoons salad dressing	is a ping-pong ball

FIGURE 10-4 *Making sense of portion sizes. Compiled by Ellen Schuster, MS, RD, Oregon State University Extension Services, March 1997. Used with permission.*

Snack Foods

1 ounce of nuts or small candies...is one handful
1 ounce of chips or pretzels ....is two handfuls
1/2 cup of potato chips, crackers or popcorn............................is one man's handful
1/3 cup of potato chips, crackers or popcorn............................is one woman's handful

Serving Dishes/Utensils

1/2 cup...is a small fruit bowl, a custard cup or mashed potato scoop
1 1/2 cups..is a large cereal/soup bowl
1 1/2 cups of pasta, noodles...is a dinner plate, not heaped
1/2 cup of pasta, noodles..is a cafeteria vegetable dish

You might want to know that...

> 1 cupped hand holds 2 tablespoons of liquid if you don't have measuring spoons
> 1 slice of bread is one ounce or 1 serving; some rolls or bagels weigh 3 to 5 ounces or more making
>   them equal to 3 to 5 servings of bread

Sources Environmental Nutrition, April 1994
First Magazine, August 30, 1993
Kansas Dept. of Health and Environment
Mademoiselle, September 1993
National Pasta Association newsletter
Nutrition Action, November 1996
Skim the Fat by the American Dietetic Association, 1995
Tufts University Diet and Nutrition Letter, September 1994

FIGURE 10-4   *Making sense of portion sizes (cont).*

requested may be inconvenient for the client; therefore full cooperation may be compromised. Clients need to be trained in how to give complete data to the interviewer. It is common to use the telephone to conduct a recall interview, thus creating a need for visual materials to facilitate communication and aid in estimating portion sizes.[23,24]

The dietary recall method has been used by many of our national surveys, where the technique has been highly refined. USDA survey workers designed a "multiple-pass" method to standardize the interview process and improve the accuracy of the data. The "passes" refer to how the interview is conducted: the first pass asks for a list of all the food and beverage consumed for the past 24 hours as a free-flowing recall. During the second pass, the interviewer repeats each food and eating occasion, asking the subject to remember anything forgotten, with specific probes for foods consumed between eating occasions and things that might be overlooked, such as beverages, condiments, and snacks. The third pass determines the time and meal name for each eating occasion; the fourth pass captures detailed information about each food—such as portion size, type, brand name, and possible additions to each food item. Then a final pass asks the subject to review each eating occasion and food and to add any forgotten details as the interviewer reads aloud the completed food list. The use of this method increased the reported intake from an average of 1,748 calories for women in the CSFII 1994–1996 survey to 2,050 calories for a representative sample in 1998.[25] Whether a survey is administered in person or by telephone, it is good to have a standard form for recording the information so that important details—such as date of the interview, person conducting the interview, whether vitamin supplements were taken, and comments about completeness of the information—will not be forgotten. The dietetics professional should thoughtfully explain the importance of the dietary information and show appreciation for the effort the patient makes to keep a detailed record. When the objective is purely research, it is important to offer some kind of compensation, because the effort required of the respondent is not trivial.

Other kinds of recall methods have been reported. Bingham described a self-recorded 24-hour dietary recall that was written from memory by subjects when they were in the research clinic.[26] The University of Minnesota Nutrition Coding Center has developed software that guides the interview and prompts the interviewer to record important information about the subject, such as name and age, as well as suggested probes for requesting details about each food. This software guarantees that appropriate details are asked about each food because the interview cannot proceed to the next food until the current food is located on the database.

FOOD FREQUENCY QUESTIONNAIRE

Both the diary and recall require considerable time and effort on the part of both client and practitioner. A busy practitioner may not have the required time to conduct the recall and thus will rely on the client to keep a food diary. If the subject does not remember to keep the diary or the record lacks adequate details for analysis, the dietetics practitioner may not have sufficient data to plan an intervention. Likewise, the researcher may not have time for the recall, and the research subject may be unwilling to record the diary. To overcome these problems, researchers have developed data collection tools based on carefully designed food lists that help the client estimate past food and beverage intake. These food lists are referred to as "food frequency questionnaires" or FFQs. The FFQ comprises a diverse group of instruments owing to the fact that each instrument is developed with a specific outcome in mind. Collectively, the objective of the FFQ is to characterize usual intake of a group of people. The intent is usually to select a list of foods that are uniquely characteristic of a specific population, whether U.S. citizens in general or specific subjects within the United States, such as Vietnamese immigrants, children, or the elderly. The intent may also be to capture intake of a particular nutrient or group of foods, such as intake of fiber, or intake of fruits and vegetables.

Four researchers—Briefel, Block, Willett, and Subar—have given detailed descriptions on how instruments have been developed. Briefel described the development of a food list for the Second National Health and Nutrition Examination Survey (NHANES II). This list was designed to capture foods containing nutrients related to risk for cancer, cardiovascular disease, and osteoporosis, such as vitamins A and C, caffeine, and calcium; it was also intended to compare these results to those from past NHANES surveys for trend analysis.[27] Block took this methodology and popularized its use in other studies. She describes the development of the list, which basically entailed selecting foods from those reported in the NHANES II survey that provided most of the nutrients of interest.[28] The Block/NCI instruments developed using this methodology were based on about 98 foods reported in NHANES II. These foods captured over 90% of energy and 17 nutrients reported in this survey. From this list, questionnaires were developed that queried subjects about their food intake over the preceding year and used this information to estimate their habitual intake. A review of this work, however, reveals that it was not

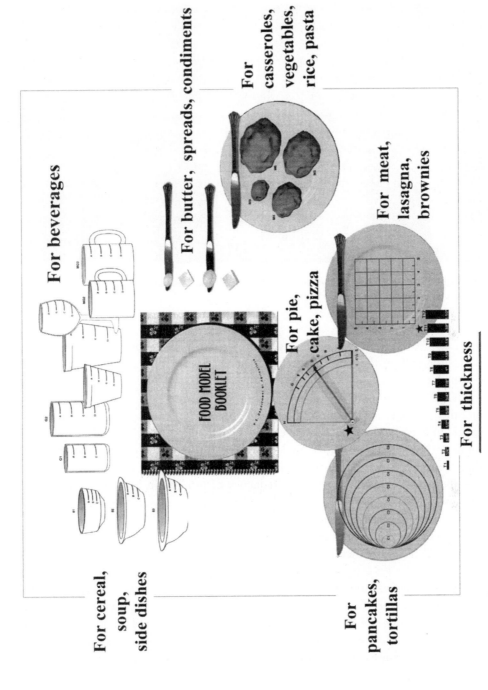

For beverages

For cereal, soup, side dishes

For butter, spreads, condiments

For casseroles, vegetables, rice, pasta

For meat, lasagna, brownies

For pie, cake, pizza

For pancakes, tortillas

For thickness

FOOD MODEL BOOKLET

FIGURE 10-5 *Selected illustrations (not to scale) from the USDA Food Model Booklet, a 26-page booklet designed for the Continuing Survey of Food Intake of Individuals. Courtesy USDA Food Survey Research Group. Available at: http://www.barc.usda.gov/bhnrc/foodsurvey/home.htm. Accessed February 26, 2006.*

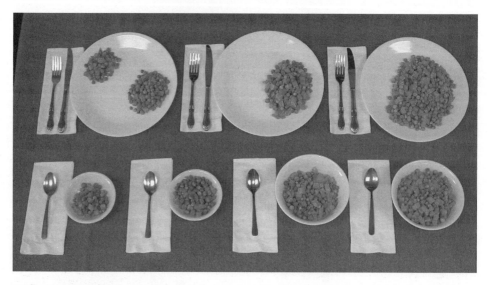

FIGURE 10-6 *Food displayed in mounds on plates and in bowls as a guide to estimating portion sizes. Amount left to right is 1/4, 1/2, 1, and 2 cups.*

precisely 98 foods but rather a less precise listing of 98 food groups that represented the bulk of the nutrient intake of survey respondents. Adding to the imprecision that comes from asking people to summarize their intake of a group of foods, FFQs also require subjects to report this intake as a daily, weekly, or monthly average. Aggregating information at this level is sometimes difficult for clients and research subjects. For example, one single entry from this list of 98 foods is "cornbread, biscuits, and crackers." From the nutritional standpoint, these items are similar, they are breads, they each contain fat, and a typical serving has about 160 calories; thus, their frequency of intake can be combined and still capture the major nutrients consumed. Although this may make sense to the dietetics practitioner, it may not be an intuitive food group for the average person, who might not consider cornbread a substitute for crackers or biscuits and who might find it very difficult to group the intake of these foods into a single frequency.

Because of these and other problems with questionnaire clarity, nutritional epidemiologists at the National Cancer Institute (NCI) used cognitive research techniques to evaluate the Block/NCI questionnaire and developed an alternate instrument.[29] The cognitive research technique involved interviewing subjects as they completed the questionnaire, asking them to talk aloud as they formulated their responses to each item on the questionnaire. This process let the developers know which items were difficult to answer and gave clues as to how they should be revised to capture the desired information. Subar led this NCI initiative; the resulting instrument is sometimes referred to as the "cognitive" questionnaire, or more officially the NCI DHQ (Diet History Questionnaire). This tool is available free on the NCI website at http://riskfactor.cancer.gov/DHQ/. Although the instrument is easily available, translating subject responses to nutrient intake values requires a complex software system. Software for analyzing the intake is also available on the NCI website, but putting the system into operation requires either a scanner and program to decode responses or some other type of coding system.

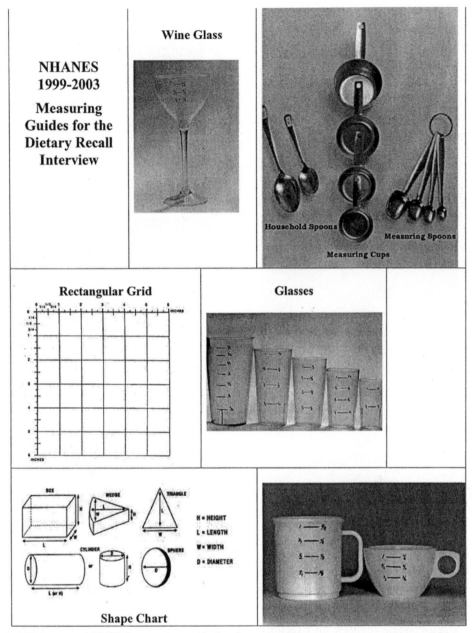

FIGURE 10-7 *NHANES measuring guide for dietary recall interview (not to scale). Available at: http://www.cdc.gov/nchs/about/major/nhanes/index. Accessed February 26, 2006.*

Rather than attempting to estimate actual intake, Willett sought to develop questionnaires that explain differences in intake among individuals in his target population. He surveyed a subset of his intended study population using a questionnaire designed around foods thought to contribute these nutrients, then conducted stepwise multiple regression analyses to identify those foods that explain the most between-person variance for each nutrient. The Willett and Block instruments have been used in numerous studies by a variety of investigators. Most investigators who select an instrument do so more on how it has performed in use rather than on how it was developed.

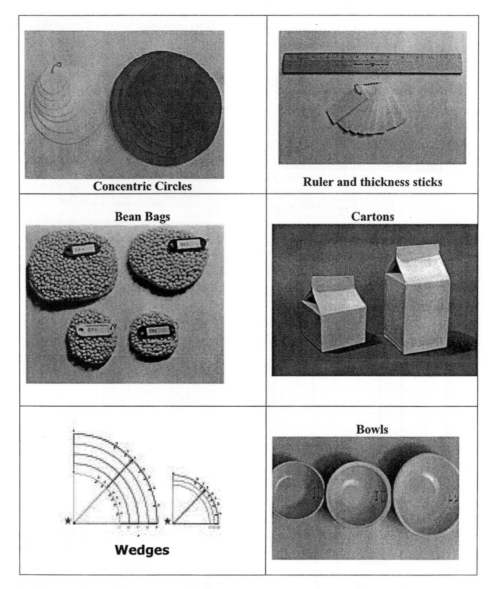

FIGURE 10-7 *NHANES measuring guide for dietary recall interview (cont). Note: not to scale.*

To validate the new NCI DHQ, Subar conducted a large study to compare the DHQ to food diaries and to the Block and Willett questionnaires. The comparison involved asking subjects to keep a food diary in each season of the year and then respond to the DHQ and either the Block or Willett questionnaires. Results from their study showed that the Block and DHQ had comparable estimates of intake and, with a calorie adjustment, the Willett questionnaire had similar results.[30]

Other validated questionnaires are also available. The Fred Hutchinson Cancer Center in Washington state has an instrument that is an adaptation of the Block/NCI questionnaire design and uses the NDS-R database.[31] The Hawaii Cancer Center questionnaire was developed to study a more ethnically diverse population.[32] Table 10-3 gives the contact information for six questionnaire developers.

Most food frequency questionnaires are summarized as average nutrient intake. The typical method for collecting FFQ data is to use a mark-sense response form,

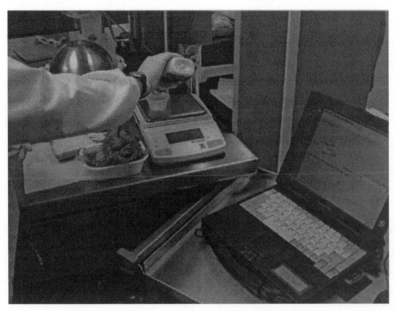

FIGURE 10-8   *ProNessy, an electronic scale connected to a computer to capture weight of food as it is portioned for service. (Courtesy of Wake Forest University Baptist Medical Center General Clinical Research Center.)*

where the subject blackens in a bubble that corresponds to his or her response. Then the questionnaire is optically scanned to obtain a file representing the responses to each questionnaire item.

This file is used to calculate the nutrient composition of the intake using a software application designed by the questionnaire developer, or the questionnaire responses may be entered by hand into spreadsheet software using a specially designed form. Developers who have made their questionnaires available to researchers typically provide an analysis service. Although these work well for the researcher who will analyze the data several months after they are collected, this method is not very useful for dietetics practitioners. Patient interactions depend on a more timely response from the dietetics professional, who needs to develop a treatment plan to coincide with other medical measurements and interventions. On-line questionnaires that offer immediate feedback promise to make these questionnaires available to the dietetics practitioner. Three such questionnaires are available: Block's questionnaire, with pricing directed to the researcher, is available at http://www.nutritionquest.com; Viocare has placed the Hutchinson FFQ, priced for individual as well as research use, at http://www.viocare.com; and the NCI DHQ has an on-line version available at http://riskfactor.cancer.gov/DHQ.

<h3>SCREENERS</h3>

The FFQ was greeted with optimism as a simpler way to obtain dietary information, but the response time to a questionnaire is still typically 30 minutes to 1 hour and many research subjects take longer, so researchers have sought to simplify this instrument. One obvious way to simplify the tool is to shorten the questionnaire by asking about fewer foods. When the research or clinical objective is limited, such as protocols where the primary interest is fat or calcium intake, it seems reasonable to

TABLE 10-3	Food Frequency Instruments Developed to Estimate Dietary Intake	
ORGANIZATION	**FEATURES**	**CONTACT INFORMATION:**
The Arizona Diet and Behavioral Assessment Center The Arizona Cancer Center 2601 N. Campbell Ave. Suite 109 Tucson, AZ 85719	General questionnaire plus specific screeners for tea, heterocyclic amines, cruciferous vegetables, citrus, arsenic or selenium, and folate	Phone: 520-626-8316 Fax: 520-626-3355 E-mail: egraver@azcc.arizona.edu Available at: http://www.azdiet-behavior.azcc.arizona.edu
Block FFQ NutritionQuest 15 Shattuck Square, Suite 288 Berkeley, CA 94704	Block questionnaires for adults in English, Spanish, Chinese; FFQs for children, physical activity; Scannable and online	Phone: 510-704-8514 Fax: 510-704-8996 E-mail: Info@Nutritionquest.com http://www.nutritionquest.com
Willett FFQ Harvard School of Public Health Department of Nutrition 651 Huntington Avenue Boston, MA 02115	Semiquantitative food frequency questionnaires for children and adults[43,44]	Phone: 617-432-4680 Fax: 617-432-0464 https://regepi.bwh.harvard.edu/health
Fred Hutchinson Cancer Research Center Nutrition Assessment Shared Resource (NASR) 1100 Fairview Ave. N. M1-B208 Seattle, WA 98109-1024	Self-administered booklet optically scanned at NASR. Analysis uses data from the University of Minnesota NDS-R[45]	Phone: 206-667-4161 E-mail: ffq@fhcrc.org http://ffq.fhcrc.org
National Cancer Institute Executive Plaza North 4005 6130 Executive Blvd-MSC 7344 Bethesda, MD 20892-7344	General questionnaire and analysis software available, both can be modified for use. Includes supplement use and is scannable. Online web-based version also available.[29]	Phone: 301-496-8500 http://riskfactor.cancer.gov/DHQ/
Cancer Research Center of Hawaii University of Hawaii 1236 Lauhala St., Suite 407 Honolulu, HI 96813	Scannable food frequency[46] validated in multiethnic populations in Hawaii, Los Angeles, and Pacific Islands.	Phone: 808-586-2987 Fax: 808-586-2982 http://www.CRCH.org/ShNutriSupport.htm

ask only about intake of foods that contribute to this single nutrient. Many such instruments have been developed, and the term "screener" is often used to describe these shortened forms. Block was one of the first to make a screener available for general use. Her first screener was designed in two parts, a fat screener and a fruit/vegetable/fiber screener. The first instruments were self-scoring (Figure 10-9); subsequent versions were placed on the Internet to be freely used by the consumer (Figure 10-10 A and B and http://www.nutritionquest.com; click on free diet analysis). The Internet versions of these screeners have an accompanying database used behind the scenes to generate nutrient intake data based on responses to the screener. Dietetics practitioners and others should contact Block for permission to reproduce this copyrighted screener.

CLINICAL QUESTIONNAIRES

Some questionnaires have a specific clinical objective. One example of this kind of questionnaire is the MEDFICTS questionnaire (Figure 10-11). This instrument was

Eating Habits Screener   **Your name:**_____   **Age:**_____   **Sex:** M   F

Think about your eating habits over the past year or so. About how often do you eat each of the following foods? Remember breakfast, lunch, dinner, snacks and eating out. Mark an 'x' in one column for each food.

Meats and Snacks	(0) 1/MONTH or less	(1) 2-3 times a MONTH	(2) 1-2 times a WEEK	(3) 3-4 times a WEEK	(4) 5+ times a WEEK	Score
Hamburgers, ground beef, meat, burritos, tacos	O	O	O	O	O	_____
Beef or pork, such as steaks, roasts, ribs, or in sandwiches	O	O	O	O	O	_____
Fried chicken	O	O	O	O	O	_____
Hot dogs, or Polish or Italian sausage	O	O	O	O	O	_____
Cold cuts, lunch meats, ham (not low-fat)	O	O	O	O	O	_____
Bacon or breakfast sausage	O	O	O	O	O	_____
Salad dressings (not low-fat)	O	O	O	O	O	_____
Margarine, butter or oil in cooking	O	O	O	O	O	_____
Eggs (not Egg Beaters or just egg whites)	O	O	O	O	O	_____
Muffins or biscuits	O	O	O	O	O	_____
Cheese, cheese spread (not low-fat)	O	O	O	O	O	_____
Whole milk	O	O	O	O	O	_____
French fries, fried potatoes	O	O	O	O	O	_____
Corn chips, potato chips, popcorn, crackers	O	O	O	O	O	_____
Dougnuts, pastries, cake, cookies (not low-fat)	O	O	O	O	O	_____
Ice cream (not sherbet or non-fat)	O	O	O	O	O	_____

Fat Score = [   ]

Fruits and Vegetables	(0) Less than 1/WEEK	(1) Once a WEEK	(2) 2-3 times a WEEK	(3) 4-6 times a WEEK	(4) Once a DAY	(5) 2+ a DAY	Score
Fruit juice, like orange, apple, grape — fresh, frozen or canned. (Not sodas or other drinks)	O	O	O	O	O	O	_____
How often do you eat any fruit, fresh or canned (not counting juice?)	O	O	O	O	O	O	_____
Vegetable juice, like tomato juice, V-8, carrot	O	O	O	O	O	O	_____
Green salad	O	O	O	O	O	O	_____
Potatoes, any kind, including baked, mashed or french fried	O	O	O	O	O	O	_____
Vegetable soup, or stew with vegetables	O	O	O	O	O	O	_____
Any other vegetables, including string beans, peas, corn, broccoli or any other kind	O	O	O	O	O	O	_____

Fruit/Vegetable Score = [   ]

Do you take vitamins, like One-a-Day or vitamin C? O Never O Once in a while O A few times a week O Almost every day

FIGURE 10-9   *Block self scoring: eating habits screener. Block Dietary Data Systems. Available at: http://www.nutritionquest.com/fv_screener.html. Reprinted with permission. The Fat Screener and Fruit/Vegetable/Fiber Screener and their associated scoring algorithms are the property of Block Dietary Data Systems, Berkeley, CA. To use these tools, permission must be obtained from the owner. Please contact vendor for licensing. Phone: 510-704-8514.*

How well are you doing?

How to score your answers:

▶ Check one column for each food.

▶ At the top of each column is a number. Write the number of the column you checked, on the right side of the page beside each food.

▶ Add up these numbers, separately for the Meat/Snacks Score and for the Fruit/Vegetable Score.

Scoring for the **Meat/Snacks section** of the screener:

If your score is:
- 0-7: Your fat intake is very low, probably less than 25% of calories. Congratulations!
- 8-14: Your fat intake is about like most Americans, probably between 30% and 35% of calories. Experts recommend that it be less than 30%. Try eating some of your high-scoring foods less often, and eat more fruits and vegetables.
- 15-22: Your diet is quite high in fat, probably higher than the U.S. average of 35% of calories. Look at the foods you scored highest on. You don't have to give up your favorites, just eat them less often or in smaller portions. Try lower-fat milk, low-fat salad dressing. And fill up on grains, fruits, and vegetables!
- 23+: Your diet is very high in fat, probably 40-50% of calories! Look at the foods you scored highest on, and eat them less often. Switch to 2% milk, and low-fat lunch meats and salad dressing. Most of the food you eat should come from bread, rice, cereals, fruits and vegetables.

Scoring for the **Fruit/Vegetables section** of the screener:

If your score is:
- 0-10: You are not eating enough fruits and vegetables! You are probably eating fewer than 3 servings a day, but experts recommend 5 or more. You may be low in important vitamins, and fiber. Pick a few fruits or vegetables you like, and eat more of them. Green salad counts, too, and fruit juice or vegetable juice.
- 11-12: Your diet is like most Americans — low in fruits and vegetables! You're eating fewer than 4 servings, but experts recommend 5 or more. Pick some you like, and eat them more often. Green salad counts, and fruit juice or vegetable juice.
- 13-15: You are doing better than most people, but you are still not eating 5 servings of fruits and vegetables every day. Try adding fruit or vegetable juice, or salad — or just any fruit or vegetable you like.
- 16+: You're doing very well in fruits/vegetables, probably around 5 servings a day! Congratulations! The best score on this screener is 19 or more. Go for it!

Eat a low-fat diet, that has five servings a day of fruits and vegetables.

For a detailed dietary analysis, see your heath care provider or dietitian, or call BDDS at 510-704-8514.

©BDDS. Scoring for 1-Page BBDS Screener dated 97a

FIGURE 10-9 *Block self scoring: eating habits screener (cont).*

developed for use in cardiovascular health screening and was validated in several clinical settings.[35]

<u>SUPPLEMENT INTAKE</u>

Nutrition assessments often ignore the contribution of dietary supplements to total intake largely because databases have not carried information on the composition of supplements. Even our national surveys have not considered supplement use until very recently. The USDA CSFII and NFCS and NHANES III report nutrient intakes from food only. This omission is gradually being corrected as supplement databases

Fruit, Vegetable, and Fiber Screener

Your Name (optional): [   ]

Age: [   ]

Sex: ○ Male ○ Female

Think about your eating habits over the past year or so. About how often do you eat each of the following foods? Remember breakfast, lunch, dinner, snacks and eating out. Check one radio button for each food.

Fruits, Vegetables, and Grains	Less than 1/WEEK	Once a WEEK	2-3 times a WEEK	4-6 times a WEEK	Once a DAY	2+ a DAY
Fruit juice, like orange, apple, grape , fresh, frozen or canned. (Not sodas or other drinks)	○	○	○	○	○	○
How often do you eat any fruit, fresh or canned (not counting juice?)	○	○	○	○	○	○
Vegetable juice, like tomato juice, V-8, carrot	○	○	○	○	○	○
Green salad	○	○	○	○	○	○
Potatoes, any kind, including baked, mashed or french fried	○	○	○	○	○	○
Vegetable soup, or stew with vegetables	○	○	○	○	○	○
Any other vegetables, including string beans, peas, corn, broccoli or any other kind	○	○	○	○	○	○
Fiber cereals like Raisin Bran, Shredded Wheat or Fruit-n-Fiber	○	○	○	○	○	○
	Less than 1/WEEK	Once a WEEK	2-3 times a WEEK	4-6 times a WEEK	Once a DAY	2+ a DAY
Beans such as baked beans, pinto, kidney, or lentils (not green beans)	○	○	○	○	○	○
Dark bread such as whole wheat or rye	○	○	○	○	○	○

FIGURE 10-10 **A.** *Block Fat and Fruit, Vegetable and Fiber Screeners. Block Dietary Data Systems. Available at http://www.nutritionquest.com/fv_screener.html. Reprinted with permission. The Fat Screener and Fruit/Vegetable/Fiber Screener and their associated scoring algorithms are the property of Block Dietary Data Systems, Berkeley, CA. To use these tools, permission must be obtained from the owner. Please contact vendor for licensing. Phone: 510-704-8514.*

Fat Screener

Your Name (optional): [   ]

Age: [   ]

Sex: ☐ Male ☐ Female

Think about your eating habits over the past year or so. About how often do you eat each of the following foods? Remember breakfast, lunch, dinner, snacks and eating out. Check one radio button for each food.

Meats and Snacks	1/MONTH or less	2-3 times a MONTH	1-2 times a WEEK	3-4 times a WEEK	5+ times a WEEK
Hamburgers, ground beef, meat burritos, tacos	☐	☐	☐	☐	☐
Beef or pork, such as steaks, roasts, ribs, or in sandwiches	☐	☐	☐	☐	☐
Fried chicken	☐	☐	☐	☐	☐
Hot dogs, or Polish or Italian sausage	☐	☐	☐	☐	☐
Cold cuts, lunch meats, ham (not low-fat)	☐	☐	☐	☐	☐
Bacon or breakfast sausage	☐	☐	☐	☐	☐
Salad dressings (not low-fat)	☐	☐	☐	☐	☐
Margarine, butter or mayo on bread or potatoes	☐	☐	☐	☐	☐
Margarine, butter or oil in cooking	☐	☐	☐	☐	☐
Eggs (not Egg Beaters or just egg whites)	☐	☐	☐	☐	☐
Pizza	☐	☐	☐	☐	☐
Cheese, cheese spread (not low-fat)	☐	☐	☐	☐	☐
Whole milk	☐	☐	☐	☐	☐
French fries, fried potatoes	☐	☐	☐	☐	☐
Corn chips, potato chips, popcorn, crackers	☐	☐	☐	☐	☐
Doughnuts, pastries, cake, cookies (not low-fat)	☐	☐	☐	☐	☐
Ice cream (not sherbet or non-fat)	☐	☐	☐	☐	☐

FIGURE 10-10 B. *Block Fat Screener. Block Dietary Data Systems. Available at http://www .nutritionquest.com/fv_screener.html. Reprinted with permission. The Fat Screener and Fruit/ Vegetable/Fiber Screener and their associated scoring algorithms are the property of Block Dietary Data Systems, Berkeley, CA. To use these tools, permission must be obtained from the owner. Please contact vendor for licensing. Phone: 510-704-8514.*

In each food category for both Group 1 and Group 2 foods check one box from the "Weekly Consumption" column (number of servings eaten per week) and then check one box from the "Serving Size" column. If you check Rarely/Never, do not check a serving size box. See last page for score.

Food Category	Weekly Consumption			Serving Size			Score
Meats ■ • Recommended amount per day:≤6 oz (equal in size to 2 decks of playing cards) • Base your estimate on the food you consume most often. • Beef and lamb selections are trimmed to 1/8" fat.	Rarely/ never	3 or less	4 or more	Small <6 oz/d 1 pt	Average 6 oz/d 2 pts	Large >6 oz/d 3 pts	
1. 10 gm or more total fat in 3 oz cooked portion							
Beef - Ground beef, Ribs, Steak (T-bone, Flank, Porterhouse, Tenderloin), Chuck blade roast, Brisket, Meatloaf(w/ ground beef), Corned beef **Processed meats** - 1/4lb burger or / lg. sandwich, Bacon, Lunch meat, Sausage/knock wurst, Hot dogs, Ham (bone-end), Ground turkey **Other meats, Poultry, Seafood** - Pork chops (center loin), / Pork roast (Blade, Boston, Sirloin), Pork spareribs, Ground pork, Lamb chops, Lamb (ribs), Organ meats*, Chicken w/ skin, Eel, Mackerel, Pompano	□	□ 3 pts	□ 7 pts	X □ 1 pt	□ 2 pts	□ 3 pts	_____
2. Less than 10 gm total fat in 3 oz cooked portion							
Lean beef - Round steak (Eye of round, Top round), Sirloin**, Tip & bottom round**, Chuck arm pot roast**, Top loin** **Low fat processed meats** - Low fat lunch meat, Canadian bacon, "Lean" fast food sandwich, Boneless ham **Other meats, Poultry, Seafood** - Chicken, Turkey (w/o skin)§, most Seafood*, Lamb leg shank, Pork tenderloin, Sirloin top loin, Veal cutlets, Sirloin, Shoulder, Ground veal, Venison, Veal chops and Ribs**, Lamb (whole leg, loin, fore-shank, sirloin)**	□	□	□	X □	□	□† 6 pts	_____
Eggs ■ Weekly consumption is the number of times you eat eggs each week				Check the number of eggs eaten each time			
1. Whole eggs, Yolks	□	□ 3 pts	□ 7 pts	≤1 x □ 1 pt	2 □ 2 pts	≥3 □ 3 pts	_____
2. Egg whites, Egg substitutes (½ c)	□	□	□	x □	□	□	_____
Dairy ■							
Milk - Average serving 1 cup 1. Whole milk, 2%milk, 2%buttermilk, Yogurt (whole milk)	□	□ 3 pts	□ 7 pts	x □ 1 pt	□ 2 pts	□ 3 pts	_____
2. Skim milk, 1% milk, Skim buttermilk, Yogurt (non-fat, 1% lowfat)	□	□	□	x □	□	□	_____
Cheese - Average serving 1 oz 1. Cream cheese, Cheddar, Monterey Jack, Colby, Swiss, American Processed, Blue cheese, Regular cottage cheese (½ c), and Ricotta (¼c)	□	□ 3 pts	□ 7 pts	x □ 1 pt	□ 2 pts	□ 3 pts	_____
2. Low-fat & fat-free cheeses, Skim milk mozzarella, String cheese, Low fat, Skim milk & Fat-free cottage cheese (½ c) and Ricotta (¼ c)	□	□	□	x □	□	□	_____
Frozen Desserts ■ Average serving ½ c							
1. Ice cream, Milk Shakes	□	□ 3 pts	□ 7 pts	x □ 1 pt	□ 2 pts	□ 3 pts	_____
2. Ice milk, Frozen Yogurt	□	□	□	□	□	□	_____

FIGURE 10-11   *MEDFICTS assessment tool. Adapted with permission from Kris-Etherton et al[33] (cont.)*

	Rarely/Never	Weekly			Serving Size			Score
Frying Foods ■ Average servings: see below. This section refers to method of preparation for vegetables and meat.								
1. French fries, Fried vegetables (½ c), Fried chicken, fish, meat (3 oz)	□	□ 3 pts	□ 7 pts	x	□ 1 pt	□ 2 pts	□ 3 pts	_____
2. Vegetables, not deep fried (½ c), Meat, poultry, or fish-prepared by baking, broiling, grilling, poaching, roasting, stewing: (3 oz)	□	□	□	x	□	□	□	_____
In Baked Goods ■ 1 Average serving								
1. Doughnuts, Biscuits, Butter Rolls, Muffins, Croissants, Sweet rolls, Danish, Cakes, Pies, Coffee cakes, Cookies	□	□ 3 pts	□ 7 pts	x	□ 1 pt	□ 2 pts	□ 3 pts	_____
2. Fruits bars, Low fat cookies/cakes/pastries, Angel food cake, Homemade baked goods with vegetable oils, breads, bagels	□	□	□	x	□	□	□	_____
Convenience Foods ■								
1. Canned, Packaged, or Frozen dinners: eg, Pizza (1 slice), Macaroni &cheese (1 c), Pot pie (1), Cream soups (1 c), Potato, rice & pasta dishes with cream/cheese sauces (½ c)	□	□ 3 pts	□ 7 pts	x	□ 1 pt	□ 2 pts	□ 3 pts	_____
2. Diet/Reduced calorie or reduced fat dinners (1), Potato, rice & pasta dishes without cream/cheese sauces (½c)	□	□	□	x	□	□	□	_____
Table Fats ■ Average serving: 1 Tbsp								
1. Butter, Stick Margarine, Regular salad dressing, Mayonnaise, Sour cream (2 Tbsp)	□	□ 3 pts	□ 7 pts	x	□ 1 pt	□ 2 pts	□ 3 pts	_____
2. Diet and tub margarine, Low fat & fat free salad dressings, Low fat & fat free mayonnaise	□	□	□	x	□	□	□	_____
Snacks ■								
1. Chips (potato, corn, taco), Cheese puffs, Snack mix, Nuts (1 oz), Regular crackers (½ oz), Candy (milk chocolate, caramel, coconut) (about 1 ½ oz), Regular popcorn (3 c)	□	□ 3 pts	□ 7 pts	x	□ 1 pt	□ 2 pts	□ 3 pts	_____
2. Pretzels, Fat free chips (1 oz), Low fat crackers (½ oz), Fruit, Fruit rolls, Licorice, Hard candy (1 med piece), Bread sticks (1-2 pc), Air-popped or low fat popcorn (3 c)	□	□	□	x	□	□	□	

† Score 6 pts if this box is checked
§ All parts not listed in group 1 have
   < 10 gm total fat.
* Organ meats, shrimp, abalone, and
   squid are low in fat but high in cholesterol
**Only lean cuts with all visible fat trimmed.
   If not trimmed of all visible fat, score as if in Group 1.

Total from page 1 _____
Total from page 2 _____
FINAL SCORE _____

To Score: For each food category, multiply points in weekly consumption box by points in serving size box and record total in score column. If group 2 foods checked, no points are scored (except for Group 2 meats, large serving = 6 pts).

Example:

□	□ 3 pts	☑ 7 pts	x □ 1 pt	□ 2 pts	☑ 3 pts	21

Add score on page 1 and page 2 to get final score.

Key:
≥ 70   Need to make some dietary changes
40-70   Step I Diet
< 40   Step II Diet

FIGURE 10-11   *MEDFICTS assessment tool (cont).*

are developed. The NHANES supplement database contains 1,600 supplement products with 914 unique supplement ingredients.[34] Because supplement products tend to be modified approximately every 2 years, maintaining an accurate database requires a continuous development effort. The myriad of products available together with the consumer's lack of specific details about products used make the accurate assessment of supplement intake very difficult.

Fortunately, competition among brand-name products has given rise to supplements that imitate the market leader, so that reasonable intake estimates are possible. For example, one familiar multiple vitamin is called One-A-Day, so a category "one-a-day type" is often listed on a database with values typical of the majority of multiple vitamins on the market. This is probably a better solution than ignoring supplements altogether, but it loses some information that could be valuable, such as recognizing intake of components thought to have a health benefit (e.g., lutein or folate) that have at one time or another been used to give individual products a market (and health) advantage.

The number of supplement formulations has exploded as products have sought a market niche with infants, the elderly, in pregnancy, for eye care, for heart health, and formulations targeted to many other market segments. Attempts to capture accurate details about supplement intake have given rise to databases with numerous entries representing generic supplements, such as alfalfa tablets, cod liver oil, or multivitamins and specific brand-name products such as Centrum and Geritol. Supplements involve much more than vitamins and minerals, as consumers are encouraged to improve health, beauty, strength, and vitality with a wide variety of herbs and botanicals. These products are difficult to characterize because formulations lack government standardization and labeling requirements are minimal. The NIH established an Office of Dietary Supplements in 1995 that is charged with the responsibility to make information about the composition, use, and physiological effect of known supplements and to encourage research to improve our knowledge about the potential health benefits of these products.

Assessing intake of dietary supplements is becoming increasingly important. Often dietetics professionals have treatment and research goals that are limited to food intake; the capturing of supplement intake is a secondary aim. Some supple-

TABLE 10-4	Institutions Providing Contract Services for Food Diary Calculations
ORGANIZATION	**CONTACT INFORMATION**
The Arizona Diet and Behavioral Assessment Center The Arizona Cancer Center 2601 N. Campbell Ave., Suite 109 Tucson, AZ 85719	Phone: 520-626-8316 Fax: 520-626-3355 E-mail: egraver@azcc.arizona.edu Available at: http://www.azdiet-behavior. azcc.arizona.edu
Nutrition Coordinating Center University of Minnesota 1300 South Second St,, Suite 300 Minneapolis, MN 55454-1015	NCC Service Center Manager Phone: 612-626-9450 Fax: 612-626-9444 E-mail: mstevens@keystone.ncc.umn.edu Available at: http://www.ncc.umn.edu
Dietary Assessment & Epidemiology Research Program Friedman School of Nutrition Science & Policy 711 Washington St. Boston, MA 02111	Phone: 617-556-3351 Fax: 617 556-3344 E-mail: Janice.Maras@tufts.edu Available at: http://www.hnrc.tufts.edu/
Department of Nutritional Sciences 5 Henderson Bldg. Pennsylvania State University University Park, PA 16802	Coordinator, Diet Assessment Center Phone: 814-863-5955 Fax: 814-835-9971 E-mail: Dcm1@psu.edu

ments, however, provide as much of some nutrients as are present in all the food consumed in one day. Thus capturing supplement intake is critical if intake data are to be valid and representative.

SOFTWARE FOR CALCULATING NUTRIENT COMPOSITION OF DIARIES AND RECALLS

Numerous applications are available for calculating composition of food records and recalls. Printed tables are useful for locating the composition of specific foods. *Pennington's Bowes and Church* food composition book[35] is updated on a regular basis and lists food by generic name and by brand. Software applications are useful for calculating the composition of a full diet. Both dietetics practitioners and researchers have used Food Processor[36] and Nutritionist PRO[37] PC programs. These are robust programs with intuitive user interfaces. They also have attractive printouts that are especially appropriate for counseling purposes. When software offers nutrient data for many foods by brand name, the database is often sparse, meaning that many of the nutrients present in the food do not have values in the database. Brand-name products are typically analyzed only for nutrients appearing on the food label. If nutrients other than those on the label are needed for a project, the database should be carefully evaluated for completeness.

Two programs often used by researchers are the University of Minnesota Nutrient Data System (NDS) developed by the Department of Epidemiology at Minnesota to analyze food intake from large intervention studies and FIAS, which is an adaptation of software used by USDA to calculate composition of their national food consumption surveys. Table 10-4 lists several organizations offering nutrient calculation services for food diaries and recalls.

NUTRIENT DATA SYSTEM (NDS)

The University of Minnesota database has evolved over the years to probably the most complete and comprehensive database available for calculation of ad libitum dietary intakes. NHLBI funded this application to support its lipid studies and so has always required detailed information about food preparation methods, especially in terms of fat usage. The database was ported to the PC in the early 1990s and called Nutrient Data System (NDS).[38] The Window's version of this application, called NDS-R (R for research) Version 31, expanded folate values to include total folate, synthetic folic acid, natural folate, and dietary folate equivalents to represent the units used for the current RDA.[39] NDS-R offers over 100 nutrients and nutrient calculations (Table 10-5). Fluoride has been added to this list and is available as a separate module. The user interface is designed to support direct entry of dietary recalls as they are being conducted. The interface provides access to nutrient values by brand name for hundreds of foods. The database is updated twice annually, making it responsive to changes in the marketplace. The most clinically useful report compares intake to the RDA; however, most printouts do not have a consumer-oriented format. Nutrient composition of intake records can be exported to files for importing into spreadsheet or statistical packages. This feature is useful for research. The cost of this program (approximately $8,000 initially with annual support costs of $2,600 per year) limits its use to well-funded research projects.

Food Intake Analysis System (FIAS)

The FIAS[40] program uses the USDA Food and Nutrient Database for Dietary Studies (FNDDS) database of over 7,300 foods and 61 nutrients and other food components. While the FNDDS database is composed mainly of generic food profiles, help in describing many brand-name products is available after the appropriate food profile is selected. For example, if a frozen chicken and vegetable entrée with noodles is chosen, FIAS assists the user to select the correct amount for a variety of frozen meal brands. Cereals and candy bars are listed by brand name, since the composition of each brand is unique. Otherwise, foods tend to be listed with their generic description. The recipe module utilizes USDA's files that have retention and yield factors that gives FIAS sophisticated recipe calculation feature. The program allows you to select retention factors for nutrients that might undergo changes during preparation and to apply a moisture and/or fat gain or loss that might occur during cooking. The cost of FIAS is $6,000, again limiting its use to well-funded projects.

Internet Applications

Several Internet applications are available for calculating nutrient intakes. The USDA Center for Nutrition Policy and Promotion offers a free analysis program called the Interactive Healthy Eating Index (IHEI), which is currently located at http://209.48.219.53/default.asp. This program uses the USDA FNDDS Database (see below) and offers the total daily intake for energy and numerous other components with several evaluations of the intake including a "Healthy Eating Index" that uses a 10-point score on several nutrient factors such as fat content and a comparison to the Food Guide Pyramid. The University of Illinois has a free calculation system based on the USDA Standard Reference Database (see below) plus commercial and fast food items. This program is called Nutrient Analysis System or NAT and is located at http://www.nat.uiuc.edu/. NAT gives the nutrient content of a diet or menu entered into the program, which includes water, energy, and 20 other nutrient components and compares nutrient totals to the Recommended Dietary Allowances (RDA). These software applications bring dietary assessment into the home and empower the consumer to monitor intake and plan interventions based on own food preferences.

Nutrient Databases

Data from food records, food recalls, and food lists or food frequency assessments are usually reported as consumption by nutrient or by food group. Thus the food composition database is a critical part of the system, determining in part the accuracy and appropriateness of the assessment. Critical aspects of a database are as follows:

1. Representativeness of foods consumed by the population being served.
2. Inclusion of an array of nutrients needed by the population.
3. "Completeness" of the database, including values for all the nutrients listed.

This last factor is especially critical when a database includes many commercial and fast-food entries, as these products may present only nutrients required for a food label.

TABLE 10-5

Comparison of USDA SR 16, USDA Survey, and U Minn NDS Databases for Selected Nutrients.

	USDA SR 16	USDA SURVEY	U MINN NDS
Water	100	100	100
Energy	100	100	100
Protein	100	100	100
Total fat	100	100	100
Total saturated fat	97	100	100
Total monounsaturated fat	94	100	100
Total polyunsaturated fat	94	100	100
Cholesterol	98	100	100
Phytosterols	9		
Sitosterol	1		
Stigmasterol	1		
Campesterol	1		
Total carbohydrate	100	100	100
Ash	100		
Dietary fiber	90	100	100
Water insoluble diet fiber			96
Water soluble diet fiber			96
Pectins			78
Alcohol	58	100	100
Caffeine	53	100	100
Theobromine	53	100	
Total vitamin A	98	100	100
Beta-carotene	55	100	100
Alpha-carotene	53	100	100
Beta-cryptoxanthin	53	100	100
Lutein + zeaxanthin	52	100	100
Lycopene	53	100	100
Retinol	89	100	100
Total alpha-toc eq			99
Alpha-tocopherol	54	100	99
Beta-tocopherol	8		99
Gamma-tocopherol	8		99
Delta-tocopherol	8		99
Vitamin D	7	100	99
Ascorbic acid	96	100	100
Thiamin	94	100	100
Riboflavin	94	100	100
Niacin	94	100	100
Pantothenic acid	84		98
Vitamin B6	92	100	99
Total folate	92	100	100
Dietary folate equivalents	89	100	100
Natural folate (food folate)	90	100	100
Synthetic folate (folic acid)	89	100	100
Vitamin K	49	100	99
Vitamin B12	92	100	100
Calcium	98	100	100
Phosphorus	95	100	100
Magnesium	94	100	100
Manganese	81		
Iron	98	100	100
Zinc	93	100	100
Copper	93	100	100
Sodium	100	100	100
Selenium	84	100	100
Potassium	96	100	100
Tryptophan	65		97
Threonine	66		98
Isoleucine	66		98

	USDA SR 16	USDA SURVEY	U MINN NDS
Leucine	66		98
Lysine	66		98
Methionine	66		98
Cystine	65		97
Phenylalanine	66		98
Tyrosine	65		97
Valine	66		98
Arginine	66		97
Histidine	66		97
Alanine	65		97
Aspartic acid	65		97
Glutamic acid	65		97
Glycine	65		97
Proline	65		97
Serine	65		97
Hydroxyproline	8		
Animal protein			100
Vegetable protein			100
Fatty acid 4:0 butyric acid	60	100	100
Fatty acid 6:0 caproic acid	61	100	100
Fatty acid 8:0 caprylic acid	62	100	100
Fatty acid 10:0 capric acid	73	100	100
Fatty acid 12:0 lauric acid	78	100	100
Fatty acid 13:0	1	100	
Fatty acid 14:0 myristic acid	84	100	100
Fatty acid 15:0	6		
Fatty acid 16:0 palmitic acid	88	100	100
Fatty acid 17:0 margaric acid	7	100	100
Fatty acid 18:0 stearic acid	88	100	100
Fatty acid 20:0 arachidic acid	8		100
Fatty acid 22:0 behenic acid	6		100
Fatty acid 24:0	3		
Fatty acid 14:1 myristoleic	8		100
Fatty acid 15:1	3		
Fatty acid 16:1 palmitoleic	84		100
Fatty acid 17:1	4		
Fatty acid 18:1 oleic	88		100
Fatty acid 20:1 gadoleic	73		100
Fatty acid 22:1 erucic	63		100
Fatty acid 24:1	1		
Fatty acid 18:2 linoleic	88		100
Fatty acid 18:3 linolenic	87		100
Fatty acid 18:4 parinaric	59		100
Fatty acid 20:2	4		
Fatty acid 20:3	5		
Fatty acid 20:4 arachidonic	73		100
Fatty acid 20:5 n-3 eicosapentaenoic	63		100
Fatty acid 22:5 n-3 docosapentainoic	62		100
Fatty acid 22:6 n-3 docosahaenoic acid	63		100
Omega-3 fatty acids			100
Trans fatty acids	2		100
Fructose	52		97
Galactose	3		98
Glucose	5		97
Lactose	5		99
Maltose	5		99
Sucose	5		98
Total sugar	61	100	
Starch	2		98
Phytic acid			99
Oxalic acid			97

USDA maintains three comprehensive nutrient databases:

1. The standard reference database (SR)
2. The FNDDS database
3. The primary data set (PDS)

The SR database is the most basic, containing the most nutrients (approximately 77) for probably the most foods (over 6,000). Most nutrient values on the SR database are analyzed values, although some nutrients may be calculated, as was done when folate values were updated in Version 12 to reflect the increased levels in grains mandated by FDA by January 1, 1998. Replacement of calculated folate values with chemically analyzed values began with Version 13.

The FNDDS database differs from the SR database in many ways.[41] First, it offers only nutrients that have values for all foods on the database (this includes about 60 nutrients). Also, the foods listed on the database are selected to represent food in the form it will likely be reported by survey respondents. For example, the SR database has over 60 separate chuck roast entries that specify the grade of beef, whether blade or arm roast, and whether raw or cooked, whereas the FNDDS database has only two roast entries, beef roast (for rib) and pot roast (for chuck). Subjects responding to questions in a survey will not likely know details about the grade or cut of the roast they consumed, and they do not consume it raw, so the added details available on the SR database are not useful for a survey. Alcoholic beverages are a good example of where the FNDDS database has more detail than the SR database. Alcoholic beverages are listed by recipe on the FNDDS database (i.e., Manhattan, daiquiri, highball), but the SR listing is primarily composed of ingredients (i.e., gin, bourbon). The FNDDS database is used to calculate consumption for NHANES. Many commercial software applications have data from both of these USDA databases and some use only one. The SR is not as well suited for calculating food diaries and recalls as is the FNDDS database, but it includes more nutrients. The FNDDS database, on the other hand, is suitable for research studies where the intention is to compare results to the CSFII and NHANES data, since it is the database used for those surveys.

The PDS is an intermediate database created from SR in the process of developing the FNDDS database. It has the 60 nutrients required on the FNDDS database and is used as an ingredient file for generating the detailed foods required for the USDA FNDDS database. Table 10-5 lists the nutrients available on the USDA and NDS databases.

The most convenient way to use the USDA databases is through a software application that contains the database. The databases are also available in searchable form on the Internet. SR may be searched at http://www.nal.usda.gov/fnic/foodcomp/ and the FNDDS by choosing the "What's in the food you eat" link at http://www.ars.usda.gov/Services_docs.htm?docid=7783. The full databases can also be downloaded from their respective website for use with a spreadsheet or database application; however, the large size of the database makes this a complex task.

Several other nutrient databases are available on the USDA Food and Nutrition Information Center's website (http://www.nal.usda.gov/fnic/foodcomp/), including choline, flavonoids, fluoride, isoflavones, oxalic acid in selected vegetables, and proanthocyanidins. These specialized databases have values for selected foods and do not necessarily correspond to foods on the larger, more comprehensive USDA databases (i.e., the SR database or the FNDDS database).

An annual nutrient databank conference features updates by USDA and by researchers developing nutrient data and applications using nutrient data. The USDA website gives information about upcoming conferences (http://www.nal.usda.gov/fnic/foodcomp/index.html). The Database Conference organizers also publish a databank directory that lists both databases and software and is updated about every 2 years. This directory is available online at http://www.medicine.uiowa.edu/gcrc/nndc/survey.html.

Food frequencies and screeners must have a corresponding database to enable nutrient intake data to be generated. These databases are in constant need of updating. Early questionnaires sought to estimate intake of 15 to 20 vitamin and mineral components, but as researchers expand their questions to encompass nutrients not part of the original database, food frequencies and their databases are expanded. Also, it is not sufficient to merely update the database; the instrument itself needs revision to keep pace with new foods on the market, such as new fat-modified foods, new vegetarian main dishes, constantly increasing serving sizes, and foods with added phytochemicals, to name a few recent changes affecting questionnaire design. As new data become available, such as choline tables, or as new research interests appear, such as the glycemic index, databases for both food frequency questionnaires and software to calculate composition of food diaries and recalls must be updated.

Issues to Ponder

- What kinds of dietary data are needed to determine past nutrition or to shape recommendations for planning future food intake? Is knowledge of specific nutrients needed or would an indication of foods consumed from major food groups suffice?

- Does the need for food consumption data justify the time required for data collection and analysis?

- Can your client reasonably be expected to provide complete and accurate information about his or her diet?

- Is a food diary the best way to collect food intake data from your client or would a food frequency questionnaire be more efficient?

- Have you adequately trained your client or research subject to provide food intake data and does he or she understand how you will use this information?

- Have you made adequate arrangements to collect and report information about supplement intake?

- If nutrient values will be reported, does your database contain foods consumed by your population? Are the nutrients provided on the database the ones you need? And are complete data available for every food on the database?

VALIDITY OF DATA COLLECTION METHODS

Researchers and others have discussed difficulties encountered in estimating an individual's habitual intake with accuracy, and numerous studies have been conducted to assess accuracy of the methods we use. It is beyond the scope of this chapter to discuss this process in detail, but no discussion of dietary intake assessment is complete without at least a brief overview of validation studies.

Researchers assess the validity and reliability of assessment methods by observing actual intake before asking subjects to recall what they have eaten as a means to judge the precision of the data-gathering process. Biological markers are also used to assess accuracy of intake assessments, including urinary excretion of nitrogen, sodium, or potassium; serum vitamin E, carotenoids, or iron; and fat composition of subcutaneous adipose tissue as compared to intake of these components. These measurements are helpful in suggesting the validity of the instrument for assessing intake, although correlations between biomarkers and intake are not high. In recent years, the use of doubly labeled water has become the gold standard for assessing validity of intakes.[42] This technique estimates actual energy expenditure. Thus the energy value of reported intakes can be compared to known energy expenditure from doubly labeled water over several days. If the subject has not gained or lost weight, then the researcher can be fairly confident that when reported intake matches energy expenditure, the other nutrients are probably well represented in the composition of the foods eaten. Biomarkers can only suggest that assessment methods are valid, but their use in carefully conducted studies has given researchers confidence that the data collection methods yield useful information. However, their variability gives a sobering message about the heterogeneity of intakes within a single individual—a warning to both dietetics practitioners and researchers about the fallibility of even the most rigorously applied method.

APPLICATIONS FOR DIETETICS PROFESSIONALS

This chapter's emphasis on assessment factors impacting the research environment is deliberate, partly because research factors are easier to access but also because the dietetics professional's practice is based on knowledge developed through research. The dietetics practitioner has a unique opportunity to develop his or her own repertory of assessment methods and tools and should not be bound by the same constraints as the researcher. By understanding why researchers adopt a particular set of tools and borrowing those that apply to clinical situations—but also freely deviating from those tools when the clinical situation requires it—the dietetics professional serves the patient best. Just as there is no "average" family of 2.3 children, there are no "average" patients; instead, there are real people with real needs that must be met in a way that is culturally, emotionally, and intellectually appropriate. If a research tool is likely to be useful, then the dietetics professional should use it, but because it is adopted in the research setting does not guarantee it will be appropriate for clinical practice. Research is better at informing us of the limits of our knowledge than it is in telling us how to perform our jobs. Successful clinical practice involves a blend of life experiences, training, and research.

Below are guidelines for gathering information about a patient's past nutrition intake for use in formulating the nutrition care plan:

- Select the least intrusive method that has the precision needed for your objective. Assessment by food groups is appropriate for most clinical objectives.
- Train subjects in the data collection technique and provide well-designed forms and materials for written records. Accurate input is needed to support realistic recommendations.
- Choose validated questionnaires and documented and complete food composition tables or software when detailed nutrient composition data are required.
- Inform the subject or client of the importance of the intake data to the treatment objective or the study purpose.
- Review diaries and questionnaires as soon as they are received and query the subject for missing details.

- Give feedback to your clients and subjects on the importance and value of their contribution to the treatment objective.

REFERENCES

1. Mertz W, Tsui JC, Judd JT, et al. What are people really eating? The relation between energy intakes derived from estimated diet records and intake determined to maintain body weight. Am J Clin Nutr 1991;54:291–295.
2. Goris AH, Meijer EP, Westerterp KR. Repeated measurement of habitual food intake increases under-reporting and induces selective under-reporting. Br J Nutr 2001;85:629–634.
3. Goris AH, Westerterp KR. Underreporting of habitual food intake is explained by undereating in highly motivated lean women. J Nutr 1999;129:878–882.
4. Johansson G, Wikman A, Ahren AM, Hallmans G, Johansson I. Underreporting of energy intake in repeated 24-hour recalls related to gender, age, weight status, day of interview, educational level, reported food intake, smoking habits and area of living. Public Health Nutr 2001;4:919–927.
5. Johansson L, Solvoll K, Bjorneboe GE, Drevon CA. Under and overreporting of energy intake related to weight status and lifestyle in a nationwide sample. Am J Clin Nutr 1998;68:266–274.
6. Johnson RK, Goran MI, Poehlman ET. Correlates of over- and underreporting of energy intake in healthy older men and women. Am J Clin Nutr 1994;59:1286–1290.
7. Klesges RC, Eck LH, Ray JW. Who underreports dietary intake in a dietary recall? Evidence from the Second National Health and Nutrition Examination Survey. J Consult Clin Psychol 1995;63:438–444.
8. Lafay L, Basdevant A, Charles MA, et al. Determinants and nature of dietary underreporting in a free-living population: The Fleurbaix Laventie Ville Sante (FLVS) Study. Int J Obes 1997;21:567–573.
9. Lafay L, Mennen L, Basdevant A, et al. Does energy intake underreporting involve all kinds of food or only specific food items? Results from the Fleurbaix Laventie Ville Sante (FLVS) Study. Int J Obes Relat Metab Disord 2000;24:1500–1506.
10. Poppitt SD, Swann D, Black AE, Prentice AM. Assessment of selective underreporting of food intake by both obese and non-obese women in a metabolic facility. Int J Obes Relat Metab Disord 1998;22:303–311.
11. Bingham SA, Cassidy A, Cole TJ, et al. Validation of weighed records and other methods of dietary assessment using the 24 h urine nitrogen technique and other biological markers. Br J Nutr 1995;73:531–550.
12. Henderson MM, Kushi LH, Thompson DJ, et al. Feasibility of a randomized trial of a low-fat diet for the prevention of breast cancer: dietary compliance in the Women's Health Trial Vanguard Study. Prev Med 1990;19:115–133.
13. Haines PS, Hama MY, Guilkey DK, Popkin BM. Weekend eating in the United States is linked with greater energy, fat, and alcohol intake. Obes Res 2003;11:945–949.
14. Basiotis PP, Welsh SO, Cronin FJ, Kelsay JL, Mertz W. Number of days of food intake records required to estimate individual and group nutrient intakes with defined confidence. J Nutr 1987;117:1638–1641.
15. National Health Video, Inc. How to keep a food diary. Los Angeles: National Health Video, 1994. Available at: http://www.nhv.com. Accessed February 26, 2006
16. Nasco Food Replicas. Available at: http://www.nascofa.com/prod/Home. Accessed September 11, 2005.
17. Measuring guides for the dietary recall interview, NHANES 1999–2003. Available at: http://www.cdc.gov/nchs/about/major/nhanes/index.htm. Accessed September 11, 2005.
18. USDA Food Survey Research Group, Food Model Booklet. Available at: http://www.barc.usda.gov/bhnrc/foodsurvey/home.htm. Accessed February 26, 2006
19. Posner B, Smigelski C, Duggal A, Morgan JL, Cobb J, Cupples LA. Validation of two-dimensional models for estimation of portion size in nutrition research. J Am Diet Assoc 1992;92:738–741.
20. Van Horn LV, Stumbo P, Moag-Stahlberg A, et al. The Dietary Intervention Study in Children (DISC): dietary assessment methods for 8- to 10-year-olds. J Am Diet Assoc 1993;93:1396–1403.
21. Kretsch MJ, Fong AK. Validation of a new computerized technique for quantitating individual dietary intake: the nutrition evaluation scale system (NESSy) vs the weighed food record. Am J Clin Nutr 1990;51:477–484.
22. Weiss R, Fong AK, Kretsch MJ. Adapting ProNutra to interactively track food weights from an electronic scale using ProNESSy. J Food Comp Anal 2003;16:305–311.
23. Van Horn LV, Gernhofer N, Moag-Stahlberg A, et al. Dietary assessment in children using electronic methods: telephones and tape recorders. J Am Diet Assoc 1990;90:412–416.

24. Tran KM, Johnson RK, Soultanakis RP, Matthews DE. In-person vs telephone-administered multi-ple-pass 24-hour recalls in women: validation with doubly labeled water. J Am Diet Assoc 2000;100:777–783.

25. Moshfegh A, Borrud L, Perloff B, and LaComb R. Improved method for the 24-hour dietary recall for use in national surveys. FASEB J 1999;13(4):A603.

26. Bingham SA, Gill C, Welch A, et al. Validation of dietary assessment methods in the UK arm of EPIC using weighed records, and 24-hour urinary nitrogen and potassium and serum vitamin C and carotenoids as biomarkers. Int J Epidemiol 1997;26(suppl 1):S137–S151.

27. Plan and operation of the Third National Health and Nutrition Examination Survey, 1988–94. National Center for Health Statistics. Vital Health Stat 1994;1(32).

28. Block G, Hartman AM, Dresser CM, Carroll MD, Gannon J, Gardner L. A data-based approach to diet questionnaire design and testing. Am J Epidemiol 1986;124:453–469.

29. Subar AF, Thompson FE, Smith AF, et al. Improving food frequency questionnaires: a qualitative approach using cognitive interviewing. J Am Diet Assoc 1995;95:781–788, quiz 789–790.

30. Subar AF, Thompson FE, Kipnis V, et al. Comparative validation of the Block, Willett, and National Cancer Institute food frequency questionnaires: the Eating at America's Table Study. Am J Epidemiol 2001;154:1089–1099.

31. Kristal AR, Shattuck AL, Williams A. Food frequency questionnaires for diet intervention research. Baltimore, MD: Proceedings of the 17th National Nutrient Databank Conference, June 10, 1992.

32. Hankin JH, Stallones RA, Messinger HB. A short dietary method for epidemiologic studies: 3 Development of Questionnaire. Am J Epidemiol 1968;87:285–298.

33. Kris-Etherton P, Eissenstat B, Jaax S, et al. Validation for MEDFICTS, a dietary assessment instru-ment for evaluating adherence to total and saturated fat recommendations of the National Cholesterol Education Program Step 1 and Step 2 diets. J Am Diet Assoc 2001;101:81–86.

34. Summary of ODS workshop—Assessment of dietary supplement use: Workshop on database needs. Available at: http://ods.od.nih.gov/news/conferences/Dietary_Supplement_Use_Summary.html. Accessed September 11, 2005.

35. Pennington JAT. Bowes and Church's Food Values of Portions Commonly Consumed, 18th Ed. New York: Lippincott Williams & Wilkins, 2004.

36. ESHA Food Processor Software, ESHA Research, PO Box 13028, Salem, OR 97309. Phone: 503-585-6242. Available at: http://www.esha.com/foodpro.htm. Accessed February 26, 2006.

37. Axxya Systems, 4035 Willowbend Blvd, Suite 410, Houston, TX 77025. Phone: 800-709-2799; E-mail: info@axxya.com. Available at: http://www.nutritionistpro.com. Accessed February 26, 2006.

38. Nutrition Coordinating Center, University of Minnesota, 1300 South Second Street, Suite 300, Minneapolis, MN 55454-1015. Phone: 612-626-9428. Available at: http://www.ncc.umn.edu. Accessed September 11, 2005.

39. Institute of Medicine. Dietary Reference Intakes for Thiamine, Riboflavin, Niacin, Vitamin B-6, Folate, Vitamin B-12, Pantothenic Acid, Biotin, and Choline. Washington, DC: National Academy Press, 2000.

40. Human Nutrition Center, University of Texas-Houston, School of Public Health, Human Nutrition Center, 1200 Herman Pressler, 6th Floor East, Houston, TX 77030. Phone: 713-500-9775; Fax: 713-500-9329; E-mail: hnc@utsph.sphuth.tmc.edu. Available at: http://www.sph.uth.tmc.edu/hnc/FIAS/software.htm. Accessed September 11, 2005.

41. Stumbo PJ. Structure and uses of USDA food composition databases. J Food Comp Anal 2001;14:323–328.

42. Subar AF, Kipnis V, Troiano RP, et al. Using intake biomarkers to evaluate the extent of dietary misreporting in a large sample of adults: The OPEN study. Am J Epidemiol 2003;158:1–13.

43. Willett WC, Sampson L, Stampfer MJ, et al. Reproducibility and validity of a semiquantitative food frequency questionnaire. Am J Epidemiol 1985;122:51–65.

44. Rockett HR, Breitenbach M, Frazier AL, et al. Validation of a youth/adolescent food frequency questionnaire. Prev Med 1997;26:808–816.

45. Patterson RE, Kristal AR, Tinker LF, Carter RA, Bolton MP, Agurs-Collins T. Measurement char-acteristics of the Women's Health Initiative food frequency questionnaire. Ann Epidemiol 1999;9:178–187.

46. Lyu LC, Hankin JH, Liu LQ, et al. Telephone vs face-to-face interviews for quantitative food fre-quency assessment. J Am Diet Assoc 1998;98:44–48.

CONDUCTING RESEARCH IN A CLINICAL PRACTICE SETTING

Esther F. Myers

The profession of dietetics needs research conducted in the clinical practice setting to clearly demonstrate the value of services provided.[1-5] A small survey of selected health plan decision makers shows greater attention to evidence-based practice and high-quality data on outcomes and effectiveness to justify health plan spending and maintenance of expanded coverage of nutrition services.[6] Healthcare decision makers, such as the Centers for Medicare/Medicaid Services, are relying increasingly on evidence-based guides for practice as the basis for coverage decisions. Evidence-based guides depend on published research to support the content and approach of the proposed nutrition care interventions as well as the frequency and duration of nutrition care appointments.[7] Accrediting agencies such as the Joint Commission on Accreditation of Healthcare Organizations (JCAHO) also require that each healthcare facility demonstrate its ability to collect, analyze, and use data to continually improve all aspects of healthcare.[8] Nutrition care outcomes data are a valuable contribution to a facility's effort to meet these accreditation standards.

The practicing dietetics professional must be a vital part of the research enterprise to fully integrate research with practice.[9,10] Eck and coworkers proposed a model articulating how to integrate research into practice. This model describes a process that begins with a question stemming from current dietetics practice, followed by a literature search to determine the availability of research to answer the question.[9] If research were not available, then the dietetics practitioner would design and conduct a study to answer the question and incorporate the findings into practice. Dwyer also identified the need to involve registered dietitians in research to enhance their ability to incorporate new findings of research into practice.[11]

Although the American Dietetic Association (ADA) has identified the importance of research through articulation of a research philosophy, dietetics leaders have identified the need to increase the quantity of research that deals with the everyday life of the practitioner.[5] Only 7 to 15% of the research published in 1996 in major nutrition journals, including the *Journal of the American Dietetic Association* (JADA), *Journal of Parenteral and Enteral Nutrition* (JPEN), and *Nutrition in Clinical Practice* (NCP), was outcomes research.[9] Only 2 to 11% of articles published in JADA were authored by clinical dietitians.[9] Persons with doctoral or medical degrees who do not have applied clinical nutrition experience frequently conduct nutrition research. This research is often planned and completed without the input of clinical dietitians; therefore, the practical situations encountered by dietetics professionals in the clinical setting are often not addressed.[12]

THE RESEARCH CONTINUUM

Dwyer defines research as the organized study of a phenomenon—at both the basic and applied levels—with the specific topics of endeavor varying between investigators and over time.[11] It is clear from this definition that research can encompass a wide variety of activities. It is beyond the scope of this chapter to completely describe all types of research; Monsen's text, *Research: Successful Approaches,* provides a comprehensive review of the many types of research used to support the dietetics profession.[13]

The ADA identified research as the "foundation of practice, education and policy" and articulated the broad categories of research commonly used by dietetics professionals (Figure 11-1).[5] Basic science, nutrition science, and food science research are infrequently conducted in the clinical practice setting, where outcomes research is more likely. Clinical, behavioral, and social sciences or management research involving studies about the implementation of interventions and the impact of healthcare management policies on dietetics services are most likely to be conducted in the practice setting. Monsen described outcomes research as that which has a unique focus on practice-related issues and tangible results.[1] Eck and coworkers further described outcomes research as that conducted in clinical settings with the goal of improving patient outcomes or documenting the outcomes of nutrition interventions.[9]

TYPES OF RESEARCH

It may be helpful to think of research on a continuum according to the level of control of confounding variables. For example, studies at one end of the continuum, randomized controlled clinical trials, have a high degree of identification and control of all potential confounding variables; large samples that are meticulously selected from the intended population; sophisticated research designs; and statistical analysis. At the other end of the continuum, performance improvement data are collected in a manner intended to answer only the question for the study population (e.g., not generalized to other populations). Since the purpose of performance improvement is to evaluate practice as it currently exists, little or no attempt is made to control the confounding variables that occur in daily practice. Although this type of data collection and analysis is commonly referred to as performance improvement or quality improvement, it is research nonetheless. Performance improvement studies may focus on process measures as well as outcomes.

TRADITIONAL RANDOMIZED CLINICAL TRIALS VERSUS PRACTICE-BASED RESEARCH

Large multicenter randomized trials are essential to clearly demonstrate that a given intervention or screening/assessment tool is effective. The decision makers in healthcare or community settings, however, want to know what kind of results can be expected in the daily practice setting. A randomized clinical trial has an emphasis on ensuring that all potential confounding elements are controlled, so that the only thing that varies is the intervention of interest. Although this is extremely important in a clinical research trial, it presents a very artificial environment; this is unlikely to be encountered in daily practice, where there will be many confounding elements in each episode of care. One might view the research conducted in the practice setting as an essential second step in demonstrating the efficacy of the interventions, which

Research: Foundation of the Dietetics Profession

The American Dietetic Association believes that research is the foundation of the profession, providing the basis for practice, education and policy.

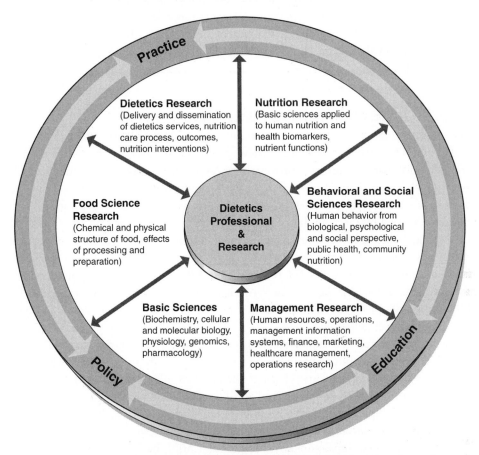

Dietetics is the integration and application of principles derived from the science of nutrition, biochemistry, physiology, food management and behavioral and social sciences to achieve and maintain people's health.

Scientists from many disciplines contribute to the categories of research used by the dietetics professional. Descriptors of each category of research found in the wedges are for illustrative purposes and not intended to be limiting, as there are other emerging areas of research.

FIGURE 11-1 *Research and the dietetics profession. Adapted with permission from Manore MM, Myers EF. Research and the dietetics profession: making a bigger impact. J Am Diet Assoc 2003;103: 108–112.*

can then be taken and delivered to diverse populations in an uncontrolled environment and still yield beneficial outcomes.

DIETETICS PROFESSIONALS AND RESEARCH

STANDARDS OF PRACTICE

Standards of Professional Performance indicate that dietetics professionals are responsible for applying findings of current research in daily practice.[14] The

Standards of Professional Performance describe the elements of practice in all areas of dietetics that are fundamental in providing quality services. Research is the second of the six key standards. The research standard states that the dietetics professional applies, participates in, or generates research to enhance practice. Standard 5, although not labeled as research, states that (dietetics professionals) systematically evaluate the quality and effectiveness of practice and revise practice as needed.[14]

WHAT ARE DIETETICS PROFESSIONALS REALLY DOING?

The practice audit conducted by the Commission on Dietetic Registration (CDR) revealed that 43 to 50% of dietitians reviewed and evaluated research, collected data, and provided data to justify nutrition services on a weekly or monthly basis.[15] Significantly fewer dietitians (4 to 16%) were involved in what may be considered more formal research activities, such as documenting measurable program outcomes, designing research studies, or serving as principal investigator.

Although the exact measures of involvement in research vary over time and by type of dietetics practice roles, the current level of involvement appears to be low in clinical practice settings. In 1988, Schiller reported that 49% of nutrition support dietitians surveyed spent some time on research.[16] A few years later, in 1993, Guyer reported that 11% of dietetics professionals spent more than 1 hour per week on research and only 5% reported spending more than 5% of their time on it.[17] In 1995, Witte and Messersmith reported that clinical managers identified conducting research as the task performed least often and perceived as being the least important task in their position; 99% reported applying new knowledge to the job, but only 23% reported using nutrition expertise in research and investigative studies in clinical dietetics.[18]

The ADA, representing over 68,000 dietetics professionals, has articulated a commitment to research, but a recent membership survey showed that a small proportion of members, approximately 2% (about 1,500), had doctoral degrees.[19] Of the 550 members likely to be researchers who responded to this survey, 70% were actively involved in conducting research. This raises the question of whether the amount and types of research needed to keep the profession vibrant can be met by these individual researchers alone.

PROFESSIONAL DEVELOPMENT IN RESEARCH SKILLS

The CDR Professional Development Portfolio process is based on the underlying principle that effective continuing professional education (CPE) involves more than information transfer alone. This process has practitioners identify the knowledge and skills needed for professional competence, use appropriate educational methods, and develop individualized strategies to implement what has been learned.[20] Research skills can be identified in this process as an area of professional development.[20] Research and grants are among the nine categories of professional skills. This category is intended to reflect skills that enable a dietetics professional to apply research findings to improve practice and professional value, to interpret research for the public, and to engage in research in a variety of settings. The "9000" category includes eight learning needs: research and grants; data analysis and statistics; evaluation and application of research; outcomes research and cost-benefit analysis;

proposal development and grant applications; publication and communication of research outcomes; research development and design; and research instruments and techniques (see Figure 11-3 on page 234). An individual can specify one of three levels to indicate the goal for professional development during a 5-year period. A research project is considered a scholarly activity suitable for CPE.[21]

OPPORTUNITIES

RESEARCH ON THE NUTRITION CARE PROCESS

The quality of patient care is considered equally as important an outcome as cost control or cost reduction. This perspective provides an ideal opportunity for dietetics practitioners to conduct research tailored to measure the quality aspects of the services that they provide. The time has never been better for the dietetics professional to consider becoming actively involved in research.

The adoption of the Nutrition Care Process by the ADA in May 2003 (see Chapter 9) provided the structure for describing and evaluating the nutrition care provided by dietetics professionals.[22] Although this may not seem to be a dramatic event, it truly will revolutionize the way dietetics professionals think about, describe, and evaluate nutrition care. For the first time, dietetics professionals will be able to use the same terms and language to describe what is occurring when they are providing nutrition care to clients/patients. The dietetics profession will have nutrition diagnosis, interventions, and nutrition monitoring as the beginnings of a unique standardized language by 2006 that can clearly link specific aspects of nutrition care outcomes. The nutrition care model provides the theoretical framework for explicit evaluation of each component of the process: nutrition assessment, nutrition diagnoses, nutrition intervention, and nutrition monitoring and evaluation (see Chapter 9).[22]

Coupled with a standardized language, the Nutrition Care Process provides the basis for a new level of research that can systematically evaluate all aspects of nutrition care provided by dietetics professionals. The ADA is actively working to develop a way to name, define, and organize both the nutrition diagnoses and nutrition interventions (Board of Directors minutes, June 2003). The intent is to create a "vocabulary" that can be used universally by dietetics practitioners and researchers to link interventions and outcomes. One of the ways to create these links is through the use of a PES statement in the nutrition diagnosis step of the nutrition care process. The "P" stands for *problem* (nutrition diagnosis), the "E" for *etiology*, and the "S" for *signs and symptoms*. This statement is generally written in the following format: "P" as related to "E" as evidenced by "S." See Table 11-1 for examples of PES statements.

In the past, even the most eloquent outcomes research studies were only able to link given outcomes to an ambiguous "nutrition visit" that provided common content and frequency of "visits" that were "minutes" long. The PES statement sets the stage for selecting an intervention to address the underlying cause (etiology) and measuring the signs and symptoms at subsequent intervals to see if the problem is being resolved. The Nutrition Care Process and standardized language should enable dietetics professionals to evaluate outcomes of care based on the same approach of providing medical nutrition therapy for a specific condition.

TABLE 11-1	Examples of PES Statements
Inadequate oral and food beverage intake R/T chewing difficulty, loss of appetite, loss of taste AEB intake of 500-calorie deficit	
Inconsistent CHO intake R/T food and knowledge deficit of CHO and insulin interactions AEB CHO intake ranging from 30 to 60 g per meal	
Low adherence to nutrition-related recommendations R/T dislike of protein drink AEB fluid intake of less than 48 oz and protein intake of less than 50 g and stated patient preferences	

AEB = as evidenced by; CHO = carbohydrate; PES = problem, etiology, signs and symptoms; R/T = related to .

EXAMPLES OF NUTRITION CARE PROCESS RESEARCH

A "standard" Nutrition Care Process implies that all patients/clients receive care provided using the same approach. This process actually allows the dietetics practitioner to more clearly delineate how he or she provides care that is tailored to the individual client/patient within each step of the process—the ultimate in client-centered care. It streamlines the way practitioners identify the nutrition diagnosis and intervention, the way care is documented and recorded, and the optimum way to collect data for outcomes research or performance improvement.

EVIDENCE-BASED GUIDES

The development of evidence-based guides for common conditions is another critical breakthrough for supporting research conducted by dietetics practitioners.[7,23–27] These guides are based on existing evidence and clearly articulate the types of outcomes that can be expected if the content of the guide is followed. Evidence-based guides can easily serve as a critical starting point for the description of the medical nutrition therapy provided and as a common protocol for data collection by multiple institutions. These guides can assist the dietetics practitioner by beginning to answer the following questions:

- What outcomes should I consider measuring?
- What outcome is considered "successful"?
- What questions require more research to be answered adequately?

Statements graded as II, III, and IV provide excellent research opportunities to strengthen clinical practice (Table 11-2).

Examples of conclusion statements that would offer good opportunities for future research are shown in Table 11-3.

Issues to Ponder

Use of the Nutrition Care Process should allow dietetics professionals to ask the following types of questions:

- Do all dietetics professionals identify the same nutrition diagnosis for a given client/patient? If not, what affects their choices? Education? Experience?
- What are the most common nutrition diagnoses for clients with a specific condition or medical diagnosis (e.g., excessive caloric consumption for patients with type 2 diabetes)?
- What is the most common nutrition intervention selected for a given nutrition diagnosis? Does the choice of nutrition intervention vary by disease/condition or is it more closely related to a nutrition diagnosis?
- What are the outcomes associated with the interventions selected?
- How does a dietetics professional's years of experience, level of education, or personal traits affect the choice of nutrition diagnosis, intervention, and ultimately the client/patient's outcome?

Evidence analysis is information that is needed to create these guides and is the first step to ensure that the guides are based on evidence. The next step is to demonstrate that the outcomes can be achieved when the guides are applied in a practice setting. The Dietetics Practice-Based Research Network is an ideal mechanism to facilitate formal field-testing in practice (see pages 231–232).

The JCAHO standards require documentation of continuous performance improvement and evidence that one standard of care exists throughout a facility. Results from outcomes research will serve to meet both of these requirements.[8] The ADA was specifically identified in one of the JCAHO publications as an example of a professional organization that had truly made strides in implementing evidence-based care.[29]

CHALLENGES IN THE RESEARCH ENVIRONMENT

While dietetics professionals and clinical dietitians express commitment and interest in research, little time is actually spent doing research. Common barriers identified are often related to the work environment or perceptions of personal competence in

TABLE 11-2		Grade Definitions: Strength of the Evidence for a Conclusion/Recommendation
GRADE	**EVALUATION**	
I	Good	The evidence consists of results from studies of strong design for answering the question addressed. The results are both clinically important and consistent, with minor exceptions at most. The results are free of serious doubts about generalizability, bias, and flaws in research design. Studies with negative results have sufficiently large sample sizes to have adequate statistical power.
II	Fair	The evidence consists of results from studies of strong design answering the question addressed, but there is uncertainty attached to the conclusion because of inconsistencies among the results from different studies or because of doubts about generalizability, bias, research design flaws, or adequacy of sample size. Alternatively, the evidence consists solely of results from weaker designs for the questions addressed, but the results have been confirmed in separate studies and are consistent, with minor exceptions at most.
III	Limited	The evidence consists of results from a limited number of studies of weak design for answering the questions addressed. Evidence from studies of strong design is either unavailable because no studies of strong design have been done or because the studies that have been done are inconclusive due to lack of generalizability, bias, design flaws, or inadequate sample sizes.
IV	Expert opinion only	The support of the conclusion consists solely of the statement of informed medical commentators based on their clinical experience, unsubstantiated by the results of any research studies.
V	Not assignable	There is no evidence available that directly supports or refutes the conclusion.

Source: Adapted with permission from the Evidence Analysis Manual. Available from the Evidence Analysis Library at http://www.adaevidencelibrary.org.

TABLE 11-3	Examples of Conclusion Statements from Evidence Analysis Library	
QUESTION	CONCLUSION STATEMENT	GRADE
What is the evidence supporting the benefit of added isoflavones on lipids?	There is sufficient evidence supporting the benefit of added isoflavones on improving total and low-density-lipoprotein cholesterol.	III
Is control of noise and light changes necessary to ensure an accurate resting metabolic rate measure by indirect calorimetry in ill adult patients?	Two narrative reviews representing expert opinions suggest that lighting and noise should be quiet for patients in critical care settings and logically extend to other settings.	IV
What evidence suggests a relationship between a patient's intake of probiotics to reduce symptoms and the reduction of symptoms associated with cancer in all cancer patients?	There is no evidence available that directly supports or refutes the relationship between a patient's intake of probiotics to reduce symptoms and the reduction of symptoms associated with cancer in all cancer patients.	V

Source: Evidence Analysis Library.[28]

research. The most commonly cited barriers are lack of financial resources and weak administrative support for research.[30] Environments most likely to support research include those with a clear emphasis on research (e.g., academic medical centers and research-oriented universities), accessible resources (particularly staff), and leadership with research expertise.[31] Gardner reported that research was more likely to be conducted in a multilevel facility or hospitals with more than 300 beds.[30] Guyer and colleagues reported that lack of resources and financial support were often cited as barriers to conducting research.[17]

Time and Priority in Daily Practice

One of the greatest challenges for dietetics professionals is incorporating the responsibility for "conducting or participating in research" into job descriptions so time and priority is given to research.[9,17] The ADA has published 30 sample position descriptions for dietetics professionals; only two of which (clinical research dietitian; research and development nutritionist) focus on research. The job descriptions for clinical nutrition manager and assistant/associate professor also include research as a primary duty and responsibility. Many position descriptions for clinical dietitians include a statement such as "participates in nutrition research studies and communicates findings through reports, abstracts, presentations, and publication." If the dietetics professional works in a JCAHO-accredited healthcare organization, there is a clear expectation that performance improvement data be collected, evaluated, and used.[8] However, more extensive research is not commonly included in position descriptions, individual performance plans, or professional development plans in many healthcare organizations other than in academic medical centers. For the approximately 65% of dietetics professionals employed in hospitals, long-term care, private practice, or community nutrition settings, little value is placed on the time and energy that is required to participate in research.[33] Despite the fact that employers have yet to recognize and compensate for research, Eck and coworkers found that 76% of a small sample of clinical dietitians/managers reported that they were willing to work extra hours to do research.[9] Clearly one way to provide adequate "resources" for research is to have it specifically identified in the expectations through the job description and associated performance evaluation systems.

The second way of expanding resources for research includes the institutional capacity to provide mentors and support staff such as statisticians and data entry personnel. If the institution is large enough and has a mission that promotes medical education, there is likely to be at least minimal support for research. Large academic medical centers have research administration departments and institutional review boards (IRBs) as well as resources for research development, training, and funding. Smaller facilities may have to rely on other institutions or universities for this support, either through affiliation agreements or informal networking. Dietetics professionals should examine where research is being conducted within their institution and meet with the principal investigators to identify any possible collaborative nutrition-related opportunities that could enhance existing projects or be incorporated into future research proposals.

RESEARCH DESIGN AND DATA ANALYSIS SKILLS

The educational standards for entry-level dietetics professionals include the basics of research.[34] Both entry-level practitioners and employers of entry-level practitioners rated research-related competencies as very important. Of the six areas where competencies required "demonstrated ability," employers rated only management lower in importance than research; practitioners rated management and food-service lower in importance. Over half of all registered dietitians have master's level education; however, clinical dietetics practitioners indicated that lack of research skills is one of the most significant barriers they face.[35]

Surveys indicated that over 80% of clinical dietetics practitioners believed they had adequate skills to participate in research and data collection, 71 to 90% reported needing additional assistance in research design, 62 to 90% felt unprepared to write a research proposal, and 90% reported inadequate skills for data analysis.[9,16,17] Despite the perceived lack of research skills, only 36% of dietetics professionals who had completed the professional development portfolio through 2003 had identified "research and grants" as a learning need they intended to pursue in the next 5 years.[5] Research accounted for only 2.3% of the total learning needs being pursued in CPE plans submitted between 2000 and 2004; outcomes research and cost-benefit analysis accounted for only 0.2% of the total (personal communication, Commision on Dietetics Registration, September 12, 2005).

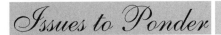

Issues to Ponder

How can barriers to conduct research in your practice setting be overcome?

- Is research a priority?
- What resources are lacking?
- Is expertise available for research design and statistical analysis?
- Who are potential collaborators?

PROTECTION OF HUMAN SUBJECTS

Regulatory requirements for protection of human subjects apply as outlined in Title 45 of the Code of Federal Regulations and the Health Insurance Portability and Accountability Act (HIPAA) when research involves human subjects.[36,37] Human subjects are "living individuals about whom a researcher obtains data through intervention or interaction with the individuals or obtains identifiable private information."[38] All institutions where research is conducted have personnel knowledgeable about the requirements for protection of patient rights and informed consent and a staff person who is designated as an expert on HIPAA. Researchers are required to demonstrate knowledge and understanding of HIPAA, protection of human subjects, and elements of informed consent. In many institutions, researchers must complete training and take an examination.

Institutional Review Boards

An IRB is a group (at least five) of "sufficiently qualified" individuals with varied backgrounds and professions who are charged with the responsibility of protecting the rights, safety, and welfare of human research participants.[38] The IRB evaluates the potential risk to the subject and the adequacy of the informed consent process for all research studies. The IRB members must have no vested interest in the research study or its outcomes. The responsibility of the IRB is to ensure that all research studies are ethical and justified.

Any research that uses personal health information (e.g., medical, family, employment, or administrative records) or tissue specimens or includes data collection from surveys, interviews, or observation is subject to protection of human subjects and must meet institution, IRB, and state and federal requirements.[38] IRBs require a fully developed research protocol. The review process may take from 3 to 9 months to gain approval. It is not uncommon to receive significant recommendations for changes in the protocol and in the informed consent process to assure that subjects are fully protected and informed about the research. The IRB will determine if a full board review is indicated or whether the research plan is exempt or qualifies for an expedited review. Examples of research that might be exempt from a full board review include secondary data analysis when data cannot be linked to subjects, educational research involving normal teaching practices, and some survey research, interviews, or observations when the information is not recorded in a way that the subject can be identified or linked to responses. It is not safe to assume that surveys or interviews will automatically fall into the category of minimal risk. Loss of confidentiality can cause harm to subjects, their relatives, and others, or sensitive questions may cause distress. Additional information on how to categorize research designs and about the IRB process can be obtained at the National Institutes of Health (NIH) website[39]: http://www.niaid.nih.gov/ncn/clinical/decisiontrees/default.htm.

Informed Consent

The basic premise behind the informed consent process for human subjects is that each person participating in research must be given sufficient information to understand the nature of the study, possible risks and benefits, and alternative options; he or she must also have the opportunity to ask questions before making a decision to participate.[40]

HIPAA Requirements

The HIPAA requirements include protection for health information about living participants or about deceased persons, any related human tissue samples, chart reviews, and/or information stored in databases or repositories. Again, the concern is about the potential disclosure of protected information that may still be linked to the person and whether the release of that information will put people at more than minimal risk. In most cases, institutions have recommended that language addressing the HIPAA requirements be included as part of the routine informed consent process.[39]

Learn More about IRBs

There are several on-line courses and references available to researchers. Those applying for federal funding must include a certificate indicating that they have completed a course and are knowledgeable of the requirements.[41,42] On-line courses offered by NIH for all investigators who are applying for funding can be found at the following website[42]: http://www.niaid.nih.gov/ncn/grants/manage/index.htm. A complete guidebook for IRBs is also available from the Office of Human Research Protections but probably provides more in-depth information than most researchers need.[36] Local IRBs frequently provide educational programs to help keep researchers up to date on requirements.

COLLABORATIVE OPPORTUNITIES AND PARTNERING

Dwyer suggests that actively involving dietetics professionals in clinical and scientific research helps to reduce the considerable time lag that often exists in applying new and existing knowledge.[11] Dwyer makes 14 suggestions for incorporating research competencies in dietetics practice:

- Urge research-oriented dietitians with advanced degrees to join relevant nutrition research societies.
- Develop more proactive programs for support of dietetics training—in particular, excellent clinical nutrition and dietetics research and training programs.
- Advocate with hospital associations, accrediting bodies, federal agencies, and others to include dietitians in practice patterns initiatives, clinical guidelines development, and research outcomes.
- Lobby for establishing dietetics research traineeships at federally funded centers.
- Begin a frank dialogue with universities about what is feasible regarding "on the job" clinical training for research careers of those not so trained at universities given the exigencies and economic stresses engendered by healthcare reform.
- Work with universities to develop doctorate-level tracks for clinical research and community service needs and foster collaboration between universities and teaching hospitals.
- Advocate and perpetuate the view that clinical nutrition involves several disciplines.
- Develop bridging schemes for enhancing research training.
- Start examining the barriers currently perceived to impede dietetics professionals whose practice focuses on scientific and clinical research aspects.
- Survey alleged inequities regarding rank, salary, course and student loads, research funding, and other problems faced by the dietetics faculty.
- Include nutrition scientists with dietetics credentials on study sections and grant review of relevant nutrition and food research.
- Recognize that "turf" problems exist and work to resolve them.
- Develop clinical research fellowships for dietetics professionals with advanced

degrees that go beyond appropriate funding for them and develop career ladders for graduates of such fellowships.

- Ensure that investigators design sound research, avoid conflicts of interest, and are not intimidated by special interest groups.

Eck and colleagues proposed a model for making outcomes research a part of standard practice in clinical dietetics.[9] Trostler and Myers proposed a mechanism of creating a dietetics practice-based research network that would allow practitioners to participate in the research process without the burden of planning and analyzing the results.[43]

COLLABORATION WITH UNIVERSITY FACULTY

University faculty members are often experienced dietetics researchers. In addition, to having conducted their own research, they may be actively mentoring graduate students who are learning about research. Undergraduate students may also be participating in research by designing, implementing, and evaluating a research project or participating in a larger research study being conducted by someone else in the department. In some instances, dietetics education programs require students to submit their research projects for IRB review as part of the learning objectives. University IRBs will be able to review the research proposal for students and faculty.

Dietetics professionals interested in conducting research need to obtain or enhance their research skills. For some dietetics practitioners, the preferred method of obtaining these skills is to collaborate with an experienced dietetics researcher.[9] Brehm and associates report that upper-level undergraduate and graduate students were given a project that allowed them to enhance their research and clinical skills by assisting in a research project of another faculty or preceptor.[49] Precepting a student requires a level of commitment that may not always result in gaining more time to work on the project but does give the satisfaction of knowing that you are helping the next generation of dietetics professionals learn about research and demystify the research process. Students participating in smaller projects can learn how to design relatively simple studies that can easily be incorporated into the daily routine.[10] Hays and colleagues identified a critical need to have entry-level dietetics professionals obtain skills to document efficacy of nutrition care.[45] Schiller and Moore identified 10 guidelines to achieve success in an outcomes research project.[46]

- Fully integrate research with practice to capitalize on familiarity with procedures and knowledge of literature in area of current practice.
- Expect that while data collection may be done on the job, other activities may need to be accomplished after hours or on days off (e.g., literature search or writing up results).
- Start with a small pilot study and use the experience to help design larger studies.
- Seek out and create a team of collaborators or mentors who are familiar with the area of practice, research design, or statistical methods.
- Lack of funding may not be a show-stopper for a small pilot study, and the pilot study results may be used to justify funding for a larger study.
- Select a manageable problem/research question in an area where you have control and where it will be possible to conduct the research and to implement the changes.

- Study an area where medical nutrition therapy is expected to make a large difference; focus on a high-risk population or a condition where nutrition will have a big payoff (i.e., decreased complications, length of stay, or cost).
- Carefully select the research sample; clearly identify inclusion and exclusion criteria to ensure that other factors do not impact results; randomly select and assign subjects to intervention or control groups when possible.
- Whenever possible, use existing data and established data collection methods and resources.
- Create a personal reference library of publications that describe outcomes evaluation and research.

From the perspective of the university faculty member, collaboration in student education and research enhances the classroom experience by adding a real-life flavor to projects and allowing the student to have contact with another mentor during their undergraduate or graduate experience. This provides a wonderful opportunity to identify the questions that are of interest to dietetics professionals and may serve as the genesis of future research studies.

COLLABORATION WITH OTHER HEALTHCARE RESEARCHERS

A multitude of collaborative opportunities exist with other healthcare researchers because of the richness of the dietetics profession and the focus on nutrition, social sciences, basic sciences (including genetics), food science, management, and public health.[5] Natural partners in dietetics-related research projects might be a psychologist working with a dietitian to address successful behavior modification strategies or measurement of quality of life in weight-management programs; a management professor working with a dietitian to address staffing and resource allocation; or a social scientist working with a dietetics professional to devise methods to evaluate the impact of socioeconomic status on adherence to diet. Gardner interviewed dietitians who had experienced multidisciplinary collaboration and identified many benefits such as gaining from each others experiences and abilities, mutual support, enhanced interdepartmental relationships, expanded influence of the dietetics profession, and the ability to incorporate outcomes research into more facets of dietetics practice.[30]

DIETETICS PRACTICE-BASED RESEARCH NETWORKS

The dietetics literature has many examples of research effectively conducted by dietetics professionals in the practice setting. Eck et al. reviewed research articles published in JADA, JPEN, and NCP and determined outcomes research comprised 6.6, 12.1, and 16.7%, respectively, of the total research articles published.[9] Informal practice-based research networks have recently formed to conduct a specific study and disband after completion of data collection.[43] The ADA has established a Dietetics Practice-Based Research Network (DPBRN) that will be able to answer research questions important to practitioners on an ongoing basis.[44] A practice-based research network is "a group of clinical practices and of individual providers within practices, devoted principally to the care of patients affiliated with each other and also perhaps with academic or governmental enterprises for the purpose of investigating the phenomena of practice impact occurring in communities."[43] In a practice-based research network, practitioners determine the research question and collect the data while the researcher facilitates the process but typically does not set the research agenda. Trostler and Myers summarized characteristics of practice-based research networks established by other professions and identified the following benefits to the dietetics profession[43]:

- Creates an organized way for practicing dietetics professionals to participate in all phases of the research process, from idea generation to translating results into practice.
- Provides support for research questions that are a priority of the practicing dietetics professional.
- Creates a new venue to enhance research capabilities of dietetics professionals
- Enhances clients' and other healthcare professionals' perception of the credibility of the dietetics professional and quality of services.
- Provides access to subject populations for collaborative translating research with academic dietetics professionals.
- Affords opportunities for initiating internal and external collaborations/partnerships.
- Contributes to the body of knowledge of outcomes from services provided by dietetics professionals.

ACTIVITIES FOR GETTING STARTED

There is no better time to initiate research than today. Establish a feasible timeline that promotes success. These activities focus on enhancing personal research skills, establishing ways to incorporate research into daily activities, networking, seeking mentors, and developing collaborative relationships. One of the key activities is to consciously pursue additional skills in research. Figures 11-2 to 11-4 illustrate how to incorporate research skill development into the Professional Development Portfolio. The learning plan can be revised or updated at any time during the 5-year period at http://www.cdrnet.org/pdrcenter. Activities for getting started are listed below:

1. Incorporate research skills in your professional development portfolio (see Figure 11-2).
2. Put an appointment on your calendar to check the Research and Professional Development section of ADA's website and CDR's website to identify opportunities for involvement or professional development offerings (http://www.eatright.org and http://www.cdrnet.org).
3. Consciously select at least one professional development or FNCE session to learn about a new research skill (look for sessions that list the 9000 series as one of the codes as well as clinical topic codes).

   - Ask a specific question about methodology of the research.
   - Ask a question about the statistical analysis completed.
   - Stay after the session or contact the researcher and ask if you could schedule a time or send an e-mail to discuss a related research question that you are interested in pursuing (or ask them to recommend someone with knowledge of the area that you are interested in).

Step 1: Professional Self-Reflection

When determining your goals, review the information about yourself and your practice that you recorded on pages 1-3.

What are my professional goals? *(e.g., stay abreast of current developments in nutrition, maintain expertise in nutrition support, consult for long term care, write for consumer publications, establish Quality Improvement policies and programs, obtain Masters in Public Health Degree)*

Short Term: (1 - 3 years)

Review the basics of research design principles for outcomes research

Long Term: (3 - 5 years)

Participate in planning and conducting a small outcomes research study

Professional Development Portfolio • Do not send to CDR • Maintain for personal reference.   Worksheet 1   4

FIGURE 11-2 *Step 1 of the Professional Development Portfolio. Modified with permission from Professional Development Resource Center. Available at: http://www.eatright.cdrnet.org/pdrcenter/ portfoliotoc.htm. Accessed May 23, 2005.*

4. Discuss with your supervisor your desire to participate in or conduct research.
   - Explain your desire for professional development in the area of research.
   - Ask if this can be incorporated as part of your position description and annual goals if your organization uses performance goals as part of its evaluation system.
   - Ask your supervisor for suggested contacts within your organization with similar interests.
   - Explain the potential benefits to the organization (improved patient care, visibility of and credibility of department, strategic goals of organization that are

Step 2:
Learning Needs Assessment

In this second step of the Professional Development Portfolio process you assess your learning needs.

1. Review the list below.

2. Darken the circle to the left of each learning need that will help you achieve the professional goals you set in Step 1.

3. Next to each learning need you select, darken a circle corresponding to the level (or levels) of CPE required to attain your goals (if appropriate, you may select more than one CPE level for any learning need).

You must use the learning need codes from this worksheet when completing your Learning Plan and your Learning Activities Log.

Level of CPE Desired

Level 1 – Assumes little knowledge of subject	Level 2 – Assumes general knowledge of the literature and practice	Level 3 – Assumes thorough knowledge of the literature and practice
Goal: increase knowledge	Goal: increase knowledge & application	Goal: synthesis of recent advances and future directions

RESEARCH AND GRANTS

Description: Skills that enable a dietetics professional to apply research findings to improve practice and document professional value, to interpret research for the public, and to engage in research in a variety of settings.

			Level 1	Level 2	Level 3
○	9000	Research and Grants	○	○	○
○	9010	Data analysis, statistics	○	○	○
○	9020	Evaluation and application of research	○	○	○
●	9030	Outcomes research, cost-benefit analysis	●	●	○
○	9040	Proposal development, grant applications	○	○	○
○	9050	Publication, communications of research outcomes	○	○	○
●	9060	Research development and design	●	○	○
●	9070	Research instruments and techniques	●	○	○

Professional Development Portfolio • Do not send to CDR • Maintain for personal reference.   Worksheet 2

FIGURE 11-3 *Step 2 of Professional Development Portfolio. Modified with permission from Professional Development Resource Center. Available at: http://www.eatright.cdrnet.org/pdrcenter/portfoliotoc.htm. Accessed May 23, 2005.*

related to research, possible contribution to accreditation processes of JCAHO or other accrediting bodies).

■ Discuss how this additional workload might be incorporated into your daily workload.

5. Contact your local university and dietetics education program directors of medical departments in an academic medical center.

■ Schedule a lunch date or telephone call with a researcher to discuss how you might become involved.

Registration No:

/	/	/	/	/	/

Make additional copies of this side if needed. Complete registration number and last name for each side completed.

Last Name:

STEP 3 - LEARNING PLAN

Goal #: 01   Review the basics of research design principles appropriate for outcomes research

Learning needs supporting goal:

Outcomes Research/CB analysis	Research Dev + Design	Research instrument + Techniques	
Print Learning Need	Print Learning Need	Print Learning Need	Print Learning Need
Learning Need Code:	Learning Need Code:	Learning Need Code:	Learning Need Code:
9 0 3 0	9 0 6 0	9 0 7 0	
Level of CPE Needed:	Level of CPE Needed:	Level of CPE Needed:	Level of CPE Needed:
Level 1 ●	Level 1 ●	Level 1 ●	Level 1 ○
Level 2 ●	Level 2 ○	Level 2 ○	Level 2 ○
Level 3 ○	Level 3 ○	Level 3 ○	Level 3 ○

Goal #: [ ][ ]

Learning needs supporting goal:

Print Learning Need	Print Learning Need	Print Learning Need	Print Learning Need
Learning Need Code:	Learning Need Code:	Learning Need Code:	Learning Need Code:
Level of CPE Needed:	Level of CPE Needed:	Level of CPE Needed:	Level of CPE Needed:
Level 1 ○	Level 1 ○	Level 1 ○	Level 1 ○
Level 2 ○	Level 2 ○	Level 2 ○	Level 2 ○
Level 3 ○	Level 3 ○	Level 3 ○	Level 3 ○

Enter this information online at www.cdrnet.org OR

1237521157   **Mail** this original form to CDR at: 120 South Riverside Plaza, Suite 2000, Chicago, IL 60606.
Questions? **Email** CDR at redesign@eatright.org. or **call** CDR at 1-800-877-1600. ext. 5500.

Page: [ ][ ]

FIGURE 11-4 *Step 3 of Professional Development Portfolio. Modified with permission from Professional Development Resource Center. Available at: http://www.eatright.cdrnet.org/pdrcenter/portfoliotoc.htm. Accessed May 23, 2005.*

- Have a list of questions that you think would help you do your everyday work better (potential research questions).
- Provide the researcher with a copy of recent practice-related studies completed that are of interest to you (e.g., studies about comparisons of protocol-driven nutrition care to usual care or studies that report results of protocol-driven care without comparison groups).
- Find out what research they are currently working on in their department and be prepared to think about how to add a nutrition component from your area if applicable.
- Be prepared to identify what you might be able to do.
  - Offer a student experience completing a research project with your collaboration.
  - Collect data for study of researcher's interest if it fits into your practice.

6. Join the ADA Research Dietetics Practice Group or other research-oriented organizations.
   - Newsletters and membership materials are easy ways to become more familiar with research projects; look for opportunities for involvement and get ideas for your own projects.
7. Collaborate with other dietetics researchers and other healthcare providers.
   - Find out who is currently conducting or planning to start research studies in your facilities.
   - Make it a point of asking them to explain their research study to you.
     - Be open to the possibility of helping them with a nutrition-related component of their current or proposed research study.
   - Ask them if there is a possibility of including nutrition components in future research studies.

CHALLENGES FOR THE FUTURE

Dietetics professionals will face a number of challenges in the future. Dietetics professionals need to truly embrace evidence-based practice by allocating time and energy to gain the additional research skills and to allocate time for participation in research. This requires a commitment from individual dietetics practitioners, supervisors, the institution, and the ADA.

As the Nutrition Care Process becomes recognized and applied in the practice setting, it will be critical that it evolves from a theory-based process into an evidence-based practice. A research-based standardized language is necessary to document the outcomes resulting from the provision of care according to the model. Dietetics practitioners need to make a firm commitment to continually improve their practice based on research. In order to be meaningful to the profession, findings must be published and disseminated to others in a timely manner. Dietetics professionals need to ascribe to a high standard for practice-based research by ensuring that the research designs selected are appropriate for the question being asked and that the data and results are accurately reported to reflect the nature of the study. The research must be hypothesis driven and follow sound research design and analysis principles. Discussion must clearly acknowledge both the strengths and limitations of the research. Practice-based research needs to be accepted as a legitimate type of research and well-respected journals must be willing to publish these studies. Funding for dietetics-specific research will continue to be a challenge. The ADA has articulated research priorities; however, these may not match funding agency agendas.[47] The American Dietetic Association Foundation (ADAF) has established a research endowment that in the future may help fund small practice–based research studies. Collaborative research endeavors need to be explored to obtain funding with other healthcare practitioners, university faculty, and industry or government partners when the goals and objectives are mutually acceptable. The agreements must be structured to maintain the independence of the investigator in creating the research design, collecting data, and analyzing the results. There must be a commitment to publish results regardless of the findings.

REFERENCES

1. Monsen ER. Outcomes research: placing a value on nutrition services. J Am Diet Assoc 1997;97:832.
2. Fitz P. President's page: show them the numbers. J Am Diet Assoc 1997;97:898.
3. Coulston AM. President's page: measuring—and increasing—our influence. J Am Diet Assoc 1999;99:404.
4. O'Sullivan Maillet J, Manore MM. Dietetics matters: demonstrating our impact. J Am Diet Assoc 2003;103:14.
5. Manore MM, Myers EF. Research and the dietetics profession: making a bigger impact. J Am Diet Assoc 2003;103:108–112.
6. Fitzner K, Myers EF, Caputo N, Michael P. Are health plans changing their views on nutrition service coverage? J Am Diet Assoc 2003;103:157–161.
7. Myers EF, Pritchett E, Johnson EQ. Evidence-based practice guides vs protocols: what's the difference? J Am Diet Assoc 2001;101:1085–1090.
8. 2004 Comprehensive Accreditation Manual for Hospitals: The Official Handbook (CAMH). Chicago: Joint Commission Resources Inc, 2003.
9. Eck LH, Slawson DL, Williams R, Smith K, Harmon-Clayton K, Oliver D. A model for making outcomes research standard practice in clinical dietetics. J Am Diet Assoc 1998;98:451–457.
10. Rinke WJ, Berry MW. Integrating research into clinical practice: a model and call for action. J Am Diet Assoc 1987;87:159–161.
11. Dwyer JT. Scientific underpinnings for the profession: dietitians in research. J Am Diet Assoc 1997;97:593–597.
12. Rose J. Research or practice? J Am Diet Assoc 1985;85:797–798.
13. Monsen ER, ed. Research: Successful Approaches. 2nd Ed. Chicago: American Dietetic Association, 2003.
14. Kieselhorst KJ, Skates J, Pritchett E. The American Dietetic Association Standards of Practice for Dietetics Professionals in Nutrition Care and Updated Standards of Professional Performance. J Am Diet Assoc 2005;105:641–645.
15. Rogers D, Leonberg BL, Broadhurst CB. Commission on Dietetic Registration Dietetics Practice Audit. J Am Diet Assoc 2002;102:270–292.
16. Schiller MR. Research activities and research skill needs of nutrition support dietitians. J Am Diet Assoc 1988;88:345–346.
17. Guyer LH, Roht RR, Probart CK, Bobroff LB. Broadening the scope of dietetic practice through research. Top Clin Nutr 1993;8:26–32.
18. Witte SS, Messersmith AM. Clinical nutrition management position: responsibilities and skill development strategies. J Am Diet Assoc 1995;95:1113–1120.
19. Myers EF, Beyer PL, Geiger CJ. Research activities and perspectives of research members of the American Dietetic Association. J Am Diet Assoc 2003;103:1235–1243.
20. Professional Development Resource Center. Available at: http://www.eatright.cdrnet.org/pdrcenter/portfoliotoc.htm. Accessed May 23, 2005.
21. Geiger CJ, Bittle CA, Gates GE, et al. Scholarship and the CDR recertification (Professional Development Portfolio) process. J Am Diet Assoc 2003;103:975–976.
22. Lacey K, Pritchett E. Nutrition Care Process and Model: ADA adopts road map to quality care and outcomes management. J Am Diet Assoc 2003;103:1061–1072.
23. Nutrition Diagnosis: A Critical Step in the Nutrition Care Process. Chicago: American Dietetic Association, 2006. Available at: http://www.eatright.org/Catalog. Accessed September 12, 2005.
24. American Dietetic Association. Medical Nutrition Therapy Evidence Based Guides for Practice. Chicago: American Dietetic Association, 2001. Available at: http://www.eatright.com/catalog. Accessed July 18, 2004.
25. Medical Nutrition Therapy Evidence-Based Guides for Practice. Nutrition Practice Guidelines for Gestational Diabetes Mellitus [CD-ROM]. Chicago: American Dietetic Association, 2002. Available at: http://www.eatright.com/catalog. Accessed July 18, 2004.
26. Medical Nutrition Therapy Evidence-Based Guides for Practice. Nutrition Practice Guidelines for Type 1 and 2 Diabetes Mellitus [CD-ROM]. Chicago: American Dietetic Association, 2002.
27. Medical Nutrition Therapy Evidence-Based Guides for Practice. Chronic Kidney Disease (non-dialysis) Medical Nutrition Therapy Protocol [CD-ROM]. Chicago: American Dietetic Association, 2002.
28. Evidence Analysis Library. Available at: http://www.adaevidencelibrary.org. Accessed September 12, 2005.
29. Putting Evidence to Work: Tools and Resources. Chicago: Joint Commission Resources Inc., 2003.

30. Gardner JK, Rall LC, Peterson CA. Lack of multidisciplinary collaboration is a barrier to outcomes research. J Am Diet Assoc 2002;102:65–71.

31. Bland CJ, Ruffin MT. Characteristics of a productive research environment: literature review. Acad Med 1992;67:385–397.

32. Hornick BA, ed. Job Descriptions: Models for the Dietetics Profession. Chicago: American Dietetic Association, 2003:99.

33. Rogers D. Report on the ADA 2002 dietetics compensation and benefits survey. J Am Diet Assoc 2003;103:243–255

34. Bruening KS, Mitchell BE, Pfeiffer MM. 2002 accreditation standards for dietetics education. J Am Diet Assoc 2002;102:566–577.

35. Bryk JA, Soto TK. Report on the 1997 Membership Database of the American Dietetic Association. J Am Diet Assoc 1999;99:102–107.

36. Office for Human Research Protections—IRB Guidebook. Available at: http://www.hhs.gov/ohrp/irb/irb_guidebook.htm. Accessed February 25, 2006.

37. Unsure how to handle HIPAA? Available at: http://www.HIPAA.org. Accessed May 23, 2004.

38. Protection of Participants in Behavior and Social Sciences Research. Available at: http://obssr.od.nih.gov/irb/protect.htm. Accessed May 23, 2004.

39. Decision Tree for HIPAA in SLU Research. Available at: http://www.niaid.nih.gov/ncn/clinical/decisiontrees/human.htm. Accessed May 23, 2004.

40. Guidance for Institutional Review Boards and Clinical Investigators 1998 Update. Available at: http://www.fda.gov/oc/ohrt/irbs/default.htm. Accessed May 23, 2004.

41. NIH Education Requirement. Available at: http://www.umresearch.umd.edu/IRB/irb_NIH.htm. Accessed February 25, 2006.

42. All About Grants Tutorials. Available at: http://www.niaid.nih.gov/ncn/grants/default.htm. Accessed February 25, 2006.

43. Trostler N, Myers EF. Blending practice and research: practice-based research networks an opportunity for dietetics professionals. J Am Diet Assoc 2003;103:626–632.

44. Brehm BJ, Rourke KM. Cassell C. Enhancing didactic education through participation in a clinical research project. J Am Diet Assoc 1999;99:1090–1093.

45. Hays JE, Peterson CA. Use of an outcomes research collaborative training curriculum to enhance entry-level dietitians' and established professionals' self-reported understanding of research. J Am Diet Assoc 2003;103:77–84.

46. Schiller MR, Moore C. Practical approaches to outcomes evaluation. Top Clin Nutr 1999;14:1–12.

47. Castellanos VH, Myers EF, Shanklin CW. The ADA's research priorities contribute to a bright future for dietetics professionals. J Am Diet Assoc 2004;104:678–681.

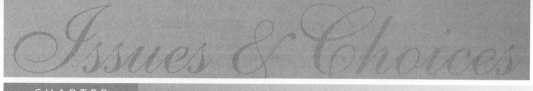

INFORMATICS IN THE NEW
HEALTHCARE ENVIRONMENT

Syed S. Haque

The invention of the computer, such as ENIAC in the mid-1950s, represented the beginning of the "information age" and the information revolution. Rapid developments in telecommunications and information technology as well as the universal availability of powerful and easy-to-use personal computers (PCs) have significantly changed our daily lives. Increasing use of PCs, coupled with the use of the Internet, has created an information explosion in our society. It has been estimated that between 1999 and 2002, the amount of new information stored on paper and magnetic storage devices grew at a rate of about 30% per year and has almost doubled every 3 years. In the year 2002 alone, the amount of new information produced was equal to 37,000 new libraries of the size of the Library of Congress, which contains 136 terabytes of information (about 20 million books and other collections). Ninety-two percent of this new information was stored mostly in hard disks. The information explosion is also having a considerable impact on the nature of work in the healthcare and biomedical fields. Consequently, computing systems and technologies have become increasingly essential for the efficient and effective management of healthcare, including dietetics and nutrition care. Although healthcare institutions in general have been slow in adopting and incorporating information technology in their specific clinical environment, information technology is already showing a profound impact in modernizing healthcare organizations and institutions in relation to the systems they use and the knowledge they produce. Healthcare professionals working in the field of dietetics and nutrition in particular need to become thoroughly familiar with the latest and most powerful information processing and management techniques available in relation to their routine and clinic-specific needs.

The delivery of healthcare, including dietetics and nutrition services, is an information-intensive process. Clinical practice itself requires the gathering, synthesizing, and use of that information in making relevant decisions. For example, high-quality patient care involves proper documentation and timely access to patients' medical history, health status, current medical conditions, and treatment plans, as well as to administrative and financial information. Dietetics professionals and food managers will need these skills to utilize the advanced communication tools necessary to their practice. In fact, the use of computers is increasing in all areas of dietetics. Other examples where dietetics professionals will find computers invaluable are for obtaining and evaluating the nutrition composition of food, departmental data processing and information management, nutrition and dietetics research, statistical analysis, nutrition assessment, inventory control, and quality assurance, to name only a few. Computers can greatly enhance patient care and improve nutrition care, clinical decision making, and operations management. Table 12-1 provides examples of computer applications in dietetics and nutrition care.

In addition to the growing need to learn and to use the ever-changing information technology within a specific healthcare setting, a host of factors are adding to the burden of dietetics professionals, including:

- Searching for information.
- Integrating disparate data points into a cohesive picture of the patient.
- Supporting treatment services and clinical decision making to improve patient outcomes.
- Developing and implementing nutrition care plans for patient health and safety.
- Improving performance in patient care and outcomes.

Dietetics professionals need to understand how various information technology solutions can be fundamental to the implementation of their care plans and critical to the workflow needs of the department.

HEALTH INFORMATICS

Increasing use of information and computing technologies—coupled with an increased awareness of the knowledge explosion in healthcare and biological sciences and the growing trend toward the use of computers for solving problems in healthcare—has changed the milieu of healthcare itself. Healthcare has now entered an era of health informatics, which takes advantage of the potentials of information tech-

TABLE 12-1	Computer Applications in Dietetics and Nutrition Care
APPLICATION CATEGORY	**EXAMPLES**
Communication	Send/receive information to and/or from other departments, e-mail, talk or chat, placing orders and verifying prices with vendors
Foodservices management	Inventory control, budgeting and financial analysis, costs control, forecasting, recipe and menu planning, production control, room services, tray assembly and delivery, menu planning and printing, computerized menu selection system, and improving patient satisfaction
Food science and technology	Computerized databases and database inquiries, library catalogues and reference documents on computer networks, diet analysis, design, analysis, and development of new food products
Public health	Collection, storage, and diet analysis of data on individual clients and programs, word processing and electronic communication relative to pertinent information from around the world, nutrition education and computer-assisted diet instructions
Clinical dietetics	Use of computers in recording nutrition care plans, calculating diets or enteral feedings, nutrient analyses, providing diet instructions, and placing diet orders, including evidence-based care and plans
Research	Determining solutions to complex problems in relation to treatment and prevention of certain diseases (e.g., high cholesterol, high blood pressure, diabetes, chronic constipation, obesity, cancers, chronic fatigue, etc.) and improving the product and process of patient care

nologies, including computer and information sciences, to solve problems associated with both the routine and complex tasks of healthcare delivery, clinical practice, education, and biomedical research. Health informatics incorporates "the use of information resource management and processing to support all health-related activities concerned with the care of the sick, disease prevention, and health promotion."[1] Thus, the goal of health informatics is to improve the efficiency and effectiveness of all the processes and tasks of healthcare.

Health informatics may be defined as a science that deals with health information and information technologies to support all healthcare activities, ranging from those pertaining to the care of the sick to healthcare promotion and disease prevention, health professions education, management of health information systems, and research and development efforts associated with healthcare. Health informatics, as a phrase, is more comprehensive and less restrictive than medical informatics. Medical informatics has been defined as "the field of study that concerns itself with the cognitive, information processing, and communication tasks of medical practice, education, and research, including the information science and technology to support these tasks."[2] Health informatics as a discipline integrates the biomedical and health sciences with the knowledge and methods of information and computer science, bioengineering, biostatistics, health services research, and bioinformatics with a focus on providing informatics solutions to problems in all aspects of healthcare. The jobs of specialists in health informatics include new titles, such as chief information officer (CIO), information architect, and database analyst; they can also involve a redefinition of work, with titles such as health information management director, medical librarian, etc. Some examples of what specialists in health informatics do include:

- Reducing diagnostic uncertainties and improving clinical decision making by using computing techniques and information technologies (e.g., development of clinical decision-making tools for determining the probability that an emergency room patient with chest pain actually has acute cardiac ischemia or should be admitted to rule out myocardial infarction).
- Designing interactive consultation systems to treat patients more efficiently and cost-effectively by using local or national databases that have referral capabilities to a broad range of clinical experiences and pertinent variables.
- Developing transportable software systems for image reconstruction and three-dimensional visualization and analysis of medical image data.
- Developing new medical applications for the methods of three-dimensional visualization and analysis, leading to improved diagnosis, treatment, understanding, and education regarding abnormalities in internal structures and in their function.
- Designing large databases of digitized medical images for use in medical decision making, teleradiology, or teleconsultation.
- Improving research designs and outcomes of clinical trials, epidemiological studies, and health services research.
- Developing computing systems and solutions that will help design more effective and more informative clinical trials, thus cutting years off of drug development processes.
- Utilizing computational approaches and modern computer-based techniques in drug design, molecular genetics, and cellular genetics to solve complex clinical problems.

- Designing and managing clinical, pharmacy, radiology, laboratory, or hospital information systems.
- Designing and implementing a system that will free more time for healthcare providers to spend on more important aspects of patient care through delegation of some information handling and processing tasks to computers.
- Designing a computer simulation suitable for analyzing medical and healthcare problems for constructing solutions to optimize decisions concerned with efficacy of information transfer, productivity and resource utilization in a healthcare facility.
- Performing quality assurance activities, inservice training, patient education software development, etc., in a healthcare facility at that facility's request.
- Designing and implementing computer-based multimedia educational/training systems (e.g., interactive CD-ROMs and web-based educational programs) for intelligent tutoring, self-paced learning, staff development, or improving clinical decision-making on selected topics.

DIETETICS OR NUTRITION INFORMATICS

Dietetics practitioners, like any healthcare specialists, analyze a situation and make recommendations or carry out actions for the betterment of their patients. Their education is focused on using bits of data as a builder uses bricks, understanding what those bits of data mean, and knowing how to apply them to the patient. Evidence-based sources of professional material such as scientific papers, practice guidelines, and research protocols that support or contraindicate courses of action are presented throughout their training and practice of the discipline. The concept of using references such as these to form opinions and guide clinical judgment is formally called evidence-based medicine. This is discussed further toward the end of the chapter.

HEALTH INFORMATION SYSTEM

The term "health information system" refers to a framework of people, procedures, knowledge resources and services, human expertise, software programs, and computer and relevant equipment designed to perform health information processing tasks. A health information system is integrated into the healthcare delivery process, designed to be a patient-oriented systemization of information involving all aspects of the patient's healthcare. A hospitalwide information system tracks health status of its patients, provision and use of services, healthcare costs, quality, utilization, and outcomes of care. Most of the functions of a hospital information system can be divided into two main groups: clinical and financial. Examples of clinical applications include laboratory automation, quality assurance, radiology, cardiology, pathology, dietetics, bedside computing, nurse scheduling, care plans, and transcription. Financial applications include patient billing, medical records and coding, patient registration, payroll, budget, and material and assets management. It is much more than a shelf with old reference books. It is a dynamic assistant to care. A state-of-the-art information system is networked throughout the institution and is expected to gradually replace older methods of collection and storage of health information. Ideally, a healthcare information system should provide a seamless flow of health information, providing the best health system for the greatest number of people at an affordable cost (see Figure 12-1).

In a fully networked information system, all of its subsystems and services are connected to each other in such a way that any information required can be accessed anywhere at any time. Dietetics information is essential to patient care helping the patient and the other healthcare providers have access to nutrition diagnoses and care. Dietetics practitioners should work with information technology staff to assure their data and services become part of the information collected. The essential data for practice and research needed to be collected and inputted will need to be determined and then collected. This chapter ends with a brief discussion of standardized language to improve data acquisition.

DATA ACQUISITION (COLLECTING AND CAPTURING DATA)

Data are nothing more than observations. The word "data" is used whether we are talking about one thing or several. Data are collected through comparison. If I look at the sky and say it is blue, I am comparing the sky to a past palette of colors and am announcing that I have matched this sky to the color blue. If I send blood to be

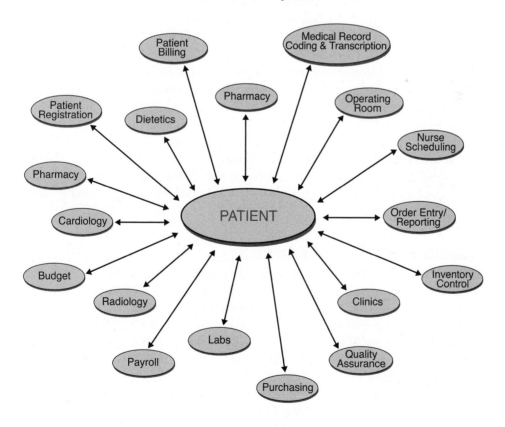

FIGURE 12-1 *Fully networked health information system.*

tested for cholesterol, a number is returned, which I can then compare to a normal level and risk ranges for that cholesterol observation. Often the process of observing and comparing is called "capturing data."

Tools used to capture data include thermometers, blood tests, scales, physical touch, sight, smell, or any other device we can use to collect an observation. Even a picture can be considered data, as in an x-ray image.

ORGANIZING DATA

Paper records have been the traditional storage devices for data. Data in the paper storage system is little more than marks on paper. To extract the information from paper, each paper must be read and interpreted. Letters, numbers, and other symbols are used to communicate the data to and from the paper. Manual review of each sheet is necessary to collect the data points needed for the creation of information. When there are many sheets of paper, the process is time-consuming. When the papers reviewed are voluminous, another piece of paper is often used to summarize the data and make the conversion to information. To compare the change in body mass index (BMI) of a patient at the beginning of a treatment, such as cancer chemotherapy, to that at the end of the therapy, reviews of paper records would be necessary to find the appropriate height and weight measurements for the analysis; these would then be used to calculate the initial and final BMIs.

ANALYZING DATA TO PROVIDE REASONING, DIAGNOSES, AND THERAPIES

Whereas data are stored in paper systems as marks of ink that are letters, numbers, or other symbols, digital computer data are stored in the form of a binary code. "Binary" means two. There are no letters, symbols, or other numbers beyond zero and one. Being machines, computers recognize a circuit as "on" or "off." Zero represents a switch being turned off and one represents a switch being turned on. A light switch can be either on or off; similarly, a single path in a computer can be considered to be on or off. A single switch is called a bit and a series of eight switches is called a byte. Depending on the pattern of these eight bits, the computer is able to express letters, numbers, and other symbols in the same way that a paper record system can. Mathematical calculations related to this binary code permit all the functions a computer is capable of carrying out and explain why the computer is called a computer.

PRESENTING INFORMATION AND KNOWLEDGE

Imagine being asked to consult on a patient who has diabetes mellitus, hyperlipidemia, hypertension, and a negative history of coronary artery disease who was recently in the hospital for acute renal failure after an alcoholic binge. The physician is requesting dietary consultation directed at compliance with a daily diet containing 2 g of sodium, 200 mg of cholesterol, and 2,000 calories. What information would you want to have available? How would you engage the patient to maximize likelihood of compliance?

Electronic medical records provide information on display screens. These can be programmed to provide structured data automatically to both the dietetics professional and patient during the evaluation. Access to laboratory records in an electronic medical record can provide the dietetics professional with the patient's name, address, date of birth, age, gender, past laboratory values, and other values in a structured way instantaneously. Estimation of cardiac risk can be based on National Cholesterol Education Program public health guidelines as a screen element that presents cardiovascular risk to the patient in his or her present state of medical health versus at goal. It can also be used to demonstrate to the patient possible benefits of behavior modifications necessary to achieve medical goals. Entry of a finding in one part of the chart appears in other parts of the chart automatically instead of requiring a repetitive entry of data, as in a paper chart. Personalized patient education aids such as handouts could be produced automatically at the end of the consultation for the patient's review at will.

These screens, however, must be programmed through collaboration between dietetics professionals and programmers. Dietetics professionals using their paper forms must explain why each element is where it is and how it interacts with other elements, so the programmer fully understands what is needed and then takes advantage of the computer's ability to manipulate data in useful ways. Designing customized patient education materials is very doable and attractive. The new food pyramid released by the U.S. Department of Agriculture[3] is a good example of broadly tailored information.

Let us take this a step further. Data, information, and knowledge are not the same. Data are nothing more than the results of observations. The patient's weight is 120 lb. The value 120 is a datum. Information is the application of that datum in a specific way. When we combine a series of observations related to the weight of a single person over time, we gain information related to that person's weight. The change of weight from 120 to 130 to 135 lb shows us that the patient is becoming heavier. Knowledge is an understanding of what information means and gives us the ability to act. It allows us to apply understanding, make predictions, and act to guide events. The first weight is recorded at the first trimester prenatal visit, the second at week 20, and the third at week 26 of a pregnancy. We would apply knowledge concerning pregnancy-related weight changes to predict whether the weight gain was appropriate and guide our recommendations related to the patient's dietary goals for the subsequent weeks of pregnancy. So data are used to provide information, which can then be analyzed and acted on in relation to the knowledge we have. Many programs are already developed, such as one that calculates and plots children's growth patterns.[4]

RESEARCH AND DEVELOPMENT

It is estimated that using computer-based medical records instead of paper-based ones could prevent half of all medical errors. Computers are becoming a fact of life in all health-related fields. They allow an extraction or harvesting of data from a few to thousands of computerized records. They can graph such data as lab values, vital signs, or changes in weight and height over short or long periods with little effort on the part of the interested person. They can automatically present data such as height and weight as a BMI. They can use the value of the BMI index as a guide to offer printable, tailored handouts designed to promote patient education. Taken to another step, this process could be used to help determine total parenteral nutrition preparations.[5] Human beings make mistakes. Computers are conceived and maintained by human beings. Errors are the eighth leading cause of death in the United States today. It is a public health initiative to move to physician computer order entry and electronic medical records at all levels of healthcare. Whereas human beings make errors due to several factors, the use of computers refines these processes continuously, thus minimizing errors.

HARDWARE AND SOFTWARE

Computers utilize hardware and software. Hardware includes the physical components of a computer, such as the keyboard, computer monitor, disk drives, motherboard, expansion cards, power supply, and so on. One of the most important pieces of hardware in any computer is its central processing unit (CPU), a highly complex silicon chip ranging from the size of a matchbook to that of a wallet. This is the computer's brain, taking requests from applications and then processing or executing actions and carrying out various operations.

The faster your processor is, the more operations it can execute per second. The more operations per second, the faster applications happen; thus, games play more smoothly and spreadsheets calculate more quickly. The software includes programs, procedures, rules, and associated documentation pertaining to the operation of a system. Software also contains the programming instructions by which a computer performs its calculations and functions. Think of software as being the path a car must take to go from one point (home) to another (work), while the hardware is the car, the road, and any traffic signals. To achieve a successful trip, there must be roads and the traveler must drive them correctly. With computers, a programmer looks at a system's hardware and determines the best way of providing it the software directions on how to reach the desired goal.

ELECTRONIC MEDICAL RECORDS: WHAT THE HEALTHCARE TEAM NEEDS TO KNOW

Due to the increasing impact of information technology in all aspects of life, almost everything is computer-based or digital: e-mail, records, images, etc. Healthcare professionals and organizations have finally begun to appreciate the potential of information technology by digitizing the healthcare environment and moving toward replacement of paper-based records to paperless or computer-based records. Although the concept of computer-based records dates back to at least the 1980s, the biggest boost for the computer-based patient record (CPR) came from the 1991 report of the Institute of Medicine (IOM). The IOM described the CPR as "an electronic patient record that resides in a system specifically designed to support users through availability of complete and accurate data, practitioner reminders and alerts, clinical decision support systems, links to bodies of medical knowledge, and other aids including the ability to provide an accurate longitudinal account of care."[6] Although the CPR provides patient information quickly, supports clinical decision making, and reduces administrative costs for the collection, storage, and retrieval of data, it was seen as a longitudinal record that captured information in an image format of the paper-based records. The electronic medical record (EMR), designed on the basis of modern systems theory coupled with advanced information technology, is seen as having the features of future healthcare systems that will improve the quality of healthcare delivery in the United States. The following is a list of basic components of the EMR:

- Health information and data repository
- Clinical documentation
- Results management
- Order entry/order management
- Decision support systems
- Electronic communication and connectivity
- Patient support
- Administrative process
- Reporting and population health management
- Clinical messaging

Electronic medical records have been around since computers were used to track laboratory results, vital signs, and other health-related information. Sometimes the system is simple, like a glucometer that has a computer in it, which tracks a series of glucose readings over a number of finger-stick blood glucose tests. Other times it may be a vast system that tracks every laboratory test, physician order, and professional progress note. There is no one producer of these systems. There is no single format for these systems. Each system is therefore different. Groups have attempted to unify these systems in design, but these efforts are voluntary at this point in time. One system may permit communication with others through an e-mail type of system while others call the same process "flags." A potassium blood test might demonstrate a critical value in blue in one system and show it in red in another. The core concept in working with an EMR system is to know that specific system. There are two critical phases for users of an electronic medical record. The first is the manipulation and presentation of stored data. The second is the input of data. Issues such as user identification, user authentication, patient privacy, and system maintenance are always present and implicit during all interactions with these systems.

HIPAA REGULATIONS: IMPLICATIONS FOR THE PRACTITIONER

With the advent of the information age and increasing access to health information due to computerized and networked health information systems, the issues relating to the privacy, security, and confidentiality of personal health information (PHI) have become increasingly important. Healthcare is an information-driven industry; information is its best asset and this valuable asset must be protected. Healthcare providers need to protect the privacy of personal and intimate details that patients share. This information is fundamental to the diagnostic and treatment process. Some people with legitimate or illegitimate access to information systems, however, could use patient data for wrong and harmful reasons. Examples would include gathering and selling PHI for personal gain, financial or otherwise, putting data in the hands of a third party who has an obvious conflict of interest, or deliberate data leaks to discredit a person or an institution without the knowledge and consent of the owner. As a result of heightened awareness of security, confidentiality, and privacy of personal health information, the U.S. Department of Health and Human Services issued the privacy rule under the Health Insurance Portability and Accountability Act (HIPAA) of 1996. Implementation and enforcement of HIPAA is having a major effect on patient privacy and security, and use of the Internet for transporting medical information. Its purpose is to assist patients with maintaining the confidentiality of their personal health information. According to the Centers for Medicare and Medicaid Services, organizations and individuals are affected in the following areas[7]:

STANDARDS FOR PRIVACY OF INDIVIDUALLY IDENTIFIABLE HEALTH INFORMATION

The Privacy Rule standards address the use and disclosure of an individual's health information—also called "protected health information"—for certain health transactions, including claims, enrollment, eligibility, payment, and coordination of benefits. These standards also address the security of electronic health information systems. Organizations covered by the Privacy Rule—also called "covered entities"—must make reasonable and appropriate administrative, technical, and physical safeguards to prevent intentional or unintentional use or disclosure of protected health information in order to avoid violation of the Privacy Rule. Some examples of identifiable health information include: name, address, names of relatives, names of employers, birth date, telephone or fax numbers, e-mail address, social security number, medical record number, health plan beneficiary number, account numbers, license numbers, vehicle identification numbers, Internet Protocol address numbers, photographs, and biometric and other unique identifiers.

The process of complying with the standards, keeping in view that highly sensitive information is stored on the networks and transmitted over the Internet between providers and payers, provides healthcare organizations opportunities to utilize most efficient e-healthcare technologies and strategies to protect privacy and confidentiality of medical records.

MANDATE ON PROVIDERS AND HEALTH PLANS, AND TIMETABLE

Providers and health plans are required to use the standards for the specified electronic transactions 24 months after they are adopted. Plans and providers may comply directly, or may use a healthcare clearinghouse. Certain health plans, in particular workers compensation, are not covered.

PRIVACY

An area under constant review, it can be looked upon in its broadest sense as preventing the sharing of health information regarding an individual patient where not expressly permitted by the patient through contract with an insurer or his or her personally expressed authorization.

PREEMPTION OF STATE LAW

The bill supersedes state laws, except where the Secretary determines that the state law is necessary to prevent fraud and abuse, to ensure appropriate state regulation of insurance or health plans, addresses controlled sub-stances, or for other purposes. If the Secretary promulgates privacy regula-tions, those regulations do not pre-empt state laws that impose more strin-gent requirements. These provisions do not limit a state's ability to require health plan reporting or audits.

<u>PENALTIES</u>

The bill imposes civil money penalties and prison for certain violations.

To be HIPAA compliant with PHI, a healthcare provider cannot discuss a specific pa-tient with any individual that does not have a legal reason to know about this per-son. This means that a provider cannot tell a husband about a wife's health condi-tion without her express permission to do so. The patient must know that when her husband asks for information regarding the areas not approved for discussion with her husband that the provider will refer the husband to the wife to discuss those is-sues. Exceptions to this include the finding of a lack of competency by a legally rec-ognized method for a given jurisdiction, such as coma in the patient and the spouse becoming the medical decision maker for the patient during the time of the patient's cognitive impairment. Look for guidance from authorities in this area regarding specific questions and issues in complying with the HIPAA standards. The Center for Medicare and Medicaid (CMS) has extensive information on line at http://www.cms.hhs.gov. Figure 12-2 is a HIPAA checklist produced by CMS.

Dietetics professionals are among the major users as well as producers of PHI. Each patient's visit contains information on symptoms, food intake, family history, physical findings, diagnosis, treatment, and outcomes. Dietetics practitioners must treat information confidentially, knowing what may be shared, the techniques to share written or electronic information, what physical safeguards need to be fol-lowed, and what software is HIPAA compliant. Implementation of HIPAA privacy and confidentiality rules within healthcare organizations should increase patients' trust that their private health information will remain confidential and only those who are permitted to know will have access to the information.

THE INTERNET: PORTALS FOR HEALTHCARE INFORMATION

Patients have traditionally discussed their healthcare needs with doctors, but they are increasingly going to the Internet as an important source of information in relation to healthcare decisions. Millions of adults go online every day to look for healthcare information. Mostly they navigate these sites using portals or search engines rather than going directly to the particular site. The Internet continues to be used by a huge and growing number of the public interested in getting information about particular diseases or treatments or staying healthy. This information can be accessed quickly and easily via search engines and portals.

A portal is an entry point, or home page, for accessing Internet content and services. Portals are single gateways to information that provide interactivity and the ability to use "technologies to transmit information to users through a stan-dardized web-based interface." A portal provides a single point of access to data

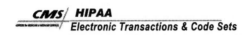

CMS/ HIPAA
Electronic Transactions & Code Sets

PROVIDER HIPAA CHECKLIST
Moving Toward Compliance

The Administrative Simplification Requirements of the Health Insurance Portability and Accountability Act of 1996 (HIPAA) will have a major impact on health care providers who do business electronically, as well as many of their health care business partners. Many changes involve complex computer system modifications. Providers need to know how to make their practices compliant with HIPAA. The Administrative Simplification Requirements of HIPAA consist of four parts:

1) Electronic transactions and code sets;
2) Security;
3) Unique identifiers; and
4) Privacy.

> **IMPORTANT:** It is up to you as the health care provider to see to it that your transactions are being conducted in compliance with HIPAA, whether or not you contract a third party biller or clearinghouse to conduct any of these transactions for you.

HIPAA does not require a health care provider to conduct all transactions listed under #1 electronically. Rather, if you are going to conduct any one of these business transactions electronically they will need to be done in the standard format outlined under HIPAA.

1. Determine if you are covered by HIPAA

Do you, or a third party billing company or clearinghouse, conduct any one of the following business transactions electronically?

➤ Claims or equivalent encounter information
➤ Payment and remittance advice
➤ Claim status inquiry/response
➤ Eligibility inquiry/response
➤ Referral authorization inquiry/response

❑ **YES** ➔ YOU ARE MOST LIKELY COVERED BY HIPAA. CONTINUE WITH THE CHECKLIST.

❑ **NO** ➔ YOU ARE MOST LIKELY NOT COVERED BY HIPAA. YOU DO NOT NEED TO CONTINUE WITH THE CHECKLIST.

2. If YES, assign a HIPAA Point Person who will be responsible for HIPAA

Your HIPAA Point Person can be your office manager or any other individual who will be responsible for HIPAA related activities. Make sure your HIPAA Point Person is given the authority, resources, and time to prepare your office staff for the impact of HIPAA on your practice. The checklist on the next page is designed to help your HIPAA person plan and prepare for HIPAA's electronic transactions and code sets requirements.

FIGURE 12-2 *Provider HIPAA checklist.*

and services that the user needs. Furthermore, information can be organized and personalized. Personalization means that users get only the information that is relevant to him or her. An interface could be called a portal if the user is able to personalize the interface manually by changing user profiles. Additionally, a portal should provide many applications, like a search-and-retrieval tool, and should help the user by providing information that might be useful.[8] An integrated healthcare portal can provide communitywide access to healthcare information and integrated services. This could include information for physicians, hospital staff, and patients. The immense flexibility of the web enables the portals to be customized to the needs of individual members.

HIPAA
Electronic Transactions & Code Sets
Provider HIPAA Checklist

Checklist for HIPAA Point Person

Familiarize yourself with the key HIPAA deadlines

☐ April 16, 2003 – TESTING: You (or your software vendors) need to start testing your software and computer systems internally no later than this date. By testing this means ensuring your software is capable of sending and receiving the transactions you do electronically in the standard HIPAA format.

☐ October 16, 2003 – COMPLIANCE DEADLINE: This is the date you must be ready to conduct transactions electronically in the standard HIPAA format with your health plans / payers.

Know how HIPAA affects your office

☐ Determine if your software is ready for HIPAA (each health care provider is responsible for making sure the software they use will be compliant with HIPAA according to the key deadlines above).

☐ Speak with your practice management software vendors (or billing agent or clearing house if you use one) to assess which items under #1 you conduct on paper and which you conduct electronically. Determine what you will need to do differently. For instance, under HIPAA additional data may be required and data fields you use now may no longer be required.

☐ Ask your vendor how and when they will be making HIPAA changes and document this in your files.

☐ Remind your vendors you must start testing your systems no later than April 16, 2003. Similarly, if you use a third party biller or clearinghouse, remind them of this testing deadline.

Talk to the health plans and payers you bill

☐ Ask them what they are doing to get ready for HIPAA and what they expect you to do.

☐ Ask them if they will have a HIPAA companion guide that specifies their coding and transaction requirements that are not specifically determined by HIPAA (while HIPAA mandates standard transactions, some health plans may not require data elements for every field). For instance, ask your payers for billing instructions on how to code for services that were previously billed using local codes (under HIPAA local codes are eliminated).

☐ Ask them whether they will have "Trading Partner Agreements" that specify transmission methods, volumes, and timelines as well as coding and transaction requirements that are not specifically determined by HIPAA. These may also specify how HIPAA compliance testing and certification are to be done.

☐ Ask them about testing your software to make sure, for instance, that they will be able to receive a claim you submit with your updated software.

☐ If you use software or systems provided by the health plan / payer (such as on-line direct data entry) to conduct transactions, ask whether they intend on continuing to support these systems.

**For more information on HIPAA please visit our website at
http://www.cms. hhs.gov/hipaa/hipaa2, send us an e-mail at
askhipaa@cms.hhs.gov, or call us at 1-866-282-0659.**

FIGURE 12-2   *Provider HIPAA checklist (cont).*

Two types of portals are available: horizontal and vertical. Horizontal portals like Yahoo are also called consumer portals, web portals, or public portals, and provide a bit of information for everyone. Vertical portals, also called enterprise information portals (EIPs) or corporate portals, provide information for a particular group with a specific interest like medicine. Both types of portals have some common features, which include single sign-on, personalization, security, organizational branding, content management and administration, and patient directory integration. Portals can be useful to healthcare institutions in improving care, reducing medical errors, increasing physician loyalty, simplifying workflow, improving access to information and current systems, and enhancing patient-physician interaction.

Dietetics professionals can use portals for improving communication while reducing paperwork. Many issues can be effectively addressed by nutrition portals, such as improving the efficiency of scheduling, workflow simplification, enhancing patient interaction, improving the quality of care, user satisfaction, policies and procedures of the department, and resource utilization. Nutrition portals can also be used for providing relevant and reliable nutrition and health information, cafeteria menus, sending reminders or alerts and specific instructions to patients, and providing online appointment settings for patients. Healthcare, as one of the largest industries, can take advantage of the tremendous potential of portals for reducing the information gap between healthcare professionals and their patients.

SEARCH ENGINES

Some websites help individuals search for information by creating a list of sites that have information indicated in the search criteria. Sites that do this are often called search engines. Search engines such as Google, Yahoo, MSN, and others do not validate the websites they provide. They simply allow a term to be entered and provide a list of websites that say something about that term. Value can be assigned to a website in several ways. First, is the site reputable? A government site will likely be freer from bias than a site a company has provided to sell its services. The National Library of Medicine (NLM) is an example of a government site that provides information on medical literature based on a process that is separate from commercial concerns. The site categorizes articles within months of their being published in certain journals that the NLM feels are focused on science. These categories are searchable using a system known as medical subject headings (MeSH). The NLM program searches its database using the MeSH terms and finds articles and abstracts about the topic. The American Dietetic Association (ADA) is an example of a website of high value for nutrition information.[9] It provides position papers, food and nutrition information both for the professional and lay public, access to continuing education, networking opportunities within specific practice areas, political advocacy, and other useful functions.

PDA PROGRAMS

Personal data assistants (PDAs) are handheld computers that fit in a pocket and provide the user with references and sometimes connectivity to larger systems. They can be programmed to perform calculations, collect data from other devices, and store notes, along with numerous other functions. Many programs are available, such as BMI calculators, nutrient analysis programs, tube-feeding algorithms, and online medical textbooks. The current estimate is that 32% of dietitians use PDAs in their practice, with an equal number considering their use.[10]

The more PDAs integrate with other systems, the more practical their use becomes. The greatest challenge with the PDA is its screen size. It can be difficult to see or to enter information by hand, but if a practitioner wants to do a quick profile based on BMI or determine the appropriate total parenteral nutrition formula, a PDA can be a quick and practical aid. Tablet personal computers (PCs) may replace PDAs in the future. HIPAA privacy issues should be addressed if patient data are on the PDA.

USING THE MEDICAL LITERATURE

About 400 BC, Hippocrates, the father of modern medicine, said "Life is short, science is long, opportunity is elusive, experimentation is dangerous, judgment is difficult."[11] More than 2,000 years later, Sir William Osler said "The desire to take medicine is perhaps the greatest feature which distinguishes man from animals."[12]

Healthcare literature supports decisions about real world issues. There are several methods for making decisions using the literature. Some are brief and focused, other are much broader. The critically appraised topic (CAT) is a literature review that is brief, relevant to the clinical issue, and evidence based. It asks a single clear question, requires a concise answer, only uses a few sources, and is not meant to be a major systematic review of the literature. The key in this type of literature review is the appraisal of the literature used. The sources must be valid and apply to the topic being reviewed.

The systematic review is more than the creation of a review article on a topic, as review articles use commentary to come to conclusions. A systematic review is fully evidence based, and comes to a blind stop when valid strong evidence is not available to go further. It starts with a clearly stated question. It has an explicit rigorous search for and appraisal of all sources of information.

Using either style of review, the individual must do five things[13]:

- Be sure to ask the right question.
- Find the evidence that applies to the question.
- Appraise how valid the evidence is for the specific question.
- Appraise the applicability of the evidence to the question.
- Reach a conclusion based on these findings.

The good question can be on any imaginable topic that is clinically important. It is based on patients' clinical needs. The answer matters to both the provider and the patient.

Assessing the evidence is like finding a needle in many haystacks. A variety of sources can be considered, such as the Internet, books, journals, libraries, and expert opinion. Once the sources of information are obtained, their relative strength should be measured. Opinion is just that and is often used where no stronger evidence is available. Case series are collections of cases with more value than a single opinion that offer a greater degree of sampling and therefore hold greater strength that a single event. Controlled trials offer a much stronger type of evidence. They compare something in one group to the same thing in another group, where a variable is purposely different. The influence of that variable is determined by what happens within the two groups.

Randomized, prospective, placebo-controlled double-blind studies are an even stronger type of evidence. These studies minimize the bias of the people conducting the study by having subjects randomly placed in each group, hiding the variable that is different between the groups, and not allowing patients or researchers to know which group had which variable until the study is over. A double-blind study exists when neither patient nor scientist knows who is getting the treatment and who is not. Meta-analysis is the analysis of groups of controlled trials in order to answer questions that each may not have completely answered. It is important to realize that, in the real world, all trials have flaws or imperfections. Depending on the topic, one must weigh the impact of the flaw on that trial's result. The applicability of the evidence found will then determine the amount of attention the reviewer should pay to the findings.

The decision reached by the review is totally dependent on the desired outcome. If the information available is very weak, the decision must reflect that. The fact that a man bought a lottery ticket from the local store and won $1 million cannot justify telling another person to buy lottery tickets as soon as possible. The fact that diabetes mellitus and high cholesterol are often found together and both can lead to early death may not necessarily justify doing a cholesterol test in another person with diabetes.

The use of evidence-based dietetics has advanced significantly in the past 5 years. The ADA's evidence analysis library (see Chapter 11) provides member practitioners with some guides but, more importantly, has an entire step-by-step evidence analysis system to help practitioners examine the evidence themselves.[14,15]

STANDARDIZED LANGUAGE FOR DATA COLLECTION

The profession of informatics deals with the sciences of managing and sharing information, but the profession of dietetics must establish what data to collect, manage, and share. The ADA is in the process of establishing a standardized language for nutrition diagnostic terminology. Chapter 9 of this book contains the 2006 version of nutrition diagnostic terminology. The purpose of creating this "controlled vocabulary"[16] is to have different practitioners use the same terminology independent of setting. To accomplish this, terms must be complete, not vague, and not redundant. The terms describe the nutrition diagnosis (problem), not the medical diagnosis. For example, medical nutrition therapy (MNT) is provided to individuals with diabetes mellitus, but the diagnosis for the registered dietitian is not diabetes, the medical diagnosis. The nutrition diagnosis would be excessive carbohydrate intake, inappropriate carbohydrate intake, obesity/overweight, low adherence to nutrition-related recommendations, or physical inactivity. The nutrition diagnosis depends on the individual person and the nutrition priorities to improve health. Much more readily than a medical diagnosis, the nutrition diagnosis (problem) may resolve.

The nutrition diagnoses being developed are similar to the nursing diagnostic codes. Nursing currently has five sets of nursing languages. The North American Nursing Diagnosis Association defined nursing diagnosis as "a clinical judgment about individual, family or community responses to actual or potential health problems/life processes. Nursing diagnosis provides the basis for selection of nursing interventions to achieve outcomes for

Issues to Ponder

- What functions do you perform that would be enhanced in quality or speed through the use of computers?

- If you were asked to define the term "dietetics informatics" what would the definition be? Do we need specialists in dietetics informatics? If so, what would they do?

- Have you started to use evidence analysis in your practice?

- What items would you want in a patient database that would allow you to customize your nutrition education materials?

- What programs could you load on a PDA or computer to facilitate your practice?

- What influence has HIPAA had on your practice? Is your work environment safeguarding PHI?

- How will standardized nutrition diagnoses assist in applying the science of informatics to dietetics?

which the nurse is accountable."[17] This concept applied to dietetics relates to the intent of the diagnoses. The diagnoses go well beyond the traditional documentation of nutrition risk status. The diagnoses are a professional shorthand for the nutrition problem and the intervention. If all or at least most dietetics professionals work to have these diagnoses fully networked into their health information systems, the nutrition diagnostic codes should facilitate information sharing and adequate information to measure desired outcomes. This structured method of collecting data that dietetics professionals have been gathering for years will document outcomes and establish standards of practice based on these findings. Over the next decade, the system will evolve and hopefully be refined to describe what nutrition diagnoses patient have, what dietetics professionals do to resolve the problems, and the success of the intervention.

CONCLUSION

Informatics is a discipline growing by leaps and bounds. It is a process for harnessing data and information in the pursuit of knowledge and the application of that knowledge. Where the previous healthcare environment had a rift between new knowledge and the patient, the 21st century is seeing attempts to bridge that gap using computers and structured processing of facts. Paper information systems cannot keep up with our new digital age. Patients' privacy can be protected by burdensome information systems such as paper records, but patient safety reports show that their lives are not as safe. Concepts taught in statistics classes can apply dynamically in daily practice when they are presented electronically.

By using modern information systems, each member of the healthcare team can be setting up the next team member to succeed. The dietetics professional can use information from physicians and nurses to define issues more quickly while providing unique insight to the healthcare team. The principle is the same as that of direct deposit in banking. Instead of needing to wait for paper and processing it at the bank in order to go to a store and purchase what you need, the money is placed directly into your account and your account can be accessed directly through a card. Savings in time is just one outcome, making jobs more efficient, easier, and more rewarding. This is the true benefit.

Today's students and professionals are preparing for a world that their teachers have just now begun to meet. This new world is based on decision support and on-demand information. The benefits should be not just to the patients but also to providers. Better patient outcomes should be the banner of the dietetics professionals of the new millennium.

....

REFERENCES
....

1. Gatewood LC. A training program for the medical school. In: Haque S, ed. Medical Informatics: Computers in Health Sciences. Proceedings of a Symposium on Computers in Health Services. November 10, 1998. Hyattsville, MD: Dependable Printing Inc., 1998:81-87.
2. Greenes RA. Academic and institutional perspectives of an emerging specialty. In: Haque S, ed. Medical Informatics: Computers in Health Services. Proceedings of a Symposium on Computers in Health Services. November 10, 1998. Hyattsville, MD: Dependable Printing Inc., 1998:1-7.
3. USDA. MyPyramid. Available at: http://mypyramid.gov. Accessed November 12, 2005.

4. Kids Nutrition.Org. Available at: http://www.kidsnutrition.org. Accessed November 12, 2005.

5. Lehmann CU, Conner KG, Cox JM. Preventing provider errors: online total parenteral nutrition calculator. Pediatrics 2004;113:748–753.

6. Simpson RL. Ensuring patient data, privacy, confidentiality and security. Nursing Management 1994;25:18–20.

7. The Centers for Medicare and Medicaid Services website. Available at http://www.cms.hhs.gov/hipaa/hipaa2/default.asp. Accessed September 16, 2004.

8. Frye C. Knowledge portals unify data streams. Application Development Trends 1999 (December). Available at: http://www.adtmag.com/pub/dec99/f9912022.shtml. Accessed March 1, 2006.

9. American Dietetic Association website. Available at: http://www.eatright.org. Accessed June 17, 2004.

10. pdaRD. The dietitian's choice for PDA products and info. Available at: http://www.pdard.com. Accessed November 12, 2005.

11. Quoted in McPhee J. Clinical unit in ethics and health law: in science we trust. Aailable at: http://www.ehlc.net/news/10_00.html. Accessed March 1, 2006.

12. Quoted in Cushing H. Life of Sir William Osler. Vol. 1. Oxford: Clarendon Press, 1925.

13. Guyatt GH, Haynes RB, Jaeschke RZ, et al. Users' Guides to the Medical Literature: XXV. Evidence-based medicine: principles for applying the Users' Guides to patient care. Evidence-Based Medicine Working Group. JAMA 2000;284:1290-1296.

14. ADA Evidence Analysis Library. The American Dietetic Association. Available at: www.eatright.org/adaevidencelibrary.com/default.cfm. Accessed November 12, 2005.

15. Myers EF, Pritchett E, Johnson, EQ. Evidence-based practice guides vs protocols: what's the difference? J Am Diet Assoc 2001;101:1085-1090.

16. Zhang J. Representations of health concepts: a cognitive perspective. J Biomed Informatics 2002;35:17-24.

17. North American Nursing Diagnosis Association (NANDA) home page. Available at: http://www.nanda.org. Accessed December 12, 2003.

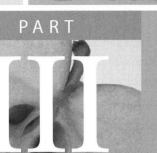

Issues & Choices

PART III

EFFECTS OF EMERGING SCIENCE AND CONTROVERSIES ON DIETETICS PRACTICE

Editor: Wanda H. Howell

GENETICS, NUTRITIONAL GENOMICS, AND DIETETICS PRACTICE: WHAT THE DIETETICS PROFESSIONAL SHOULD KNOW

Gail P.A. Kauwell

April 2003 marked two momentous occasions in science—the 50th anniversary of Watson and Crick's publication of the structure of DNA and completion of a high-quality reference sequence of the human genome. Sequencing of the human genome, the major goal of the Human Genome Project (HGP), has paved the way for an unprecedented level of understanding of the molecular functioning of organisms and the influence that environmental factors such as nutrition have on risk reduction and expression of disease. Although improvement of human health through the widespread application of genome-based knowledge is still several years away,[1] it is incumbent on dietetics and nutrition professionals to educate themselves about genomics now. An understanding of the basic principles and issues related to genetics and genomic healthcare will provide practitioners with a base for interpreting and applying the outcomes of this research and for delivering maximally effective intervention strategies once genomic healthcare is feasible on a wider scale.

To address the need for practitioners who are adequately prepared to integrate genetics into their practice, the National Coalition for Health Professional Education in Genetics (NCHPEG) developed a set of core competencies in genetics. These competencies represent the minimal knowledge, skills, and attitudes necessary for health professionals from all disciplines (see Appendix A).[2] Aspects of these competencies that are most relevant for dietetics practice include understanding basic genetics terminology and concepts, understanding the implications of genetic testing results, knowing how to elicit and use a family history, recognizing when nutrition may play a role in modifying disease risk for common chronic diseases with a genetic basis, and using the results of genomic research to individualize care. Dietetics professionals also need to understand the social and psychological implications of genetic services, appreciate the limitations of their genetics expertise, and recognize when to make referrals to genetics professionals. This chapter provides dietetics professionals and students with an overview of genetics-related topics and issues and their implications for nutrition practice. A glossary of terms appears at the end of this chapter (see Appendix B).

THE HUMAN GENOME PROJECT AND BEYOND

The Human Genome Project (HGP) was an international collaborative research program that officially began in 1990 with the goal of sequencing all of the genes that comprise a human being (i.e., the human genome) by 2005. Other goals included sequencing the genomes of model organisms (e.g., *Escherichia coli*, *Saccharomyces*

259

cerevisiae, Caenorhabditis elegans, and *Drosophila melanogaster*), developing new technologies to study whole genomes, and examining the ethical, legal, and social implications (frequently referred to as ELSI) of genomic research.

The foundation for this project was laid by the cooperative efforts of the National Human Genome Research Institute (NHGRI) of the National Institutes of Health (NIH) and the U.S. Department of Energy (DOE). The project grew to include participation by scientists at universities and research facilities from around the world, collectively referred to as the International Human Genome Sequencing Consortium.

In February 2001, the International Human Genome Sequencing Consortium published a series of papers in *Nature,* including the first draft of the sequence of the human genome.[3] Concurrently, Celera Genomics, a private for-profit company, published its version of the human genetic code in *Science.*[4] Despite the fact that the private and publicly funded versions were constructed using different techniques, they were remarkably similar.

A little over 2 years later, in April 2003, the International Human Genome Sequencing Consortium announced the successful completion of all of the HGP goals, including a finished sequence (i.e., highly accurate, contiguous sequence) of the blueprint for human life.[5] A series of news stories, viewpoints, and articles celebrating the 50th anniversary of the discovery of DNA and the achievements of the HGP appeared in the April 11 and April 24, 2003, issues of *Science* and *Nature,* respectively.[6,7] This remarkable achievement was accomplished more than 2 years in advance of the proposed completion date and under budget.

One of the unique aspects of this project was the worldwide accessibility and immediate release of new segments of DNA sequence data made available through a free public database. The rapid pace of new discoveries since the initiation of the HGP has been credited to the widespread availability of these data and the development of new tools and technologies. For example, prior to 1990, the genes associated with fewer than 100 human diseases had been discovered, but by the time completion of the HGP was announced, more than 1,400 disease-associated genes had been identified. Another unique aspect of this project was that funding was set aside to address the ethical, legal, and social implications of genomic research. Examples of such implications presented by the availability of genetic information are listed in Table 13-1. A significant accomplishment related to these issues was the adoption of genetic nondiscrimination laws related to health insurance in 41 states,[9] although the protections afforded by these laws are highly variable.[10]

Some of the interesting findings of the HGP include the discovery that only 2 to 5% of human DNA codes for genes and that the human genome consists of only 20,000 to 25,000[11] genes, not many more than the common roundworm and some plant species, which have about 18,000 and 26,000 genes, respectively. Previously, it was estimated that the human genome included anywhere from 50,000 to 140,000 genes.[12]

Recognizing that the end of the HGP was really only the beginning of the next phase of genomic research, the NHGRI initiated an international public-private venture focused on speeding the discovery of genes related to common illnesses such as diabetes, heart disease, and cancer. This effort, initiated in October 2002 and dubbed the International HapMap Project (i.e., haplotype map—a map of closely linked segments of DNA markers), is focused on charting genetic variation within the human genome by comparing genetic differences among individuals.[13] The first draft of the human HapMap (Phase I) was finished in March 2005. Phase II of the project is nearing completion and will increase the amount of information and detail provided in Phase I.[14] This research venture capitalizes on the fact that at the genome level, humans are 99.9% identical and 0.1% different. The 0.1% difference between any two individuals is believed to explain why some individuals are more susceptible to common illnesses than others. Scientists believe that comparing the haplotype patterns of groups of people with and without a particular disease will help them identify genetic variants that influence risk for common chronic diseases. These findings will also increase the likelihood of understanding the environmental contributions of illness and ultimately usher in the era of personalized medicine.

Concurrent with the announcement of the completion of the HGP, the NHGRI outlined its vision for the future of genomic research as a series of "grand challenges."[1] These challenges are aimed at stimulating scientists to advance the findings from the HGP to combat disease and improve human health. The major challenges outlined in this vision include elucidating the structure and function of the human

TABLE 13-1	Ethical, Legal, and Social Issues Surrounding the Availability of Genetic Information
GENERAL CONCERNS	**SPECIFIC CONCERNS AND IMPLICATIONS**
Fairness	Access—who should have access to personal genetic information (e.g., employers, schools, insurance agencies, courts)?
	Use—how will genetic information be used? Genetic discrimination issues
Privacy and confidentiality	Ownership/control of genetic information
Stigmatization and psychological impact	Impact of knowing one's personal genetic information
	Perceptions of individual by society
Reproductive issues	Use in reproductive decision making and reproductive rights
	Societal issues associated with reproductive technologies
	Adequacy of informed consent regarding risks/limitations of procedures
	Reliability of fetal genetic testing
Clinical issues	Adequacy of preparation/education of healthcare professionals for "new" genetics
	Evaluation and regulation of genetic tests (i.e., reliability, accuracy, utility)
	Degree to which the public is prepared to make informed choices
	Balance of limitations and social risk with long-term benefits
Uncertainties	Decisions regarding genetic testing when no treatment is available
	Decisions regarding testing of children for adult-onset diseases
Conceptual and philosophical implications	Issues related to free will versus genetic determinism: is behavior related to genes?
	Boundary issues: medical treatment versus enhancement
	Reliability of genetic tests and ability of medical community to interpret
Health and environmental issues	Safety of genetically modified foods and microbes
	Dependence of developing nations on Western technologies
Commercialization of products	Copyright and patenting issues related to genes and DNA sequences
	Accessibility of data for development into useful products

Source: Adapted from the US Department of Energy website.[8]

genome, translating genome-based knowledge into health benefits, and promoting the use of genomics to maximize benefits and minimize harms.[1] It is anticipated that this next phase of genomic research will build on the findings of the HGP to provide researchers with unprecedented opportunities for developing new preventive and therapeutic options.

THE BASICS

Genetics is the study of heredity—in particular, how qualities or traits are transmitted from parents to offspring. Genes are the basic physical and functional units of heredity. Genes normally come in pairs, with one copy of each pair located on homologous (i.e., identical) chromosomes and originating from the egg or the sperm. Chromosomes are physically separate molecules that vary in length and in the number of genes they contain. The DNA segments representing genes consist of nucleotides (i.e., adenine, cytosine, guanine or thymine attached to deoxyribose and a phosphate group) (Figure 13-1). Nucleotide sequences within the gene form discrete

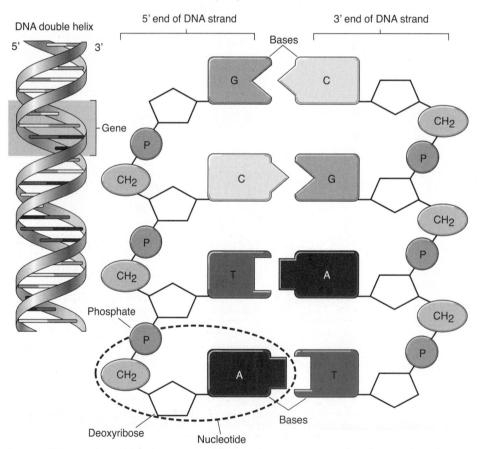

FIGURE 13-1 *DNA structure. DNA segments representing genes comprise nucleotides (see dashed circle). Each nucleotide consists of phosphate (P), deoxyribose, and one of four bases: adenine (A), cytosine (C), guanine (G) or thymine (T). Complementary base pairing occurs between adenine and thymine and cytosine and guanine. The sequence of nucleotides in the gene codes for proteins and protein products. Adapted from Kauwell[15] with permission from the American Society for Parenteral and Enteral Nutrition (ASPEN). ASPEN does not endorse the use of this material in any form other than its entirety.*

regions that play important roles in gene transcripton. These regions include the promoter, introns, exons and the termination sequence (Figure 13-2).

The complete set of DNA of an organism is referred to as its *genome*. The human genome is arranged on 24 chromosomes (i.e., 22 autosomes and 2 sex chromosomes, X and Y). Each human cell usually contains 23 pairs of chromosomes (i.e., 46 total), with 22 pairs of autosomes and 1 pair of sex chromosomes (i.e., XX or XY).

Transcription and translation are the processes whereby information contained in the DNA sequence of a specific gene is used to synthesize a protein (Figure 13-3**A**). For transcription to occur, RNA polymerase II (i.e., a transcription enzyme) must be positioned on the promoter region that precedes the gene sequence. This requires binding of regulatory proteins, referred to as transcription factors, to RNA polymerase II and to specific DNA sequences in the promoter region. The transcription factor-RNA polymerase complex initiates gene transcription by unwinding the DNA double helix (Figure 13-3**B**). During this process, one strand of the exposed DNA serves as a template (i.e., template strand) for base pairing with RNA nucleotides (i.e., nucleotides containing ribose instead of deoxyribose and uracil instead of thymine). Transcription is terminated by a special sequence of nucleotides referred to as a termination sequence (i.e., identical nucleotide sequences located on the DNA template and nontemplate strands pointing in opposite directions). The primary messenger RNA (mRNA) transcript synthesized represents a complementary copy of the specific DNA segment represented by the gene (Figure 13-3**C**).

Transcription can be influenced by environmental factors, including nutrients, which can turn gene expression on and off. Identifying the effects of various nutrients and food components on gene expression holds promise for interventions that may prevent disease or reduce disease risk.

Certain regions within the mRNA molecule do not code for protein synthesis. These noncoding regions are referred to as introns. Special enzymes remove these introns from the primary mRNA transcript and join the remaining coding sequences (i.e., exons) to form mature mRNA (Figure 13-4). Thus, in most cases, only exons are used to encode the amino acid product during translation. A single gene can give rise to more than one protein product as a result of alternative gene splicing (i.e., selective inclusion or exclusion of genetic information in the final mRNA transcript) (see Figure 13-4), posttranslational modification(s) (i.e., chemical modification after translation of the protein), or altered rates of synthesis or degradation.

Messenger RNA is translated into proteins by reading the RNA code three nucleotides at a time. Each triplet, or codon, codes for a specific amino acid, but there

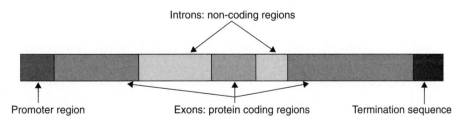

Introns: non-coding regions

Promoter region   Exons: protein coding regions   Termination sequence

FIGURE 13-2 *Components of genes. Nucleotide sequences within a gene form discrete regions that play important roles in gene transcription. These regions include the promoter, introns, exons and the termination sequence. Reprinted from Kauwell[15] with permission from the American Society for Parenteral and Enteral Nutrition (ASPEN). ASPEN does not endorse the use of this material in any form other than its entirety.*

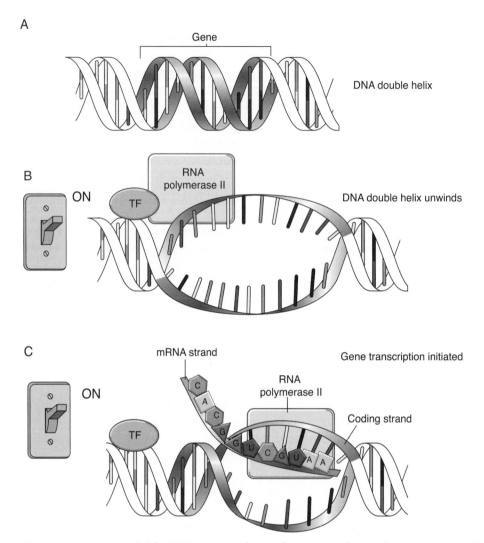

FIGURE 13-3 *Initiating transcription.* **A.** *The DNA sequence of a specific gene is used to synthesize a protein.* **B.** *To initiate transcription, RNA polymerase II must be positioned on the promoter region, a process that requires transcription factors (TF). The transcription factor–RNA polymerase complex initiates gene transcription by unwinding the DNA double helix.* **C.** *The primary mRNA transcript synthesized represents a complementary copy of the specific DNA segment represented by the gene. Adapted with permission from Kauwell GPA. Nutrition and Disease 2 Course Packet, Gainesville, FL, 2005.*

is more than one codon for each of the 20 amino acids (i.e., GCC and GCA both code for alanine—similar to having two words that have the same meaning). Since different codons can specify the same amino acid, the genetic code is said to be degenerate.

The codon sequence determines the amino acid sequence of the final protein, and the amino acid sequence of a protein affects its shape and function. The fact that the genetic code is degenerate partly explains why mutations (i.e., alterations) in the nucleotide sequence may be benign or pathogenic. Changing a single nucleotide of the codon may result in a sequence that codes for an entirely different amino acid than what is usually present in the protein product (Figure 13-5).

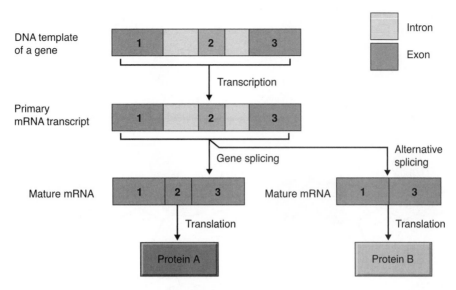

FIGURE 13-4 *Transcription and translation. During transcription, one strand of DNA, the template strand, is used to produce the primary mRNA transcript, which represents a complementary copy of the noncoding DNA strand. Special enzymes remove the introns to produce mature mRNA. The message contained in the mature mRNA is translated into a protein. Some genes produce more than one protein product as a result of alternative splicing (lower right). Adapted from Kauwell[15] with permission from the American Society for Parenteral and Enteral Nutrition (ASPEN). ASPEN does not endorse the use of this material in any form other than its entirety.*

Alternatively, the nucleotide substitution may result in a different codon that specifies the same amino acid. As a simple analogy of this concept, think of the word "gray." Changing the letter "a" to "e" (i.e., grey) does not change the meaning of the word; however, changing the letter "g" to a "t" (i.e., tray) gives it a very different meaning.

Alternate forms of a gene at a particular locus (i.e., location) on a chromosome are referred to as alleles. Allelic (i.e., different; variant) forms of the same gene produce variations in inherited characteristics, such as eye color. The term homozygous is used to describe the situation in which both copies of the gene at a particular locus on a chromosome are identical. More specifically, the term homozygous "wild" or "wild-type" (Figure 13-6**A**) is used to refer to the situation in which both copies represent the version of the gene that occurs in the majority of individuals. When an individual has two different versions (i.e., alleles) of the same gene, the condition is described as heterozygous (Figure 13-6**B**). The term homozygous mutant or homozygous variant (Figure 13-6**C**) denotes the situation in which both copies of the gene represent the allelic variant. Homozygote and heterozygote are terms used to refer to individuals with respect to their homozygosity or heterozygosity for a particular trait or condition.

Genes can have many different versions or alleles. The specific set of alleles inherited at a locus on the chromosome pair (i.e., remember, genes come in pairs, one on each chromosome) is referred to as an individual's genotype, although genotype also can refer to an individual's overall genetic makeup. In contrast, phenotype refers to the observable traits (i.e., physical, biochemical, physiological) resulting

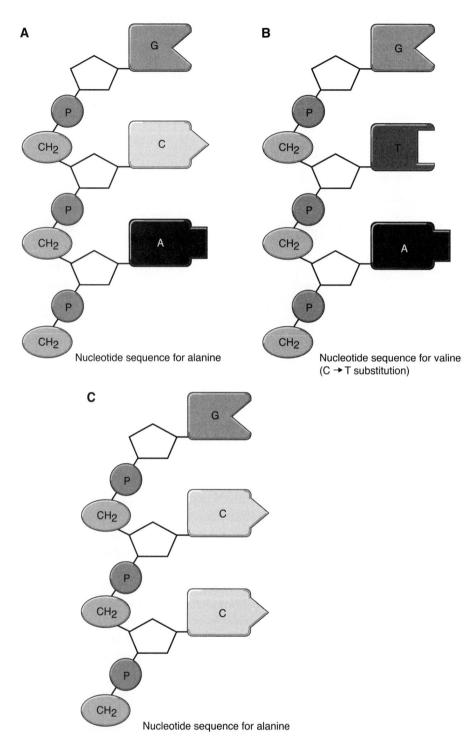

A Nucleotide sequence for alanine

B Nucleotide sequence for valine (C → T substitution)

C Nucleotide sequence for alanine

FIGURE 13-5 *Nucleotide sequence variation. A. GCA (i.e., guanine, cytosine, adenine) is one of the triplet sequences (i.e., codon) that codes for the amino acid alanine. B. A change in one base pair of the codon may or may not change the amino acid inserted into the final protein product. GTA (i.e., guanine, thymine, adenine) represents the code for valine, which results from a cytosine-to-thymine base pair substitution. C. GCC (i.e., guanine, cytosine, cytosine) represents the code for alanine. In this case, the adenine-to-cytosine substitution does not affect the final amino acid sequence of the protein product. The word "polymorphism" is used to refer to a common variation (i.e., a frequency of >1%) in the DNA nucleotide sequence. A single-nucleotide polymorphism (SNP, pronounced "snip") refers to the situation in which the DNA sequence varies by just one nucleotide, as shown in this figure. Single-nucleotide polymorphisms are the major kind of variation in the human genome. Adapted with permission from Kauwell GPA. Nutrition and Disease 2 Course Packet, Gainesville, FL, 2005.*

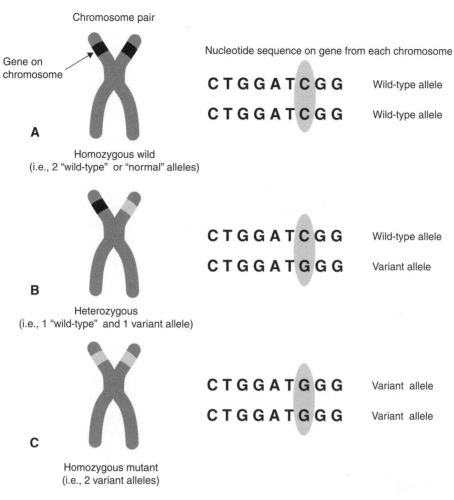

FIGURE 13-6 *Genetic variation. The corresponding genes on each chromosomal locus may have different versions. The typical version of a gene is referred to as the "normal" or "wild-type" allele; the altered allele is called the "mutant" or "variant" allele. A. Homozygous wild: both copies of the prevailing version of a gene are present. B. Heterozygous: one wild-type allele and one variant allele are present. C. Homozygous mutant: both copies of the gene are altered. Adapted from Kauwell[15] with permission from the American Society for Parenteral and Enteral Nutrition (ASPEN). ASPEN does not endorse the use of this material in any form other than in its entirety.*

from interactions among genes and the environment. Two people with the same genotype for alleles at a specific genetic locus may have different phenotypes (i.e., variable expression of the genotype) depending on the environment to which they are exposed (i.e., sun, smoking, nutrient intake, etc.) and/or other genes in their makeup. For example, suppose that both copies of the gene that codes for a particular enzyme are the same for Karla and Jaimie (i.e., same genotype), but this enzyme is fully functional only when intake of a particular nutrient is adequate. When intake of this nutrient is adequate, the enzyme functions properly and a particular "trait" is observed. If Karla's intake of the nutrient is adequate but Jaimie's is not, only Karla will express the trait (i.e., different phenotypes).

Mendelian inheritance patterns are described according to the dominance and recessivity of traits. Dominant alleles prevail, whereas recessive alleles are expressed only when the corresponding allele on the matching chromosome is recessive. The chromosome locus of the gene also is used to describe the inheritance pattern, which may be autosomal (i.e., located on an autosome) or X-linked (i.e., located on the X chromosome). Autosomal dominant disorders are expressed when a dominant disease-causing allele is inherited, even though the corresponding allele on the other chromosome may be "normal." Examples of autosomal dominant diseases include familial hypercholesterolemia, Huntington disease, and polycystic kidney disease. Autosomal recessive disorders occur only when an individual inherits a recessive disease-causing allele from both parents. Cystic fibrosis, Tay-Sachs disease, and sickle cell anemia are examples of autosomal recessive diseases. X-linked *dominant* disorders are expressed in heterozygous females (i.e., one copy of the X-linked disease-causing gene and one copy of the "normal" version of the gene are inherited) and males (i.e., the affected gene is carried only on the X chromosome, and males have only one X chromosome). X-linked *recessive* traits are expressed in males who inherit a copy of the recessive allele on their single X chromosome, while females must inherit two copies of the X-linked recessive allele, one from each parent, to express the recessive trait. Females who are *carriers* of X-linked recessive mutations (i.e., heterozygotes) do not usually express the phenotype associated with the genetic mutation, although varying degrees of clinical expression can occur. Vitamin D–resistant rickets and hemophilia A are examples of X-linked dominant and recessive disorders, respectively. Diseases and disorders with a genetic component that do not follow classic Mendelian inheritance patterns include multifactorial and mitochondrial diseases, both of which are discussed later in this chapter.

A polymorphism or polymorphic allele is a common variation in the DNA sequence of a gene. These occur fairly frequently in the general population (i.e., >1% of the population for a given polymorphism). A single nucleotide polymorphism (SNP, pronounced "snip") is one type of polymorphic change in which a single base is substituted with another (e.g., cytosine replaced with thymine; C→T). Single nucleotide polymorphisms are the major kind of variation in the human genome, and as in the example given above (i.e., gray-grey-tray), may or may not affect the amino acid sequence of the gene product. Single nucleotide polymorphisms are the underlying genetic cause of some diseases/conditions, such as sickle cell disease, or they may play a role in disease susceptibility. Researchers are anxious to identify as many SNPs as possible because they hold the keys for discovering the genetic contribution(s) to common chronic diseases such as diabetes and heart disease.[16]

When used broadly, the term "mutation" implies an alteration in a gene that may be benign, pathogenic, or of unknown significance. More strictly, the word is used to describe a change in the DNA sequence that results in significantly deleterious functional consequences. Examples of types of mutations are categorized and defined in Table 13-2.

GENETIC DISORDERS

Genetic disorders arise in whole or in part from chromosomal abnormalities and alterations or mutations in genes. Genetic disorders are generally categorized as chromosomal disorders, single-gene disorders, multifactorial inheritance disorders, and mitochondrial disorders.

TABLE 13-2	Types of Mutations[17,18]
TYPE OF MUTATION	**DESCRIPTION**
Nucleotide substitutions	
Missense	Substitution of a single base with another in the DNA sequence that results in replacement of one amino acid by another in the protein product.

	Original	Missense mutation
DNA sequence:	GCT	G**T**T
DNA template:	CGA	CA**A**
RNA sequence:	GCU[a]	GUU
Amino acid:	alanine	valine

Nonsense	Substitution of a single base with another in the DNA sequence that results in replacement of the usual codon with a stop codon. The premature stop codon results in a shortened protein. Nonsense mutations are often fatal.

	Original	Nonsense mutation
DNA sequence:	TGC	TG**A**
DNA template:	ACG	AC**T**
RNA sequence:	UGC	UG**A**
Amino acid:	cysteine	stop code

Silent	A mutation that has no observable (i.e., phenotypic) effect on cell function.

	Original	Silent mutation
DNA sequence:	AAA	AA**G**
DNA template:	TTT	TT**C**
RNA sequence:	AAA	AA**G**
Amino acid:	lysine	lysine

RNA processing	Substitutions that result in abnormal splicing sites (i.e., excision of introns from exons) or other changes in the way the RNA is processed.

(continues next page)

A = adenine, C = cytosine, G = guanine, T = thymine, U = uracil.
[a]Remember that uracil is substituted for thymine in RNA.

Sources: Adapted with permission from Nussbaum et al.[17] and Mueller and Young.[18]

CHROMOSOMAL DISORDERS

Extra or missing copies of chromosomes are almost always associated with an abnormal phenotype. Chromosomal rearrangement or translocation (i.e., attachment of all or part of a chromosome to another chromosome or interchanging of genetic material among chromosomes) may or may not result in abnormal phenotype expression depending on where the breakpoints in the translocation occur and whether or not the translocations are balanced (i.e., no loss or gain of genetic material). Collectively, chromosomal disorders are relatively common, affecting 1 in 160 live births and 50% of first-trimester spontaneously aborted fetuses.[19]

Down syndrome is an example of a chromosomal disorder. Most cases of Down syndrome result from maternal nondisjunction of chromosome 21 during meiosis. Chromosome nondisjunction is the failure of a chromosome pair to separate during meiosis (i.e., during the formation of the egg or sperm), an error that results in one daughter cell with an extra chromosome and one daughter cell with no copy of that particular chromosome. When a daughter cell with an extra copy of chromosome 21 is fertilized, the offspring will have three copies of chromosome 21 (i.e., trisomy 21), producing the phenotype associated with Down syndrome.

TABLE 13-2   Types of Mutations (*cont*)

TYPE OF MUTATION	DESCRIPTION
Deletions/insertions	
Frameshift	A mutation that changes the reading frame (i.e., sequence of mRNA translated into an amino acid sequence) of the protein encoded by the gene by inserting or deleting a number of base pairs that is not a multiple of three. The size (i.e., number of base pairs) of the insertion or deletion can vary, with whole genes being deleted in some situations.
	mRNA Amino acid sequence Original: CGUGCCGGC ... Arg-Val-Gly Frameshift insertion: CGU**AA**GCCGGC... Arg-Lys-Pro... Frameshift deletion: CGU**GC**CGGC... Arg-Arg....
In frame	Insertions or deletions that occur in multiples of three do not cause a frameshift; rather, they result in the addition or deletion of amino acids in the translated protein product. These insertions or deletions may or may not affect protein function depending on the size of the insertion/deletion and where they occur in the protein.
Inversions/translocations	
Inversions	Removal and reinsertion of a segment of DNA in the opposite direction (i.e., backwards) at the original breakage site. Inversions are a type of chromosomal rearrangement. Balanced inversions (i.e., no net loss or gain of genetic material) are not usually associated with an altered phenotype unless the breakage site occurs at the site of a gene. Unbalanced inversions are almost always associated with an abnormal phenotype. mRNA amino acid sequence Original: CGGUACCA<u>GGUUGAC</u> Arg-Tyr-Gln-Val-Asp Inverted: CGGUACCA<u>CAGUUGG</u> Arg-Tyr-His-Ser-Trp
Translocation	Removal and reinsertion of a segment of DNA in a different place. Reinsertion can occur on the same or a different chromosome. Balanced translocations (i.e., no net loss or gain of genetic material) are not usually associated with an altered phenotype unless the breakage/reinsertion site occurs at the site of a gene. Unbalanced translocations are almost always associated with an abnormal phenotype.
Trinucleotide repeat	Gene expansion characterized by sequences of three nucleotides repeated in tandem (i.e., CAGCAGCAGCAG). Expansion occurs from generation to generation and can lead to abnormal gene expression and function.

SINGLE-GENE DISORDERS

As the name implies, single-gene (i.e., monogenic) disorders result from a mutation(s) in one or both alleles at a single locus on a chromosome pair. The pattern of inheritance is similar to those described by Mendel, hence the term Mendelian inherited diseases. Over 6,000 single-gene disorders have been identified,[20] and the defective genes for more than 1,000 of these disorders have been isolated and molecularly identified.[21]

A catalogue of human genes and inherited or heritable genetic diseases is continuously updated in an online database called Online Mendelian Inheritance in Man (OMIM™).[22] Over 16,246 entries appear in this database.

Although single-gene disorders are limited to one gene, there may be more than one version of the mutant allele. This is the case for cystic fibrosis (CF), an autosomal recessive disease, for which there are over 1,000 known mutant alleles for the cystic fibrosis transmembrane conductance regulator gene (CFTR gene). The severity of CF symptoms (i.e., phenotype) is affected by the individual's genotype.

Individuals may inherit one or more of the same mutation on each copy of the CFTR gene (i.e., they may be homozygotes), or they may have different mutations on homologous genes (i.e., they may be compound heterozygote). Predicting the clinical outcome of CF is difficult due to the diversity of CF mutations and the complexity of their interactions. For example, while the majority of patients with CF manifest exocrine pancreatic insufficiency, a small percentage of patients exhibit exocrine pancreatic sufficiency, even though both groups have mutations of the CFTR gene. In other words, the combination of specific genetic mutations occurring on both alleles of the CFTR gene alters the severity of disease expression (i.e., phenotype).[23]

Although CF is considered a typical monogenic disease, other genes may also modify clinical expression. Searching for modifier genes is a relatively new area of research that has the potential to affect intervention strategies and practice standards used by the healthcare team.[23] The importance of nutrition in the treatment of single-gene disorders such as phenylketonuria, maple syrup urine disease, and galactosemia has been recognized for many years. Dietetics professionals will continue to play an important role in providing care for individuals with these disorders, but advances in genomic research will broaden the scope of practice to include the integration and application of genetics and nutrition to the prevention of disease conditions and the treatment of individuals with common chronic diseases.

MULTIFACTORIAL INHERITANCE DISORDERS

Multifactorial inheritance disorders are not inherited per se (i.e., they do not show a specific inheritance pattern); rather, they result from the interplay of genes with the environment. The underlying genetic mechanisms of these disorders are generally not well understood, although it is thought that the genetic component involves multiple genes (i.e., is polygenic). These disorders tend to cluster in families, and a positive family history is considered the strongest predictor of risk. Susceptibility for these disorders can be modified positively or negatively by other factors, including the environment. Examples of diseases/disorders that show multifactorial inheritance include obesity, type 1 and 2 diabetes, cancer, asthma, Parkinson's disease, Alzheimer's disease, hypertension, and heart disease.

Understanding the genetic contributions to common diseases will improve our ability to identify the role(s) played by nongenetic factors,[16] including nutrition. A particularly valuable research tool in this regard is the identification of SNPs. These common variations of the human genome hold much promise in helping to uncover the genetic basis of common diseases and to study the modifying effects of nutrition and other environmental stimuli. Ultimately, this research will allow dietetics professionals to tailor nutrition therapy based on an individual's genetic uniqueness. This is one of the reasons why an understanding of genetics and an appreciation for the applications and implications of genomic healthcare are critical for dietetics professionals.

MITOCHONDRIAL DISORDERS

Mitochondrial disorders are the result of inheriting mutations in genes contained in the mitochondria (i.e., mitochondrial DNA, or mtDNA). Although mitochondrial DNA is a relatively small component of our genome, it is unique in that it is solely of maternal origin. Mitochondrial DNA is located in the cytoplasm, and sperm cells contain little cytoplasm and only a few mitochondria that are not released during fertilization. Thus, all offspring of a female carrying mutated mtDNA will inherit the mutation, but none of the offspring of a male carrying the same mtDNA will inherit the mutation.

EVOLVING SCIENCE: NEW FRONTIERS FOR NUTRITION

GENETICS AND GENOMICS

Genetics is the study of the principles and mechanics of heredity, and in the traditional sense focuses on identifying single genes responsible for given traits. In contrast, genomics is the study of the structure and function of genes and how they interact with each other and with the environment.[24] Compared to genetics, genomics takes a broader, more integrated approach to examining the complex molecular aspects of living organisms. The genomic view of genetics recognizes that not all traits are inherited and expressed in a predictable manner that follows the basic laws of inheritance described by Mendel. Instead, genomics builds on the foundation of what is already known about genes, the genetic code, and inheritance patterns with the goal of identifying how interactions among genes (i.e., gene-gene interactions) and genes and the environment (i.e., gene-environment interactions) contribute to multifactorial traits and diseases.

PROTEOMICS AND OTHER EMERGING AREAS

Although genes specify the chemistry and behavior of proteins from a genomic point of view, proteins also are impacted by the quantity and types of other proteins synthesized in the same cell at the same time and by intra- and extracellular environmental signals. Proteomics, the study of proteins and how they collaborate to carry out cellular processes,[25] represents the next step in advancing our understanding of the molecular basis of health and disease. This includes understanding the subtle or not so subtle changes that occur in response to protein modification (i.e., glycosylation, phosphorylation, etc.), localization of proteins within a cell, and interactions with each other and the environment. Proteomic research is expected to accelerate the development of diagnostic and therapeutic products by elucidating the protein products of genes and their functions and by untangling the complexities of the effects of the internal and external cellular environments.

Other emerging areas of research stemming from the technological tools, techniques, and findings of the HGP also will contribute to our understanding of the molecular complexities of life and the impact of nutrition. These include transcriptomics (i.e., study of the complete collection of gene transcripts in a cell or tissue at a given time) and metabolomics (i.e., study of the entire metabolic content of a cell at a given time).[26,27] The discipline that incorporates genomics and proteomics, in tandem with genotype determination, transcriptomics, metabolomics, and bioinformatics, is referred to as functional genomics, or systems biology.[28]

NUTRITIONAL GENOMICS—NUTRIGENOMICS AND NUTRIGENETICS

"Nutritional genomics" is an umbrella term that encompasses the areas of nutrition research focused at the genome (i.e., nutrigenomics) and the gene (i.e., nutrigenetics) levels.[29] Nutritional genomic research has the potential to revolutionize dietetics practice by enhancing the scientific evidence for clinical practice; improving the ability to tailor nutrition intervention strategies, thereby improving patient/client outcomes; and expanding career opportunities.[30]

Nutrigenomics combines the tools and techniques of functional genomics to identify and understand the genome-wide effects of nutrients and bioactive food components.[26] This area of research views nutrients as dietary signals that are detected by nutrient sensor systems (i.e., sensors that alter the extent of DNA transcription in response to changes in nutrients). The aim of nutrigenomics is to define the ways in which nutrients and bioactive food components influence metabolic pathways and homeostatic control at the molecular level, specifically how they affect patterns of gene expression, protein expression, and metabolite production.[26] This is a whole-systems approach that considers multiple aspects of cellular/organ function simultaneously. In other words, it would be like having a detailed snapshot of what is happening in cells, tissues, or organisms at a given moment when an individual is exposed to certain nutrients or bioactive food components. Discovery of how regulation is disturbed early in the history of diet-related illness and the contribution of predisposing genotypes to the disease process is predicted to lead to the development of early biomarkers of disease and effective dietary intervention strategies to restore normal homeostasis as well as prevent diet-related diseases.[26]

Nutrigenomics is an emerging area of research, so specific applications to practice, based on research findings, are not well defined at this point. One potential strategy for studying the nutrigenomic effects of nutrients and dietary factors is to compare the "dietary signatures"[26] produced under homeostatic conditions, including perhaps a specific genotype(s) associated with health, to the response when homeostasis is perturbed by stressors associated with disease (i.e., proinflammatory stress, metabolic stress) and/or a genotype(s) associated with increased risk for disease. As an example, one might examine the impact of exposure to a specific type of fatty acid on gene transcription (mRNA levels), translation (protein products), and metabolism (metabolites produced) of the organism under normal and perturbed homeostatic conditions to compare the "dietary signatures" produced. Identifying the differences between these "signatures" in response to different nutrient environments (e.g., different types of fatty acids) may help elucidate early biomarkers of disease and may lead to the development of dietary intervention strategies capable of preventing or reversing the processes associated with disease in individuals at risk.

In contrast to nutrigenomics, nutrigenetics takes a narrower approach that focuses specifically on nutrient-gene interactions and how they may impact risk for multifactorial diseases or nutrient requirements.[26] Single nucleotide polymorphisms are known to contribute to disease risk for several common diet-related diseases, and nutrition may modify disease risk positively or negatively, or may influence nutrient requirements. Identifying the specific SNPs linked to altered disease risk or sensitivity to diet could lead to the development of dietary recommendations based on genotype.

As an example of the application of nutrigenetics to nutrition practice, consider the effect of a SNP in the gene that codes for methylenetetrahydrofolate reductase (MTHFR). Methylenetetrahydrofolate reductase is an important folate enzyme involved in one-carbon metabolism. Substitution of cytosine with thymine (i.e., C→T substitution) at base pair 677 (MTHFR 677C→T) in both copies of the MTHFR gene produces the TT genotype. This genotype is associated with reduced enzyme activity *in vitro*[31] and may modulate risk for several chronic diseases and conditions including vascular, neoplastic and neurological disease, neural tube defects (NTDs), and other congenital abnormalities.[32] Individuals with the TT genotype are hypothesized to have higher folate requirements,[33,34] a hypothesis that is supported by small-scale intervention studies.[35,36] Unlike single gene disorders that are relatively rare, the TT variant of the MTHFR 677C→T polymorphism is fairly common, with a population frequency (in the United States) of approximately 12% for Caucasians, 21% for Hispanics, and 1% for African Americans.[37] Given the population frequency of the MTHFR 677 TT variant, it is likely that dietetics professionals will encounter patients with this genotype or other genotypes related to common diseases in their practice, especially since it is predicted that widescale, low-cost genotyping services will be available in the near future.

It is important to recognize that an altered genotype may confer greater risk or may be associated with disease risk reduction at a given level of nutrient intake. For example, in the Physicians' Health Study, men with the TT genotype for MTHFR 677C→T had a 55% lower risk for colorectal cancer compared to men with either the CC (i.e., reference genotype; homozygous "normal" or "wild-type") or CT (i.e., heterozygous) genotype; however, the protective effect associated with this genotype appeared to be lost with low folate status.[38] Furthermore, in the Health Professionals Follow-up Study[39] and two case control studies,[40,41] alcohol consumption also appeared to negate the protection associated with the TT genotype. Although these observations need further confirmation, they provide provocative examples of how nutrient-gene interactions may alter disease risk. Interestingly, the MTHFR 677 TT genotype also has been associated with lower risk for acute lymphocytic leukemia.[42,43]

In contrast to the potential protective effect observed for certain types of cancer, the TT genotype has been associated with an increased risk for NTDs*,[37,45,46] although it only accounts for a small percentage of NTD cases.[37] Neural tube defect risk associated with this genotype may be related to nutrition status, although the data are inconclusive. For example, one retrospective study observed a weak association between maternal vitamin use and NTD risk reduction in infants with the TT genotype; however, they did not examine the genotype status of the mothers, and it is possible that a protective effect is conditional on maternal genotype.[47] In another study, the combination of low red blood cell folate concentration (folate status indicator) and the MTHFR 677 TT variant conferred higher risk for being an NTD case or having an NTD-affected infant,[48] suggesting an interactive effect between nutrition status and genotype with regard to NTD risk.

Higher homocysteine concentrations also have been associated with the TT variant and low folate intake/status.[33,49] Although elevated homocysteine is a risk factor for vascular disease, the data do not consistently support a higher rate of vascular disease in individuals with the TT genotype.[50] Examples of known nutrient-gene interactions and those under investigation are outlined in Table 13-3.

EPIGENETICS

Another type of nutrient-gene interaction that may alter cancer risk occurs independently of changes in the DNA nucleotide sequence. Nonsequence modifications

---

*Practitioners should recognize that all women of reproductive potential, regardless of genotype status, should be encouraged to consume 400 mcg of folic acid daily to reduce their risk of an NTD-affected pregnancy.[44]

TABLE 13-3	Examples of Nutrient (Diet)-Gene Interactions		
GENOTYPE/POLYMORPHISM	**GENE PRODUCT OR FUNCTION**	**NUTRIENT/DIETARY FACTOR(S)**	**CONDITION, DISEASE, OR FINDINGS**
Confirmed nutrient-gene interactions			
282YY genotype for HFE gene (i.e., hemochromatosis gene), C282Y allele (most common)	Regulation of iron absorption	Iron	Type 1—hereditary hemochromatosis[52,53]
Phenylalanine hydroxylase gene (multiple allelic variants)	Phenylalanine metabolism	Phenylalanine exposure	Phenylketonuria[54]
Nutrient-gene interactions under investigation (not definitive)			
APOA1 -75 GA and GG genotypes	Major protein in HDL cholesterol	Polyunsaturated fatty acid (PUFA) intake	HDL concentration higher in women (gender-specific) with GA allele when PUFA intake >8% of total calories; higher in women with GG allele when PUFA intake <4%[55]
APOE: E2, E3, E4 genotypes	Lipoprotein: determinant of LDL size	Quantity and quality of dietary fat	Effect of Mediterranean type diet compared to carbohydrate diet on LDL size dependent on apo-E genotype[56]
Apolipoprotein A-IV alleles	Postprandial lipoprotein metabolism	Dietary fatty acid composition	Modulation of cholesterol absorption[57]
CYP1A1 variant of a cytochrome P450 enzyme	Estradiol 2 hydrolase activity	Indole-3-carbinol (Brussels sprouts, cabbage, cauliflower)	Reduced estrogen-related cancer risk[58]
LIPC -514 TT genotype	Hepatic lipase: lipoprotein binding and uptake	High fat intake (animal fat)	HDL concentration lower than other genotypes with intake ≥30% of calories from fat of animal origin; HDL concentration highest in this genotype group when intake was <30% of calories[59]
NAT1*11 allele of N-acetyltransferase 1	Activation of aromatic and heterocyclic amines	High consumption of well-done red meat	Increased breast cancer risk[51]
PLIN 11482 G→A	Major protein in adipocytes	Energy restriction	Weight-loss resistance to energy-restricted diet in PLIN 11482A carriers (i.e., GA or AA)[61]
677 TT genotype for methylenetetrahydrofolate reductase (MTHFR)	Folate coenzyme involved in one-carbon metabolism	Adequate folate intake/status: protective; low folate intake/status or moderate alcohol consumption: loss of protection	Altered colon cancer risk[38–41]
		Low folate intake/status	Elevated homocysteine[33,39] (vascular disease risk factor)
		Low folate intake/status	Higher neural tube defect risk[47,48]

Source: Adapted from Patterson et al.[51] For a more comprehensive list of nutrient-gene interactions under investigation, refer to Corella and Ordovas.[62]

of mitotically heritable changes (i.e., passed on to daughter cells during mitosis) provide cells with additional instructions on how, when and where genetic information should be used.[63] Consequently, epigenetic changes (e.g., hypo- or hypermethylation) can modify gene expression (Figure 13-7). Methylation usually occurs on the cytosine residues located in a specific sequence of bases of the DNA molecule. Altered methylation patterns may occur at specific sites (i.e., gene-specific) or may develop globally. Hypomethylated genes are more likely to be turned "on," and global DNA hypomethylation is a common characteristic of cancer cell DNA, although methylation patterns may vary depending on cancer type.[64] Nutrients, such as folate, vitamin B_{12}, choline, and methionine, affect the supply of methyl groups and thereby have the potential to influence gene expression. Controlled feeding studies[65,66] have observed an association between moderately low folate intake and hypomethylation in postmenopausal women.

Chromatin remodeling is another form of epigenetic modification. Chromatin, a combination of nucleic acids and histones that make up chromosomes, can be chemically modified by the addition of various groups (i.e., phosphate, methyl, acetyl) to protruding histone tails. Many different combinations of patterns are produced by these chemical alterations, which have the net effect of modulating gene expression. Parental imprinting (i.e., situation in which a gene's activity depends on whether it is of maternal or paternal origin) and controlling which copy of the X chromosome is shut off in females are genetic phenomena attributed to epigenetic modification. Some researchers believe that these changes may explain why many diseases appear later in life and may even play a role in common chronic diseases such as diabetes.[67]

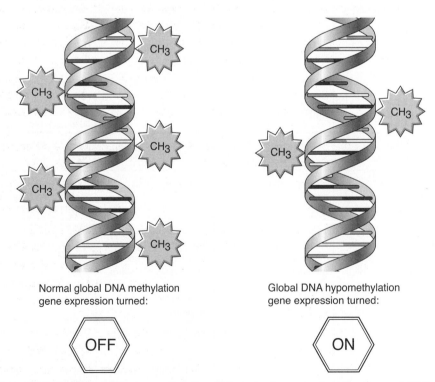

Normal global DNA methylation
gene expression turned:

OFF

Global DNA hypomethylation
gene expression turned:

ON

FIGURE 13-7   *Epigenetic modification: methylation. Epigenetic changes such as the degree of DNA methylation can modify gene expression. Although exceptions exist, hypermethylation of DNA within the promoter region is usually associated with gene repression, whereas hypomethylation is associated with gene expression. Adapted with permission from Kauwell GPA. Nutrition and Disease 2 Course Packet, Gainesville, FL, 2001.*

DISRUPTION OF DNA INTEGRITY AND REPAIR

Gene expression and stability also can be altered by misincorporation of uracil into the DNA molecule (Figure 13-8). Because of its role in the synthesis of deoxythymidine monophosphate (i.e., dTMP; thymine-containing nucleotide required for DNA synthesis) from deoxyuridine monophosphate (i.e., dUMP; uracil-containing nucleotide), folate deficiency generates an imbalance in nucleotide pools (i.e., excess dUMP compared to dTMP). Most DNA polymerase enzymes (i.e., enzymes involved in DNA replication) do not distinguish between dTMP and dUMP. Consequently, the imbalance in the nucleotide pool results in misincorporation of uracil into DNA. Another process that can cause uracil to be present in the DNA molecule is the spontaneous deamination of nonmethylated cytosine. Although cellular repair mechanisms can remove the uracil and replace it with thymine, if the repair process is overloaded (partly due to the diminished thymine pool), it can leave nicks or create strand breaks that compromise the integrity and stability of the DNA molecule.[68] Increased DNA uracil misincorporation and chromosomal damage have been reported in folate deficient individuals.[69]

GENETIC TESTING AND SCREENING

Advances in genetic research have led to an expansion of the number of disease-related genes that have been identified and the number of genetic tests available for the detection of disease or disease risk. As counselors and educators, dietetics professionals must be prepared to respond to the questions and concerns raised by their patients/clients, including those that relate to genetic health issues such as genetic testing and screening. Understanding the types, uses, benefits, and limitations of

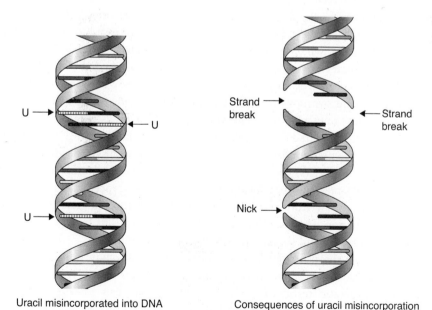

Uracil misincorporated into DNA   Consequences of uracil misincorporation

FIGURE 13-8 *Uracil misincorporation. Under normal circumstances, DNA does not contain uracil. An imbalance of nucleotide pools (i.e., deficiency of thymine), may result in the synthesis of DNA containing uracil in place of thymine. Cellular repair processes remove uracil and replace it with thymine, but if the thymine pool is limited, this repair process can result in nicks or strand breaks in the DNA molecule. Adapted with permission from Kauwell GPA. Nutrition and Disease 2 Course Packet, Gainesville, FL, 2001.*

genetic testing and knowing where to find reliable information for professionals and consumers will be increasingly important for dietetics practitioners.

Genetic testing applications fall into several general categories. These include testing to confirm a suspected diagnosis, predict the possibility of future illness, identify carrier status in unaffected individuals, and predict the response to therapy. Genetic testing is used as a means for identifying newborns who may benefit from early identification of inherited conditions (i.e., newborn screening) or, in some cases, to potentially prevent the inheritance of a genetic mutation (i.e., preimplantation testing). Specific types of genetic testing are described in Table 13-4. Detailed information about genetic tests and services is available on the GeneTests website (www.geneclinics.org/) supported by the NIH.

Genetic testing is more complex than what it may seem. The results may not always provide clear-cut "answers." Take the example of cystic fibrosis (CF). As discussed earlier in this chapter, CF results from a mutation(s) of the CFTR gene. The CFTR gene codes for a protein that transports fluids and salts across epithelial cell membranes. The defective gene product results in the production of cellular secretions that are viscous and salty, causing damage to many organ systems, including the lungs and pancreas. Over 1,400 mutations of the CFTR gene are listed in the CF Mutation Database.[72] Some of these mutations are more common than others, with variation among racial/ethnic groups in terms of which defects are most common.[23,73] The minimum standard test recommended for assessing CF carrier status includes a screening panel of 25 common mutations,[74] leaving the possibility that the more rare mutations will be missed. Thus, a negative test result is not absolute, because a rare mutation will not be identified using standard carrier testing. There are also differences in the ability to detect mutations in different racial/ethnic groups using current genetic tests. For example, the detection rate using the basic CF carrier-screening panel is approximately 90% for a non-Hispanic Caucasian couple, whereas the detection rate for an African American couple is only 69%.[75]

Tests that predict disease susceptibility are expressed in terms of probabilities, not certainties, which may be confusing to patients/clients. For example, testing for two hereditary forms of breast cancer, BRCA1 (chromosome 17) and BRCA2 (chromosome 13), is currently available to families where there is a strong history of breast and ovarian cancer. Even though both genes are expressed dominantly, a positive test does not automatically predict that breast/ovarian cancer will occur. Other factors related to the environment, or perhaps the influence of other genes, may affect expression of the disease. Similarly, a negative test does not guarantee a life free from breast cancer, since it is likely that other unidentified breast cancer genes exist and, more importantly, most breast cancer cases are not inherited; rather, they arise from sporadic mutations. Additionally, genes are often only part of the equation. Diseases that run in families may result from a combination of genetic influences and shared environmental conditions.

One of the potential benefits of genetic testing may be the relief of knowing your risk status. Discovering that your risk status is relatively low or negative (e.g., presymptomatic testing for Huntington disease) can provide a sense of relief. Individuals handle information about their genetic test results differently, so some individuals may be relieved even if they test positive because it may help them make

TABLE 13-4	Types of Genetic Testing/Screening[70,71]	
CATEGORY	**PURPOSE**	**EXAMPLE**
Diagnostic testing	Confirm or rule out a suspected genetic disorder in a symptomatic individual. Useful in determining prognosis, treatment, and risk to blood relatives.	Hereditary hemochromatosis
Prenatal testing	Type of diagnostic testing performed during pregnancy when the risk for a genetic condition in the fetus is increased because of family history or maternal age.	Down syndrome
Predictive testing	Available to asymptomatic individuals to assess potential risk for developing the disorder in the future.	(see presymptomatic and predispositional testing) Huntington disease Breast cancer
Preimplantation testing	Used to reduce the chance of passing on a particular inherited condition by testing cells of embryos conceived using *in vitro* fertilization and implanting only those embryos that are free of the gene mutation of concern.	Spinal muscular atrophy
Prenatal screening	Screening test(s) performed during pregnancy to detect the infant's risk for certain genetic diseases/disorders.	Down syndrome
Newborn screening	Completed within the first few days of life to identify infants with genetic disorders that require immediate intervention. Specific disorders for which screening is performed vary from state to state.	Phenylketonuria
Carrier screening	Detect gene mutations for autosomal recessive or X-linked recessive disorders in healthy/asymptomatic individuals belonging to at risk populations.	Cystic fibrosis, sickle cell trait
Pharmacogenomic testing	Predict effectiveness of a particular drug in the management of a particular disease.	Estrogen receptor–positive breast tumors

plans and give them a sense of control. Other individuals may feel devastated by a positive test result, particularly if no treatment exists. A positive test also may present new dilemmas related to reproductive decisions, implications for other family members, decisions related to informing relatives, and the impact on family dynamics and social relationships. Disclosure of genetic test results may have consequences for the individual or family in terms of discriminatory practices in the workplace, by insurers, and in schools. The potential psychological consequences of genetic testing are not limited to those who test positive for genetic mutations. Although a positive test may invoke feelings of fear of the unknown, guilt, and shame, those who test negative or have a low risk for a particular disease/disorder may experience survivor guilt. The risks, benefits, limitations, and ethical, legal, and social implications of genetic testing are important considerations and should be weighed before the decision to be tested is made. Discussing these points is part of the informed consent process, and informed consent should be obtained prior to testing. Dietetics professionals should be knowledgeable regarding the implications of genetic testing, and should be prepared to answer questions, make referrals, and suggest appropriate resources for their patients/clients.

FAMILY MEDICAL HISTORY AND GENETIC COUNSELING

A family medical history and pedigree analysis traditionally have been used in clinical genetics settings to identify risk for inherited diseases and disorders. A family medical history includes medical and health information and should include ethnic origin, since it is a factor related to variation in disease frequency. Pedigree analysis, a graphic representation of a family's medical history that uses standard symbols (Figure 13-9, Table 13-5), can help the practitioner visualize how traits cluster within families and move through generations.

Although not traditionally used in public health and preventive medicine settings, incorporating a family medical history into routine practice can benefit the patient/client. Considering that almost every common illness is thought to result from a combination of genetic and environmental influences,[77] integrating the family medical history with information about other known risk factors (e.g., diet, exercise patterns, smoking, and alcohol consumption) has the potential to provide more personalized information about an individual's disease risk. It also could be useful in improving early detection, making decisions about genetic testing, and developing targeted intervention and prevention strategies.[78,79]

As the application of genetics to healthcare becomes more pervasive, the family medical history will no longer be construed as a tool of the geneticist or genetic counselor; rather, it will be regarded as a tool to be used by all healthcare practitioners to provide improved patient care.[80] Dietetics professionals will need to understand, use, and contribute to the information recorded in the family medical history of their patients/clients; appreciate the limits of their genetic expertise; recognize when and how to make referrals; and understand the ethical, legal, social, and psychological implications of genetic services.[2,80] This view is supported by the NCHPEG Core Competencies[2] (Appendix A).

Conducting a nutrition assessment with a genetic focus is a logical way to begin incorporating genetics into practice. Much of the information available in the medical record and commonly elicited during a nutrition interview can be used to provide clues about the patient's/client's genetic risk status. Most authorities recommend obtaining a three-generation family history (i.e., patient, patient's parents and grandparents). Examples of types of information to inquire about for each person identified in the family medical history include age of onset of serious illnesses and chronic conditions; cause of death and age at the time of death; information about family members with birth defects, mental retardation, common diseases or disorders (i.e., asthma, diabetes, heart disease, cancer—specify location and age of diagnosis); reproductive history (i.e., miscarriages, stillbirths, gestational diabetes, maternal phenylketonuria); maternal age; and ethnicity.[19,73] A standardized family history questionnaire targeting those common diseases associated with the greatest national health burden is under development by the Centers for Disease Control and Prevention.[80]

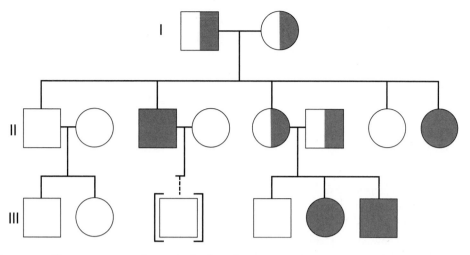

FIGURE 13-9   *Three-generation pedigree of a family with an autosomal recessive trait.*

TABLE 13-5	Standard Pedigree Nomenclature (does not represent a complete set of symbols)		
SYMBOL	**INTERPRETATION**	**SYMBOL**	**INTERPRETATION**
□	Male	□—○	Marriage/mating
○	Female	□—⁄—○	Divorced
◇	Unknown gender	□══○	Consanguinity
■ ●	Affected male/female	□—⊤—○	No offspring
◨ ◐	Male/female, heterozygous for autosomal recessive trait	⌂ ⌂	Monozygotic twins
▨ ∅	Deceased male/female	⌂ ⌂	Dizygotic twins
⌂ᴏᴏ	Siblings	[□]	Male adopted into family
■ ● ↗ ↗	Proband or index case	[□]	Male adopted out of family
□ ○ ↗ ↗	Consultand (person initiating workup)	◇ P	Pregnancy (gender unknown)
⊡	Male carrier	△	Miscarriage (spontaneous abortion)

Source: Adapted from Bennett et al.[76]

GENETIC COUNSELING: A POTENTIAL MODEL FOR DIETETICS PRACTITIONERS IN THE GENOMIC AND POSTGENOMIC ERAS

Genetic counseling is defined by the American Society of Human Genetics as "a communication process that deals with human problems associated with the occurrence, or risk of occurrence, of a genetic disorder in a family."[81] Through this counseling process, genetic counselors help the individual or family understand aspects of their diagnosis or the diagnosis for which they are at risk, including the probable course of the disease/disorder, therapeutic options, the contributions of heredity, and the implications for other family members. This process also involves helping the individual/family understand their options and choose a course of action consonant with family goals, ethics, and religious beliefs.[80] Counseling is conducted in a nondirective manner that supports autonomous decision making, and is expected to provide complete disclosure of all relevant information.[82] Confidentiality of information is also important, since information may be revealed that is not known to all family members (e.g., nonpaternity), and some information has the potential to be used in a discriminatory manner.

Unlike traditional nutrition counseling, which is largely prescriptive in nature due to its treatment orientation, information about nutrient-gene interactions will be based on probabilities. These probabilities will be expressed in terms of the chance of developing a certain disease within a given time frame and the degree to which initiating dietary changes may alter disease risk.[51] Consideration needs to be given to the model that would be most appropriate for this type of nutrition counseling.[30,51,83] Drawing

Issues to Ponder

- How will nutritional genomic research impact dietetics practice? What opportunities will it bring and how will these opportunities affect the scope of dietetics practice?
- What skills and knowledge will dietetics practitioners need in order to be competent to practice in the era of nutritional genomics? What changes are needed in dietetics education to prepare practitioners for roles they will be expected to play in the era of nutritional genomics? How will this affect entry-level education of dietetics practitioners?
- What types of tools and technologies will facilitate communication, education, and understanding about complex nutrient-genome interactions and disease risk to clients and patients?
- What are the ethical, legal, and social implications of genomic research as they relate to dietetics practitioners and dietetic practice?
- What are the psychological/social implications or ramifications of knowing your genetic profile and related disease risk?
- What, if any, boundaries should be put in place with regard to the application of genomic medicine and healthcare? What approach should be used to define these boundaries?
- What are the potential benefits of nutritional genomic research for patients/clients? For dietetics practitioners?
- What are the potential impacts of nutritional genomic research on public health policy?
- What are the potential impacts and implications of nutritional genomic research with regard to the functional food and nutrition supplement industries?
- What new employment opportunities do you envision for dietetics professionals related to nutritional genomics?
- Where can dietetics practitioners find credible genetics-related information for themselves and their clients?
- What are the risks of nutritional genomic research to consumers in terms of health fraud and quackery? What safeguards could be instituted to protect consumers from unscrupulous practices and products?

from the basic premises set forth in the model used by genetic counselors offers a good starting point for dietetics professionals.

GENOMIC NUTRITION: THE ROLE OF THE DIETETICS/NUTRITION PROFESSIONAL

The advent of the genomic era of medicine calls for dietetics and nutrition professionals to retool their skill set and to start incorporating "genetic thinking" and genetic principles into practice. The broad range of applications and implications across the lifespan (i.e., preconception to the end of life) related to disease prevention and treatment underscores the need for all dietetics professionals to develop genetic literacy.[83]

As food and nutrition experts, dietetics professionals are in a position to make unique contributions to genomic healthcare.[83] To provide leading-edge, high-quality services, dietetics and nutrition professionals will need to keep pace with genetics-related scientific advances and discoveries and to incorporate these findings into practice. For example, dietetics professionals will need to recognize when genetic factors play a role in disease risk, especially those that can be modified by nutrients or other dietary factors, and respond by making appropriate recommendations. In their roles as counselors and educators, dietetics professionals must be prepared to help patients comprehend the implications of genetic information; answer questions and address concerns related to genetic health issues; and provide appropriate resources and referrals.[83] They also will need to be prepared to evaluate the appropriateness of foods/products and edible vaccines (i.e., genetically engineered edible plants that produce vaccine antigens)[84] marketed to consumers with a particular genotype(s) or a particular family medical history and environmental risk factors. Examples of other tasks are listed in Table 13-6. Many of these roles are a logical extension of current dietetics practice, although some of them are likely to require more extensive education and training in order for dietetics professionals to achieve the desired level of competence. These roles will need to be assumed with attention to privacy and confidentiality, ethical issues, and sensitivity to the impact this information may have on patients and their families from the psychological, social, economic, and legal perspectives.[83]

TABLE 13-6 Genetics-Based Roles for Dietetics/Nutrition Professionals
1. Conduct a genetics-specific risk assessment that includes assessment of environmental risk factors, ethnicity, and cultural health beliefs and practices.
2. Explain and discuss nutrient-gene interactions and their impact on disease risk.
3. Evaluate and recommend nutrition intervention/prevention strategies based on a health risk appraisal that includes assessment of genetic, environmental, and ethnic risk factors, and cultural health beliefs and practices.
4. Obtain and interpret family medical history and construct/interpret a pedigree.
5. Understand and explain genetic test results.
6. Provide anticipatory guidance regarding the impact of genetic susceptibility for the patient and family members.
7. Foster informed decision making.
8. Recognize the indications for appropriate referrals for genetic testing/counseling.
9. Demonstrate an understanding of the social, psychological, economic, legal, and ethical issues of genetic services.

Source: Reprinted with permission from Kauwell.[83]

TABLE 13-7	Web Addresses (URL) for Genetics-Based Information and Resources (abbreviated list)
Human genome sequence data and related information	
Oak Ridge Genome Channel	http://compbio.ornl.gov/channel/
Online Mendelian Inheritance in Man	http://www.ncbi.nlm.nih.gov/Omim/omimhelp.html
Clinical and public health genetics	
Human Genome Epidemiology Network	http://www.cdc.gov/genomics/hugenet/default.htm
Office of Rare Diseases, National Institutes of Heath	http://rarediseases.info.nih.gov
National Cancer Institute, National Institutes of Health	http://www.cancer.gov/cancertopics/prevention-genetics-causes/genetics
National Newborn Screening & Genetics Resource Center	http://genes-r-us.uthscsa.edu
Support and advocacy groups	
National Organization for Rare Disorders	http://www.rarediseases.org/
National Partnership for Women and Families	http://nationalpartnership.org
Genetics education for health professionals	
HuGEM II	http://www.georgetown.edu/research/gucchd/hugem/
Genetics Education Program for Nurses	http://www.cincinnatichildrens.org/ed/clinical/gpnf/default.htm
Genetics Education Center, University of Kansas Medical Center	http://www.kumc.edu/gec/
National Coalition for Health Professional Education in Genetics	http://www.nchpeg.org/
Genetics education for the general public	
Genetic Science Learning Center	http://gslc.genetics.utah.edu/
Ethical, legal, and social implications	
The Communities of Color & Genetics Policy Project	http://www.sph.umich.edu/genpolicy/index.html
Genome Technology and Reproduction: Values and Public Policy	http://www.sph.umich.edu/genpolicy/initial/policyreport.html
National Information Resource on Ethics & Human Genetics	http://georgetown.edu/research/nrcbl/nirehg/
Ethical, Legal and Social Issues—DOE, NIH	http://www.ornl.gov/sci/TechResources/Human_Genome/elsi/elsi.html http://www.genome.gov/PolicyEthics/
Bioethics	http://www.nih.gov/sigs/bioethics/index.html http://www.nih.gov/sigs/bioethics/grow.html
Genetics professionals groups	
American Society of Human Genetics	http://www.ashg.org/genetics/ashg/ashgmenu.htm
International Society of Nurses in Genetics	http://www.isong.org/
Genetics Society of America	http://www.genetics-gsa.org/
U.S. government genetics agencies	
National Human Genome Research Institute	http://www.genome.gov/
Department of Energy HGP Information	http://www.ornl.gov/sci/TechResources/Human_Genome/project/hgp.shtml
Centers for Disease Control and Prevention, Office of Genomics & Disease Prevention	http://www.cdc.gov/genomics/default.htm
Sites that track or report what's new in genetics	
Genetics and Molecular Medicine Front Page (American Medical Association)	http://www.ama-assn.org/ama/pub/category/1799.html

Source: Adapted with permission from the Annual Review of Genomics and Human Genetics, Volume 2. ©2001 by Annual Reviews www.annualreviews.org.[86]

PROFESSIONAL AND CONSUMER RESOURCES

The Internet provides access to a wealth of reputable genetics-related resources for both professionals and consumers. The sites range from highly technical sites that catalogue and describe the specific molecular basis of diseases (e.g., OMIN) to those that provide basic tutorials (e.g., the U.S. Department of Energy) or information about support and advocacy groups (e.g., the National Organization for Rare Disorders). Unfortunately there also are websites that promote claims and services that are unfounded.[85] An abbreviated list of credible websites is included in Table 13-7. Dietetics professionals are encouraged to browse these sites to learn more about genetics and to familiarize themselves with sites that may provide valuable and reliable information for their patients/clients.

REFERENCES

1. Collins FS, Green ED, Guttmacher AE, Guyer MS. A vision for the future of genomics research: a blueprint for the genomic era. Nature 2003;422:835–847.
2. Core Competencies Working Group. Recommendations of core competencies in genetics essential for all health professionals. Genet Med 2001;3:155–159.
3. International Human Genome Sequencing Consortium. Initial sequencing and analysis of the human genome. Nature 2001;409:860–921.
4. Venter JC, Adams MD, Myers EW, et al. The sequence of the human genome. Science 2001;291:1304–1351.
5. NIH News. US Department of Health and Human Services. International consortium completes human genome project: all goals achieved; new vision for genome unveiled. April 14, 2003. Available at: http://www.nih.gov/news/pr/apr2003/nhgri-14.htm. Accessed September 24, 2005.
6. Science 2003;300:197–376.
7. Nature 2003;422:787–929.
8. US Department of Energy. Human Genome Project Information: ethical, legal and social issues. Available at: http://www.ornl.gov/sci/techresources/Human_Genome/elsi/elsi.shtml. Accessed September 24, 2005.
9. National Human Genome Research Institute. Genetic discrimination in health insurance. Available at: http://www.genome.gov/page.cfm?pageID=10002328. Accessed September 24, 2005.
10. US Department of Energy. Human Genome Project Information: genetics privacy and legislation. Available at: http://www.ornl.gov/sci/techresources/Human_Genome/elsi/legislat.shtml. Accessed September 24, 2005.
11. International Human Genome Sequencing Consortium. Finishing the euchromatic sequence of the human genome. Nature 2004:431, 931–945.
12. National Human Genome Research Institute. About the Human Genome Project. Available at: http://genome.gov/10001772. Accessed September 24, 2005.
13. NIH News Advisory. National Human Genome Research Institute. International consortium launches genetic variation mapping project. October 2002. Available at: http://www.genome.gov/page.cfm?pageID=10005336. Accessed September 24, 2005.
14. National Human Genome Research Institute. International HapMap consortium expands mapping effort. NIH News Release February 7, 2005. Available at: http://www.genome.gov/13014173. Accessed October 1, 2005.
15. Kauwell GPA. Emerging concepts in nutrigenomics: a preview of what is to come. Nutr Clin Pract 2005;20:75–87.
16. Collins FS, Guyer MS, Chakravarti A. Variations on a theme: cataloging human DNA sequence variation. Science 1997; 278:1580–1581.
17. Nussbaum RL, McInnes RR, Willard HF. Genetic variation in individuals: mutation and polymorphism. In: Thompson and Thompson Genetics in Medicine. 6th Ed. Philadelphia: Saunders, 2001:80–84.
18. Mueller RF, Young ID. The cellular and molecular basis of inheritance. In: Emery's Elements of Medical Genetics. 11th Ed. New York: Churchill Livingstone, 2001:21–24.
19. Lea DH. What nurses need to know about genetics. Dimens Crit Care Nurs 2002;21:50–60.
20. US Department of Energy. Human Genome Project Information: genetic disease information. Available at: http://www.ornl.gov/sci/techresources/Human_Genome/medicine/assist.shtml. Accessed September 24, 2005.

21. Hamosh A, Scott AF, Amberger J, Bocchini C, Valle D, McKusick VA. Online Mendelian Inheritance in Man (OMIM), a knowledge base of human genes and genetic disorders. Nucl Acids Res 2002;30:152–155.

22. Online Mendelian Inheritance in Man–NCBI GenBan. OMIM statistics. Available at: http://www3.ncbi.nlm.nih.gov/Omim/mimstats.html. Accessed September 23, 2005.

23. Luder E. Cystic fibrosis: the influence of the genotype and phenotype relationship on nutritional status. Top Clin Nutr 2003;18:92–99.

24. Guttmacher AE, Collins FS. Genomic medicine–a primer. N Engl J Med 2002;347:1512–1520.

25. Fields S. Proteomics: proteomics in genomeland. Science 2001;291:1221–1224.

26. Müller M, Kersten S. Nutrigenomics: goals and strategies. Nat Rev Genet 2003;4:315–322.

27. German JB, Watkins SM, Fay LB. Metabolomics in practice: emerging knowledge to guide future dietetic advice toward individualized health. J Am Diet Assoc 2005;105:1425–1432.

28. van Ommen B, Stierum R. Nutrigenomics: exploiting systems biology in the nutrition and health arena. Curr Opin Biotechnol 2002;13:517–521.

29. Ordovas JM, Mooser V. Nutrigenomics and nutrigenetics. Curr Opin Lipidol 2004;15:101–108.

30. Debusk RM, Fogarty CP, Ordovas JM, Kornman KS. Nutritional genomics in practice: where do we begin? J Am Diet Assoc 2005;105:589–598.

31. Frosst P, Blom HJ, Milos R, et al. A candidate genetic risk factor for vascular disease: a common mutation in methylenetetrahydrofolate reductase. Nat Genet 1995;10:111–113.

32. Schwahn B, Rozen R. Polymorphisms in the methylenetetrahydrofolate reductase gene: clinical consequences. Am J Pharmacogenom 2001;1:189–201.

33. Jacques PF, Bostom AG, Williams RR, et al. Relation between folate status, a common mutation in methylenetetrahydrofolate reductase, and plasma homocysteine concentrations. Circulation 1996;93:7–9.

34. Rosenberg IH, Rosenberg LE. The implications of genetic diversity for nutrient requirements: the case of folate. Nutr Rev 1998;56:S47–S53.

35. Ashfield-Watt PAL, Pullin CH, et al. Methylenetetrahydrofolate reductase 677C→T genotype modulates homocysteine responses to a folate-rich diet or a low-dose folic acid supplement: a randomized controlled trial. Am J Clin Nutr 2002;76:180–186.

36. Malinow MR, Nieto FJ, Kruger WD, et al. The effects of folic acid supplementation on plasma total homocysteine are modulated by multivitamin use and methylenetetrahydrofolate reductase genotypes. Arterioscler Thromb Vasc Biol 1997;17:1157–1162.

37. Botto LD, Yang Q. 5,10-Methylenetetrahydrofolate reductase gene variants and congenital anomalies: A HuGE review. Am J Epidemiol 2000;151:862–877.

38. Ma J, Stampfer MJ, Giovannucci E, et al. Methylenetetrahydrofolate reductase polymorphism, dietary interactions, and risk of colorectal cancer. Cancer Res. 1997;57:1098–1102.

39. Chen J, Giovannucci E, Kelsey K, et al. A methylenetetrahydrofolate reductase polymorphism and the risk of colorectal cancer. Cancer Res 1996;56:4862–4864.

40. Slattery ML, Potter JD, Samowitz W, Schaffer D, Leppert M. Methylenetetrahydrofolate reductase, diet, and risk of colon cancer. Cancer Epidemiol Biomarkers Prev 1999;8:513–518.

41. Levine AJ, Siegmund KD, Ervin CM, et al. The methylenetetrahydrofolate reductase 677C→T polymorphism and distal colorectal adenoma risk. Cancer Epidemiol Biomarkers Prev 2000;9:657–663.

42. Skibola CF, Smith MT, Kane E, et al. Polymorphisms in the methylenetetrahydrofolate reductase gene are associated with susceptibility to acute leukemia in adults. Proc Natl Acad Sci USA 1999;96:12810–12815.

43. Franco RF, Simões BP, Tone LG, Gabellini SM, Zago MA, Falcao RP. The methylenetetrahydrofolate reductase C677T gene polymorphism decreases the risk of childhood acute lymphocytic leukaemia. Br J Haematol 2001;115:616–618.

44. Institute of Medicine, Food and Nutrition Board. Folate. In: Dietary Reference Intakes for Thiamin, Riboflavin, Niacin, Vitamin B$_6$, Folate, Vitamin B$_{12}$, Pantothenic Acid, Biotin, and Choline. Washington DC: National Academy Press, 1998:196–305.

45. van der Put NMJ, Steegers-Theunissen RPM, Frosst P, et al. Mutated methylenetetrahydrofolate reductase as a risk factor for spina bifida. Lancet 1995;346:1070–1071.

46. van der Put NMJ, Eskes TKAB, Blom HJ. Is the common 677C→T mutation in the methylenetetrahydrofolate reductase gene a risk factor for neural tube defects? A meta-analysis. QJM 1997;90:111–115.

47. Shaw GM, Rozen R, Finnell RH, Wasserman CR, Lammer EJ. Maternal vitamin use, genetic variation of infant methylenetetrahydrofolate reductase, and risk for spina bifida. Am J Epidemiol 1998;148:30–37.

48. Christensen B, Arbour L, Tran P, et al. Genetic polymorphisms in methylenetetrahydrofolate reductase and methionine synthase, folate levels in red blood cells, and risk of neural tube defects. Am J Med Genet 1999;84:151–157.

49. Kauwell GPA, Wilsky CE, Cerda JJ, et al. Methylenetetrahydrofolate reductase mutation (677C→T) negatively influences plasma homocysteine response to marginal folate intake in elderly women. Metabolism 2000;49:1440–1443.

50. Brattström L, Wilcken DE, Ohrvik J, Brudin L. Common methylenetetrahydrofolate reductase gene mutation leads to hyperhomocysteinemia but not to vascular disease: the result of a meta-analysis. Circulation 1998;98:2520–2526.

51. Patterson RE, Eaton DL, Potter JD. The genetic revolution: change and challenge for the dietetics profession. J Am Diet Assoc 1999;99:1412–1420.

52. Feder JN, Gnirke A, Thomas W, et al. A novel MHC class-I-like gene is mutated in patients with hereditary haeomochromatosis. Nat Genet 1996;13:399–408.

53. Bomford A. Genetics of haemochromatosis. Lancet 2002;360:1673–1681.

54. Online Mendelian Inheritance in Man (OMIN). Available at: http://www3.ncbi.nlm.nih.gov/entrez/dispomim.cgi?id=261600. Accessed September 24, 2005.

55. Ordovas JM, Corella D, Cupples LA, et al. Polyunsaturated fatty acids modulate the effects of the APOA1 G-A polymorphism on HDL-cholesterol concentrations in men: The Framingham Offspring Study. Am J Clin Nutr 2002;75:38–46.

56. Moreno JA, Perez-Jimenez F, Marin C, et al. The effect of dietary fat on LDL size is influenced by apolipoprotein E genotype in healthy subjects. J Nutr 2004;134:2517–2522.

57. Weinberg RB, Geissinger BW, Kasala K, et al. Effect of apolipoprotein A-IV genotype and dietary fat on cholesterol absorption in humans. J Lipid Res 2000;41:2035–2041.

58. Michnovicz JJ. Increased estrogen 2-hydroxylation in obese women using oral indole-3-carbinol. Int J Obes Relat Metab Disord 1998;22:227–229.

59. Ordovas JM, Corella D, Serkalem D. Dietary fat intake determines the effect of a common polymorphism in the hepatic lipase gene promoter on high-density lipoprotein metabolism. Circulation 2002;106:2351–2321.

60. Zheng W, Deitz AC, Campell DR, et al. N-acetyltransferase 1 genetic polymorphism, cigarette smoking, well-done meat intake, and breast cancer risk. Cancer Epidemiol Biomarkers Prev 1999;8:233–239.

61. Corella D, Qi L, Sorli JV, et al. Obese subjects carrying the 11482G>A polymorphism at the perilipin locus are resistant to weight loss after dietary energy restriction. J Clin Endocrinol Metab 2005;90:5121–5126.

62. Corella D, Ordovas JM. Single nucleotide polymorphisms that influence lipid metabolism: interaction with dietary factors. Annu Rev Nutr 2005;25:341–390.

63. Verma M, Dunn BK, Ross S, et al. Early detection and risk assessment: proceedings and recommendations from the Workshop on Epigenetics in Cancer Prevention. Ann NY Acad Sci 2003;983:298–319.

64. Johanning GL, Heimburger DC, Piyathilake CJ. DNA methylation and diet in cancer. J Nutr 2002;132:3814S–3818S.

65. Jacob RA, Gretz DM, Taylor PC, et al. Moderate folate depletion increases plasma homocysteine and decreases lymphocyte DNA methylation in postmenopausal women. J Nutr 1998;128:1204–1212.

66. Rampersaud GC, Kauwell GPA, Hutson AD, Cerda JJ, Bailey LB. Genomic DNA methylation decreases in response to moderate folate depletion in elderly women. Am J Clin Nutr 2000;72:998–1003.

67. Dennis C. Epigenetics and disease: altered states. Nature 2003;421:686–688.

68. Choi S-W, Mason JB. Folate and carcinogenesis: an integrated scheme. J Nutr 2000;130:129–132.

69. Blount BC, Mack MM, Wehr CM, et al. Folate deficiency causes uracil misincorporation into human DNA and chromosome breakage: implications for cancer and neuronal damage. Proc Natl Acad Sci USA 1997;94:3290–3295.

70. National Human Genome Research Institute. Health: frequently asked questions about genetics. Available at: http://www.genome.gov/10001191. Accessed September 24, 2004.

71. US Department of Energy. Human Genome Project Information: gene testing. Available at: http://www.ornl.gov/TechResources/Human_Genome/medicine/genetest.html. Accessed September 24, 2005.

72. Cystic fibrosis mutation database. Available at: http://www.genet.sickkids.on.ca/cftr. Accessed September 25, 2005.

73. Cardeiro D. Ethnicity and the family history. The Genetic Family History in Practice. 2003;1(Summer):2. Available at: http://www.nchpeg.org/newsletter/inpracticesum03pdf. Accessed September 24, 2005.

74. Grody WW, Desnick RJ. Cystic fibrosis population carrier screening: here at last—are we ready? Genet Med 2001:3:149–154.

75. Richards CS, Bradley LA, Amos J, et al. American College of Medical Genetics—technical standards and guidelines for CFTR mutation testing (2005 edition). Available at: http://www.acmg.net/Pages/ACMG_Activities/stds-2002/cf.htm. Accessed September 25, 2005.

76. Bennett RL, Steinhaus KA, Uhrich SB, et al. Recommendations for standardized human pedigree nomenclature. Am J Hum Genet 1995;56:745–752.
77. Collins FS. Shattuck lecture: medical and societal consequences of the Human Genome Project. N Engl J Med 1999;341:28–37.
78. Yoon PW, Scheuner MT, Peterson-Oehlke KL, Gwinn M, Faucett A, Khoury MJ. Can family history be used as a tool for public health and preventive medicine? Genet Med 2002;4:304–310.
79. Yoon PW, Scheuner MT, Khoury MJ. Research priorities for evaluating family history in the prevention of common chronic diseases. Am J Prev Med 2003;24:128–135.
80. NCHPEG Family History Working Group. Not just for geneticists. The Genetic Family History in Practice 2003;1(Spring):1. Available at: http://www.nchpeg.org/newsletter/inpracticespr03.pdf. Accessed September 24, 2005.
81. Ad Hoc Committee on Genetic Counseling. Genetic counseling. Am J Hum Genet 1975;27:240–242.
82. Walker A. The practice of genetic counseling. In: Baker D, Schuette J, Uhlmann W, eds. A Guide to Genetic Counseling. New York: Wiley-Liss, 1998.
83. Kauwell GPA. A genomic approach to dietetic practice: are you ready? Top Clin Nutr 2003;18:81–91.
84. Poland GA, Murray D, Bonilla-Guerrero R. New vaccine development. BMJ 2002;324:1315–1319.
85. Guttmacher AE, Collins FS. Welcome to the genomic era. N Engl J Med 2003;349:996–998.
86. Guttmacher AE. Human genetics on the web. Annu Rev Genomics Hum Genet 2001; 2:213–233.

BIBLIOGRAPHY FOR BASIC GENETICS SECTION

Clark DP, Russell LD. Molecular Biology Made Simple and Fun. 2nd Ed. Vienna, IL: Cache River Press, 2000.
Gelehrter TD, Collins FS, Ginsburg D. Principles of Medical Genetics. 2nd Ed. Baltimore: Williams & Wilkins, 1998.
Jorde LB, Carey JC, Bamshad MJ, White RL. Medical Genetics. 2nd Ed. St. Louis: Mosby, 2000.
Mueller RF, Young ID. Emery's Elements of Medical Genetics. 11th Ed. New York: Churchill Livingstone, 2001.
Nussbaum RL, McInnes RR, Willard HF. Thompson and Thompson Genetics in Medicine. 6th Ed. Philadelphia: Saunders, 2001.
Raineri D. Introduction to Molecular Biology. Malden, MA: Blackwell Science, 2001.

APPENDIX A   Core Competencies in Genetics Essential for All Healthcare Professionals

The National Coalition for Health Professional Education in Genetics (NCHPEG) is an "organization of organizations" committed to a national effort to promote health professional education and access to information about advances in human genetics. NCHPEG's publication of the second edition of the Core Competencies in January 2005 provides basic guidance to a broad range of individuals and groups as they plan educational initiatives in genetics and genetically based health care.

PURPOSE

. . . The long-term goal for development of the ideal competencies in genetics is to encourage clinicians and other professionals to integrate genetics knowledge, skills, and attitudes into routine health care, thereby providing effective and comprehensive services to individuals and families. . . .

NCHPEG recommends that all health professionals possess the core competencies in genetics identified in this report so they can integrate genetics effectively and responsibly into current practice. Competence in these areas represents the minimum knowledge, skills, and attitudes necessary for health professionals from all disciplines to provide patient care that incorporates genetic perspectives and reflects sensitivity to related ethical, legal, and social concerns.

Each health-care professional should at a minimum be able to

- appreciate limitations of his or her genetics expertise,
- understand the social and psychological implications of genetic services, and
- know how and when to make a referral to a genetics professional.

BACKGROUND

. . . The sheer volume of new information now at the disposal of biomedical researchers and health-care providers is transforming our understanding of disease processes—including those of common, chronic diseases such as cancer, diabetes, and mental illness—and is changing the delivery of health care.[1–5] Public health agencies increasingly will apply genetic insights to the analysis of disease in populations and to the targeted introduction of strategies for disease prevention,[6–8] and will continue to work with the private sector to ensure the quality, efficacy, and safety of genetic tests.[9,10] The general public, empowered by access to information on the World Wide Web, grows better informed each day about genetics and genetically based health care, and health-care providers—regardless of specialty, role, or practice setting—will face questions about the implications of genetics and genomics for their patients.

IMPLEMENTATION

It is essential that individuals and groups responsible for continuing education, curriculum development, licensing, certification, and accreditation of health professionals adopt these recommendations and integrate genetics content into ongoing education.

. . . Enhanced competence in genetics will help health professionals and the public respond to the changing demands of the health-care system and will promote human welfare as a result of progress in genetics and genomics. No one can predict with certainty how genetically based health care will be organized or who will provide the bulk of genetic services when genetics is fully integrated into the health-care system. Nonetheless, many people recognize that health professionals involved in the direct provision of genetic services may require additional training to achieve an appropriately higher level of competence. Indeed, there are a number of examples of specific recommendations for training of professionals who require specialized knowledge of genetics.[7,11–20]

. . . There is, of course, no final resolution at this time to the questions of who will provide genetic services, in what settings, and under what financial structures. Indeed, there is as yet no clear answer to the question of how genetic services will be defined in the future, and that answer is unlikely to emerge any time soon. It is crucial, however, that all health professionals incorporate genetic and genomic knowledge so they are well informed about the ways in which that information can enhance patient outcomes.

. . . This document remains a work in progress, because it is virtually certain that new knowledge produced by the Human Genome Project and related activities will create an ongoing need to assess and revise expectations. Although the core competencies are challenging, NCHPEG believes it is important to prepare professionals for the health care of the future, as well as for today's reality.

THE CORE COMPETENCIES

Note: Throughout this document, the term "clients" includes individuals and their sociological and biological families.

KNOWLEDGE

All health professionals should understand:

1.1   basic human genetics terminology
1.2   the basic patterns of biological inheritance and variation, both within families and within populations
1.3   how identification of disease-associated genetic variations facilitates development of prevention, diagnosis, and treatment options
1.4   the importance of family history (minimum three generations) in assessing predisposition to disease
1.5   the role of genetic factors in maintaining health and preventing disease

1.6   the difference between clinical diagnosis of disease and identification of genetic predisposition to disease (genetic variation is not strictly correlated with disease manifestation)

1.7   the role of behavioral, social, and environmental factors (lifestyle, socioeconomic factors, pollutants, etc.) to modify or influence genetics in the manifestation of disease

1.8   the influence of ethnoculture and economics in the prevalence and diagnosis of genetic disease

1.9   the influence of ethnicity, culture, related health beliefs, and economics in the clients' ability to use genetic information and services

1.10   the potential physical and/or psychosocial benefits, limitations, and risks of genetic information for individuals, family members, and communities

1.11   the range of genetic approaches to treatment of disease (prevention, pharmacogenomics/prescription of drugs to match individual genetic profiles, gene-based drugs, gene therapy)

1.12   the resources available to assist clients seeking genetic information or services, including the types of genetics professionals available and their diverse responsibilities

1.13   the components of the genetic counseling process and the indications for referral to genetic specialists

1.14   the indications for genetic testing and/or gene-based interventions

1.15   the ethical, legal, and social issues related to genetic testing and recording of genetic information (e.g., privacy, the potential for genetic discrimination in health insurance and employment)

1.16   the history of misuse of human genetic information (eugenics)

1.17   one's own professional role in the referral to genetics services, or provision, follow-up, and quality review of genetic services

SKILLS

All health professionals should be able to:

2.1   gather genetic family history information, including an appropriate multigenerational family history

2.2   identify clients who would benefit from genetic services

2.3   explain basic concepts of probability and disease susceptibility, and the influence of genetic factors in maintenance of health and development of disease

2.4   seek assistance from and refer to appropriate genetics experts and peer support resources

2.5   obtain credible, current information about genetics for self, clients, and colleagues

2.6   use effectively new information technologies to obtain current information about genetics

2.7   educate others about client-focused policy issues

2.8   participate in professional and public education about genetics

Skills 2.9 to 2.17 delineate the components of the genetic-counseling process and are not expected of all healthcare professionals. However, health professionals should be able to facilitate the genetic-counseling process and prepare clients and families for what to expect, communicate relevant information to the genetics team, and follow up with the client after genetics services have been provided. For those health professionals who choose to provide genetic-counseling services to their clients, all components of the process, as delineated in 2.9 to 2.17, should be performed.

2.9   educate clients about availability of genetic testing and/or treatment for conditions seen frequently in practice

2.10   provide appropriate information about the potential risks, benefits, and limitations of genetic testing

2.11   provide clients with an appropriate informed-consent process to facilitate decision making related to genetic testing

2.12   provide, and encourage use of, culturally appropriate, user-friendly materials/media to convey information about genetic concepts

2.13   educate clients about the range of emotional effects they and/or family members may experience as a result of receiving genetic information

2.14   explain potential physical and psychosocial benefits and limitations of gene-based therapeutics for clients

2.15   discuss costs of genetic services, benefits and potential risks of using health insurance for payment of genetic services, potential risks of discrimination

2.16   safeguard privacy and confidentiality of genetic information of clients to the extent possible

2.17   inform clients of potential limitations to maintaining privacy and confidentiality of genetic information

ATTITUDES

All health professionals should:

3.1   recognize philosophical, theological, cultural, and ethical perspectives influencing use of genetic information and services

3.2   appreciate the sensitivity of genetic information and the need for privacy and confidentiality

3.3   recognize the importance of delivering genetic education and counseling fairly, accurately, and without coercion or personal bias

3.4   appreciate the importance of sensitivity in tailoring information and services to clients' culture, knowledge, and language level

3.5   seek coordination and collaboration with interdisciplinary team of health professionals

3.6   speak out on issues that undermine clients' rights to informed decision making and voluntary action

3.7   recognize the limitations of their own genetics expertise

3.8   demonstrate willingness to update genetics knowledge at frequent intervals

3.9   recognize when personal values and biases with regard to ethical, social, cultural, religious, and ethnic issues may affect or interfere with care provided to clients

3.10   support client-focused policies

REFERENCES

1. Dumont-Driscoll M. Genetics and the general pediatrician: where do we belong in this exploding field of medicine? Current Problems in Pediatric and Adolescent Health Care 2002;32:6–28.
2. Hayflick SJ, Eiff MP. Will the learners be learned? Genetics in Medicine 2002;4:43-44.
3. Wright JT, Hart TC. The genome projects: implications for dental practice and education. Journal of Dental Education 2002;66:659–671.
4. Kirklin D. Responding to the implications of the genetics revolution for the education and training of doctors: a medical humanities approach. Medical Education 2003;37:168–173.
5. Jenkins J, Lea DH. Nursing Care in the Genomic Era: A Case Based Approach. Boston: Jones and Bartlett Publishers, 2005.
6. Khoury MJ, Burke W, Thomson EJ, eds. Genetics and Public Health in the 21st Century: Using Genetic Information to Improve Health and Prevent Disease. New York: Oxford University Press, 2000.
7. Centers for Disease Control and Prevention (CDC). 2001. Genomic competencies for the public health workforce. Available at: http://www.cdc.gov/genomics/training/competencies/comps.htm.
8. Centers for Disease Control and Prevention (CDC). Harnessing Genetics to Prevent Disease and Improve Health: A State Policy Guide. Atlanta, GA: Centers for Disease Control and Prevention, 2003.
9. Burke W. Genetic testing in primary care. Annual Review of Genomics and Human Genetics 2004;5:1–14.
10. Burke W, Zimmern R. Ensuring the appropriate use of genetic tests. Nature Reviews Genetics 2004;5:955–959.
11. American Society of Human Genetics Information and Education Committee (ASHG). ASHG report from the ASHG Information and Education Committee: medical school curriculum in genetics. American Journal of Human Genetics 1995;56:535–537.
12. Fine B, Baker D, Fiddler M. ABGC Consensus Development Consortium. Practice-based competencies for accreditation of and training in graduate programs in genetic counseling. Journal of Genetic Counseling 1996;5:113–121.
13. Association of Professors of Human and Medical Genetics (APHMG). Clinical objectives in medical genetics for undergraduate medical students. Genetics in Medicine 1998;1:54–55.
14. American Society of Clinical Oncologists (ASCO). 1997. Cancer genetics curriculum. Available at: http://www.asco.org.
15. Hayflick S, Eiff, M. Role of primary care providers in the delivery of genetic services. Community Genetics 1998;1:18–22.
16. Stephenson J. Group drafts core curriculum for "What docs need to know about genetics." Journal of the American Medical Association 1998;279:735–736.
17. Taylor-Brown S, Johnson, A. 1998. Genetics practice. Update available at: www.naswdc.org.
18. Reynolds P, Benkendorf J. Genes and generalists: why we need professionals with added competencies. Western Journal of Medicine 1999;171:375–379.
19. Jenkins J, Dimond E, Steinberg S. Preparing for the future through genetics nursing education. Journal of Nursing Scholarship 2001;33:191–195.
20. Wormington CM. The genomics revolution and molecular optometry: educational implications. Optometry Education 2004;29:43–48.

Note: A complete copy of the Core Competencies and related materials can be obtained from the NCHPEG website at http://www.nchpeg.org. Competencies and related materials adapted with permission from the National Coalition for Health Professional Education in Genetics.

APPENDIX B   Glossary of Terms

Allele: Any one of a number of variant forms of a gene at a particular locus on a chromosome; allelic (i.e., different; variant) forms of the same gene can produce variations in inherited characteristics.

Alternative splicing: Selective inclusion or exclusion of genetic information in the final mRNA transcript resulting in different protein products from the same gene.

Autosomal dominant allele: Gene on one of the non–sex chromosomes that prevails when the corresponding allele on the matching chromosome is recessive.

Autosomal dominant disorder: Disorder that is expressed when a dominant disease-causing allele of a non–sex chromosome (autosome) is inherited.

Autosomal recessive allele: Gene on one of the non–sex chromosomes that prevails only when the corresponding allele on the matching chromosome also is recessive.

Autosomal recessive disorder: Disorder that is expressed only when both disease-causing alleles of a non–sex chromosome (autosome) is inherited.

Chromosomal disorders: Disorders resulting from abnormalities in chromosome number or structure.

Chromosome: In eukaryotic cells, thread-like, linear strands of DNA and associated proteins located in the nucleus of cells that contain the hereditary information packaged in genes.

Chromosome nondisjunction: Failure of a chromosome pair to separate during meiosis (i.e., during the formation of the egg or sperm), an error that results in one daughter cell with an extra chromosome, and one daughter cell with no copy of that particular chromosome.

DNA: Abbreviation for deoxyribonucleic acid; a nucleic acid comprising a double helix strand of nucleotides joined by hydrogen bonds formed as a result of complementary base pairing (i.e., adenine and thymine, cytosine, and guanine).

ELSI: Abbreviation used to refer to the ethical, legal, and social implications of genetic research.

Epigenetics: Study of mitotically heritable changes in gene function that occur independent of changes in the DNA nucleotide sequence; nonsequence modifications that provide additional instructions on how, when, and where genetic information is to be used; includes the study of how environmental factors that affect a parent lead to changes in gene expression in the offspring.

Exon: Coding region of a gene; the regions of a gene's DNA that comprise mature mRNA and are used to encode the amino acid product during translation.

Family history –3 generation: Family history that includes medical history information of individuals from three generations (i.e., patient, patient's parents, and patient's grandparents).

Gene: Basic physical and functional unit of heredity consisting of a segment of DNA arranged along a chromosome that encodes a protein(s).

Genetics: Study of heredity, in particular, how qualities or traits are transmitted from parents to offspring.

Genome: Complete collection of genetic information of a species or individual.

Genotype: Specific set of alleles inherited at a locus on the chromosome pair; specific genetic makeup of an individual.

Haplotype: A set of closely linked alleles (of different genes) that tend to be inherited together. Haplotypes contain common sequence variants (i.e., single nucleotide polymorphisms, or SNPs). These variants serve as genetic markers and are being used to learn more about patterns of genetic variation associated with risk for common chronic diseases.

HapMap: Shortened term for haplotype map, a resource being developed by the International HapMap Project that will identify and catalog similarities and differences in humans using closely linked segments of DNA markers on different genes. The goal is to link genetic variants to the risk for specific diseases/conditions.

Heterozygous: Term used to describe the case in which the genes occurring at the same locus of a homologous chromosome pair are different (i.e., variant).

Homologous: Having the same form/structure and linear sequence of gene locations as another chromosome.

Homozygous: Term used to describe the case in which both copies of a gene at a particular locus of a homologous chromosome pair are identical.

Human Genome Project (HGP): An international, collaborative research program officially initiated in 1990 with the goal of sequencing all of the genes that comprise a human being by 2005.

Intron: Noncoding region of a gene that is usually removed from the primary mRNA transcript to produce the mature mRNA.

Locus (plural, loci): Position/location of a gene on a chromosome.

Meiosis: Process of cell division occurring in sexually reproductive organisms in which the number of chromosomes in reproductive cells is reduced from diploid (i.e., a pair of each chromosome) to haploid (i.e., single set of chromosomes).

Mendelian inheritance: Inheritance patterns that follow the principles of Mendel's laws.

Metabolomics: Study of the entire metabolic content of a cell (i.e., metabolites) at a given time for the purpose of identifying each metabolic pathway, its metabolites, and their functional roles.[24]

Mitochondrial disorder: A disorder that arises as a result of inheriting a mutation in a gene contained in mitochondrial DNA (mtDNA).

mRNA: Abbreviation used to refer to messenger RNA. The primary mRNA transcript refers to the complementary sequence of bases transcribed from DNA; removal of introns from the primary mRNA transcript produces mature mRNA, which is translated into proteins.

Multifactorial inheritance diseases/disorders: Diseases/disorders that result from the interplay of genes with the environment; they are not inherited per se. The underlying genetic mechanisms of these disorders are generally not well understood, although it is thought that the genetic component involves multiple genes (i.e., the causes are polygenic); susceptibility for these disorders can be modified positively or negatively by other factors, including the environment.

Mutation: Permanent alterations in the genetic material of a cell that may be benign, pathogenic, or of unknown significance; germline mutations can be passed on to offspring; somatic mutations are not transmissible but can result in malfunction or death of a cell; basic types of mutations are described in Table 13-2.

Nucleotide: Structural unit of DNA and RNA consisting of a sugar (deoxyribose or ribose, respectively), phosphate, and base (adenine, cytosine, guanine, thymine, or uracil).

Nutrigenetics: Study of the interactions between nutrients/bioactive components and genetic variation, with particular interest in how these interactions may affect risk for multifactorial diseases and nutrient requirements of an individual.

Nutrigenomics: Study of the genomewide effects of nutrients and bioactive food components in terms of their influence on metabolic pathways and homeostatic control at the molecular level with specific attention to how they affect patterns of gene expression, protein expression, and metabolite production.[24]

Nutritional genomics: Umbrella term that encompasses the areas of nutrition research referred to as nutrigenomics and nutrigenetics.

Pedigree analysis: Graphic representation of a family's medical history that uses standard symbols that can help the practitioner visualize how traits cluster within families and move through generations.

Phenotype: Observable traits (i.e., physical, biochemical, physiological) resulting from interactions among genes and the environment.

Polymorphism: Variation in the DNA nucleotide sequence that occurs with a frequency of more than 1%.

Posttranslational modification: Chemical modification (i.e., phosphorylation, acetylation, etc.) that occurs after translation of the protein.

Promoter region: Area of a gene upstream from the coding region that contains the information enabling gene transcription; area of the gene in which transcription is initiated.

Proteomics: Study of the identity, structure, and function of all the proteins expressed by a genome.

RNA: Abbreviation for ribonucleic acid, a nucleic acid comprising a single strand of nucleotides (i.e., ribose sugar, phosphate and one of four bases: adenine, cytosine, guanine, and uracil). In eukaryotes, RNA carries genetic information transcribed from DNA in the cell's nucleus to the cytoplasm of the cell where it used to assemble proteins by way of the process known as translation.

RNA polymerase: Enzyme that binds to the promoter region of a gene to initiate transcription.

Single-gene disorders: Disorders resulting from a mutation(s) in one or both alleles at a single locus on a chromosome pair

Single-nucleotide polymorphism (SNP, pronounced "snip"): Type of polymorphic change in which a single base is substituted with another (e.g., cytosine replaced with thymine; C→T); SNPs that occur fairly frequently in the general population may or may not affect the amino acid sequence of the gene.

Systems biology (functional genomics): Discipline that incorporates genomics and proteomics, in tandem with genotype determination, transcriptomics, metabolomics to study the behavior of constituents present under defined conditions and the interactions that occur among the constituents in the system.

Termination sequence: A nucleotide sequence that signals the end of transcription.

Transcription: Process whereby the DNA sequence of a gene is copied to produce a complementary copy of itself in the form of messenger RNA.

Transcriptomics: Study of the complete collection of gene transcripts in a cell or tissue at a given time.[24]

Translation: Process by which the information contained in the mature messenger RNA transcript is decoded to produce a polypeptide chain by reading the RNA code three letters at a time.

Translocation: Transfer of a chromosome or chromosomal segment of DNA to new location; reinsertion of a chromosomal segment of DNA can occur on the same or a different chromosome.

Triplet: A codon; three adjacent nucleotides in a molecule of DNA or RNA that code for a specific amino acid or a stop codon.

Uracil misincorporation: Incorporation of uracil into the DNA molecule; uracil is not a usual component of DNA.

Wild-type: Referring to the prevailing or typical form of an organism, strain, gene, or characteristic as it occurs in nature.

X-linked: Refers to genes located on the X chromosome or characteristics or conditions of genes located on the X chromosome.

HYPERTENSION AND CLINICAL NUTRITION PRACTICE

Jennifer Muir Bowers

Hypertension affects 32% of Americans over the age of 20 years.[1] It accounts for 10.4 million visits to physicians' offices and 3.2 million hospital outpatient clinic visits.[2] Hypertension is the cause of death in over 19,000 Americans each year and is the most common cause of cardiovascular and cerebrovascular complications.[3] Certain subgroups, including blacks and individuals over the age of 55 years, are at higher risk for hypertension.[4] Other risk factors for hypertension include a positive family history, overweight status, increased alcohol consumption, and physical inactivity.[5]

Traditional medical nutrition therapy for hypertension includes a low-sodium diet, weight reduction, decreased alcohol consumption, reduction of dietary saturated fat, and increased physical activity.[6] High sodium intake has long been linked to hypertension, and a decrease in dietary sodium is what most clinicians emphasize in patient education. Although traditional nutrition and dietetics textbooks still emphasize this medical nutrition therapy, this treatment is now under closer scrutiny. More recent research is revealing that it is more than just one nutrient that affects blood pressure in patients with hypertension. In fact, multiple nutrients, certain foods, and whole food groups are being studied to learn whether they have any impact on blood pressure.

SODIUM AND POTASSIUM

Sodium is the mineral most widely associated with effects on blood pressure. It has been directly correlated with mean blood pressure levels as well as the prevalence of hypertension in a multitude of studies including humans and animals.[7,8] Public health recommendations for dietary sodium intake have been recommended by one group as 5 g/day, regardless of medical history.[8] Moderate salt restriction (6 g of salt per day or 2,400 mg of sodium per day) has been recommended for the treatment of hypertension.[6]

Conversely, potassium intake has been shown to be inversely correlated with blood pressure in diverse populations.[7] Further, depletion of serum potassium exacerbates hypertension.[9] This has prompted research on the effect of potassium supplementation on blood pressure. Although some studies have shown that potassium supplements can reduce blood pressure in normotensive and hypertensive subjects, these supplements have also been linked to the incidence of stroke.[10,11] Supplementation with potassium has been suggested only for patients who are unable to reduce their intake of sodium.[12] Potassium supplementation in the range of 94 to 406 mg/day in hypertensive subjects has been shown to improve blood pressure by 4.4 mm Hg systolic and 2.5 mm Hg diastolic.[8] A more beneficial approach to the dietary treatment of hypertension is an increased intake of fruits and vegetables, which will naturally increase the dietary consumption of potassium.[8]

DIETARY APPROACHES TO STOP HYPERTENSION—THE "DASH" STUDY

Perhaps the most comprehensive and well-known study on dietary factors related to hypertension is the Dietary Approaches to Stop Hypertension (DASH) study. This multicenter, randomized feeding project studied the blood pressure response of 459 subjects after consuming one of three diets: a control diet (a "typical" American diet), a diet high in fruits and vegetables, or a "combination" diet that was high in fruits, vegetables, low-fat dairy products, whole grains, poultry, fish, and nuts but was reduced in red meat, fats, and sugars.[13] DASH subjects were free-living nonobese adults over the age of 22 years, with a mean blood pressure of 120 to 159 systolic and 80 to 95 mm Hg diastolic, who were not taking antihypertensive medication.[13] To account for the disproportionately higher incidence of hypertension in minority populations, two-thirds of the participants were African Americans.[14] Exclusion criteria included diabetes mellitus, hyperlipidemia, a cardiac event within 6 months of the study, pregnancy or lactation, renal insufficiency, intake of > 14 alcoholic beverages per week, unwillingness to discontinue use of vitamins or minerals, and any chronic disease that would interfere with study participation.[13] Interestingly, the participants' prestudy diets were determined to be "typical" of Americans of similar age and ethnicity.[14] The DASH study researchers prepared foods in metabolic kitchens and participants ate lunch or dinner on site on weekdays for 8 weeks; their breakfasts and weekend meals were provided for participants to take home. Weight was intentionally kept constant to eliminate weight loss as a contributor to changes in blood pressure.[15] For similar reasons, sodium intake was also held constant at 3 g/day between the three groups of subjects.[13,16]

Compliance with the protocols of the DASH feeding study was deemed excellent by the researchers.[17] Blood pressure was significantly reduced in both groups who were given an intervention diet. The participants following the diet rich in fruits and vegetables had a mean reduction in blood pressure of 2.8 mm Hg systolic and 1.1 mmHg diastolic, while those eating the combination diet had a mean reduction in blood pressure of 11.4 mm Hg systolic and 5.5 mm Hg diastolic.[15] Subgroup analyses demonstrated that subjects with higher blood pressures at baseline experienced the greatest reduction in blood pressure after dietary intervention.[18] Minority participants showed statistically greater reductions in blood pressure than did Caucasians, potentially reflecting a greater response to dietary interventions.[15] Further, when subjects were fed a reduced-sodium (1,100 to 2,300 mg/day) version of the DASH diet, an even greater reduction in blood pressure was noted.[19,20]

That the combination diet showed almost twice as great a reduction in blood pressure as the diet rich in fruits and vegetables has drawn significant attention from clinicians and researchers. The dietary pattern that the DASH combination diet followed is outlined in Table 14-1.[16,21] The combination diet is now referred to as the DASH diet by most dietetics professionals and clinicians. Further, it appears that the synergy between the combination diet and a reduction of dietary sodium has the best potential effect on the blood pressure of hypertensive patients.[22]

The increased intake of foods rich in magnesium and calcium in the DASH combination diet is notable. Research has demonstrated that blood pressure is inversely associated with potassium, calcium, and magnesium intakes[7,8] Further analysis of calcium supplementation and blood pressure revealed modest effects.[23] Magnesium studies have been inconclusive to date.[24] Although current literature does not support supplementation with these nutrients at this point, further investigation into these minerals and their effect on blood pressure in hypertensive individuals is warranted.[8,25] Research studies inquiring into the potential mineral-mineral synergistic effects, or antagonizing effects, would be of great interest.

PREMIER

The PREMIER study attempted to compare traditional medical nutrition therapy for hypertension (low sodium, low alcohol, and weight reduction) with the DASH diet approach. PREMIER was a multicenter randomized trial to determine the effects of multicomponent lifestyle interventions on blood pressure.[26] Subjects

TABLE 14-1   Sample DASH Diet

FOOD GROUP	SERVINGS PER DAY	SERVING SIZES	IMPORTANT NUTRIENTS
Grains	7–8	1 slice bread 1/2 cup dry cereal 1/2 cup cooked rice, pasta, or cereal	Energy Fiber
Vegetables	4–5	1 cup raw leafy vegetables 1/2 cup cooked vegetables 6 oz vegetable juice	Potassium Magnesium Fiber
Fruits	4–5	6 oz fruit juice 1 medium fruit 1/2 cup dried fruit 1/2 cup fresh, frozen, or canned fruit	Potassium Magnesium Fiber
Low-fat or fat-free dairy foods	2–3	8 oz milk 1 cup yogurt 1.5 oz cheese	Calcium Protein
Meats, poultry, and fish	<2	3 oz cooked meats, poultry, or fish	Protein Magnesium
Nuts, seeds, dry beans, and peas	4–5 per week	1.5 oz or 1/3 cup nuts 1/2 oz or 2 tbsp seeds 1/2 cup cooked dry beans and peas	Energy Magnesium Potassium Protein Fiber
Fats and oils	2–3	1 tsp soft margarine 1 tbsp low-fat mayonnaise 2 tbsp light salad dressing 1 tsp vegetable oil	Adds satiety (DASH diet had only 27% of kcal from fat)
Sweets	5 per week	1 tbsp sugar 1 tbsp jelly or jam 1/2 oz jelly beans 8 oz lemonade	None

Source: Adapted from Windhauser MM, Ernst DB, Karanja NM, et al. Translating the Dietary Approaches to Stop Hypertension diet from research to practice: dietary and behavior change techniques. J Am Diet Assoc 1999;99(8 suppl):S90–S95.

included over 800 males and females of various ethnicities over the age of 25 years who had a baseline blood pressure of 120 to 159 mm Hg systolic and 80 to 95 mm Hg diastolic. Medication-related exclusion criteria included regular use of antihypertensive medications, insulin, antidiabetes drugs, antipsychotics, weight-loss medications, or other drugs that raise or lower blood pressure. Medical exclusions included cardiovascular events, congestive heart failure, angina, peripheral vascular disease, cancer, renal insufficiency, hyperglycemia, or psychiatric hospitalizations. Three experimental interventions were studied: (1) an "advice only" group, where subjects received two 30-minute individualized counseling sessions addressing weight reduction, healthy eating (low sodium, low alcohol, and the DASH diet), and physical activity; (2) an "established intervention" group where individual and group sessions included information and behavioral counseling about traditional medical nutrition therapy (low sodium and weight reduction); (3) an "established intervention plus DASH" group where the structure was the same as the second group but the nutrition information focused on the multiple dietary aspects of the DASH diet. Both established intervention groups received group interventions for nearly a year. Outcomes included blood pressure, weight, and biochemical values (homocysteine, lipids, glucose, and insulin).

Results from the PREMIER study demonstrated that both nutrition interventions were successful in reducing blood pressure and weight.[27] The "established intervention plus DASH" group, however, had the greatest decrease in blood pressure (from 38 to 12% prevalence) when compared to the "established intervention" (from 38 to 17% prevalence) and the "advice only" groups (from 38 to 26% prevalence).[28] The DASH diet led to a more significant reduction in blood pressure than traditional medical nutrition therapy alone. Another conclusion to draw from the PREMIER trial is that patients are able to make multiple lifestyle changes over a relatively short period of time, which can optimize their overall health.

DIET, EXERCISE, AND WEIGHT LOSS INTERVENTION TRIAL (DEW-IT)

In contrast to the PREMIER study, the DEW-IT incorporated both traditional medical nutrition therapy for hypertension (low sodium, weight reduction) and the DASH diet as well as regular aerobic exercise.[29] This experimental group was compared to a control group who received no intervention until the study was complete. The objective was to determine if a group of overweight hypertensive patients would have a reduction in blood pressure and other cardiovascular risk factors with a comprehensive lifestyle intervention. The uniqueness of the DEW-IT trial was the simultaneous implementation of several lifestyle recommendations. Participants included 45 overweight or obese adults with hypertension, who were stable on a single antihypertensive medication. The 9-week intervention comprised supervised aerobic exercise (three times a week) and provided meals. Those in the experimental group had substantially lower blood pressure after the intervention and lost an average of 5.5 kg, compared to the 0.6 kg loss in the control group. Blood pressure reductions were similar to those seen with pharmacologic therapy.[29] Although this is an impressive and comprehensive nutrition intervention, participants were not free-living, nor were they studied after the trial to determine if the reduction in blood pressure was maintained. A longer experiment with lifestyle training for the hypertensive patients would be ideal.

OTHER NUTRIENTS AND FOODS

Certain nutrients and even particular foods have been studied specifically to determine whether they have any effects on blood pressure. Vitamin C may also play a role in the regulation of blood pressure. Plasma vitamin C was inversely related to diastolic blood pressure in a trial that incorporated vitamin C depletion and repletion diet phases.[30] In this study, those subjects with the lowest blood levels of vitamin C had the highest blood pressure. This raises the question whether vitamin C affects blood pressure directly, or whether other nutrients commonly found in vitamin C–rich foods (potassium, phytochemicals, fiber, etc.) have this effect, or whether this reduction in blood pressure is the synergistic effect of a combination of nutrients. Further research can help to address and answer these questions.

The effect of oats has been studied, with conflicting results. One investigation found that a group of hypertensive men and women had a significant reduction in both systolic and diastolic blood pressure after a 6-week trial of an oat-rich diet.[31] In this study, the oat-rich diet contained 5.52 g of beta-glucan per day in the form of oat cereal, while the control group consumed a diet of less than 1.0 g of total fiber per day. These results, however, were not duplicated by another group of researchers who found no changes in blood pressure in hypertensive men who consumed an oat-rich diet (5.5 g of beta-glucan per day) for 12 weeks.[32] Both of these studies were small (comprising 18 to 36 subjects) and may need to be incorporated into a larger trial looking at more foods and a combination of nutrients in order to determine interactions.

Soy milk has demonstrated some potential in the dietary treatment of hypertension. One study compared skimmed cow's milk to soy milk in hypertensive men and women.[33] These investigators found that after 3 months of consuming 1 L/day of soy milk, blood pressure was decreased. The soy milk provided to the subjects contained the isoflavones genistein and daidzein. Similar effects have not been shown with supplemental tablets containing these isoflavones.[34] It can be speculated that some sort of interaction between the isoflavones, protein, or certain amino acids (arginine) in soy foods may play a role in the hypotensive effects.

The relationship between fatty acid intake and blood pressure has been of interest because of the interaction between prostaglandins and enzymes that induce either vasodilation or vasoconstriction and can affect platelet aggregation.[3,8] Eicosapentaenoic acid (EPA) and docosahexaenoic acid (DHA) have been shown to lower blood pressure by inhibiting thromboxane A_2 formation and enhancing PGI_3, with a net result of vasodilation and reduced platelet aggregation.[3] Gamma linolenic acid supplementation increases the production of the vasodilator PGE_1, decreases aldosterone, and reduces density and affinity of the adrenal angiotensin II receptor, thus potentially reducing blood pressure.[3]

Linolenic acid can be converted to gamma linolenic acid in the body, and there is some evidence that certain dietary factors such as magnesium, calcium, potassium, sodium, and vitamins A and C may act as cofactors in this conversion.[3] This appears to support the emerging belief that it is a synergy of a variety of nutrients that ultimately determines blood pressure. The most effective amounts of polyunsaturated, monounsaturated, and saturated fatty acids in the diet for optimum blood pressure improvement have not yet been identified.

Finally, certain herbal supplements have been recommended in the treatment of hypertension. Although many of these preparations do not have published clinical results, one type of unicellar freshwater green alga, *Chlorella pyrenoidosa*, does. Doses of 10 g/day of this alga in the tablet and extract form have been shown to reduce blood pressure in hypertensive subjects after 2 months.[35] Pycnogenol has been shown to demonstrate some hypotensive effects by inhibiting the angiotensin converting enzyme.[36] Other herbal supplements commonly used by those with hypertension—with sometimes dangerous consequences—include garlic, ephedra or ma huang, St. John's wort, yohimbine, and licorice.[37,38] Potential problems from these are summarized in Table 14-2.[39] Clinicians should be aware of what their patients may be taking as supplemental therapies and ask questions regarding this.

FUTURE CONSIDERATIONS

Advances in genetic research have uncovered provocative discoveries in the areas of disease prevention and management (see Chapter 13 for more explanations and definitions). Hypertension is an area that is of increasing interest in this regard. One gene of interest is the angiotensinogen M235T locus. There is evidence that a sodium-reduced diet has a significant lowering effect on systolic and diastolic blood pressure for individuals with the TT and MT genotypes of the 235T allele but not in persons with the MM genotype.[40] No association between the angiotensin-converting enzyme genotype and blood pressure response was found in DASH study participants, but significant reductions in both systolic and diastolic blood pressure were seen in certain genotypes of the angiotensinogen gene.[41] These researchers reported that DASH study subjects with the angiotensinogen genotype

TABLE 14-2	Popular Herbal Supplements Taken for Hypertension and Their Possible Adverse Effects
HERB	**POSSIBLE EFFECTS**
Garlic	Garlic juice may cause stomach ulceration and decreased serum protein and albumin Raw garlic can increase clotting time Effect on platelet aggregation; contraindicated in presurgery patients Undesirable body odor can result
Ephedra sinica or ma huang	Heart attack, hemorrhagic stroke, death Tremors Insomnia Nephrolithiasis Should not be combined with MAO inhibitors, pseudoephedrine, or caffeine
St. John's wort	"Serotonin syndrome" with flushing, confusion, tremors, agitation, and lethargy Gastrointestinal symptoms Fatigue, dizziness Photosensitivity Chronic administration has shown slight histopathological changes in the livers and kidneys of animals
Yohimbine	Hypertension, hypotension, tachycardia Anxiety, nervousness, insomnia Bronchospasm
Licorice	Hypertension, cardiac arrest Sodium and water retention Excessive potassium excretion

Source: Sarubin A. The Health Professional's Guide to Popular Dietary Supplements. Chicago: American Dietetic Association, 2000.

AA were more responsive to the DASH diet than the GG genotype. In elderly hypertensive subjects, it appears that certain angiotensinogen genotypes are more responsive to sodium reduction than others.[42] Additionally, certain angiotensin-converting enzyme genotypes appear to be more responsive to weight-loss programs and subsequent blood pressure reduction.[43] Further, some research has shown an increase in frequency of a particular allele of the aldosterone synthase gene in hypertensive individuals when compared to normotensive individuals.[44] A German group, however, has published findings that do not support the link between the aldosterone synthase gene and increased salt sensitivity.[45] Certain variants of the angiotensinogen core promoter are associated with a blunted aldosterone response, which may make individuals less responsive to nutrition or pharmaceutical therapies for hypertension.[46]

Clinicians may see the use of plasma $ProANP_{1-30}$, a biomarker, in predicting whether or not a patient will respond to a sodium-reduced diet. Plasma concentration of $ProANP_{1-30}$, a fragment of the atrial natriuretic peptide prohormone, has been found to be closely correlated to salt sensitivity in healthy subjects with a familial history of hypertension.[47] Identifying patients who are more likely to respond to traditional sodium restriction could be a useful tool in medical nutrition therapy. Biomarkers or genetic information may eventually play a role in all nutrients involved in the diet therapy of hypertension.

Issues to Ponder

- What additional skills or skill sets should dietitians acquire to better diagnose, prevent, and treat hypertension?
- What additional outcome studies should be performed to demonstrate the effect of diet, certain food groups, or specific nutrients on blood pressure? How should these studies be designed?
- How could a healthcare team approach prevention and treatment of hypertension from a multidisciplinary perspective?
- How can the dietitian's effectiveness be documented in the care of the hypertensive patient? What studies should be conducted and what outcomes should be measured?
- What public health messages should be presented and disseminated regarding diet and blood pressure?
- Should nutrition advice addressing hypertension be different for patients based on their gender, race, ethnicity, age, and cultural background?
- What will the field of nutritional genomics uncover regarding nutrition therapy for hypertension? How will this change traditional medical nutrition therapy for hypertension?
- How can dietitians be more effective in the prevention and treatment of hypertension in public health venues, ambulatory care clinics, and inpatient settings?
- How will the obesity epidemic affect medical nutrition therapy and the dietitian's role in the care of the hypertensive adult and pediatric patient?

IMPLICATIONS FOR CLINICAL PRACTICE

An integrative nutrition therapy approach appears to be the most effective for the dietary treatment of hypertension. Clinicians should keep themselves abreast of new published research literature. See Table 14-3 for a comprehensive review of current nutrition recommendations for the prevention and treatment of hypertension. It seems somewhat clear at this point that the focus on an overall healthy diet, with an

TABLE 14-3	Nutrition Recommendations for the Prevention and Treatment of Hypertension	
NUTRIENT/FOOD/FOOD GROUP/LIFESTYLE ISSUE	**RECOMMENDATIONS FOR PREVENTION8**	**RECOMMENDATIONS FOR TREATMENT**
Sodium or sodium chloride	2 g sodium (5 g salt) per day[8] 2.4 g sodium (6 g salt) per day[6]	1.7 g sodium (4 g salt) per day[8] 2.4 g sodium (6 g salt) per day[6]
Potassium	273–312 mg per day[8] 350 mg/day[6]	4,700 mg/day[13]
Calcium	"Adequate intake for general health"[6]	1,000–2,000 mg/day [6] 1250 mg/day[13]
Magnesium	"Adequate intake for general health"[6]	500 mg/day[13]
Vitamin C	Recommended dietary allowance (90 mg/day)[30]	No specific recommendations for treatment at this time
Oats or fiber	No specific recommendations for prevention at this time	5.52 g of beta-glucan per day[31] 31 g fiber per day[13]
Total fat	< 15–30% total calories [8]	< 30% total calories[6] < 27% total calories[13]
Saturated fat	< 7% total calories [8]	< 10% total calories6 < 6% total calories[13]
Monounsaturated fat	< 10% total calories[8]	~ 10% total calories[6] < 13% total calories[13]
Omega-3 fatty acids	200 mg/day of DHA and EPA[8] 1–2% total calories [8]	3.7 g/day of fish oil supplement[6]
Soy	No specific recommendations for prevention at this time	500 mL soy milk twice daily[33]
Alcohol	Limit to 1 oz of ethanol per day for men and 0.5 oz per day for women[6]	Limit to 1 oz of ethanol per day for men and 0.5 oz per day for women[6]
Fruits and vegetables	"Adequate quantity (400–500 g/day)" [8]	8–10 servings per day[6]
Weight	Lose weight if overweight[6]	Weight reduction if > 115% ideal body weight[6] Weight reduction improves blood pressure[29]
Physical activity	Aerobic activity 30–45 min/day on most days [6]	Aerobic activity 30–45 min/day on most days [6]
Tobacco	Stop smoking [6]	Stop smoking [6]

increased consumption of fruits, vegetables, nuts, whole grains, low-fat dairy products, and lean protein sources, as well as a reduction in the amount of salty and high-sodium foods, red meats, and saturated fats, is the best approach in hypertension. Simply concentrating on one nutrient, whether it be sodium or potassium, or on one particular food would be narrow-minded at this point. Until specific interactions—synergistic or antagonistic—are better understood, this well-rounded, healthy diet approach is optimal. Finally, genetic markers and biochemical indices that assist in the individualized medical nutrition therapy of patients are on the horizon. Clinicians need to be aware of these diagnostic and therapeutic tools and understand them as they become more widely utilized and available in healthcare.

REFERENCES

1. National Center for Health Statistics (NCHS). Health, United States 2002. With Chartbook on Trends in the Health of Americans. Hyattsville, MD: US Department of Health and Human Services, Centers for Disease Control and Prevention, 2002.
2. Centers for Disease Control and Prevention (CDC). National hospital ambulatory medical care survey: 2001 outpatient department summary. Advance Data from Vital and Health Statistics 2003;338:1–32.
3. Das UN. Nutritional factors in the pathobiology of human essential hypertension. Nutrition 2001;17:337–346.
4. National Center for Health Statistics (NCHS). Health, United States 2003. With Chartbook on Trends in the Health of Americans. Hyattsville, MD: US Department of Health and Human Services, Centers for Disease Control and Prevention, 2003.
5. National High Blood Pressure Education Program (NHBPEP) Working Group. Report on primary prevention of hypertension. Ann Intern Med 1993;153:186.
6. Krummel DA. Medical nutrition therapy in hypertension. In: Mahan K, Escott-Stump E, eds. Krause's Food, Nutrition and Diet Therapy. 11th Ed. Philadelphia: Saunders, 2004.
7. INTERSALT Cooperative Research Group. INTERSALT: an international study of electrolyte excretion and blood pressure. Results for 24 hr urinary sodium and potassium excretion. BMJ 1998;297:319–328.
8. Reddy KS, Katan MB. Diet, nutrition and the prevention of hypertension and cardiovascular diseases. Public Health Nutr 2004;7(1A):167–186.
9. Coruzzi P, Brambilla L, Brambilla V, et al. Potassium depletion and salt sensitivity in essential hypertension. J Clin Endocrinol Metab 2001;86:2857–2862.
10. Whelton PK, He J, Cutler JA, et al. Effects of oral potassium on blood pressure: meta-analysis of randomized controlled clinical trials. JAMA 1997;277:1624–1632.
11. Khaw KT, Barrett-Connor E. Dietary potassium and stroke-associated mortality. A 12-year prospective population study. N Engl J Med. 1987;316:235–240.
12. Whelton PK, He J. Potassium in preventing and treating high blood pressure. Semin Nephrol 1999;19:494–499.
13. Vogt TM, Appel LJ, Obarzanek E, et al. Dietary approaches to stop hypertension: rationale, design and methods. J Am Diet Assoc 1999;99(8 suppl):S12–S18.
14. Karanja NM, McCullough ML, Kumanyika SK, et al. Pre-enrollment diets of Dietary Approaches to Stop Hypertension trial participants. J Am Diet Assoc 1999;99(8 suppl):S28–S34.
15. Harsha DW, Lin P, Obarzanek E, Karanja NM, Moore TJ, Caballero B. Dietary Approaches to Stop Hypertension: a summary to study results. J Am Diet Assoc 1999;99(8 suppl):S35–S39.
16. Karanja NM, Obarzanek E, Lin P, et al. Descriptive characteristics of the dietary patterns used in the Dietary Approaches to Stop Hypertension trial. J Am Diet Assoc 1999;99(8 suppl):S19–S28.
17. Windhauser MM, Evans MA, McCullough ML, et al. Dietary adherence in the Dietary Approaches to Stop Hypertension trial. J Am Diet Assoc 1999;99(8 suppl):S76–S83.
18. Conlin PR, Chow D, Miller ER, et al. The effect of dietary patterns on blood pressure control in hypertensive patients: results from the Dietary Approaches to Stop Hypertension (DASH) trial. Am J Hypertens 2000;13:949–955.
19. Sacks FM, Svetkey LP, Vollmer WM, et al. Effects on blood pressure of reduced dietary sodium and the Dietary Approaches to Stop Hypertension (DASH) diet. N Eng J Med 2001;344:3–10.
20. Vollmer WM, Sacks FM, Ard J, et al. Effects of diet and sodium intake on blood pressure: subgroup analysis of the DASH-Sodium trial. Ann Intern Med 2001;135:1019–1028.
21. Windhauser MM, Ernst DB, Karanja NM, et al. Translating the Dietary Approaches to Stop Hypertension diet from research to practice: dietary and behavior change techniques. J Am Diet Assoc 1999;99(8 suppl):S90–S95.
22. Vollmer WM, Sacks FM, Svetkey LP. New insights into the effects on blood pressure of diets low in salt and high in fruits and vegetables and low-fat dairy products. Curr Control Trials Cardiovasc Med 2001;2:71–74.
23. Griffith LE, Guyatt GH, Cook RJ, Bucher HC, Cook DJ. The influence of dietary and nondietary calcium supplementation on blood pressure: An updated metaanalysis of randomized controlled trials. Am J Hypertens 1999;12(1 Pt 1):84–92.
24. Mizushima S, Cappuccio FP, Nichols R, Elliott P. Dietary magnesium intake and blood pressure: a qualitative overview of the observational studies. J Hum Hypertens 1998;12:447–453.
25. Suter PM, Sierro C, Vetter W. Nutritional factors in the control of blood pressure and hypertension. Nutr Clin Care 2002;5:9–19.

26. Svetkey LP, Harsha DW, Vollmer WM, et al. PREMIER: a clinical trial of comprehensive lifestyle modification for blood pressure control: rationale, design and baseline characteristics. Ann Epidemiol 2003;13:462–471.

27. Appel LJ, Champagne CM, Harsha DW, et al.; writing group for the PREMIER Collaborative Research Group. Effects of comprehensive lifestyle modification on blood pressure control: main results of the PREMIER clinical trial. JAMA 2003;289:2082–2093.

28. McGuire HL, Svetkey LP, Harsha DW, Elmer PJ, Appel LJ, Ard JD. Comprehensive lifestyle modification and blood pressure control: a review of the PREMIER trial. J Clin Hypertens (Greenwich) 2004;6:383–390.

29. Miller ER III, Erlinger TP, Young DR, et al. Results of the diet, exercise and weight loss intervention trial (DEW-IT). Hypertension 2002;40:612–618.

30. Block G. Ascorbic acid, blood pressure and the American diet. Ann NY Acad Sci 2002;959:180–187.

31. Keenan JM, Pins JJ, Frazel C, Moran A, Turnquist L. Oat ingestion reduces systolic and diastolic blood pressure in patients with mild or borderline hypertension: a pilot trial. J Fam Pract 2002;51:369.

32. Davy BM, Melby CL, Beske SD, Ho RC, Davrath LR, Davy KP. Oat consumption does not affect resting casual and ambulatory 24-h arterial blood pressure in men with high-normal blood pressure to stage I hypertension. J Nutr 2002;132:394–398.

33. Rivas M, Garay RP, Escanero JF, Cia P JR, Cia P, Alda JO. Soy milk lowers blood pressure in men and women with mild to moderate essential hypertension. J Nutr 2002;132:1900–1902.

34. Hodgson JM, Puddey IB, Beilin LJ, et al. Effects of isoflavonoids on blood pressure in subjects with high-normal ambulatory blood pressure levels: a randomized controlled trial. Am J Hypertens 1999;12:47–53.

35. Merchant RE, Andre CA. A review of recent clinical trials of the nutritional supplement Chlorella pyrenoidosa in the treatment of fibromyalgia, hypertension and ulcerative colitis. Alt Ther Health Med 2001;7:79–91.

36. Rohdewald P. A review of the French maritime pine bark extract (pycnogenol), an herbal medication with a diverse clinical pharmacology. Int J Clin Pharmacol Ther 2002;40:158–168.

37. Mansoor GA. Herbs and alternative therapies in the hypertension clinic. Am J Hypertens 2001;14(9 Pt 1):971–975.

38. Goertz CH, Grimm RH, Svendsen K, Grandits G. Treatment of Hypertension with Alternative Therapies (THAT) study: a randomized clinical trial. J Hypertens 2002;20:2063–2068.

39. Sarubin A. The Health Professional's Guide to Popular Dietary Supplements. Chicago: American Dietetic Association, 2000.

40. Hunt SC, Geleijnse JM, Wu LL, Witteman JC, Williams RR, Grobbee DE. Enhanced blood pressure response to mild sodium reduction in subjects with the 235T variant of the angiotensinogen gene. Am J Hypertens 1999;12:460–466.

41. Svetkey LP, Moore TJ, Simons-Morton DG, et al. Angiotensinogen genotype and blood pressure response in the Dietary Approaches to Stop Hypertension (DASH) study. J Hypertens 2001;19:1949–1956.

42. Johnson AG, Nguyen RV, Davis D. Blood pressure is linked to salt intake and modulated by the angiotensinogen gene in normotensive and hypertensive elderly subjects. J Hypertens 2001:19:1053–1060.

43. Kostis JB, Wilson AC, Hooper WC, et al; TONE Cooperative Research Group. Association of angiotensin-converting enzyme DD genotype with blood pressure sensitivity to weight loss. Am Heart J 2002;144:625–629.

44. Tiago AD, Badenhorst D, Nkeh B, et al. Impact of renin-angiotensin-aldosterone system gene variants on the severity of hypertension in patients with newly diagnosed hypertension. Am J Hypertens 2003;16:1006–1010.

45. Brand E, Schorr U, Ringel J, Beige J, Distler A, Sharma AM. Aldosterone synthase gene (CYP11B2) C-344T polymorphism in Caucasians from the Berlin Salt-Sensitivity Trial (BeSST). J Hypertens 1999;17:1563–1567.

46. Hilgers KF, Delles C, Veelken R, Schmieder RE. Angiotensinogen gene core promoter variants and non-modulating hypertension. Hypertension 2001;38:1250–1254.

47. Melander O, Frandsen E, Groop L, Hulthen UL. Plasma ProANP(1-30) reflects salt sensitivity in subjects with heredity for hypertension. Hypertension 2002;39:996–999.

Issues & Choices

CHAPTER

NUTRITION AND CORONARY ARTERY DISEASE

Wanda H. Howell

D ietary intervention efforts to reduce morbidity and mortality from coronary artery disease (CAD) have traditionally focused on efforts to control blood lipid concentrations. Specifically, the time-honored diet–heart disease hypothesis maintained that increased dietary levels of saturated fatty acids, total fat, and cholesterol promote hyperlipidemia, which, in turn, increases the risk of developing CAD. This hypothesis continues to be the foundation for the National Cholesterol Education Program (NCEP) Adult Treatment Panel guidelines.[1] Considerable evidence is now emerging to indicate that hyperlipidemia is only one among several diet-related CAD risk factors.

According to the response-to-injury hypothesis, CAD is caused by atherosclerosis, which is initiated by endothelial dysfunction in association with hypertension, diabetes mellitus, smoking, and elevated homocysteine concentrations. This endothelial dysfunction promotes cholesterol deposition in macrophages and smooth muscle cells in the arterial wall as a result of elevated plasma concentrations of low-density lipoprotein cholesterol (LDL-C), lipoprotein(a), and remnant lipoproteins as well as decreased concentrations of high-density lipoprotein (HDL). Subsequent events leading to vessel occlusion include inflammation and thrombosis, both of which have been shown to be affected by a variety of dietary factors.

The nutrition care professional is continually challenged to incorporate into practice new evidence from research relating diet and CAD. The practitioner must look beyond the antiatherogenic (lipid-lowering) properties of dietary components to other mechanisms of protection against CAD. Various nutrient factors have been shown to exhibit antithrombogenic, anti-inflammatory, and antioxidant properties. The range of potential mechanisms is presented in Table 15-1 and discussed below.

ANTIATHEROGENIC DIETARY FACTORS

FORMER NCEP STEP 1 AND 2 DIETS

The NCEP targets lowering LDL-C concentrations via a diet reduced in total fat, saturated fatty acids, and cholesterol. The former Step 1 diet recommended < 30% of total kilocalories from total fat, < 10% from saturated fatty acids, and < 300 mg cholesterol.[2] The former Step 2 diet further restricted saturated fatty acids to < 7% of total kilocalories and cholesterol to < 200 mg.[3] The NCEP III guidelines replace

308

TABLE 15-1	CAD-Protective Nutrition Factors

Antiatherogenic (cholesterol lowering)
      PUFA (omega-6 fatty acids)
      Viscous (soluble) fiber—oat (beta-glucan) products
      Plant sterols/stanols
      Soy protein

Antithrombogenic/anti-inflammatory
      PUFA (omega-3 fatty acids)
      Folate, vitamin B_{12}, vitamin B_6 (homocysteine reduction)
      Polyphenols/flavonoids

Antioxidant
      Vitamin E (alpha-tocopherol)
      Vitamin A (beta-carotene)
      Vitamin C (ascorbic acid)
      Polyphenols/flavonoids

CAD = coronary artery disease; PUFA = polyunsaturated fatty acids.

the step diets with the Therapeutic Lifestyle Changes (TLC) approach.[1] The TLC diet recommends the same restrictions for saturated fatty acids and cholesterol as the Step 2 diet, with the total fat specified at 25 to 35% of total kilocalories. This diet, along with encouragement of moderate physical activity, constitutes the first step of the TLC approach. If the LDL-C goal is not reached, step two is initiated, which incorporates 2 g/day of plant stanols/sterols and 10 to 15 g/day of viscous (soluble) fiber as dietary enhancements for lowering LDL-C concentrations. In addition to the levels of total fat, saturated fatty acids, and cholesterol mentioned above, the nutrient composition of the recommended TLC diet includes up to 10% polyunsaturated fatty acids, up to 20% monounsaturated fatty acids, 60% carbohydrate, 15% protein, 20 to 30 g/day of total dietary fiber, and energy intake balanced with expenditure to maintain desirable body weight.

Although no data are yet available to evaluate the TLC approach, several studies have reported outcomes related to the use of the NCEP Step 1 and 2 diets.[4–6] Considerable variability is seen in the reported data, with the percent decrease in LDL-C concentrations in response to the Step 1 diet ranging from 4.5 to 10%, and that for the Step 2 diet ranging from 7.7 to 12%. Variability also exists in the data related to the individual components of these diets. Virtually all studies confirm the efficacy of restricting saturated fatty acids to control LDL-C concentrations. Specifically, for each percent decrease in saturated fatty acid in the diet, a corresponding reduction in LDL-C concentration of 1.8 mg/dL is predicted; a 10% reduction of saturated fatty acid intake would result in a lowering of LDL-C of 18 mg/dL.[4] Evidence also suggests that there are differential lipid-raising effects among the types of saturated fatty acids. Stearic acid (C18:0) intake has been shown to actually decrease plasma total cholesterol and LDL-C concentrations.[7,8] Only three SFAs appear to elevate plasma cholesterol concentration: lauric acid (C12:0); myristic acid (C14:0); and palmitic acid (C16:0). These fatty acids constitute approximately 26% of the total dietary fat consumed in the United States.[9]

In contrast to the effects of saturated fatty acids, a comprehensive meta-analytic study did not find a significant effect of reducing total dietary fat or cholesterol intake on LDL-C concentrations.[4] Furthermore, decreasing total dietary fat intake has consistently been shown to deleteriously reduce plasma high-density-lipoprotein cholesterol (HDL-C) and increase triacylglycerol (TG) concentrations.[10–12] This effect is likely due to the usual practice of substituting carbohydrate for fat in isocaloric diets. It has also prompted a renewed focus on the type rather than the total amount of dietary fat.[13]

MONOUNSATURATED FATTY ACIDS

Oleic acid makes up approximately 93% of the cis-monounsaturated fatty acid intake in the United States, with an average total intake of 13 to 14% of total energy. This is in contrast to the typical Mediterranean diet, in which monounsaturated fatty acids account for 16 to 29% of the total energy intake.[14] Epidemiologic studies suggest that this diet, comprising high levels of monounsaturated and low levels of saturated fatty acids, with olive oil as the primary fat source, is associated with the relatively low prevalence of CAD in some Mediterranean countries. Data from the longitudinal Nurses' Health Study in the United States also suggest that intake of monounsaturated fatty acid is protective against CAD.[15] It is important to note that the protective effect of monounsaturated fatty acid is seen only with a concomitant reduction in the dietary intake of saturated fatty acid. Otherwise monounsaturated fatty acids are considered cardioneutral.

To encourage a reduction in the intake of dietary saturated fatty acids, most dietary guidelines emphasize the substitution of complex carbohydrates. Evidence from the DELTA (Dietary Effects on Lipoproteins and Thrombogenic Activity) Study suggests, however, that the substitution of monounsaturated fatty acid instead of carbohydrates may protect against the significant reduction in HDL-C and the increase in TG seen as a consequence on a low-fat/carbohydrate-rich diet.[16]

Contrasting data are reported for the trans-monounsaturated fatty acids, of which elaidic acid (C18:1 trans) represents the most common form. Estimated U.S. dietary intake ranges from 2.6 to 12.8 g/day.[17] Trans-monounsaturated fatty acids are the result of anaerobic bacterial fermentation in ruminant animals and thus are introduced into human diets in the form of meat and dairy products (C16:1 trans). The primary sources, however, are products containing hydrogenated vegetable or fish oils. Clinical studies have demonstrated that consumption of trans- compared to cis-fatty acids results in higher plasma cholesterol levels. Relative to saturated fatty acids, consumption of trans-monounsaturated fatty acids results in lower plasma cholesterol concentrations.[18] Research involving trans-fatty acids has been hampered by limitations and inconsistencies in food composition data in nutrient data banks. As of January 2006, food labels are required to include entries for trans-fatty acids.

POLYUNSATURATED FATTY ACIDS (OMEGA-6)

The protective effects of polyunsaturated fatty acids on CAD risk reduction have generally been attributed to the omega-6 fatty acids, whose parent member, linoleic acid, is found in highest concentrations in vegetable oils such as safflower, sunflower, and corn oils. An increase in the dietary intake of polyunsaturated fatty acids, unlike saturated fatty acids, has been shown to reduce plasma LDL-C concentrations. For each 1% increase in intake, plasma LDL-C concentration is predicted to decrease by 0.50 mg/dL.[4] An upper limit of 10% of total energy from polyunsaturated fatty acids has been recommended, because diets very high in linoleic acid have been shown to reduce HDL-C as well as LDL-C concentrations.[19] Diets high in linoleic acid (omega-6 fatty acid) have also been associated with immunosuppression and increased thrombogenicity because of their effect on eicosanoid metabolism, which is discussed below.[20]

VISCOUS (SOLUBLE) FIBER

Oat products have a greater proportion of soluble fiber than any other grain. The LDL-C–lowering effect is attributed to beta-glucan, their main soluble fiber component. Several mechanisms of action for the hypocholesterolemic effect of soluble fiber have been proposed.[21] Soluble fiber may act as a bile acid sequestrant, increasing the hepatic conversion of cholesterol to bile acids. It may also impose a physical barrier to reduce the absorption of bile acids and cholesterol by creating a viscous food mass in the small intestine. Finally, the production of short-chain fatty acids after fermentation of soluble fiber inhibits hepatic cholesterol synthesis.

Epidemiologic studies of the effect of soluble fiber consumption on the primary endpoint of CAD mortality have not reported significant reductions beyond what could be attributed to decreased dietary saturated fatty acid intake. Clinical trials of secondary endpoints have produced conflicting results, with the most consistent but modest reductions in LDL-C concentrations being seen in hypercholesterolemic subjects.[22] This modest reduction in LDL-C is estimated to be about 2 to 3 mg/dL after accounting for decreased intake of saturated fatty acid.

Despite these findings, in 1997 the U.S. Food and Drug Administration (FDA) approved a health claim for oat products that, in combination with a diet low in saturated fatty acids and cholesterol, they may reduce the risk of heart disease. At least 3 g/day of beta-glucan was specified to achieve the desired effect. This claim was recently tested in mildly to moderately hypercholesterolemic subjects fed 3 g/day of beta-glucan for 8 weeks in the form of oat bran.[23] No beneficial effects were shown for any of the blood lipids.

PLANT STEROLS/STANOLS

A variety of food products enriched with plant sterols and stanols are now available to consumers. Plant sterols—of which campesterol, beta-sitosterol and stigmasterol are the most abundant in nature—are structurally related to dietary cholesterol. Unlike cholesterol, however, plant sterols are not synthesized by the human body and are very poorly absorbed by the human intestine. Saturation of sterols with hydrogen leads to the formation of plant stanols, such as campestanol and sitostanol. For incorporation into foods, plant sterols and stanols are often esterified with fatty acids to improve their fat solubility, thus allowing maximal incorporation into a limited amount of fat. The specific plant sterols currently incorporated into foods to lower blood cholesterol concentrations are extracted from soybean or tall (pine tree) oil.[24]

The LDL-C–lowering effect of plant sterols is attributed to inhibited exogenous and endogenous cholesterol absorption. This inhibition may be due to the creation of mucosal barriers to cholesterol transport or to alterations in rates of cholesterol esterification in the intestinal wall. Although the magnitude of the decreased rate of cholesterol absorption is reported to be 33 to 60%, LDL-C reductions are much lower because of compensatory increases in endogenous cholesterol production.[25]

The predicted LDL-C reduction as a result of consuming approximately 2 g/day of plant sterols or stanols is 9 to 14%, according to a meta-analysis of 14 studies. Little or no effect on HDL-C or TG concentrations has been reported. Furthermore, in contrast to the data reported for oat fiber, this effect is independent of baseline LDL-C concentrations or the composition of the background diet.

Another positive feature of plant sterols and stanols is their lack of adverse effects, based on extensive short-term safety evaluation studies. Longer-term studies are needed, however, to determine the extent to which the absorption of fat-soluble components other than cholesterol is affected. These dietary components include vitamins and antioxidants.

SOY PROTEIN

The interest in the LDL-C–lowering potential of soy protein has been stimulated by the epidemiologic observation that Asian populations that consume it in large quantities have also been found to have a lower prevalence of CAD. Several components of soy protein have been implicated in the cholesterol-lowering effect.[26] Phytic acid is known to interfere with zinc absorption, creating a high ratio of zinc to copper, which tends to result in a rise in blood cholesterol. Soy foods contain enough copper in addition to phytic acid to normalize the zinc-to-copper ratio and prevent this rise in plasma cholesterol. Isoflavones are phytoestrogens, which have been shown to decrease LDL-C and increase HDL-C. It is important to note that the potential protective effect depends on the composition of soy protein products, which varies widely. No single component has been consistently shown to confer the LDL-C–lowering effect. This has led many to question the health claim approved by the FDA in 1999 that "25 g of soy protein a day, as part of a diet low in saturated fat and cholesterol, may reduce the risk of heart disease."[21]

The American Heart Association Nutrition Committee indicates that several clinical trials have demonstrated that consuming 25 to 50 g/day of soy protein is safe and effective in reducing LDL-C by 4 to 8%, with the greatest reduction seen in subjects with hypercholesterolemia.[26] This is a considerably smaller effect than that reported in a meta-analysis of 38 studies, which predicted a 12.9% decrease in LDL-C.[27]

ANTITHROMBOGENIC DIETARY FACTORS

POLYUNSATURATED FATTY ACIDS (OMEGA-3)

As mentioned above, thrombosis is an important terminal event in the development of symptomatic CAD. The coagulation system, which includes platelets and coagulation proteins, plays a role in the evolution of thrombotic lesions. Omega-3 fatty acids have been shown to reduce platelet aggregation.[28] This effect is postulated to be a result of their competitive inhibition of thrombogenic eicosanoid thromboxane

(TXA$_2$) production via cycloogenase[29] (see Figure 15-1). TXA$_2$ is derived from arachidonic acid, the chief metabolite of linoleic acid. Dietary increases in omega-3 fatty acids inhibit TXA$_2$ production while increasing the availability of the prostanoid PGI$_3$, a potent platelet antiaggregator. PGI$_3$ is derived from eicosapentaenoic acid (EPA), a chief metabolite of alpha-linolenic acids. EPA also reduces the production of the 2-series prostaglandins and prostacylins and the 4-series leukotrienes. Thus, decreasing the ratio of linoleic acid to alpha-linolenic acid in the diet (currently estimated at 10:1) may decrease thrombogenicity, inflammation, and vasoconstriction.

Early evidence of a link between the intake of omega-3 fatty acid and prevalence of CAD came from a study comparing Danes (high prevalence) and Eskimos (low prevalence).[30] The linoleic acid content of the Eskimo diet is half that of the Danes, whereas the EPA (C20:5n-3) and docosahexaenoic acid (DHA) (C22:6n-3) content in the diet of the Eskimos is almost five times that found in the Danish diet. This very high intake of EPA and DHA is due to regular consumption of oily fish, such as herring, sardines, mackerel, tuna, trout, and salmon. Feeding on plants that contain alpha-linolenic acid (C18:3n-3), such as phytoplankton, allows these fish to produce concentrated sources of EPA and DHA. Plant sources of alpha-linolenic acid, although far less concentrated, are linseed, canola or rapeseed, walnut, and soybean oils.

Subsequent clinical trials have evaluated the efficacy of dietary and supplemental omega-3 fatty acids. The Indian Experiment of Infarct Survival[31] and the Lyon Heart Study[32] provided evidence in support of a beneficial effect of plant-based alpha-linolenic acid on primary and secondary outcomes, respectively. The positive role of marine-based EPA and DHA in secondary prevention has been shown in several trials. The data have been summarized in a recent meta-analysis, which reported a risk ratio for nonfatal myocardial infarction (MI) at 0.8, for fatal MI at 0.7, and for sudden death at 0.7.[33]

Based on the available evidence, the current Dietary Reference Intakes (DRIs) for energy and macronutrients indicates an acceptable macronutrient distribution range for alpha-linolenic acid of 0.6 to 1.2%, or 1.3 to 2.7 g/day on the basis of a 2,000-calorie diet. This is about 10 times the current intake but can be met by

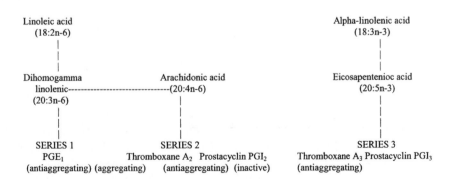

FIGURE 15-1 *Comparative effects of linoleic and alpha-linolenic acids on eicosanoid metabolism. Reprinted with permission from Howell WH. Diet and blood lipids. Nutr Today 1997;32:3.*

consuming two fatty-fish meals per week and by using liquid vegetable oils containing alpha-linolenic acid.[34]

Supplement use for primary prevention of CAD is unnecessary and may be related to increased clotting time and excessive bleeding. Nonetheless, the FDA has ruled that intakes of up to 3 g/day are generally recognized as safe and has approved a qualified health claim for EPA and DHA in dietary supplements.[35]

FOLATE, VITAMIN B_{12}, VITAMIN B_6

Considerable interest in plasma homocysteine as a possible marker for the development of CAD has been generated based on evidence from several case-control and prospective studies. A meta-analysis of many of these investigations indicated that as much as 10% of CAD risk could be attributed to hyperhomocysteinemia.[36] Furthermore, this study suggested that an increase in plasma homocysteine of 5 mmol/L could increase CAD risk to a similar degree as an increase of 20 mg/dL in plasma total cholesterol.

In contrast to these findings, the Multiple Risk Factor Intervention Trial and the Atherosclerosis Risk in Communities Study have not confirmed a relationship between homocysteine and CAD risk.[37,38] Given the importance of these reports and the absence of clinical trial data, the nutrition committee of the American Heart Association has indicated that it may be premature to conclude that homocysteine levels are predictive of the development of CAD.[39] Complicating this issue is the lack of clearly defined physiologic mechanisms by which homocysteinemia influences the development of CAD. Current theories center on platelet and endothelial dysfunction.

Data from the Framingham Heart Study provided early evidence of an association between the status of folate and vitamins B_{12} and B_6 in relation to plasma homocysteine concentrations.[40] Specifically, two-thirds of the subjects with hyperhomocysteinemia had a deficiency of folate, B_{12}, or B_6. Adequate clinical trial data are currently lacking to guide dietary or supplement recommendations for the control of homocysteine concentrations and thus for the purpose of primary CAD prevention. It may be prudent to supplement folate (1 mg/day), vitamin B_{12} (0.4 mg/day, and vitamin B_6 (10 mg/day) in those with multiple CAD risk factors and with mild to moderate elevations in plasma homocysteine (15 to 100 mmol/L).[39] For the significant portion of the population who do not meet the current recommended intake of folate, dietary counseling to increase the intake of leafy green vegetables, fortified cereals, fruits, and legumes is certainly advisable.

C-REACTIVE PROTEIN (CRP) AND INFLAMMATION

CRP is recognized as a key clinical marker of inflammation and an independent predictor of risk for CAD. A recent report from the Women's Health Study compared the predictive value of plasma CRP concentration to that of LDL-C.[41] These data indicate that having a low LDL-C and a high CRP value results in a greater absolute risk than a high LDL-C and low CRP. The authors concluded that the CRP level is a stronger predictor of CAD events than the LDL-C level. Although these results await confirmation, they suggest an important new CAD risk factor that should be monitored by the nutrition care professional.

ANTIOXIDANT DIETARY FACTORS

ANTIOXIDANT VITAMINS

It is well accepted that free-radical oxidation of LDLs is a key factor in the pathogenesis of CAD. Oxidation of LDL lipids leads to the production of a diverse array of biologically active compounds that affect endothelial cell-surface adhesion molecules, which facilitate the mobilization and uptake of circulating inflammatory cells,[42] thus defining the interrelationship between oxidation and inflammation. The exogenous antioxidant defense system includes three well-investigated diet-derived compounds: vitamin C (ascorbic acid); vitamin E (alpha-tocopherol); and beta-carotene (preformed vitamin A).

Epidemiologic studies consistently indicate that greater dietary and supplemental intake of antioxidants is associated with lower CAD risk. The preponderance of evidence from primary prevention trials does not support a beneficial effect of dietary antioxidants. In fact, supplementation with beta-carotene and alpha-tocopherol in male and female smokers resulted in increases in mortality from lung cancer (beta-carotene) and stroke (alpha-tocopherol).[43,44] Furthermore, data from the Cholesterol Lowering Atherosclerosis Study (CLAS) secondary prevention trial suggest the positive effect of alpha-tocopherol may be in inhibiting lesion progression, not in its role as an antioxidant.[45] High alpha-tocopherol intakes (800 to 1200 mg/day) have also been associated with hemorrhage secondary to antiplatelet effects. It should be noted that ascorbic acid testing has been limited to a few small intervention trials, with negative results. Several large clinical trials involving dietary antioxidant cocktails are ongoing and may alter the current view that it is of no benefit. These trials include the Women's Health Study[46]; the Women's Antioxidant Cardiovascular Disease Study[47]; the Supplemental Vitamin, Minerals, and Antioxidant (SU.VI.MAX) trial[48]; and the Physicians' Health Study.[49]

POLYPHENOLS/FLAVONOIDS

Observational studies of polyphenolic flavonoid intake from fruits, vegetables, red wine, and tea have provided mixed results. Overall, the

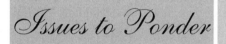

Issues to Ponder

- Why is it important for nutrition care professionals to develop the skills necessary to effectively evaluate scientific publications?

- In providing nutrition education or counseling, how do you reconcile the different conclusions proposed by the "experts"?

- Should dietitians and other health care professionals feel compelled to follow national nutrition guidelines that may be based on controversial interpretations of the scientific data?

- How would you interpret findings from a meta-analytic investigation differently as compared to results from a single study? Should one type of investigation carry more weight?

- What are the similarities and differences in the nutrition recommendations for the prevention and management of coronary artery disease, obesity, and diabetes mellitus? Would it be useful to think and educate in terms of a "good health" diet approach rather than a disease approach?

- How much of the incidence of these chronic diseases can be attributed to poor weight management and physical inactivity?

evidence suggests that individuals with the highest intake have a moderately reduced CAD risk.[50] Secondary prevention trials have generally found no relationship between flavonoid intake and CAD outcomes. One meta-analysis of studies involving tea consumption, however, did suggest a reduction in CAD risk of 11% with the consumption of three cups per day.[51]

Although the antioxidant properties of flavonoids are generally accepted, evidence of their effects on endothelial and platelet function and on inflammation has recently been reviewed.[52] In addition to these effects, alcohol consumption of one to two drinks per day has been shown to increase HDL-C by approximately 12% on average[53] and to reduce platelet aggregation in a manner similar to that of aspirin therapy.[54]

CONCLUSION

Alternative diet–heart disease hypotheses suggest that nutrition intervention can play a more influential role in managing heart disease risk than was traditionally thought. Moreover, this new perspective calls for a shift toward adding beneficial factors to the diet rather than simply eliminating "bad foods."

CAD risk is not related to any single dietary component. Many of the effects are interactive; some dietary elements promote or attenuate the effects of others. Research has shown that maintaining desirable body weight through hypocaloric diets and increased physical activity produces an important and comprehensive effect on reducing overall CAD risk. Weight control combined with increased dietary intake of fresh fruits and vegetables, whole grains, and high-omega-3 fish form the foundation of an appropriate dietary approach.

REFERENCES

1. Third Report of the Expert Panel on Detection, Evaluation, and Treatment of High Blood Cholesterol in Adults. NIH Pub 01-3095. Washington, DC: US Department of Health and Human Services, Public Health Service, 2001.
2. Report of the National Cholesterol Education Program Expert Panel on Detection, Evaluation, and Treatment of High Blood Cholesterol in Adults. The Expert Panel. Arch Intern Med 1988;148:36–69.
3. Summary of the second report of the National Cholesterol Education Program (NCEP) Expert Panel on Detection, Evaluation, and Treatment of High Blood Cholesterol in Adults (Adult Treatment Panel II). JAMA 1983;269:3015–3023.
4. Howell WH, McNamara DJ, Tosca MA, Smith BT, Gaines, JA. Plasma lipid and lipoprotein response to dietary fat and cholesterol: a meta-analysis. Am J Clin Nutr 1997;65:1747–1764.
5. Yo-Poth S, Zhao G, Etherton T, et al. Effects of the National Cholesterol Education Program's Step I and Step II dietary intervention programs on cardiovascular disease risk factors: a meta-analysis. Am J Clin Nutr 1999;69:632–646.
6. Jenkins DJ, Kendall CW, Marchie D, et al. The effect of combining plant sterols, soy protein, viscous fibers, and almonds in treating hypercholesterolemia. Metabolism 2003;52:1478–1483.
7. Ginsberg HN, Kris-Etherton P, Dennis B, et al. The effects of reducing saturated fatty acids on plasma lipids and lipoproteins in healthy subjects. Arterioscler Thromb Vasc Biol 1998;18:441–449.
8. Bonanome A, Grundy SM. Effect of dietary stearic acid on plasma cholesterol and lipoprotein levels. N Eng J Med 1988;318:1244–1248.
9. McNamara DJ. Cardiovascular disease. In: Shils ME, Olson JA, Shike M, eds. Modern nutrition in health and disease. 8th Ed. Philadelphia: Lea & Febiger, 1994:1533–1544.

10. Mensink RP, Katan MB. Effect of monounsaturated fatty acids versus complex carbohydrates on high-density lipoproteins in healthy men and women. Lancet 1987;1:122–125.

11. Mensink RP, de Groot MJ, van den Broeke LT, et al. Effects of monounsaturated fat v complex carbohydrates on serum lipoproteins and apolipoproteins in healthy men and women. Metabolism 1989;38:172–178.

12. Ginsberg HN, Barr SL, Gilbert A, et al. Reduction of plasma cholesterol levels in normal men on an American Heart Association Step I diet or a Step II diet with added monounsaturated fat. N Eng J Med 1990;322:574–579.

13. Willet WC, Stampfer MJ. Rebuild the food pyramid. Sci Am 2003;64–71.

14. Kris-Etherton P. Monounsaturated fatty acids and risk of cardiovascular disease. Circulation 1999;100:1253–1258.

15. Hu FB, Stampfer MJ, Manson JE, et al. Dietary fat intake and the risk of coronary heart disease in women. N Engl J Med 1977;337:1491–1499.

16. Kris-Etherton PM, for the DELTA Investigators. Effects of replacing saturated fat with monounsaturated fat or carbohydrate on plasma lipids and lipoproteins in individuals with markers for insulin resistance (abstr). FASEB J 1996;10:2666.

17. Emken EA. Physicochemical properties, intake, and metabolism: trans fatty acids and coronary heart disease risk: report of the expert panel on trans fatty acids and coronary heart disease. Am J Clin Nutr 1995;62:659S–669S.

18. Lichtenstein AH. Trans fatty acids, plasma lipid levels, and risk of developing cardiovascular disease. Circulation 1997;95:2588–2591.

19. Mattson FH, Grundy SM. Comparison of effects of dietary saturated, monounsaturated, and polyunsaturated fatty acids on plasma lipids and lipoproteins in man. J Lipid Res 1985;26:194–202.

20. Lagaarde M. Metabolism of omega-3/omega-6 fatty acids in blood and vascular cells. Biochem Soc Trans 1990;18:770–772.

21. Kerckhoffs DAJM, Brouns F, Hornstra G, Mensink RP. Effects on the human serum lipoprotein profile of beta-glucan, soy protein and isoflavones, plant sterols and stanols, garlic and tocotrienols. J Nutr 2002;132:2494–2505.

22. Ripsin CM, Keenan JM, Jacobs DR, et al. Oat products and lipid lowering: a meta-analysis. JAMA 1992;267:3317–3825.

23. Lovegrove JA, Clohessy A, Milton H, Williams CM. Modest doses of beta-glucan do not reduce concentrations of potentially atherogenic lipoproteins. Am J Clin Nutr 2000;72:49–55.

24. Lichtenstein AH, Deckelbaum MD. Stanol/sterol ester-containing foods and blood cholesterol levels. Circulation 2001;103:1177–1179.

25. Jones PJ, Raeine-Sarjaz M, Ntanios FY. Modulation of plasma lipid levels and cholesterol kinetics by phytosterol versus phytostanol esters. J Lipid Res 2000;41:697–705.

26. Erdman JW. Soy protein and cardiovascular disease. Circulation 2000;102:2555–2559.

27. Anderson JW, Johnstone BM, Cook-Newell ME. Meta-analysis of the effects of soy protein intake on serum lipids. N Eng J Med 1995;333:276–282.

28. Agren JJ, Vaisanen S, Hanninen O. Hemostatic factors and platelet aggregation after a fish-enriched diet or fish oil or docosahexaenoic acid supplementation. Prostaglandins Leukot Essent Fatty Acids 1997;17:279–286.

29. Uauy R Mena P, Valenzuela A. Essential fatty acids as determinants of lipid requirements in infants, children and adults. Eur J Clin Nutr 1999;53(suppl 1):S66–S77.

30. Bang HO, Dyerberg J, Sinclari HM. The composition of the Eskimo food in northwestern Greenland. Am J Clin Nutr 1980;33:2657–2661.

31. Singh RB, Niaz MA, Sharma JP. Randomized, double-blind, placebo-controlled trial of fish oil and mustard oil in patients with suspected acute myocardial infarction; the Indian experiment of infarct survival-4. Cardiovasc Drugs Ther 1997;11:485–491.

32. de Lorgeril M, Renaud S, Mamelle N. Mediterranean alpha-linolenic acid-rich diet in secondary prevention of coronary heart disease. Lancet 1994;343:1454–1459.

33. Bucher HC, Hengstler P, Schindler C. N-3 polyunsaturated fatty acids in coronary heart disease: a meta-analysis of randomized controlled trials. Am J Med 2002;112:298–304.

34. Kris-Etherton, PM, Harris WS, Appel LJ. Fish consumption, fish oil, omega-3 fatty acids, and cardiovascular disease. Circulation 2002;106:2747–2757.

35. Office of Nutritional Products, Labeling, and Dietary Supplements, Center for Food Safety and Applied Nutrition, US Food and Drug Administration. Letter responding to a request to reconsider the qualified health claim for a dietary supplement health claim for omega-3 fatty acids and coronary heart disease. Docket No. 91N-0103. February 8, 2002. Available at: http://www.cfsan.fda.gov/-dms/ds-ltr28.html.

36. Boushey CJ, Beresford SA, Omenn GS. A quantitative assessment of plasma homocysteine as a risk factor for vascular disease: probable benefits of increasing folic acid intakes. JAMA 1995;274:1049–1057.

37. Evand RW, Shaten BJ, Hempel JD. Homocysteine and risk of cardiovascular disease in the Multiple Risk Factor Intervention Trial. Arterioscler Thromb Vasc Biol 1997;17:1947–1953.

38. Folsom AR, Nieto FJ, McGovern PG. Prospective study of coronary heart disease incidence in relation to fasting total homocysteine, related genetic polymorphisms, and B vitamins: the Atherosclerosis Risk in Communities (ARIC) study. Circulation 1998;98:204–210.

39. Malinow MR, Bostom AG, Krauss RM. Homocysteine, diet, and cardiovascular diseases. Circulation 1999;99:178–182.

40. Selhub J, Jacques PF, Wilson PW. Vitamin status and intake as primary determinants of homocysteinemia in an elderly population. JAMA 1993;270:2693–2698.

41. Ridker PM, Rifal N, Rose L. Comparison of C-reactive protein and low-density lipoprotein cholesterol levels in the prediction of first cardiovascular events. N Engl J Med 2002;347:1557–1565.

42. Navab M, Berliner JA, Watson AD, et al. The yin and yang of oxidation in the development of the fatty streak. Arterioscler Thromb Vasc Biol 1996;16:831–842.

43. The Alpha-Tocopherol, Beta-Carotene Cancer Prevention Study Group. The effect of vitamin E and beta-carotene on the incidence of lung cancer and other cancers in male smokers. N Eng J Med 1994;330:1029–1035.

44. Omenn GS, Goodman GE, Thornquist MD, et al. Effects of a combination of beta-carotene and vitamin A on lung cancer and cardiovascular disease. N Eng J Med 1996;334:1150–1155.

45. Azen SP, Qian D, Mack WJ, et al. Effect of supplementary antioxidant vitamin intake on carotid arterial wall intima-media thickness in a controlled clinical trial of cholesterol lowering. Circulation 1996;94:2369–2372.

46. Hoffman RM, Garewal HS. Antioxidants and the prevention of coronary heart disease. Arch Intern Med 1995;155:241–246.

47. Manson JE, Gaziano JM, Spelsberg A. A secondary prevention trial of antioxidant vitamins and cardiovascular disease in women. Rationale, design, and methods. The WACS Research Group. Ann Epidemiol 1955;5:333–335.

48. Hercberg S, Prezlosi P, Briancon S. A primary prevention trial using nutritional doses of antioxidant vitamins and minerals in cardiovascular diseases and cancers in a general population: the SU.VI.MAX study-design, methods, and participant characteristics. Control Clin Trials 1998;19:336–351.

49. Christen WG, Gaziano JM, Hennekens CH. Design of Physician's Health Study II: a randomized trial of beta-carotene, vitamins E and C, and multivitamins in prevention of cancer, cardiovascular disease, and eye disease, a review of completed trials. Ann Epidemiol 2000;10:125–134.

50. Yochum L, Kushi LH, Meyer K, Folsom AR. Dietary flavonoid intake and risk of cardiovascular disease in postmenopausal women. Am J Epidemiol 1999;149:943–949.

51. Peters U, Poole C, Arab L. Does tea affect cardiovascular disease? A meta-analysis. Am J Epidemiol 2001;154:495–503.

52. Vita JA. Polyphenols and cardiovascular disease: Effects on endothelial and platelet function. Am J Clin Nutr 2005;81(suppl):292S–297S.

53. Linn S, Carroll M, Johnson C. High-density lipoprotein cholesterol and alcohol consumption in US white and black adults: data from NHANES II. Am J Pub Health 1993;83:811–816.

54. Hendriks HF, van der Gang MS. Alcohol, coagulation and fibrinolysis. Novartis Found Symp 1998;216:111–120; discussion 120–124.

CHAPTER

16

OBESITY: THE CHALLENGE FOR THE HEALTHCARE PROFESSIONAL

Abby S. Bloch

One cannot open a newspaper, listen to the TV, or attend a conference without the topic of obesity—its causes and its effects on the individual and society—being raised. For healthcare professionals in general and dietetics professionals specifically, weight management is of major import. In May 2005, in response to this growing concern, the *Journal of the American Dietetic Association* published a supplement devoted entirely to obesity.[1] What becomes obvious to healthcare professionals who seek scientific support or clinical direction in structuring a nutrition care plan is that there is no consistency of approach or successful model from which to choose. The impact of obesity and its clinical and economic implications, however, can no longer be ignored. Figure 16-1 outlines the massive scope and complexity involved in addressing this problem.

PREVALENCE OF OBESITY IN THE UNITED STATES

In a survey by the Trust for America's Health (TFAH), obesity levels rose in 2005 as compared with 2004 in every state except Oregon, where the level remained the same.[2] In this survey, adult obesity levels were 16% higher or more in every state. In fact, 20% or more of adults were obese in 41 states and the District of Columbia (based on the average of the most recent 3 years of data). Ten states had levels exceeding 25%. Seven of these were in the southeastern United States.[2] Colorado had the lowest levels, at 16.4%, based on the average of the most recent 3 years of data.

In addition, over 52% of adults were either obese or overweight in every state. Twenty-three states had obese-plus-overweight levels of adults exceeding 60%. Mississippi had the highest combined level of obese-plus-overweight adults at 64.5% based on the average of the most recent 3 years of data. Colorado had the lowest, at 52.6%.[2]

An estimated 119 million American adults are overweight or obese.[3] Adult obesity rates have risen significantly, from 15% in 1980[3] to 19.4% in 1997, to 23.7% in 2003, and to 24.5% in 2004.[4] More than 9 million children, or 15%, are either overweight or obese. The rate of childhood obesity more than doubled from 1980 to 2000.[5] It is projected that 73% of American adults could be overweight or obese by 2008.[6] According to the National Institutes of Health (NIH) and the Centers for Disease Control and Prevention (CDC), being overweight or obese increases an individual's risk for developing over 35 major diseases, including type 2 diabetes, heart disease and stroke, cancer, sleep apnea, osteoarthritis, gallbladder disease, and fatty liver disease.[7] According to the CDC, "obesity contributes to about . . .

Framework for addressing obesity

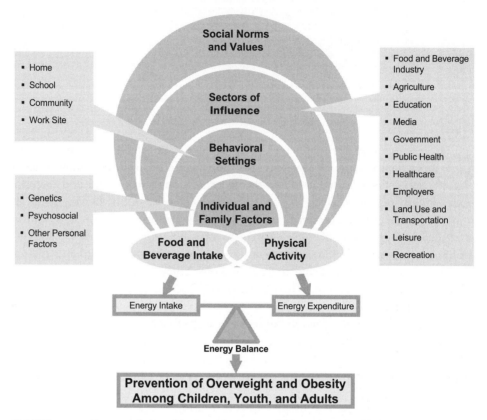

FIGURE 16-1 *Framework for addressing obesity. Available at: http://healthyamericans.org/reports/ obesity2005/Obesity2005Report.pdf; Accessed March 1, 2006. Adapted with permission from Trust for America's Health[2] from Preventing Childhood Obesity. Washington, DC: Institute of Medicine, 2005.*

two-thirds of heart disease, 20% of cancer in women, and 15% of cancer in men."[8] Based on recent scientific findings, fitness may matter more than weight in some individuals. Therefore obesity and overweight should be evaluated within the context of an individual's overall health.

The direct and indirect costs of obesity, including medical costs and lost productivity, amount to more than $117 billion each year, according to estimates from the U.S. Department of Health and Human Services (HHS).[9] This includes $61 billion in direct medical costs for the treatment of related diseases and $56 billion in indirect costs, such as lost productivity. A 2002 study published in *Health Affairs* found that obesity increases healthcare costs for inpatient ambulatory care by 36% and medication costs by 77% compared to the normal weight range.[10] Employers and businesses bear a sizable portion of the costs associated with treating obesity-related conditions.[11] These costs are primarily for lost productivity, paid sick leave, and the increased costs of health, life, and disability insurance.

In a 2003 study, Finkelstein and colleagues stated that annual U.S. obesity-attributable medical expenditures are estimated at $75 billion, half of which are financed by Medicare and Medicaid.[12] They cite 80,000 bariatric surgeries performed on obese patients in 2002, costing between $15,000 and $30,000 per patient. In a 2004 review article in the *Journal of the American Medical Association*, Mokdad and associates concluded that smoking remains the leading cause of mortality.[13] Poor diet and physical inactivity, however, may soon overtake tobacco as the leading cause of death. These findings, along with escalating healthcare costs and an aging population, are compelling reasons for U.S. healthcare and public health systems to establish a more effective preventive approach to this epidemic. In April 2005, an article by officials from CDC and NIH concluded that obesity was the attributable cause of approximately 112,000 deaths annually.[14] This generation might well be the first in history to die younger than their parents.

In their study, Mokdad and colleagues found that overweight and obesity were significantly associated with diabetes, high blood pressure, high cholesterol, asthma, arthritis, and poor health status. Compared with adults of normal weight, adults with a body mass index (BMI) of 40 or higher had the following increased risk: 7.37 for diagnosed diabetes, 6.38 for high blood pressure, 1.88 for high cholesterol levels, 2.72 for asthma, 4.41 for arthritis, and 4.19 for fair or poor health. The authors concluded that obesity and diabetes are escalating among U.S. adults in both sexes, all ages, all races, all educational levels, and all smoking levels.[15]

To assess trends in intake of energy, protein, carbohydrate, total fat, and saturated fat during 1971–2000, the CDC analyzed data from four National Health and Nutrition Examination Surveys (NHANES): NHANES I (conducted during 1971–1974), NHANES II (1976–1980), NHANES III (1988–1994), and NHANES IV (1999–2000). The analysis indicated that, during 1971–2000, increases occurred in mean energy intake in total calories and mean percentage of calories from carbohydrate; decreases occurred in mean percentage of calories from total fat and saturated fat.[16]

During an interview in March 2004, Tommy G. Thompson, Secretary of the U.S. Department of Health and Human Services, stated: "Americans need to understand that overweight and obesity are literally killing us. To know that poor eating habits and inactivity are on the verge of surpassing tobacco use as the leading cause of preventable death in America should motivate all Americans to take action to protect their health. We need to tackle America's weight issues as aggressively as we are addressing smoking and tobacco."[17]

In June 2004, the CDC issued a report on the prevalence and economic impact of obesity. From 1999 to 2002, height and weight data showed that the prevalence of overweight and obesity among adults rose from 64.5 to 65.7%, and the prevalence of overweight among children aged 6 to 19 rose from 15 to 16.5%. The CDC authors concluded: "Substantial progress will need to be made in the efforts to lower the prevalence of overweight and obesity if the goals of Healthy People 2010 are to be met."[16] The NHANES results indicate continuing disparities by gender and between racial/ethnic groups in the prevalence of overweight and obesity. This report concluded that there is no indication that the prevalence of obesity among adults and overweight among children is decreasing. The high levels of overweight among children and obesity among adults remain a major public health concern.[18]

An interesting outcome of the 2004 annual conference of the American Medical Association (AMA) was the focus on overweight and obesity, especially in those papers that addressed the physician's own weight problems to set an example for patients. The new AMA policy highlights racial and ethnic differences due to the rates of obesity and its related conditions—such as coronary heart disease, stroke, cancer, and diabetes—among minority populations. Racial and ethnic minorities are at greater risk for obesity, with nearly twice as many African American women being obese as white women. Dietetics practitioners and other healthcare professionals could include or adapt a number of the AMA policies, which comprise the following:

- Physicians [all healthcare professionals] should use culturally responsive care to improve treatment and management of obesity and should take cultural and socioeconomic factors into consideration in conducting nutrition-related research.
- Culturally effective guidelines that include ethnic food staples and multicultural symbols should be included in the revised Dietary Guidelines for Americans and the Food Guide Pyramid.
- Restaurants with multiple locations should be required to provide information on the nutritional content of food items. School and work cafeterias should have ingredients lists for all menu items. Healthy foods should be made available at hospitals as well.

APPROACHES USED IN WEIGHT MANAGEMENT

Prevention, management, and reversal of overweight and obesity present the dietetics professional with great challenges. If ever there was a topic that elicited controversy and disparate approaches, obesity treatment has to be near the top. The array of options vary from nutritional interventions, behavioral therapy, pharmacotherapy, surgical intervention, to the more unorthodox treatments and procedures such as the recently popular liposuction and ultrasound techniques to dispel adipose tissue from truncal fat stores. Programs that focus on the individual, family, school, workplace, and community are all being developed and implemented in an effort to reverse the continuing trend toward weight gain among the majority of the U.S. population and now globally (see Figure 16-1). Options other than those involving nutrition interventions are beyond the scope of this chapter. Dietetics professionals, however, should work with bariatric surgeons and the multidisciplinary team to assure that individuals undergoing bypass surgery are optimally nourished

Issues to Ponder

- Where does your state rank in obesity? Where does it rank in medical costs? What strategies and community efforts might be implemented to bring a change in this ranking? See http://healthyamericans.org/ See State Maps or F as in Fat Report, October 2005, pp. 16–17.
- Are you familiar with the cultural, ethnic, and socioeconomic diversity of your community? Are dietary and nutritional tools and information reflective and responsive to this diversity? If not, do you have any ideas as to how to provide such material?
- Looking at Figure 16-1, where would you focus your efforts and funds based on your experience and knowledge?

both before and after the procedure as well as to prevent long-term malnutrition, specific deficiencies, and other complications from occurring.

LOW-FAT , LOW-CALORIE, PORTION-CONTROLLED REGIMENS

The scientific rationale, physiology, and metabolic consequences of obesity and weight loss should be understood when the nutritional options for therapy are being considered. The low-fat (< 30% of total calories), low-calorie, portion-controlled approach has been the gold standard for weight management for several decades. Along with the dietary guidelines and the food-guide pyramid, low-fat regimens have prevailed as the diets of choice. Such regimens, however, have clearly not succeeded in controlling the weight of the majority of adults and, more recently, of children and adolescents. Whether the limitation is in the method of teaching and counseling individuals to implement the program, the individual's ability to adhere to the food choices, or environmental and societal influences that undermine the inherent discipline and control needed to succeed, this approach has not been widely successful.

In a recent critique in the *Journal of the American College of Cardiology*, Dr. Sylvan Weinberg, Director of Medical Education at the Dayton Heart Hospital and Clinical Professor of Medicine at the Wright State University School of Medicine as well as former president of the American College of Cardiology, stated:

> The low-fat "diet–heart hypothesis" has been controversial for nearly 100 years. The low-fat–high-carbohydrate diet, promulgated vigorously by the National Cholesterol Education Program, National Institutes of Health, and American Heart Association since the Lipid Research Clinics–Primary Prevention Program in 1984, and earlier by the U.S. Department of Agriculture food pyramid, may well have played an unintended role in the current epidemics of obesity, lipid abnormalities, type II diabetes, and metabolic syndromes. This diet can no longer be defended by appeal to the authority of prestigious medical organizations or by rejecting clinical experience and a growing medical literature suggesting that the much-maligned low-carbohydrate–high-protein diet may have a salutary effect on the epidemics in question.[19]

For those wishing to explore these issues, Dr. Weinberg provides several interesting points in his critique about the supporting documentation concerning low-fat recommendations and the need to revisit the science surrounding our current recommendations and practices.[19]

In a 2004 commentary, German and Dillard expressed concern about the potential risks of advocating a low-fat—especially a low-saturated-fat—intake without better evidence indicating which types of saturated fatty acids and in what amounts are optimal for health.[20] They state:

> Fatty acids are required not only for membrane synthesis, modifications of proteins and carbohydrates, construction of various structural elements in cells and tissues, production of signaling compounds, and fuel, but also for solubilizing a variety of nonpolar and poorly soluble cellular and extracellular constituents.

They go on to point out that

> studies on the long-term health benefits of consuming a low-fat diet—particularly after variation in human responses is taken into account—are lacking, and low-fat diets have been shown to exert a potentially deleterious effect on lipoprotein profiles in some persons. .... These differences in response are examples of why it is important to take into account individual differences in response to both dietary fat and carbohydrates when studies of the effects of either low-fat diets or diets with reduced saturated fat or studies of the effects of specific dietary saturated fatty acids are pursued.[20]

Issues to Ponder

- With these concerns being expressed by numerous well-respected clinicians and researchers, the dietetics professional and other healthcare professionals may want to revisit the literature and evaluate the strengths and weaknesses of this approach to weight management.
- What should we, as healthcare professionals, do in advising or counseling individuals about their fat intake?

This same commentary states: "Perhaps it is ironic that diets enriched in saturated fat and cholesterol increase LDL-cholesterol concentrations but also increase HDL-cholesterol concentrations. The lack of a scientific, mechanistic understanding of these relations should be a warning that population-wide recommendations for all persons at all ages and circumstances to reduce their intake of saturated fats may be premature."[20]

MEAL REPLACEMENT AND STRUCTURED MEAL PLANS

Other options have been studied and have potential. The use of meal replacements over a 6-month study period was found to be as effective as a structured low-fat diet for weight loss.[21] A systematic evaluation of randomized controlled trials utilizing partial meal replacement plans for weight management found that this approach safely and effectively produced significant sustainable weight loss at both the 3-month and 1-year evaluation time points and improved weight-related risk factors for disease.[22] In another study, 100 patients were randomly assigned to one of two dietary interventions for 3 months. Group A was prescribed an energy-restricted diet of 1,200 to 1,500 kcal/day and group B was given an isocaloric diet, replacing two out of three meals with nutrient-fortified liquid meal replacements. After 3 months, all the subjects were given the same caloric reduction and used once-daily replacements for a total of 4 years. The study showed that providing a structured meal plan with liquid meal replacements could be an effective treatment for obese subjects. The study also showed that long-term maintenance of weight loss with meal replacements improves biomarkers of disease risk.[23] A prospective randomized controlled clinical trial was also done in which 100 obese volunteers between the ages of 35 and 65 years were randomized to either the meal replacement group (n = 50; 240 g/day, 1,200 kcal/day) or the control group (n = 50) for 12 weeks. Of the total number of participants, 74 completed the trial. The soy-based meal replacement formula used in this trial was effective in lowering body weight and fat mass as well as reducing LDL cholesterol.[24]

An earlier study looked at structured meal plans in a randomized controlled study, with 163 overweight women assigned to one of four conditions: (1) a standard behavioral treatment program (SBT) with weekly meetings for 6 months; (2) SBT plus structured meal plans and grocery lists; (3) SBT plus meal plans plus food provision, with subjects sharing the cost; or (4) SBT plus meal plans plus free food provision. Group 1 lost significantly less weight than the other three groups with significant differences in weight loss between groups 2 to 4. The researchers suggested that the success of these groups was due to the provision of highly structured meal plans and grocery lists. Subjects receiving meal plans were more likely to exhibit an eating pattern of three meals per day, had more definite plans regarding what to eat, and reported more favorable changes in foods stored in their homes and in perceived barriers to weight loss. The authors concluded that providing structured meal plans and grocery lists improved the outcome in a behavioral weight control program; no further benefit was seen by actually giving food to patients.[25]

Behavior Modification

Behavior modification has been used in both clinical practice and research settings by many clinicians and researchers. In a review article, Brownell stated that the failure to properly address behavioral modification is part of the reason why so many weight-loss programs cannot sustain long-term weight loss, even though initial weight loss is often achieved with relative ease. Brownell focuses on lifestyle changes: exercise, relapse prevention, and the concept of a reasonable weight. He stresses the importance of integrating behavioral therapy into a multifaceted approach for managing obesity and associated conditions, such as type 2 (non-insulin-dependent) diabetes.[26]

Another review article, written after the National Institute of Diabetes and Digestive and Kidney Diseases conference on behavioral science research in diabetes, identified four key topics related to obesity and physical activity that should be given high priority in future research efforts: (1) environmental factors related to obesity, eating, and physical activity; (2) adoption and maintenance of healthful eating, physical activity, and weight; (3) etiology of eating and physical activity; and (4) multiple behavior changes.[27]

One group that has studied and published extensively on behavior modification programs is Wadden and colleagues at the University of Pennsylvania. Among their most interesting and challenging studies was one that investigated whether informing obese individuals that they would lose only modest amounts of weight would help them to adopt more realistic weight-loss expectations. At a screening interview, 53 obese women reported that they expected to lose the equivalent of 28% of their initial weight during 1 year of treatment with the medication sibutramine. Prior to beginning treatment, participants were informed, both verbally and in writing, that they could expect to lose 5 to 15% of their initial weight, the loss typically accepted by current behavioral and pharmacologic approaches. This information, however, had little impact on their weight-loss expectations when these were assessed during the program and at its completion.[28]

Another study by Foster and coworkers examined ways to reduce the contrast between treatment expectations and subsequent outcomes by looking at the role of physical characteristics, treatment setting, and mood in patients' evaluations of treatment outcomes. A total of 394 obese individuals seeking weight loss by a variety of modalities were given the Beck Depression Inventory and the Goals and Relative Weight Questionnaire prior to treatment. Perceptions of their own "dream," "acceptable," "happy," and "disappointed" weights were requested from each subject prior to starting the study. Initial body weight was the strongest predictor of the ratings of disappointed, acceptable, and happy obtained from the subjects. Sex and height were the strongest determinants of stated dream weight. Heavier participants chose higher absolute weights, but the weight loss required to reach each of the outcomes was greater for heavier than for lighter patients. The authors make a compelling point that presents a therapeutic dilemma for the practitioner: the amount of weight loss produced by the best behavioral and/or pharmacologic treatments is less than the "disappointing" weight level stated by the patient. Patients with the highest pretreatment weights are likely to have the most unrealistic expectations for success.[29] Those practitioners working with individuals in weight-loss programs need to be sensitive to and aware of such unrealistic expectations when counseling their patients.

COMMERCIAL WEIGHT-LOSS PROGRAMS

Another approach is commercial weight-loss programs. Some benefits of these programs are planned menus and psychological support via group participation. Cost, sales promotions that encourage on-the-spot commitment to prepaid contracts, and the cost of program food and additional vitamins may deter some individual from participating.[30]

A study looking at various programs was undertaken with overweight and obese men (n = 65) and women (n = 358) with a BMI of 27 to 40. Roughly half (or 212) of the participants were randomized to either a self-help program (consisting of two 20-minute counseling sessions with a nutritionist and provision of self-help resources). The remaining 211 subjects were placed in a commercial weight-loss program (consisting of a food plan, an activity plan, and a cognitive restructuring behavior modification plan delivered at weekly meetings). After 2 years, 150 participants (71%) in the commercial group and 159 (75%) in the self-help group completed the study. The structured commercial weight-loss program resulted in modest but greater weight loss than that achieved by the self-help group over a 2-year period.[31]

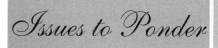

Issues to Ponder

- Would you be comfortable using one or more of these approaches in managing or counseling an individual wishing to lose weight?
- How would you deal with an individual's expectations, goals, and level of progress during a weight-loss regimen?

LOW/CONTROLLED-CARBOHYDRATE REGIMENS

Despite the popularity of the low-carbohydrate approach to weight management, many healthcare professionals continue to be skeptical or opposed to this method owing to their concerns about its safety, efficacy, and long-term success. Based on the successful experiences of many individuals who have limited their carbohydrate intake as well as emerging scientific evidence supporting beneficial clinical outcomes—such as improved lipid and glucose parameters—this approach is a potentially viable option in dealing with the obesity crisis. The following section, in which this approach is more extensively discussed than the others, is intended to give the reader who might not be familiar with emerging research in this area some basic background. Once this approach is understood, the practitioner might be less skeptical in considering it as a potential option to the management of individuals with weight problems.*

Numerous studies lasting from 3 months to 1 year have given rise to safety and efficacy data for weight loss as well as improved health parameters, improved cardiovascular lipid levels, stable blood glucose levels, and improved markers of metabolic syndrome with lower carbohydrate intake.[32-48] The amount of carbohydrate in a low-carbohydrate regimen varies from 20 to 50 or 60 g. A controlled carbohydrate intake may range from 60 to 75 to 150 g or more, depending on the caloric intake and the individual's ability to metabolize carbohydrates. These levels are significantly lower than the 300 g of carbohydrates recommended in most dietary guidelines (55 to 65% carbohydrate on a 2,000-calorie regimen will equal 275 to 325 g of carbohydrate).

Clinical Risk Factors

Concerns about the dangers of developing increased risk factors for heart disease, kidney disease, loss of muscle mass, and bone loss have not been adequately supported by scientific evidence. Emerging research shows clinical benefits when carbohydrate intake is decreased and healthy fats are increased as well.[19,49-71] A common concern is the level of carbohydrate required for healthy brain and organ function. Beneficial uses of ketones for brain function have been known and well documented since the 1960s. The human body has an essential nutrient requirement for both protein (amino acids) and fats (free fatty acids) but no essential requirement for carbohydrate. The liver endogenously produces whatever glucose is required for metabolic needs without needing exogenous carbohydrates. Therefore, as long as caloric requirements are met through protein, fatty acids, and minimal carbohydrates, preserving lean body mass, the essential carbohydrate requirements of the brain, red blood cells, retina, etc. need not be derived from food sources, especially simple carbohydrate sources, despite the recent Institute of Medicine recommendation for dietary carbohydrate (130 g or 26% of a 2,000-kcal diet).[64]

The Role of Carbohydrate Restriction for Individuals with Type 2 Diabetes

The controlled carbohydrate regimen could be one viable alternative dietary approach considered by clinicians managing overweight patients with type 2 diabetes. This can be achieved by restricting carbohydrates initially and carefully monitoring blood glucose and insulin levels and adjusting medications to needs. Hypertensive medications would need to be monitored as well. This approach appears to result in better blood glucose control than the current standard of care, with associated decreases in medication regimens. Numerous studies looking at various scientific questions related to carbohydrate intake and type 2 diabetes management are in progress. Findings from studies are emerging to validate the benefit of controlling carbohydrates in individuals with type 2 diabetes.[33,40,42,51,52]

---

*For an opposing presentation of this issue, an article by Robert F. Kushner, MD, is suggested. See Kushner RF. Low-carbohydrate diets, con: the mythical phoenix or credible science? Nutr Clin Pract 2005;20:13–16.

Cardiovascular Responses to Controlled Carbohydrate Intakes

Will this dietary alternative increase patients' potential risk of heart disease? These at-risk individuals are frequently obese, with hyperinsulinism, insulin resistance, or prediabetes, and/or may have metabolic syndrome, or elevated serum glucose levels with a concomitant elevation of serum insulin. The Harvard Nurses Health Study found that when glycemic load was measured against the risk of coronary heart disease (CHD) in 75,000 women, those who consumed more carbohydrates and a greater glycemic load had significantly more coronary events.[65] The authors concluded that "a high intake of rapidly digested and absorbed carbohydrate increases the risk of CHD independent of conventional coronary disease risk factors. These data add to the concern that the current low fat, high carbohydrate diet recommended in the United States may not be optimal for the prevention of CHD and could actually increase the risk in individuals with degrees of insulin resistance and glucose intolerance."[65]

Hypertriglyceridemia has been shown to be an independent risk factor for coronary heart disease as well as strokes.[66] A study by Tanne and associates showed that high serum triglycerides and fractionated cholesterol levels were associated with increased risk of ischemic stroke/transient ischemic attack in a large cohort (over 11,000) men and women with coronary heart disease.[67] The increased risk associated with high triglycerides was found across subgroups of age, gender, patient characteristics, and cholesterol fractions. The researchers concluded that high serum triglycerides constitute an independent risk factor for ischemic stroke, whereas high HDL levels were an independent protective factor among patients with coronary heart disease.[67] This link between triglyceride levels and heart disease is modifiable by dietary intervention. High triglyceride and low HDL levels can be improved by decreasing simple sugars and refined carbohydrates as well as the total amount of carbohydrate consumed.[32,34,36,37,42–44,47,48]

When carbohydrates are controlled, lipid levels improve, as seen in another study done in adolescents comparing a low-fat, calorie-controlled diet to a low-carbohydrate diet involving an unrestricted calorie intake (carbohydrates equaling 8% of total caloric intake). The investigators found that all lipid parameters improved on the controlled carbohydrate diet even though the caloric intake was over 700 calories more than that in the low-fat diet.[68] These results have been repeated in several other studies that arrived at a similar conclusion when the carbohydrate level was adequately reduced. Recent dietary studies in adults showed that the controlled carbohydrate diet resulted in greater weight loss, better compliance, and improved overall lipid profiles.[34,36,37,39,69,70] Preliminary reports also show that C-reactive protein, a marker of inflammation, is stable or decreased on a low-carbohydrate intake versus a low-fat intake.[47,58]

Body Composition, Ketosis, Hepatic, and Renal Concerns of Low-Carbohydrate Regimens

What about the impact of restricting carbohydrates on lean body mass versus fat mass? Studies have shown that lean body mass is preserved and fat mass lost on this regimen.[34,36,41,70–72] In one study, 12 healthy normal-weight men (to remove weight loss as a confounding variable) on a carbohydrate-restricted diet (8% carbohydrate) for 6 weeks were compared to 8 men consuming their normal diet. A significant reduction in fat mass and a concomitant increase in lean body mass occurred on the carbohydrate-restricted diet compared to the controls, improving both body composition and hormonal balance.[72]

Many concerns such as ketosis or hepatic and renal damage caused by limiting carbohydrates are not well substantiated in the scientific literature. Ketosis is tightly regulated in healthy individuals. In dietary ketosis, or physiologic ketosis, the body's tight regulation of pH levels is similar to its control of temperature fluctuations, or regulation of serum glucose levels. Ketoacidosis, an abnormal metabolic response, which is not the same as the ketosis that occurs from normal fatty acid oxidation, should not be confused with normal physiologic ketosis, which is benign. Similarly misunderstood is the brain's ability to effectively utilize ketones for energy.[73–75] Cahill, one of the original researchers in ketone body metabolism, writes: "D-beta-hydroxybutyrate, the principal 'ketone' body in starving man, displaces glucose as the predominating fuel for brain, decreasing the need for glucose synthesis in liver (and kidney) and accordingly spares its precursor, muscle-derived amino acids."[75]

Similar concerns have been raised about hepatic or renal damage caused by high protein regimens but not documented in normal subjects.[57,63,76] In a recent review, Dr. A.H. Manninen, from the department of physiology, Faculty of Medicine, University of Oulu, Finland, summarized these concerns by stating:

> There is no scientific evidence whatsoever that high-protein intake has adverse effects on liver function. Relative to renal function, there are no data in the scientific literature demonstrating that healthy kidneys are damaged by the increased demands of protein consumed in quantities 2-3 times above the Recommended Dietary Allowance (RDA). In contrast with the earlier hypothesis that high protein intake promotes osteoporosis, some epidemiological studies found a positive association between protein intake and bone mineral density. Further, recent studies suggest, at least in the short term, that RDA for protein (0.8 g/kg) does not support normal calcium homeostasis. Finally, a negative correlation has been shown between protein intake and systolic and diastolic blood pressures in several epidemiological surveys. In conclusion, there is little if any scientific evidence supporting the above mentioned statement. Certainly, such public warnings should be based on a thorough analysis of the scientific literature, not unsubstantiated fears and misrepresentations. For individuals with normal renal function, the risks are minimal and must be balanced against the real and established risk of continued obesity.[53]

Numerous studies support clinical observations that a low-carbohydrate high-protein intake does not compromise calcium excretion or bone metabolism despite the prevailing belief.[54–56,59,60,62] A study by Dawson-Hughes and coworkers concluded that: "In contrast to the widely held belief that increased protein intake results in calcium wasting, meat supplements, when exchanged isocalorically for carbohydrates, may have a favorable impact on the skeleton in healthy older men and women."[54]

Cancer Risk or Benefit?

An emerging area of interest is the possible role of low-carbohydrate regimens, both preventatively and to avoid the recurrence of cancer. Many healthcare professionals question both the fat content as well as the fruit/vegetable intake of a low-carbohydrate regimen and the potential increased risk of cancer. Interestingly, research over the past 5 or more years has begun to focus on insulin and insulin-like growth factors as affecting cancer risk as well as survival.[77–80] The relationship between dietary carbohydrate, glycemic load, hyperinsulinemia, and cancer risk has recently been recognized. Fat as an independent nutrient has not been convincingly implicated in cancer risk or mortality.[81–84] The cancer connection to fat is its potential role in contributing to obesity and excess caloric intake, which does increase the risk of developing cancer in certain sites as well as the risk of mortality.

Vegetables are encouraged in every phase of the low-carbohydrate program, including the most restrictive phase. The reason that 20 to 25 g of carbohydrate was originally established for the carbohydrate-restricted program was to allow the individual to consume three to five servings of healthy vegetables along with healthy protein and fat selections. As the individual progresses through the diet, more vegetables along with low-glycemic fruits, nuts/seeds, whole grains, and legumes are encouraged. Many individuals find that they consume more vegetables on the low-carbohydrate program than they did while following their normal eating patterns.

Application of Low/Controlled-Carbohydrate Regimens

Many versions of the low/controlled-carbohydrate regimen exist. The low-carbohydrate approach has individuals reduce their carbohydrate intake to 20 to 25 g initially for several weeks, choosing carbohydrates predominantly in the form of leafy greens or low-glycemic vegetables. The remaining foods consist of healthy fats, proteins, and adequate fluids (water preferred) along with exercise and a complete multivitamin/mineral supplement to obtain optimal nutrition. Interestingly, emerging research is raising questions about saturated fats in relation to risk factors as well as their metabolic activity.[20,85] One can just as easily select fish, chicken, nuts/seeds, peanut butter, legumes, olive oil, and many other choices that would fit into a healthy dietary selection while lowering carbohydrate consumption. It should be noted, however, that the studies done to date did not restrict the high-fat/high-cholesterol foods, yet the subjects still improved their lipid profiles.[32,34–37,39,41–45,47,48]

Many dietetics professionals prefer to eliminate carbohydrates gradually until individuals reach their appropriate threshold for carbohydrates that will not induce weight gain. This approach will be slower in achieving weight loss but is also a successful strategy for those uncomfortable with the restrictions required by reducing carbohydrates initially and then adding them back into the diet slowly. Current research, more sophisticated than that previously available, is corroborating the metabolic rationale for a low-carbohydrate approach.

Issues to Ponder

- What are your concerns about this approach? Are they supported by scientific findings?
- How does one sort out the various issues concerning low-carbohydrate regimens: low carbohydrate, controlled carbohydrate, glycemic index, glycemic load, simple sugars, refined carbohydrate foods, complex carbohydrates—and make them understood by those wishing to lose weight?

POTENTIAL FACTORS LEADING TO INCREASES IN OBESITY RATES

ENVIRONMENTAL INFLUENCES

According to Wadden and Brownell and more recently Bray and Champgne, the marked increase in prevalence of obesity appears to be attributable to what they call a "toxic environment" that implicitly discourages physical activity while explicitly encouraging the consumption of supersized portions of high-fat, high-sugar foods.[86,87] Wadden and Brownell offer a two-pronged approach to the management of the obesity epidemic. The first approach calls for better treatments, including behavioral, pharmacologic, and surgical interventions, for individuals who are obese. The second and potentially more promising approach is the prevention of obesity by tackling the toxic environment. The authors challenge legislators to enact bold public policy initiatives such as regulating food advertising directed at children or providing community play spaces or walking/bicycle paths. They would like to see obesity viewed as a public health problem, which would allow it to become a central focus of future research.[87]

ENERGY DENSITY AND PORTION SIZING

Increases in both the portion size and energy density of food have been shown to increase energy intake, but the combined effects of such increases have only recently been investigated. One study determined the combined effects of energy density and portion size on energy intake in women. Increases in portion size and energy density led to statistically significant independent and additive increases in energy intake. Subjects consumed 56% more energy when served the largest portion of the higher-energy-dense entree than when served the smallest portion of the lower-energy-dense entree. Subjects did not compensate for the additional intake by eating less at the subsequent meal. The authors concluded that the energy density and the portion size of a food act independently to affect energy intake. The findings indicate that large portions of foods with a high energy density may facilitate the overconsumption of energy.[88]

In another study looking at food consumption from fast foods of both overweight and lean adolescents, the researchers found that adolescents overconsumed fast food regardless of body weight, although this was more pronounced in overweight participants. In addition, they found that overweight adolescents were less likely than their lean counterparts to compensate for the energy consumed in fast food by adjusting energy intake throughout the day.[89]

GENETIC INFLUENCES

Research in the past decade has shown that genetic influences clearly predispose some individuals to obesity. Mulch and Williamson provide a review of this emerging field:

> The recognition that nutrients have the ability to interact and modulate molecular mechanisms underlying an organism's physiological functions has prompted a revolution in the field of nutrition. Performing population-scaled epidemiological studies in the absence of genetic knowledge may result in erroneous scientific conclusions and misinformed nutritional

recommendations. To circumvent such issues and more comprehensively probe the relationship between genes and diet, the field of nutrition has begun to capitalize on both the technologies and supporting analytical software brought forth in the post-genomic era. The creation of nutrigenomics and nutrigenetics, two fields with distinct approaches to elucidate the interaction between diet and genes but with a common ultimate goal to optimize health through the personalization of diet, provide powerful approaches to unravel the complex relationship between nutritional molecules, genetic polymorphisms, and the biological system as a whole. Reluctance to embrace these new fields exists primarily due to the fear that producing overwhelming quantities of biological data within the confines of a single study will submerge the original query; however, the current review aims to position nutrigenomics and nutrigenetics as the emerging faces of nutrition that, when considered with more classical approaches, will provide the necessary stepping stones to achieve the ambitious goal of optimizing an individual's health via nutritional intervention.[90]

This emerging area of work is beyond the scope of this chapter other than to recognize its importance for future dietary recommendations (see Chapter 13).

Issues to Ponder

If we accept the statement that "one diet does not fit all," how should dietetics and healthcare professionals approach the management of weight, both in preventing overweight/obesity and maintaining fitness and health as well as weight-loss regimens?

CONCLUSION

We are not solving the obesity problem with our current methods and recommendations. A new paradigm is needed. Individual requirements and clinical parameters—such as metabolic syndrome, lipoprotein subclass patterns, or other genetic determinants of an individual's predisposition to nutrient metabolism—are becoming the wave of the future for providing dietary recommendations.[91,92]

An array of exciting possibilities lie ahead of us with more options and greater potential to improve the quality of life and the health of at-risk individuals who are overweight and obese while lessening the economic burden of healthcare costs. An individualized diet and nutritional care plan optimally suited to a given individual can be implemented. One diet will not fit all patients. Some individuals might do best on a diet that is very low in fats and high in carbohydrates. Others might respond favorably to a vegetarian or vegan-type approach. Behavior modification or meal replacements might be the best approach for some individuals, while controlling carbohydrates might be the easiest technique of weight management and managing health parameters for others. Identifying specific needs and conditions is key to successful application for the best approach and management of each individual. Hopefully, emerging science will allow this type of dietary planning—a plan specific to each phenotype or eventually each genotype. Health professionals need to be knowledgeable about and comfortable with all options for the most effective management of individuals who continue to struggle with their health, weight, and eating issues.

REFERENCES

1. Obesity: etiology, treatment, prevention, and application in practice. J Am Diet Assoc 2005;105(5 suppl).
2. F as in fat: how obesity policies are failing in America. Washington, DC: Trust for America's Health, August 2005. Available at: http://healthyamericans.org/reports/obesity2005/Obesity2005Report.pdf. Accessed October 2005.
3. Health, United States, 2003. Atlanta: Centers for Disease Control and Prevention, National Center on Vital Statistics, 2003: table 68.
4. Schiller JS, Martinez M, Hao C, Barnes P. Early release of selected estimates based on data from the January–September 2004 National Health Interview Survey. National Center for Health Statistics, 2005. Available at: http://www.cdc.gov/nchs/nhis.htm. Accessed March 1, 2006.
5. Serdula MK, Ivery D, Coates RJ, et al. Do obese children become obese adults? A review of the literature. Prev Med 1993;22:167–177.
6. The public health effects of sprawl. Congressional Briefing Summary. Washington, DC: Environmental and Energy Study Institute, October 2, 2003. Available at: http://www.eesi.org/publications/Briefing%20Summaries/10.2.03%20Briefing%20Summary.pdf. Accessed March 1, 2006.
7. Weight-Control Information Network, National Institute of Diabetes and Digestive and Kidney Diseases (NIDDK). Do you know the health risks of being overweight? Available at: http://win.niddk.nih.gov/publications/health_risks.htm. Accessed June 6, 2005.
8. Centers for Disease Control and Prevention. Overweight and obesity consequences. Available at: http://www.cdc.gov/nccdphp/dnpa/obesity/consequences.htm. Accessed March 1, 2006.
9. Wechsler H. HHS efforts to combat the obesity epidemic among children and adolescents. Testimony before the Subcommittee on Oversight and Investigations, Committee on Energy and Commerce, U.S. House of Representatives. Available at: http://www.hhs.gov/asl/testify/t040616.html. Accessed June 16, 2004.
10. Strum R. The effects of obesity, smoking, and drinking on medical problems and costs. Health Affairs 2002;21:245–253.
11. Fitch K, Pyenson B, Abbs S, Liang M. Obesity: A big problem getting bigger. Milliman Consultants and Actuaries, 2004. Available at http://milliman.com/services/healthcare.researchreports.asp?id=1373. Accessed March 1, 2006.
12. Finkelstein EA, Fiebelkorn JC, Wang G. State-level estimates of annual medical expenditures attributable to obesity. Obes Res 2004;12:18–24.
13. Mokdad AH, Marks JS, Stroup DF, Gerberding JL. Actual causes of death in the United States, 2000. JAMA 2004;291:1238–45.
14. Flegal KM, Graubard BI, Williamson DF, Gail MH. Excess deaths associated with underweight, overweight, and obesity. JAMA 2005;293:1861–1867.
15. Mokdad AH, Ford ES, Bowman BA, et al. Prevalence of obesity, diabetes, and obesity-related health risk factors, 2001. JAMA 2003;289:76–79.
16. Centers for Disease Control and Prevention. Trends in intake of energy and macronutrients— United States, 1971–2000. MMWR 2004;53:80–82.
17. Stein R. Obesity rivals tobacco for most U.S. deaths: CDC predicts inactivity, unhealthy eating to overtake cancer by 2005. Washington Post, Tuesday, March 9, 2004.
18. Hedley AA, Ogden CL, Johnson CL, Carroll MD, Curtin LR, Flegal KM. Prevalence of overweight and obesity among US children, adolescents, and adults, 1999–2002. JAMA 2004;291:2847–2850.
19. Weinberg SL. The diet-heart hypothesis: a critique. J Am Coll Cardiol 2004;43:731–733.
20. German JB, Dillard CJ. Saturated fats: what dietary intake? Am J Clin Nutr 2004;80:550–559.
21. Clifton PM, Noakes M, Keogh J, Foster P. How effective are meal replacements for treating obesity? Asia Pac J Clin Nutr. 2003;12(suppl):S51.
22. Heymsfield SB, van Mierlo CA, van der Knaap HC, Heo M, Frier HI. Weight management using a meal replacement strategy: meta and pooling analysis from six studies. Int J Obes Relat Metab Disord 2003;27:537–549.
23. Ditschuneit HH, Flechtner-Mors M. Value of structured meals for weight management: risk factors and long-term weight maintenance. Obes Res 2001;9(suppl 4):284S–289S.
24. Allison DB, Gadbury G, Schwartz LG, et al. A novel soy-based meal replacement formula for weight loss among obese individuals: a randomized controlled clinical trial. Eur J Clin Nutr 2003;57:514–522
25. Wing RR, Jeffery RW, Burton LR, Thorson C, Nissinoff KS, Baxter JE. Food provision vs structured meal plans in the behavioral treatment of obesity. Int J Obes Relat Metab Disord 1996;20:56–62.

26. Brownell KD. Diet, exercise and behavioural intervention: the nonpharmacological approach. Eur J Clin Invest 1998;28(suppl 2):19–21; discussion 22.

27. Wing RR, Goldstein MG, Acton KJ, et al. Behavioral science research in diabetes: lifestyle changes related to obesity, eating behavior, and physical activity. Diabetes Care 2001;24:117–123.

28. Wadden TA, Womble LG, Sarwer DB, Berkowitz RI, Clark VL, Foster GD. Great expectations: "I'm losing 25% of my weight no matter what you say." J Consult Clin Psychol 2003;71:1084–1089.

29. Foster GD, Wadden TA, Phelan S, Sarwer DB, Sanderson RS. Obese patients' perceptions of treatment outcomes and the factors that influence them. Arch Intern Med 2001;161:2133–2139.

30. Witherspoon B, Rosenzweig M. Industry-sponsored weight loss programs: description, cost, and effectiveness. J Am Acad Nurse Pract 2004;16:198–205.

31. Heshka S, Anderson JW, Atkinson RL, et al. Weight loss with self-help compared with a structured commercial program: a randomized trial. JAMA 2003;289:1792–1798.

32. Yancy WS Jr, Olsen MK, Guyton JR, Bakst RP, Westman EC. A low-carbohydrate, ketogenic diet versus a low-fat diet to treat obesity and hyperlipidemia: a randomized, controlled trial. Ann Intern Med 2004;140:769–777.

33. Boden G, Sargrad K, Homko C, Davis E, Mozzoli M, Stein TP. Effects of the Atkins diet in type 2 diabetes: metabolic balance studies. Diabetes 2004;53(S2): A75.

34. Brehm BJ, Seeley RJ, Daniels SR, D'Alessio DA. A randomized trial comparing a very low carbohydrate diet and a calorie-restricted low fat diet on body weight and cardiovascular risk factors in healthy women. J Clin Endocrinol Metab 2003;88:1617–1623.

35. Dansinger ML, Gleason JL, Griffith JL, Li W, Selker, HP, Schaefer EJ. One year effectiveness of the Atkins, Ornish, Weight Watchers, and Zone diets in decreasing body weight and heart disease risk. Presented at the American Heart Association Scientific Sessions, November 12, 2003, Orlando, Florida.

36. Farnsworth E, Luscombe ND, Noakes M, Wittert G, Argyiou E, Clifton PM. Effect of a high-protein, energy-restricted diet on body composition, glycemic control, and lipid concentrations in overweight and obese hyperinsulinemic men and women. Am J Clin Nutr 2003;78:31–39.

37. Foster GD, Wyatt HR, Hill JO, et al. A randomized trial of a low-carbohydrate diet for obesity. N Engl J Med 2003;348:2082–2090.

38. Nickols-Richardson SM, Volpe JM, Coleman MM. Premenopausal women following a low-carbohydrate/high-protein diet experience greater weight loss and less hunger compared to a high-carbohydrate/low-fat diet. Presented at Experimental Biology 2004, Washington, DC. FASEB J 2004:abstr 8519.

39. Greene P, Willett W, Devecis J, Skaf A. Pilot 12-week feeding weight-loss comparison: low-fat vs low-carbohydrate (ketogenic) diets. Presented at the North American Association for the Study of Obesity Annual Meeting 2003. Obes Res 2003;11S:95OR.

40. Gutierrez M, Akhavan M, Jovanovic L, Peterson CM. Utility of a short-term 25% carbohydrate diet on improving glycemic control in type 2 diabetes mellitus. J Am Coll Nutr 1998;17:595–600.

41. Hays JH, DiSabatino A, Gorman RT, Vincent S, Stillabower ME. Effect of a high saturated fat and no-starch diet on serum lipid subfractions in patients with documented atherosclerotic cardiovascular disease. Mayo Clin Proc 2003;78:1331–1336.

42. Meckling KA, O'Sullivan C, Saari D. Comparison of a low-fat diet to a low-carbohydrate diet on weight loss, body composition, and risk factors for diabetes and cardiovascular disease in free-living, overweight men and women. J Clin Endocrinol Metab 2004;89:2717–2723.

43. Sharman MJ, Kraemer WJ, Love DM, et al. A ketogenic diet favorably affects serum biomarkers for cardiovascular disease in normal-weight men. J Nutr 2002;132:1879–1885.

44. Sharman MJ, Gomez AL, Kraemer WJ, Volek JS. Very low-carbohydrate and low-fat diets affect fasting lipids and postprandial lipemia differently in overweight men. J Nutr 2004;134:880–885.

45. Volek JS, Gomez AL, Kraemer WJ. Fasting lipoprotein and postprandial triacylglycerol responses to a low-carbohydrate diet supplemented with n-3 fatty acids. J Am Coll Nutr 2000;19:383–391.

46. Volek JS, Westman EC. Very-low-carbohydrate weight-loss diets revisited. Cleve Clin J Med 2002;69:849–862.

47. Volek JS, Sharman MJ, Gomez AL, Scheett TP, Kraemer WJ. An isoenergetic very low carbohydrate diet improves serum HDL cholesterol and triacylglycerol concentrations, the total cholesterol to HDL cholesterol ratio and postprandial lipemic responses compared with a low fat diet in normal weight, normolipidemic Women. J Nutr. 2003;133:2756–2761.

48. Volek JS, Sharman MJ, Gomez AL, et al. Comparison of a very low-carbohydrate and low-fat diet on fasting lipids, LDL subclasses, insulin resistance, and postprandial lipemic responses in overweight women. J Am Coll Nutr. 2004;23:177–184.

49. Westman EC, Yancy WS, Edman JS, Tomlin KF, Perkins CE. Effect of 6-month adherence to a very low carbohydrate diet program. Am J Med. 2002;113:30–36.

50. Westman EC, Mavropoulos J, Yancy WS, Volek JS. A review of low-carbohydrate ketogenic diets. Curr Atheroscler Rep. 2003;5:476–483.

51. Yancy WS, Vernon MC, Westman EC. A pilot trial of a low-carbohydrate, ketogenic diet in patients with type 2 diabetes. Metab Syndr Rel Disord 2003;1:239–243.

52. Stern L, Iqbal N, Seshadri P, et al. The effects of low-carbohydrate versus conventional weight loss diets in severely obese adults: one-year follow-up of a randomized trial. Ann Intern Med 2004;140:778–785.

53. Manninen AH. High-protein weight loss diets and purported adverse effects: where is the evidence? Sports Nutr Rev J 2004;1:45–51.

54. Dawson-Hughes B, Harris SS, Rasmussen H, Song L, Dallal GE. Effect of dietary protein supplements on calcium excretion in healthy older men and women. J Clin Endocrinol Metab 2004;89:1169–1173.

55. Hannan MT, Tucker KL, Dawson-Hughes B, Cupples LA, Felson DT, Kiel DP. Effect of dietary protein on bone loss in elderly men and women: the Framingham Osteoporosis Study. J Bone Min Res 2000;15:2504–2512.

56. Heaney RP. Dietary protein and phosphorus do not affect calcium absorption. Am J Clin Nutr 2000;72:758–761.

57. Knight EL, Stampfer MJ, Hankinson SE, Spiegelman D, Curhan GC. The impact of protein intake on renal function decline in women with normal renal function or mild renal insufficiency. Ann Intern Med 2003;138:460–467.

58. O'Brien KD, Brehm BJ, Seeley RJ. Greater reduction in inflammatory markers with a low carbohydrate diet than with a calorically matched low fat diet. Presented at the American Heart Association's Scientific Sessions, November 19, 2002. abstr 2081.

59. Promislow JH, Goodman-Gruen D, Slymen DJ. Barrett-Connor E. Protein consumption and bone mineral density in the elderly: the Rancho Bernardo Study. Am J Epidemiol 2002:155:636–644.

60. Roughead Z, Johnson L, Lykken G, Hunt JR. Controlled high meat diets do not affect calcium retention or indices of bone status in healthy postmenopausal women. J Nutr 2003;133:1020–1026.

61. Samaha FF, Iqbal N, Seshadri P, et al. A low-carbohydrate as compared with a low-fat diet in severe obesity. N Engl J Med 2003;348:2074–2081.

62. Skov AR, Haulrik N, Toubro S, Molgaard C, Astrup A. Effect of protein intake on bone mineralization during weight loss: a 6-month trial. Obes Res 2002;10:432–438.

63. Skov AR, Toubro S, Bulow J, Krabbe K, Parving HH, Astrup A. Changes in renal function during weight loss induced by high vs low-protein low-fat diets in overweight subjects. Int J Obes Relat Metab Disord 1999;23:1170–1177.

64. Food and Nutrition Board, Institute of Medicine. Dietary Reference Intakes for Energy, Carbohydrate, Fiber, Fat, Fatty Acids, Cholesterol, Protein, and Amino Acids (Macronutrients). Washington, DC: National Academy Press, 2002.

65. Liu S, Willett WC, Stampfer MJ, et al. A prospective study of dietary glycemic load, carbohydrate intake, and risk of coronary heart disease in US women. Am J Clin Nutr 2000;71:1455–1461.

66. Austin MA, Hokanson JE, Edwards KL. Hypertriglyceridemia as a cardiovascular risk factor. Am J Cardiol 1998;81(4A):7B–12B.

67. Tanne D, Koren-Morag N, Graff E, Goldbourt U. Blood lipids and first-ever ischemic stroke/transient ischemic attack in the Bezafibrate Infarction Prevention (BIP) registry: high triglycerides constitute an independent risk factor. Circulation 2001;104:2892–2897.

68. Sondike SB, Copperman N, Jacobson MS. Effects of a low-carbohydrate diet on weight loss and cardiovascular risk factors in overweight adolescents. J Pediatr 2003;142:253–258.

69. Stadler D, Burden V, McMurry M, Gerhard G, Connor W, Karanja N. Impact of 42-day Atkins diet and energy-matched low-fat diet on weight and anthropometric indices. Abstract of the 12th Annual FASEB Meeting on Experimental Biology: Translating the Genome, San Diego, CA, April 11–15, 2003. FASEB J 2003;17(4–5):abstr 453.3.

70. Layman DK, Boileau RA, Erickson DJ, et al. A reduced ratio of dietary carbohydrate to protein improves body composition and blood lipid profiles during weight loss in adult women. J Nutr 2003;133:411–417.

71. Layman DK, Baum JI. Dietary protein impact on glycemic control during weight loss. J Nutr 2004;134:968S–973S.

72. Volek JS, Sharman MJ, Love DM, et al. Body composition and hormonal responses to a carbohydrate-restricted diet. Metabolism 2002;51:864–870.

73. Veech RL. The therapeutic implications of ketone bodies: the effects of ketone bodies in pathological conditions: ketosis, ketogenic diet, redox states, insulin resistance, and mitochondrial metabolism. Prostaglandins Leukot Essent Fatty Acids 2004;70:309–319.

74. Veech RL, Chance B, Kashiwaya Y, Lardy HA, Cahill GF Jr. Ketone bodies, potential therapeutic uses. IUBMB Life 2001;51:241–247.

75. Cahill GF Jr, Veech RL. Ketoacids? Good medicine? Trans Am Clin Climatol Assoc 2003;114:149–161; discussion 162–163.

76. Phinney SD, Bistrian BR, Wolfe RR, Blackburn GL. The human metabolic response to chronic ketosis without caloric restriction: physical and biochemical adaptation. Metabolism 1983;32:757–768.

77. Romieu I, Lazcano-Ponce E, Sanchez-Zamorano LM, Willett W, Hernandez-Avila M. Carbohydrates and the risk of breast cancer among Mexican women. Cancer Epidemiol Biomarkers Prev 2004;13:1283–1289.

78. Lawlor DA, Smith GD, Ebrahim S. Hyperinsulinaemia and increased risk of breast cancer: findings—British Women's Heart/HealthStudy. Cancer Causes Control 2004;15:267–275.

79. Cho E, Spiegelman D, Hunter DJ, Chen WY, Colditz GA, Willett WC. Premenopausal dietary carbohydrate, glycemic index, glycemic load, and fiber in relation to risk of breast cancer. Cancer Epidemiol Biomarkers Prev 2003;12:1153–1158.

80. Borugian MJ, Sheps SB, Kim-Sing C. Insulin, macronutrient intake/physical activity: are potential indicators of insulin resistance associated with mortality from breast cancer? Cancer Epidemiol Biomarkers Prev 2004;13:1163–1172.

81. Holmes MD, Colditz GA, Hunter DJ, et al. Meat, fish and egg intake and risk of breast cancer. Int J Cancer 2003;104:221–227.

82. Holmes MD, Hunter DJ, Colditz GA, et al. Association of dietary intake of fat and fatty acids with risk of breast cancer. JAMA 1999;281:914–920.

83. Brown JK, Byers T, Doyle C, et al. Nutrition and physical activity during and after cancer treatment: an American Cancer Society guide for informed choices. American Cancer Society. CA: Cancer J Clin 2003;53:268–291.

84. Kushi L, Giovannucci E. Dietary fat and cancer. Am J Med 2002;113(suppl 9B):63S–70S.

85. Mozaffarian D, Rimm EB, Herrington DM. Dietary fats, carbohydrate, and progression of coronary atherosclerosis in postmenopausal women. Am J Clin Nutr 2004;80:1175–1184.

86. Wadden TA, Brownell KD, Foster GD. Obesity: responding to the global epidemic. J Consult Clin Psychol 2002;70:510–525.

87. Bray GA, Champagne CM. Beyond energy balance: there is more to obesity than kilocalories. J Am Diet Assoc 2005;105:S17–S23.

88. Kral TV, Roe LS, Rolls BJ. Combined effects of energy density and portion size on energy intake in women. Am J Clin Nutr. 2004;79:962–968.

89. Ebbeling CB, Sinclair KB, Pereira MA, Garcia-Lago E, Feldman HA, Ludwig DS. Compensation for energy intake from fast food among overweight and lean adolescents. JAMA 2004;291:2828–2833.

90. Mutch DM, Wahli W, Williamson G. Nutrigenomics and nutrigenetics: the emerging faces of nutrition. FASEB J 2005;19:1602–1616.

91. Dreon DM, Fernstrom HA, Williams PT, Krauss RM. A very-low-fat diet is not associated with improved lipoprotein profiles in men with a predominance of large, low-density lipoproteins. Am J Clin Nutr 1999;69:411–418.

92. Krauss RM. Atherogenic lipoprotein phenotype and diet-gene interactions. J Nutr 2001;131:340S–343S.

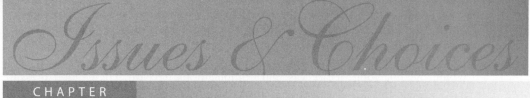

CHAPTER

17

NUTRITIONAL APPROACHES TO DIABETES MELLITUS

Judith Wylie-Rosett

Multiple metabolic disorders associated with a defect in insulin secretion, insulin action, or both play a role in the development of diabetes mellitus.[1] Research continues to identify more pathways involved in glucose uptake by cells and the utilization of glucose within them. The etiology of diabetes involves a more general dysregulation of fuel metabolism, including abnormalities in the cellular uptake of amino acids and fatty acids as well as of glucose.[2] Many factors are associated with the dramatic rise in diabetes worldwide.[3–6] Recent definitions of the metabolic syndrome from the World Health Organization (WHO) and National Cholesterol Education Program (NCEP) are helpful in assessing the prevalence of the metabolic syndrome and the risks it poses for cardiovascular disease and type 2 diabetes.[4] Hypertriglyceridemia is a common clinical comorbidity of diabetes, especially when the blood glucose level is elevated. High levels of postprandial free fatty acids, which also appear to be highly atherogenic, are not measured in clinical practice.

The development of diabetes involves a complex interaction of environmental and genetic factors. Diabetes, a common endocrine problem in dogs and cats as well as humans, usually develops when the expression of genes regulating pathways involved in energy metabolism are altered by environmental factors.[7] For example, insulin deficiency can develop as the result of pancreatic beta cell failure due to autoimmune or viral destruction. Insulin resistance can ultimately lead to a relative insulin deficiency, even in the presence of high insulin levels, if requirements exceed production capacity. The multiple causes of insulin resistance include obesity (particularly the accumulation of visceral, intrahepatic, and intramuscular fat), genetic factors, aging, and medications such as steroids. Antiretroviral therapy and novel antipsychotic agents [e.g., olanzapine (Zyprexa) and risperidone (Risperdal)] can also cause the accumulation of visceral fat and an increased risk of diabetes.

The historic debate over the importance of metabolic control was resolved over a decade ago with evidence that improving glycemic control could prevent diabetic microvascular and neurological complications, notably nephropathy, retinopathy, and neuropathy.[1,8] Improved glycemic control can reduce the burden of diabetes as a leading cause of adult blindness, nontraumatic lower limb amputation, and end-stage renal disease. Diabetic macrovascular disease develops as a result of the synergistic interaction of several metabolic abnormalities. The so-called "ABCs of diabetes" focus on rigorous control of hemoglobin A1c (HbA1c), blood pressure, and low-density-lipoprotein (LDL) cholesterol to reduce the impact of diabetes on large arteries. Elevated HbA1c appears to be a biomarker for the glycosylation of other proteins in the body, and elevation of glucose per se is associated with impaired wound healing long before vascular complications develop. High blood pressure may precede the development of diabetes as part of the metabolic syndrome. The control of blood pressure reduces risk of renal microvascular disease as well as cardiac complications.[1,8] Although current guidelines focus on the control of LDL cholesterol, measurement of the small, dense LDL lipoprotein subfraction is of increasing interest in diabetes-related risk for cardiovascular disease (CVD).[1,8]

If the medication used in diabetes management increases insulin production by the pancreas, hypoglycemia may occur. The risk of hypoglycemia, however, is not due to diabetes per se. Professional and patient education must emphasize the hypoglycemic risk associated with exogenous insulin or medications that stimulate endogenous insulin production. Although hypoglycemia can cause dramatic impaired cognitive functioning, permanent neurological impairment is rare.

PUBLIC HEALTH PERSPECTIVE

Diabetes is increasing at an epidemic rate in the United States and worldwide.[3] An estimated 20 million adults in the United States have diabetes, although one-third have not been diagnosed with the disease. Despite the strong link between diabetes and obesity, populations that have been exposed to famine and individuals who have suffered from early undernutrition appear to have disproportionately high rates of diabetes.[2-7] The estimated proportion of the U.S. population between 40 and 74 years of age with diabetes increased by 49%, or from 8.9 to 12.3%, between the first and second National Health and Nutrition Examination Surveys (NHANES).[3] The prevalence of diabetes can rise dramatically with industrialization in developing countries as the result of obesity and a sedentary lifestyle. Ironically, both low- and high-birth-weight infants can be at increased risk for developing diabetes later in life. The global health burden of diabetes will present major challenges as obesity becomes more common than starvation in developing economies. India and China have the highest prevalence of diabetes in the world, and the United States has the third highest.[3] The economic burden of obesity has risen to equal that of smoking in the United States. CVD and diabetes account for much of this excess cost. Public health measures are needed to lessen the economic burden as well as the excess morbidity and mortality associated with obesity. The worldwide per capita intake of sugars (high-fructose syrups as well as sucrose) increased by ~32% between 1962 and 2000.[6] This increase was primarily accounted for by beverages and foods from fast-food outlets that were consumed between meals. The consumption of high-fructose syrup from soft drinks has doubled during the past 20 years and accounts for more than 100 calories per capita daily. Other dietary changes associated with the rise in obesity and an increasingly younger age for developing diabetes include supersizing of portions and an increased intake of energy-dense snacks. Reducing obesity can delay or perhaps prevent the development of diabetes.[8-10]

DIABETES SCREENING

Diagnostic criteria for diabetes are established on the basis of blood glucose levels associated with the risk of developing complications.[1,8] HbA1c is not used to diagnose diabetes because of the lack of laboratory standardization, although it is the measure used to assess glycemic control. The American Diabetes Association has recommended screening of all adults > 45 years of age using fasting glucose levels and repeat screening every 3 years if the results are normal.[1] Diabetes is usually diagnosed on the basis of having a fasting plasma glucose level > 7.0 mmol/L (126 mg/dL) on two occasions or a random glucose level of > 11.1 mmol/L (200 mg/dL) in conjunction with symptoms of diabetes mellitus.[1] Oral glucose tolerance tests are not used routinely because of the time and expense involved, even though elevation of postprandial glucose may develop before fasting glucose levels are abnormal. Diabetes is present when the 2-hour postprandial glucose is > 11.1 mmol/L (200 mg/dL) after a 75-g glucose challenge. A glucose tolerance test in patients at risk for CVD can help identify those who may have diabetes based on postprandial values but whose fasting glucose levels are below the threshold for the diagnosis of diabetes. Such patients should have more rigorous treatment of the CVD risk factors associated with diabetes even though being labeled as having diabetes earlier may result in emotional distress.

In 2003, a fasting glucose level between 5.5 and 6.9 mmol/L (100 and 125 mg/dL) became the criterion for diagnosing impaired fasting glucose (IFG). Having IFG clearly warrants checking fasting glucose levels more frequently than every 3 years.[1] Diabetes screening should occur before 45 years of age and more frequently in patients with obesity, a family history of diabetes (i.e., parent or sibling), dyslipidemia with a high-density-lipoprotein (HDL) cholesterol level < 0.90 mmol/L (35 mg/dL) and/or triglyceride level > 2.82 mmol/L (250 mg/dL), hypertension > 140/90 mm Hg, gestational diabetes or delivery of babies > 4.09 kg (9.0 lb), and being from an ethnic/racial group with a high prevalence of diabetes (e.g., African Americans, Hispanic Americans, Native Americans, Asian Americans, and Pacific Islanders).[1]

PREDIABETES

Increased risk for cardiovascular disease develops in the prediabetic state, which is considered to be either impaired fasting glucose or impaired glucose tolerance (after a glucose load). Prospective cohort data indicate that impaired glucose tolerance is associated with more than a doubling of cardiovascular risk.[16] The identification of impaired fasting glucose is more readily achieved, but it may be less predictive than impaired glucose tolerance with respect to CVD risk. An estimated 20 million adults in the United States have impaired fasting glucose with a level of 5.5 to 6.9 mmol/L (100 to 125 mg/dL).[1,5] Efforts to reduce the public health burden focus on reducing glycemic exposure by intervening in individuals at high risk for developing diabetes with impaired fasting or glucose tolerance.

CLASSIFICATION OF DIABETES

Diabetes is classified into two basic categories, one for the inability to produce insulin and the other for defects in insulin utilization; this typology, however, does not fully characterize the etiology of blood glucose elevation.[1] Advances in human genomics have broadened our understanding of the wide array of genes expressed in the multiple steps of blood glucose regulation. Such genes may regulate one of the many steps involved in metabolism before or after glucose reaches cells to be utilized for energy. An individual with diabetes may have a defect in expression in one or more of these genes.

TYPE 1 DIABETES MELLITUS

About 5 to 10% of individuals known to have diabetes are characterized as being ketosis-prone because their inability to produce insulin results in an absolute insulin deficiency.[1] Without exogenous insulin to facilitate the entry of glucose into cells, the body must use fat for energy. Polyuria, polydipsia, and polyphasia develop as classic symptoms of an absolute insulin deficiency. Ironically, almost half of new cases are diagnosed after 20 years of age, even though type 1 diabetes is usually associated with diagnosis during childhood or adolescence and was historically known as juvenile-onset diabetes. Type 1 diabetes is considered to be a T-cell–mediated autoimmune disease affecting the beta cells in the pancreatic islets of Langerhans. Viruses such coxsackie, mumps, and rubella can trigger an autoimmune response to the beta cells; heavy metals and other toxins can directly damage them.

Aggregation of type 1 diabetes in families led to identification of histocompatibility leukocyte antigen (HLA) alleles. The autoantibodies to islet cells and insulin are specific, while the glutamic acid decarboxylase (GAD) may represent a more generalized autoimmunity.[1] A wide array of dietary factors may interact with other environmental factors, which results in the development of antibodies. This process is partially genetically modulated in the development of type 1 diabetes.[7] A remission or "honeymoon" period of up to 12 months may occur after the clinical onset of type 1 diabetes and the initiation of insulin therapy, but this remission ends with a gradual permanent loss of the capacity to produce insulin. Current research is focusing on genetic linkage studies and antibody biomarkers in individuals at high risk for type 1 diabetes. Research studies are also focusing on intensive insulin and other interventions, such as immunosuppressive therapy, to prevent the development or delay the onset of overt type 1 diabetes in high-risk individuals.

TYPE 2 DIABETES MELLITUS

Type 2 diabetes, which accounts for 80 to 95% of all cases, is linked to insulin resistance, obesity, and inadequate compensatory production of insulin by the pancreatic beta cells.[1,8–10] The initial symptoms in type 2 diabetes may unfortunately be secondary to the development of complications and include poor wound healing, blurred vision, recurrent gum or bladder infections, and changes in hand or foot sensation. Many individuals with type 2 diabetes have asymptomatic glucose elevations, which can readily be detected by a routine blood test but may go undetected until complications develop.

When indigenous populations are lean, the rates of diabetes are low; but the rate of diabetes and obesity dramatically increases with industrialization, which is often accompanied by urban poverty.[3,5,6,8,12–15] Reduced physical activity and increased intake of energy-dense processed foods are environmental triggers for the expression of genetic predisposition. Compared to Caucasians, the risk for developing type 2 diabetes is twofold greater in African Americans, 2.5-fold greater in Hispanic Americans, and fivefold greater in Native Americans.[3,5,9,16] Other population groups at high risk for developing type 2 diabetes include Asian Indians and Pacific Islanders. Vulnerable population groups appear to have an even greater risk of developing diabetes with the relatively rapid lifestyle changes, often occurring within a generation. Epidemiological and experimental animal data suggest that overcompensation for early undernutrition during fetal development or early infancy may increase insulin resistance beyond what would be expected from obesity alone and may also alter beta-cell insulin production.

The endocrine functions of fat tissue play an important role in insulin resistance and diabetes risk. Android fat distribution is associated with greater insulin resistance than gynoid fat distribution.[9] Fat tissue, especially visceral fat, can secrete hormones that signal a wider range of reactions involved in energy metabolism. Leptin was the first hormone identified in adipose tissue and may play a less important role in diabetes than more recently identified ones. These hormones include tumor necrosis factor alpha, which plays a key role in insulin resistance; adiponectin, which is a collagen-like protein that appears to improve insulin sensitivity; and resistin, which appear to counterregulate adiponectin and increase insulin resistance.[2,4,6] Visceral fat accumulation [usually assessed based on a waist of > 89 cm (35 inches) in women and > 102 cm (40 inches) in men] is associated with increased insulin resistance and a metabolic syndrome characterized by increased risk of diabetes, hypertension, and dyslipidemia.[9]

The lipid disorder associated with insulin resistance is characterized by elevated triglyceride levels, reduced HDL cholesterol levels, and higher concentrations of the highly atherogenic small, dense LDL cholesterol particles. Visceral fat is associated with intrahepatic and intramuscular fat deposition, which also appears to play an important role in the secretion of the hormones involved in insulin sensitivity and resistance.

A number of genetic mutations appear to play a role in the development of the metabolic alterations associated with type 2 diabetes. Linkage studies of families with maturity-onset diabetes of the young (MODY), a rare disorder, has led to identification of the glucokinase gene, which is involved in glucose sensing, and three additional genetic mutations.[1] The risk of developing type 2 diabetes is associated with the mutation of several genes involved in energy metabolism. These genes include those involved in the regulation of glucose transport (glut1-4), glycogen synthetase, the beta 3 adrenergic receptor, lipoprotein lipase, fatty acid binding protein 2, apolipoprotein E, and insulin receptor substrate 1.[1,12] Genetic mutations associated with efficient energy utilization, which would permit survival during famine, have been termed the thrifty genotype. These genetic mutations, however, appear to increase risk of developing obesity and diabetes in population groups such as the Pima Indians when they are exposed to a calorically dense diet and a sedentary lifestyle. Diabetes is occurring at a younger age, often during or even before puberty, in the very overweight youth of African, Hispanic, Asian, and Pacific Islander descent as well as in Native Americans.[11]

NUTRITION AND TREATMENT GOALS

Medical nutrition therapy (MNT) is important in diabetes prevention, from reducing the risk of developing overt diabetes (primary prevention) to preventing and controlling complications (secondary and tertiary prevention). Weight loss is the key strategy for preventing conversion to overt diabetes in high-risk individuals. The treatment goals for overt diabetes are to prevent complications through metabolic control and reduce end-organ damage through early detection of complications and their treatment. Treatment approaches to diabetes vary considerably and often fail to achieve goals for metabolic control. Glycemic control is central to preventing retinopathy and nephropathy, which are the primary diabetic microvascular complications. Large-vessel diabetic complications—which become manifest as cardiac, cerebral, and peripheral vascular disease—are associated with dyslipidemia and hypertension as well as hyperglycemia.

Neuropathic complications of diabetes can affect virtually all body systems. Neuropathy can lead to orthostatic hypotension, with a rapid fall in blood pressure on standing, gastric paresis leading to vomiting or lower bowel dysfunction, and sensory loss. When loss of protective sensation leads to undetected injuries, peripheral vascular disease (PVD) can readily result in the amputation of a lower limb. The assessment of nutrition and physical activity must address the way in which diabetic complications have affected activities of daily living, with emphasis on exercise and dietary habits.

Clinical trials in both type 1 and type 2 diabetes indicate that the improvement of glycemic control greatly reduces the development and progression rates for microvascular and neuropathic complications and may improve beta-cell function.[18–25] In the Diabetes Control and Complications Trial (DCCT), which was conducted in 1,441 patients with type 1 diabetes, intensive treatment achieved an HbA1c of 7.2%, compared to 9% with conventional treatment.[18] The reduction in HBA1c was associated with a 76% age-adjusted risk reduction for retinopathy and a 54% reduction for renal disease progression. Intensive treatment also reduced the occurrence of clinical albuminuria (urinary albumin excretion > 3,000 mg/24 hr) by 54% and clinical neuropathy by 60%.[18] The reduction in the risk of complications was proportional to the decrease in HbA1c, with a reduction in complications being seen before reaching the normal glycemic range.[21] The United Kingdom Prospective Diabetes Study (UKPDS) provided evidence that improvements in glycemic control and blood pressure in newly diagnosed patients with type 2 diabetes can reduce the risk of macrovascular complications.[22–25]

WEIGHT-LOSS TREATMENT AND PREDIABETES

The evidence from multiple research studies suggests that addressing obesity and overweight is the most effective strategy for treating impaired fasting glucose or impaired glucose tolerance.[26–28] This research continues to examine how weight loss will affect concomitant cardiovascular risk. The Da Quing IGT and Diabetes study provided preliminary evidence that diet and exercise intervention lowered the conversion to overt diabetes over a 6-year period.[28] The Diabetes Prevention Program (DPP), a randomized controlled clinical trial conducted in 3,234 individuals with impaired glucose tolerance, demonstrated that the incidence of diabetes could be reduced by 58% over a 3-year period with a 7% weight loss.[17] The 3-year reduction in diabetes incidence with weight loss was almost double the 31% reduction achieved with metformin, a medication that increases insulin sensitivity.[17] The Finnish Diabetes Prevention Study also achieved a 58% reduction in the incidence of type 2 diabetes with lifestyle intervention.[27]

DIABETES MEDICATIONS

The pharmaceutical industry is actively pursing the development of medication to improve metabolic control.[29] Table 17-1 lists insulin preparations and provides an overview of the option with respect to the onset, peak, and duration of action of each drug. Newer insulin preparations are designed to reduce the risk of hypoglycemia. New rapid-acting insulin can be taken when food is eaten rather than trying to judge how long before a meal insulin should be taken. Some of the very long-acting preparations are designed to have no peak and can thereby better mimic the effects on basal insulin secretion.

A growing number of oral pharmaceutical agents are available as antidiabetic drugs. Table 17-2 provides an overview of the oral medications used in type 2 diabetes. These include sulfonylureas, biguanides, thiazolidinediones, meglitinides, and alpha-glucosidase inhibitors. An increasing number of patients are on two or more of these medications so as to address the multiple defects involved in type 2 diabetes. MNT can help optimize metabolic control and reduce potential medication side effects.

Sulfonylureas are widely used and, until recently, were the only class of anti-hyperglycemia agents available in the United States. Sulfonylureas enhance insulin secretion; they include tolbutamide, chlorpropamide, tolazamide, glipizide, glipizide-XL, glyburide, glyburide-micronized, and glimepiride. The most common side effects of sulfonylureas are hypoglycemia and weight gain.

Meglitidines can lower glucose by stimulating insulin secretion, but they are not sulfonylureas. Insulin is secreted in the presence of glucose; therefore, the instructions for use include taking meglitidines with meals.

Biguanides reduce hepatic glucose output; metformin is the only one currently available in the United States. The most common side effects of metformin are transient gastrointestinal discomfort, diarrhea, and nausea, which can be reduced by taking it with meals. Lactic acidosis is a rare but potentially fatal side effect because biguanides impair clearance of lactate and may also increase lactate production.

TABLE 17-1	Action Patterns of Insulins			
INSULINS	**BRAND NAME**	**ONSET OF ACTION**	**PEAK ACTION**	**DURATION OF ACTION**
Very rapid acting				
Insulin aspart analogue	NovoLog	10–20 min	0.5–2.5 hr	3–5 hr
Insulin lispro analogue	Humalog	10–20 min	0.5–2.5 hr	3–5 hr
Regular insulin	Humulin R Novolin R	30–40 min	2–4 hr	5–7 hr
Intermediate-acting				
NPH insulin	Humulin N Novolin N	1–3 hr	4–10 hr	14–24 hr
Lente insulin	Humulin L	2–4 hr	4–15 hr	16–24 hr
Long-acting				
Ultralente insulin	Humulin U	3–4 hr	8–14 hr	18–24 hr
Insulin glargine	Lantus	1–2 hr	No peak	~ 24 hr

TABLE 17-2   Oral Antidiabetic Medications: Mechanisms of Action and Side Effects

MEDICATION CLASS AND MECHANISM OF ACTION	GENERIC NAME	BRAND NAME	COMMENTS AND SIDE EFFECTS
Sulfonylureas: Stimulate the pancreatic beta cell to produce more insulin	Chlorpropamide, first-generation	Diabinese	Use with caution in the elderly. May cause hypoglycemia.
	Tolazamide, first-generation	Tolinase	May cause hypoglycemia.
	Glyburide, second-generation	Micronase Diabeta Glynase Pres Tab	Take 1 to 2 times a day. May cause hypoglycemia.
	Glipizide, second-generation	Glucotrol Glucotrol XL	Take 2 times a day or once with XL. May cause hypoglycemia.
	Glimepiride, third-generation	Amaryl	Take 1 time a day. May cause hypoglycemia.
Biguanides: Reduce output of glucose from the liver.	Metformin	Glucophage	Contraindicated in patients with congestive heart failure or renal/liver problems. Check creatinine clearance if over 65 years of age.
Alpha-glucosidase inhibitors: Delay and blocks absorption of carbohydrate containing foods	Acarbose Miglitol	Precose Glyset	May have side effects in the gastrointestinal tract.
Thiazolidinediones: Enhance insulin sensitivity	Rosiglitazone Pioglitazone	Avandia Actos	Fluid retention, which can lead to congestive heart failure in the elderly or other high-risk patients. Reduced effectiveness of birth control pills. Contraindicated in liver disease. Liver enzymes must be checked on an ongoing basis.
Meglitinides: Enhance insulin secretion in the presence of glucose.	Repaglinide	Prandin	Take with each meal. May cause hypoglycemia.

Metformin is contraindicated for patients with moderate renal insufficiency (serum creatinine > 0.16 mmol/L), but there is some risk of lactic acid accumulation in more moderate renal disease. Lactic acid levels are likely to be increased when excessive alcohol is consumed and also during acute illness. Physical activity can increase lactate levels, but normally functioning kidneys can generally excrete the lactate produced. Omitting metformin for a day or more during acute illness or if a large quantity of alcohol has been consumed reduces the risk of developing lactic acidosis. A small weight loss may occur with metformin therapy; this may be accompanied by a modest decrease in triglyceride, LDL cholesterol, and total cholesterol levels and a modest rise in HDL cholesterol level.

Thiazolidinediones, which enhance insulin sensitivity without directly affecting insulin secretion, include rosiglitazone and pioglitazone. Weight gain has been reported with thiazolidinedione therapy, even though insulin secretion is not enhanced. Fluid retention and weight gain are common in patients on thiazolidinedione therapy. In some cases, the fluid retention can result in congestive heart failure. Patients most at risk for this adverse affect are elderly, insulin-treated patients.

The alpha-glucosidase inhibitors lower blood glucose by inhibiting glucose absorption from the gut after meals; they also reduce postprandial hyperglycemia. Acarbose and miglitol are currently available in the United States. Absorption of dextrins, maltose, sucrose, and starch is reduced, but there is no effect on lactose and glucose absorption. Flatulence, abdominal pain, and diarrhea are common side effects that can be reduced by beginning therapy at a low dose, slowly titrating the dosage, and decreasing carbohydrate intake.

Insulin is also often used in type 2 diabetes as adjunctive therapy when the use of oral agents does not lead to glycemic control. A bedtime dose of long-acting insulin is frequently used to help reduce fasting glucose levels.

DIABETES MEDICAL NUTRITION THERAPY

MNT should begin with an assessment of how lifestyle influences metabolic measures related to diabetes and its comorbidities.[1,30,31] This assessment also addresses the interrelationship of lifestyle and medications as they affect the metabolic parameters. The concept of instructing patients to follow the diabetic diet is clearly outdated and grossly oversimplifies the issues that must be addressed in MNT. Medicaid, Medicare, and other third-party payers cover MNT provided by registered dietitians.[1] A wide variety of educational tools are used in conjunction with MNT. The diabetes exchange system was the primary tool used in teaching patients for many years, but carbohydrate counting and other tools are widely used today in MNT for diabetes mellitus.

MNT APPROACH IN TYPE 1 DIABETES

MNT for type 1 diabetes focuses on matching insulin treatment to usual lifestyle and the pattern of normal endogenous insulin secretion. The potential to match insulin action to lifestyle has vastly improved with increasingly sophisticated blood glucose monitoring and insulin delivery systems.[1,30,31] Nutrition counseling in the DCCT intensively treated group was highly individualized, and dietary behaviors associated with better glycemic control included adherence to overall meal plan (timing and amount of carbohydrate); appropriate treatment of hypoglycemia (avoiding excessive consumption of carbohydrate to treat symptoms); prompt intervention for hyperglycemia (more insulin and/or less food); and consistent consumption of planned evening snacks.[33] MNT guidelines for tailoring intervention in type 1 diabetes are available.[34] The initial insulin dose in type 1 diabetes is often calculated on the basis of body weight, with approximately 0.5 to 0.6 units of insulin per kilogram per day, approximately half for basal needs and half as boluses for meals and snacks; the amount needed for boluses would be reduced if an individual ate very little carbohydrate. The exact needs are estimated by evaluating blood glucose patterns with a consistent lifestyle to the extent feasible while focusing on carbohydrate intake (eating time and amounts), physical activity (time, duration, and intensity), insulin (time and dosage), and other factors that may influence blood glucose. The blood glucose patterns can then be used to better estimate insulin requirements and to adjust insulin to lifestyle changes. Gradually, algorithms can be developed to adjust insulin for changes in carbohydrate intake or physical activity.

MNT APPROACH IN TYPE 2 DIABETES

Reducing cardiovascular risk is a primary goal for MNT in type 2 diabetes.[1,30,31] Diet and exercise are considered to be the cornerstones of diabetes management, with emphasis on improving the dyslipidemia associated with diabetes as well as other cardiovascular risk factors associated with overweight and obesity.[35] The Look-AHEAD (Action for Health in Diabetes) trial is an ongoing study to determine how much intensive lifestyle intervention and weight loss add to the risk reduction in patients with type 2 diabetes.[36] An earlier meta-analysis of lifestyle intervention weight-loss studies in type 2 diabetes indicated that dietary intervention (often very low-calorie diets) achieved weight loss and improved glycemic control.[37] Data from randomized, controlled clinical trials indicate that combining physical activity, dietary change, and behavioral strategies achieves the best long-term weight loss. A modest weight loss of 5 to 10% of body weight has been associated with improvements in glycemic control and cardiovascular risk factors.[9,30,31]

A multinational observational study, which did not evaluate lifestyle, found no improvement in morbidity or mortality associated with weight loss in individuals with type 2 diabetes.[38] It is not known if undetected illness or unhealthy dietary habits may have affected the study results. An evidence-based review concluded undertaking lifestyle changes to lose a modest amount of weight could improve health outcomes.[9]

There is considerable interest in how dietary composition affects weight loss and health outcomes. A study that evaluated the effects of a 381-J (1,600 kcal) isocaloric diet utilizing a 12-week parallel study found that energy restriction independent of dietary composition achieved weight loss and improved glycemic control.[39] Increases in monounsaturated fatty acids and carbohydrate were both effective as substitutes for saturated fat in lowering LDL cholesterol levels. The high-carbohydrate diet reduced HDL cholesterol levels at weeks 4 and 8, but the HDL cholesterol level had returned to the baseline level by week 12. A study by Samaha and colleagues that compared a very low carbohydrate diet with ketosis induction to a low-fat diet included a subset of patients with type 2 diabetes. After 6 and 12 months on the diet, the diabetic patients in the low-carbohydrate arm required less antidiabetes medications and tended to have better HbA1c levels than those in the low-fat arm.[40,41] Additional studies with a larger sample of diabetic patients and a longer follow-up period are needed to assess the long-term efficacy and safety of very low carbohydrates in diabetes management.

Much of the emphasis in type 2 diabetes is on controlling dyslipidemia and hypertension, which are common comorbidities that are linked to cardiovascular risk. Various combinations of antihyperglycemic agents are being used to improve blood glucose levels because monotherapy is usually inadequate.[1] More that one antihypertensive medication is usually needed to control blood pressure. Angiotensin-converting enzyme inhibitors are used in patients who have microalbuminuria. MNT guidelines for the management of type 2 diabetes have been developed and tested in a clinical trial.[42–44]

DIET AND NUTRITION COMPOSITION

Nutrition has been considered important in diabetes management, but specific dietary recommendations have been debated for over 3,500 years. The first diabetes dietary recommendation from Papyrus Ebers in 1550 BC focused on eating carbohydrate-containing foods. Restriction of carbohydrate-containing foods emerged in the sixth century AD. During the 17th and 18th centuries, recommendations varied from replacing sugar loss with a high-carbohydrate diet to eating meat and fat and "avoiding" carbohydrate. During the 19th and early 20th centuries, fasting and measured diabetic diets that limited carbohydrate were widely used, but some patients were treated with higher-carbohydrate diets that focused on potatoes or oatmeal. High-carbohydrates became the preparatory diet for glucose tolerance tests during the 1930s.

By the 1950s the macronutrient goals were 20% protein, 40% fat, and 40% carbohydrate.[26,27] Gradually, recommendations focused on decreasing dietary fat and increasing carbohydrate up to 60% of calories, with a focus on the differing needs of type 1 and 2 diabetes. By 1994, the American Diabetes Association's recommendations began to emphasize the importance of individualization based on dietitian assessment, with no specific recommendations for the balance between total fat and carbohydrate intake.[30,31]

PROTEIN

Decision making about how much protein is desirable in diabetes management is complex. The adult Recommended Dietary Allowance for protein intake (0.8 g/kg per day) is approximately 10% of total daily energy needs, but many adults in the United Stated consume 20 to 30% of calories as protein intake.[30,31,45] Interest is increasing in the role of protein in weight loss, which is vitally important in diabetes management. Some individuals who are trying to lose weight prefer a higher protein intake to reduce the sense of hunger, and the American Diabetes Association has reviewed issues relating weight loss to the intake of protein and other macronutrients.[46] The utilization of protein as energy is less efficient than that of carbohydrate and fat; therefore, an increased intake of protein could theoretically have a metabolic advantage with regard to weight loss.

The risk of renal complications also needs to be addressed. The renal solute load is increased when protein is metabolized as an energy source, but a higher protein intake may be associated with better metabolic control for many patients with diabetes. The Modification of Diet in Renal Disease (MDRD) study evaluated the effects of dietary protein restriction and strict blood pressure control in patients with both advanced and moderate renal disease, but the study did not focus on diabetic nephropathy.[47–50] Although the overall results of the MDRD study were inconclusive, secondary analyses suggested that reducing protein intake by 0.2 g/kg per day was associated with a reduction of 1.15 mL/min per year in the decline of the glomerular filtration rate (GFR), thus prolonging the time to renal failure by 41%. When patients with diabetes exhibit renal insufficiency, reducing protein intake to 0.6 g/kg per day in selected high-risk patients may slow the rate of GFR decline, which is consistent with the conclusions of the MDRD study.[50]

OVERALL DISTRIBUTION OF CALORIES, FAT, AND CARBOHYDRATE

The macronutrient distribution in diabetes management can be fairly fluid, and monitoring glucose and lipid levels can help guide recommendations for individual patients.[30,31] Monitoring carbohydrate intake is usually needed to control postprandial glycemic excursions in type 1 diabetes and gestational diabetes. In type 2 diabetes, monitoring postprandial glucose can also help determine the level of emphasis that should be placed on carbohydrate intake.[1,30,31] Decreasing dietary fat and increasing carbohydrate intake can potentially worsen the dyslipidemia of type 2 diabetes by lowering HDL-cholesterol levels and increasing the level of very low density lipoprotein (VLDL) cholesterol, triglyceride, and small, dense, LDL cholesterol particles.[27,35,51,52] Increasing fat intake, however, especially from fast foods and snack foods, can easily result in a higher calorie intake. In an isocaloric feeding study, feeding a diet higher in monounsaturated fatty acids and a higher-carbohydrate diet rich in fiber had similar effects on the lipid profile and lipoprotein subfractions.[51] An energy-restricted dietary comparison of these approaches yielded similar results.[38]

TYPE OF FAT

Fatty-acid double bonds are important in lipid metabolism, and selected omega-3 fatty acids appear to play a key role in cardiac electrophysiology. Both monounsaturated and polyunsaturated fatty acids reduce LDL cholesterol levels, but they may differ with respect to their effects on HDL cholesterol level. Reducing intake of total fat, and saturated fatty acids in particular, tends to further reduce the low HDL cholesterol level associated with insulin resistance and diabetes.[27] Weight loss may ameliorate this effect. Reducing saturated fat intake and increasing polyunsaturated fat tends to reduce HDL cholesterol as well. Monounsaturated fat may have a lesser tendency for reducing HDL cholesterol. A metaanalysis of dietary intervention studies in type 2 diabetes found that diets rich in highly monounsaturated fats reduced VLDL cholesterol and triglyceride levels without adversely affecting body weight or other lipids.[52] However, a direct comparison of monounsaturated fatty acids with polyunsaturated fatty acids was beyond the scope of the analyses. One review suggests that all unsaturated fatty acids are efficacious in lowering LDL cholesterol and that the lowering of HDL cholesterol is related to a reduction in total dietary fat and saturated fatty acid.[53]

Hydrogenization of the cis isomer of fatty acids in oils creates trans isomers that function more like saturated fatty acids in food products and potentially in the human body. Individuals with diabetes and/or other CVD risk factors should consider trans fatty acid intake as part of saturated fatty acid intake because of the similarity in their effects on CVD risk.[54]

Omega-3 fatty acids from fish may play an important role in reducing cardiovascular complications of diabetes. Population groups that have a high fish intake have lower rates of diabetes and cardiovascular disease. Fatty acids from fish and other sources such as flax seed that have the double bond in the omega-3 position reduce triglyceride production.[55] Omega-3 fatty acids also appear to reduce risk of arrhythmias and sudden death. Early feeding studies raised questions about the potential of omega-3 fatty acids to raise blood glucose levels and LDL cholesterol levels.[30,31] A metaanalysis of diabetes-related clinical trials has indicated that omega-3 fatty acids can reduce fasting triglyceride levels by 39%, with a slight increase (~ 2%) in LDL cholesterol and no change in HbA1c levels.[55]

TYPE OF CARBOHYDRATE AND CALORIC SWEETENERS

The type of dietary carbohydrate should be examined with respect to how it affects overall dietary intake and the results of blood glucose monitoring. Postprandial hyperglycemia is a major concern in the management of diabetes.[1,6,30,31] Based on studies conducted in the 1970s and 1980s, the American Diabetes Association concluded that mono- and disaccharides did not result in higher postprandial glycemic response than polysaccharides.[30,31,56] The glycemic effect of carbohydrate-containing foods has been studied extensively and is the source of considerable debate.[57,58] Although the American Diabetes Association's nutrition recommendations indicate that sugar consumption should be based on overall nutrition considerations,[30,31] the American Heart Association has raised concerns that consumption of large quantities of sugar-containing soft drinks and other beverage products is a major cause of obesity and can also present challenges with respect to balancing insulin action to the carbohydrate load.[56] The dramatic increase in the consumption of sugared beverages is of concern in the development of obesity and diabetes as well as in diabetes management. The federal 2005 Dietary Guidelines[59] recommend choosing carbohydrate wisely and suggest that consumption of excess sweets may contribute to the rise in obesity; the guidelines, however, also allow for discretional calories as sugar, with the amount varying on the basis of calorie needs.

Advanced glycosylation end products (AGEs) are associated with increases in factors associated with an increased risk of diabetes complications, AGEs can result from poor diabetes control or, through nonenzymatic glycosylation, from heating foods.[56,60,61] One feeding study using an experimental diet high in AGEs has demonstrated higher circulating levels of AGEs and an increase in inflammatory mediators associated with diabetic complications.[60] In this study, the high-AGE foods were created by browning and other methods of high-temperature cooking. Fats used in frying or exposed to high heat had the highest AGE content, with a mean of 100 ± 19 kU/g. Meat and meat substitutes also had high levels, especially when they were broiled, with an average AGE level of 43 ± 7 kU/g for the meat group. Foods that were predominately carbohydrate contained the lowest values of AGEs at 3.4 ± 1.8 kU/g.[61] The amount of AGEs present in all food categories was related to cooking temperature, length of cooking time, and presence of moisture. Although only about 10% of ingested advanced glycation end products enter the circulation, they are excreted slowly, especially in diabetes.[60] Research is needed to determine whether dietary changes to reduce AGE intake can actually reduce the risk of diabetic complications.

Fructose, mannitol, and sorbitol are often substituted for sucrose in "sugar-free" products. They can shift the balance from oxidation of fatty acids to esterification of fatty acids in the liver, which can in turn increase the synthesis of very low density lipoprotein.[56] The effects on lipids appear to be inconsistent, but susceptible individuals may have a worsening of dyslipidemia. These sweeteners appear to offer no advantage in the management of diabetes over other carbohydrate sources, especially with respect to calorie control.

Considerable debate exists over the clinical importance of the postprandial glycemic effects of carbohydrate-containing foods.[6,57,58] The glycemic index refers to the rise in plasma glucose after a 50-g carbohydrate load from the food or from a reference carbohydrate source (initially oral glucose and subsequently using white bread as the reference food). Food processing decreases particle size and thereby increases the glycemic index of a food. The chemical complexity of the carbohydrate is not related to the postprandial glycemic response. For example, many starches, which are polysaccharides, have higher glycemic indices than sugars, which are disaccharides or monosaccharides. The type of starch also affects the glycemic index. Amylose has a lower glycemic index than amylopectin because the amylose is a straight chain glucose molecule that is not as readily gelatinized as the highly branched glucose chains in amylopectin. Legumes, which are high in amylose and soluble fiber, have a lower glycemic index. The glycemic indices of mixed foods are also tested, and the glycemic load of a meal or the diet is sometimes calculated by multiplying the glycemic index by the number of grams of carbohydrate in the serving, meal, or day's intake of food.[62,63]

Prospective cohort data from the Nurses and the Physician Health Studies suggest that eating a diet that has a lower glycemic load is associated with a lower risk of developing diabetes.[64,65] Preliminary evidence suggests that foods with a lower glycemic index may provide greater satiety and reduce energy intake in obese individuals. Some studies suggest that the effects of lowering the glycemic load extend to improving lipid levels and potentially to other indices of cardiovascular risk, such as fibrinolytic activity.[62,63] Additional research is needed to assess the long-term clinical significance of these studies. Public awareness is growing of the glycemic index, and glycemic index rating systems are being incorporated into food labels in Australia and elsewhere.[63]

The term "net" carbohydrate is used to describe the metabolically available carbohydrate in food products. Net carbohydrate, which may appear on the front of the food package label rather than as part of the nutrition facts panel, is calculated by subtracting the grams of fiber and in some cases the sugar alcohols from the total carbohydrate content.[6,68] The Office of Policy and Program Development of the U.S. Department of Agriculture's (USDA) Food Safety and Inspection Service issued an interim policy on carbohydrate labeling in 2003.[68] The text of the interim policy states that the USDA:

> does not object to terms such as "Net Carbs," "Effective Carbs," and "Net Impact Carbs" when used in a manner that is truthful and not misleading. Because there are no regulatory definitions for these terms, they must be accompanied by specific information informing the consumer of the meaning of the use of such terms on labeling and providing the calculation necessary to determine the number of carbohydrates included by the term. Furthermore, terms such as "Low Carbohydrate" may be used in ad copy on labeling in conjunction with terms used to describe a diet or lifestyle (not a particular food or product), provided they are used in a manner that is truthful and not misleading.

Although fructose, sorbitol, and mannitol are alcohol sweeteners used in products promoted as "sugar free," they are not calorie free. As the cost of fructose has decreased, high-fructose syrups have been widely used as sweeteners in soft drinks, fruit drinks, etc. The low cost of such products appears to play a role on the dramatic rise in the intake of sweetened beverages, which is linked to the obesity epidemic. Alternately, high-intensity sweeteners are considered virtually noncaloric; they include aspartame, saccharin, acesulfame potassium, sucralose, and neotame. These products can be readily used to control energy and carbohydrate intake from beverages and other sweetened food products.

FAT SUBSTITUTES

Reduced-fat and fat-free products were widely promoted during the 1990s after a variety of fat substitutes were approved by the FDA.[69,70] These fat substitutes mimic one or more of the roles of fat in a food. They may be protein-based (usually from egg white or whey), carbohydrate-based (from modified starches, dextrins, or maltodextrins), or fat-based (from emulsifiers replacing triglycerides with mono- or disaccharides or from modification to achieve a partially absorbable or nonabsorbable fat). Issues to consider in diabetes management include the calorie content and energy density of food products that contain fat substitutes. Some food products containing fat substitutes are higher in energy density than the original full-fat product.[69]

ETHANOL

Intake of alcohol can lower or raise blood glucose based on the availability of insulin. The overall recommendations with regard to alcohol intake for people with diabetes are consistent with general health recommendations.[1] Alcohol can inhibit hepatic glucose production and cause hypoglycemia if it is consumed without food, especially by individuals who are treated with insulin or sulfonylureas. Alcohol can therefore increase the risk of hypoglycemia. Hypoglycemia is also a manifestation of hepatic failure because of failure of gluconeogenesis and depletion of glycogen stores.

Consumption of large quantities of alcohol can increase insulin resistance and result in hyperglycemia if the pancreas cannot produce enough insulin to compensate for the insulin resistance. In individuals with diabetes, hyperglycemia can occur acutely after binge drinking; it is a common manifestation of early chronic liver disease due to increased insulin resistance.[70] Alcohol intake can also increase risks associated with pancreatitis, hypertriglyceridemia, neuropathy, myocardiopathy, and renal failure.

MICRONUTRIENTS

The role of micronutrients in diabetes management warrants careful consideration.[71–82] The interrelationship between diabetes and micronutrients is reciprocal. Poorly controlled diabetes can alter vitamin and mineral status, and alterations in micronutrients can affect glucose and overall energy homeostasis.[74,75]

Chromium is found in tissues throughout the body. A chromium-containing compound commonly known as glucose tolerance factor is involved in glucose homeostasis. Severe chromium deficiency is associated with glucose intolerance.

In a randomized controlled clinical trial conducted in patients with type 2 diabetes in China, supplemental chromium reduced fasting glucose, HbA1c, insulin, and cholesterol levels.[72] In an uncontrolled study of 13 patients treated with corticosteroids, chromium picolinate supplementation reduced the rise in fasting glucose and the need for antihyperglycemic medication.[73] Most patients with diabetes do not appear to be chromium deficient, however, and further studies are needed to determine for whom chromium supplementation could improve carbohydrate metabolism.

Magnesium modulates glucose transport across cell membranes. Poorly controlled diabetes can induce hypomagnesemia by increasing urinary excretion, and hypomagnesemia can increase insulin resistance. The clinical usefulness of supplementation, which is usually by intake of magnesium-based antacids, for patients with type 2 diabetes and insulin resistance is not established.

The B vitamin group, particularly thiamine, riboflavin, niacin, and vitamin B_6, are involved in glucose metabolism. Requirements of these may be altered by excess excretion in poorly controlled diabetes. Nicotinic acid can worsen glycemic control when it is used to treat hyperlipidemia, but uncontrolled studies suggest that it may also potentially help protect beta-cell function from autoimmune destruction. Zinc and antioxidant requirements increase during wound healing. Assessment of zinc status is needed for patients with poor wound healing, and supplementation may be clinically indicated.

Antioxidants such as vitamin E, beta-carotene, and vitamin C could potentially play a role in preventing diabetic complications. One small study found that vitamin E supplementation improved retinal blood flow and creatinine clearance but did not improve indices of metabolic control.[76] More research is needed to thoroughly evaluate the potential risk as well as benefits of vitamin E and other antioxidant supplementation for reducing oxidative stress and protein glycosylation associated with diabetic complications. The American Diabetes Association recommends individualizing assessment to determine who may need vitamin or mineral supplements.[1] The potential role of antioxidants in insulin resistance is unclear. Recent data from the NHANES III suggest that serum beta-carotene and lycopene levels may be inversely related to glucose tolerance and fasting insulin levels.[77] Vitamin C appeared to have a similar relationship, which was largely accounted for on the basis of dietary intake and other covariates.[78] Elevated fasting homocysteine levels appear to be a biomarker for macrovascular but not for microvascular complications of diabetes.[79] Folate and vitamin B_{12} levels play a role in homocysteine metabolism, and plasma levels of these nutrients are inversely related to homocysteine levels. The 2005 Dietary Guidelines emphasize the importance of vegetables, fruits, whole grains, and enrichment/fortification of grains for disease prevention in the general population.[59] In NHANES III, an elevated serum ferritin level was associated with an increased risk of diabetes. This observed relationship may be an indication of inflammation or possibly of a potential role of excess body iron stores in diabetes pathophysiology.

Poorly controlled diabetes and diabetic complications can affect micronutrient requirements. Fluid loss associated with hyperglycemia is associated with increased excretion of water-soluble vitamins. Wound healing can increase requirements for zinc and vitamins A, C, and E. Data from a recent randomized controlled clinical trial indicate that a daily multivitamin mineral supplement decreased the infection rate and lost days of productivity for patients with diabetes.[71]

CHALLENGES FOR THE FUTURE

Medical and technological advances have shifted much of the decision making and care responsibility to patients. Changes in third-party reimbursement have expanded access to MNT, blood glucose monitoring supplies, and diabetes self-management training (DSMT). Patients are increasingly assuming responsibility for treatment intensification to control blood glucose and other metabolic abnormalities, such as dyslipidemia and high blood pressure. Multiple medications are usually used to achieve the treatment goals of a HbA1c of < 7%, LDL cholesterol of < 100 mg/dL, and blood pressure of 120/80 mm Hg. Advocacy has continued to improve third-party coverage of diabetes care and education, but reimbursement policy cannot meet the emerging diabetes-related public health burden.

Current research has advanced understanding of the mechanisms of pharmacological agents, and a growing number of products derived from plants are being explored for their potential medicinal value. Traditional herbal products from China, India, and elsewhere are being evaluated to isolate the biochemical components that have medicinal properties.[81-94] As scientific knowledge advances, a growing number of these isolated compounds are being patented to protect the potential profits that may be gained from new pharmacological agents derived from these compounds.

The National Institutes of Health and other agencies are studying how the herbal and other traditional remedies of indigenous cultures may be helpful in preventing diabetes and other chronic diseases. Streptozotocin, which destroys the beta cells in the islet of the pancreas, is often used to create animal models of diabetes and to evaluate compounds isolated from a plant that may have pharmacological benefits for diabetes treatment or prevention.

Pharmacological agents are expected to play an important role in the treatment of diabetes, but the needs for those at risk for diabetes are beyond the potential of a medical approach. Therefore, there is a need to address the potential benefits of traditional remedies rather than assuming that a medical approach alone can address diabetes risk.

SUMMARY

Obesity and a sedentary lifestyle are associated with a worldwide increase in the prevalence of diabetes. Government and voluntary agencies in the United States and

Issues to Ponder

- What are the roles of public health and MNT in preventing diabetes?
- How can dietetics professionals help individuals with diabetes use monitoring of postprandial glucose levels to develop strategies for improving glycemic control?
- What is the role of diabetes MNT in addressing medication side effects?
- What are the potential effects of complementary and alternative medicine in diabetes prevention and management?
- What strategies can facilitate patient communication with the diabetes care team in addressing the complex care needs related to preventing diabetes complications?
- What MNT strategies can be used to help achieve diabetes A (HbA1c), B (blood pressure), and C (cholesterol) goals without adversely affecting the patient's quality of life due to medication side effects or dietary restrictions?
- What measures can be applied across the continuum of diabetes care, from preventing diabetes (primary prevention) to preventing and controlling complications (secondary and tertiary prevention)?
- How will the development of medications and monitoring techniques affect MNT in diabetes?

elsewhere are focusing on obesity, diabetes, and sedentary lifestyle as public health problems.

The long-term goal of MNT in diabetes is to prevent and/or delay diabetic complications by restoring metabolism as close to normal as possible. The focus is on adjusting energy intake and expenditure to achieve a modest weight loss of approximately 10% and reducing the impact of CVD risk factors such as hypertension and dyslipidemia. The distribution of macronutrient intake may vary based on a number of factors, including matching insulin to lifestyle in type 1 diabetes and reducing cardiovascular risk factors in type 2 diabetes. An assessment of micronutrient status is needed for patients in poor control, with complications, or with other evidence of being at risk.

There is no one diabetic diet. MNT should be based on individual assessment and the development of a treatment plan. Ideally, a dietetics professional consults with the healthcare team and the patient, assesses need, and develops an individualized treatment plan that considers overall health needs as well as amelioration of the metabolic effects of diabetes and its complications.

The risk for developing diabetes is closely linked to lifestyle and obesity. Lifestyle is also important in achieving metabolic control. Lifestyle issues must be addressed to reduce the growing global public health burden of diabetes.

REFERENCES

1. American Diabetes Association Position Statement: Standards of Medical Care. Diabetes Care 2005;28:S4–S36.
2. Dago-Jack S. Ethnic disparities in type 2 diabetes: pathophysiology and implications for prevention and management. J Natl Med Assoc 2003;95:774, 779–789.
3. Wild S, Roglic G, Green A, Sicree R, King H. Global prevalence of diabetes: estimates for the year 2000 and projections for 2030. Diabetes Care 2004;27:1047–1053.
4. Laaksonen DE, Niskanen L, Lakka HM, Lakka TA, Uusitupa M. Epidemiology and treatment of the metabolic syndrome. Ann Med 2004;36:332–346.
5. Vinicor F. The public health burden of diabetes and the reality of the limits. Diabetes Care 1998; 21(suppl 3):C15–C18.
6. Wylie-Rosett J, Segal-Isaacson CJ, Segal-Isaacson A. Carbohydrates and increases in obesity: does the type of carbohydrate make a difference? Obes Res 2004;12(suppl 2):124S–129S.
7. Rand JS, Fleeman LM, Farrow HA, Appleton DJ, Lederer R. Canine and feline diabetes mellitus: nature or nurture? J Nutr 2004;134(suppl):2072S–2080S.
8. National Diabetic Education Program. Making systems changes for better diabetes care: executive summary. Available at: http://betterdiabetescare.nih.gov/. Accessed January 14, 2005.
9. Obesity Education Initiative Expert Panel. Clinical guidelines on the identification evaluation, and treatment of overweight and obesity in adults: The evidence report. Washington, DC: US Department of Health and Human Services, Public Health Service, National Institutes of Health, National Heart Lung and Blood Institute. Available at: http://www.nhlbi.nih.gov/guidelines/ obesity/ob_home.htm. Accessed January 14, 2005.
10. Diabetes Prevention Program Research Group. Reduction in the incidence of type 2 diabetes with lifestyle intervention or metformin. N Engl J Med 2002;346:393–403.
11. Rosenbloom AL, Joe JR, Young RS, Winter WE. Emerging epidemic of type 2 diabetes in youth. Diabetes Care 1999;22:345–354.
12. Lobstein T, Baur L, Uauy R. IASO International Obesity Task Force. Obesity in children and young people: a crisis in public health. Obes Rev Obes Rev 2004;5(suppl 1):4–104.
13. Centers for Disease Control and Prevention (CDC). Self-reported concern about food security associated with obesity. Washington, 1995–1999. MMWR 2003;52:840–842.
14. French SA. Pricing effects on food choices. J Nutr 2003;133:841S–843S.
15. Drewnowski A, Specter DE. Poverty and obesity. The role of energy density and energy costs. Am J Clin Nutr 2004;79:6–16.
16. Wei M, Gaskill SP, Haffner SM, Stern MP. Effects of diabetes and level of glycemic control on all-cause mortality. The San Antonio Heart Study. Diabetes Care 1998;21:1167–1172.
17. Poplin BM, Neilson SJ. The sweetening of the world's diet. Obes Res 2003;11:1325–1332.

18. Diabetes Control and Complications Trial Research Group The effect of intensive treatment of diabetes on the development and progression of long-term complications in insulin dependent diabetes mellitus. N Engl J Med 1993;329:977–986.

19. Implications of the Diabetes Control and Complications Trial. Diabetes Control and Complications Trial Research Group. Weight gain associated with intensive therapy in the Diabetes Control and Complications Trial. Diabetes Care 1998;11:567–573.

20. Klein RL, McHenry MB, Lok KH, et al; DCCT/EDIC Research Group. Apolipoprotein C-III protein concentrations and gene polymorphisms in type 1 diabetes: associations with lipoprotein subclasses. Metabolism 2004;53:1296–304.

21. Eastman RC, Harris MI. Is there a glycemic threshold for mortality risk? Diabetes Care 1998;21: 331–333.

22. UK Prospective Diabetes Study Group. Effect of intensive blood-glucose control with metformin on complications in overweight patients with type 2 diabetes (UKPDS 34). Lancet 1998;352:8354–8365.

23. UK Prospective Diabetes Study Group. Tight blood pressure control and risk of macrovascular and microvascular complications in type 2 diabetes (UKPDS 38). BMJ 1998;317:703–713.

24. UK Prospective Diabetes Study Group. Intensive blood-glucose control with sulphonylureas or insulin compared to conventional treatment and risk of complications in patients with type 2 diabetes (UKPDS 33). Lancet 1998;352:837–853.

25. Song SH, Brown PM. Coronary heart disease risk assessment in diabetes mellitus: comparison of UKPDS risk engine with Framingham risk assessment function and its clinical implications. Diabetes Med 2004;21:238–245.

26. Knowler WC, Barrett-Connor E, Fowler SE, et al. Diabetes Prevention Program Research Group. Reduction in the incidence of type 2 diabetes with lifestyle intervention or metformin. N Engl J Med 2002;346:393–403.

27. Tuonilehto J, Lindstrom J, Ericksson JG, et al. for the Finnish Diabetes Study Group. Prevention of type 2 diabetes mellitus by changes in lifestyle among subject with impaired glucose tolerance. N Engl J Med 2001;344:1343–1350.

28. Pan XR, Hu YH, Wang JX, et al. Effect of diet and exercise in preventing NIDDM in people with impaired glucose tolerance. The DaQing IGT and Diabetes Study. Diabetes Care 1997;20: 537–544.

29. Campbell RK, White J, White J Jr. Medications for the Treatment of Diabetes. Alexandria, VA: American Diabetes Association, 2003.

30. American Diabetes Association Position Statement. Nutrition recommendations and principles for people with diabetes mellitus. Diabetes Care 2004;27(suppl 1)S36–S46.

31. Franz MJ, Bantle JP, Beebe CA, et al. Evidence-based nutrition principles and recommendations for the treatment and prevention of diabetes and related complications (technical review). Diabetes Care 2002;25:148–198.

32. Diabetes Control and Complications Trial Research Group. Expanded role of the dietitian in the Diabetes Control and Complications Trial; implications for clinical practice. J Am Diet Assoc 1993;93:758–764.

33. Delehanty L, Halford BH. The role of diet behaviors in achieving improved glycemic control in intensively treated patients in the Diabetes Control and Complications Trial. Diabetes Care 1993;16:1453–1458.

34. Kulkarni K, Castle G, Gregory R, et al. Nutrition Practice Guidelines for type 1 diabetes mellitus positively affect dietitian practice and patient outcomes. The Diabetes Care and Education Dietetic Practice Group. J Am Diet Assoc 1998;98:62–70.

35. American Diabetes Association Position Statement. Management of dyslipidemia in adults with diabetes. Diabetes Care 2004;27(suppl 1):S68–S71.

36. Ryan DH, Espeland MA, Foster GD, et al; Look AHEAD Research Group. Look AHEAD (Action for Health in Diabetes): design and methods for a clinical trial of weight loss for the prevention of cardiovascular disease in type 2 diabetes. Control Clin Trials 2003;24:610–628.

37. Brown AS, Upchurch S, Anding R, Winter M, Rameriz G. Promoting weight loss in type II diabetes. Diabetes Care 1996;19:613–624.

38. Chaturvedi N, Fuller JH. Mortality risk by body weight and weight change in people with NIDDM. The WHO Multinational Study of Vascular Disease in Diabetes. Diabetes Care 1995;18:766–774.

39. Heibronn LK, Noakes M, Clifton PM. Effects of energy restriction, weight loss, and dietary composition on plasma lipids and glucose in patients with type 2 diabetes. Diabetes Care 1999; 22:889–895.

40. Samaha FF, Iqbal N, Seshadri P, et al. Low-carbohydrate as compared with a low-fat diet in severe obesity. N Engl J Med 2003;348:2074–2081.

41. Stern L, Iqbal N, Seshadri P, et al. The effects of low-carbohydrate versus conventional weight loss diets in severely obese adults: one-year follow-up of a randomized trial. Ann Intern Med 2004; 140:778–785.

42. Franz MJ. Practice guidelines for nutrition care by dietetics practitioners for outpatients with non-insulin dependent diabetes mellitus: consensus statement. J Am Diet Assoc 1992;92:1136–1139.

43. Franz MJ, Splett PL, Monk Barry B, et al. Cost-effectiveness of medical nutrition therapy provided by dietitians for persons with non-insulin dependent diabetes mellitus. J Am Diet Assoc 1995;95:1018–1024.

44. Monk A, Barry B, McClain K, Weaver T, Cooper N, Franz MH. Practice guidelines for medical nutrition therapy provided by dietitians for persons with non-insulin dependent diabetes mellitus. J Am Diet Assoc 1995;95:999–1006.

47. Levey AS, Green T, Beck GJ, et al. Dietary protein restriction and the progression of chronic renal disease: what have all of the results of the MDRD study shown? Modification of Diet in Renal Disease Study Group. J Am Soc Nephrol 1999;10:2426–2439.

48. Modification of Diet in Renal Disease Study Group. Effects of dietary protein restriction on the progression of moderate renal disease in the Modification of Diet in Renal Disease Study. J Am Soc Nephrol 1996;7:2616–2626.

49. Menon V, Wang X, Greene T, et al. Relationship between C-reactive protein, albumin, and cardiovascular disease in patients with chronic kidney disease. Am J Kidney Dis 2003;42:44–52.

50. Levey AS, Adler S, Caggiula AW, et al. Effects of dietary protein restriction on the progression of advanced renal disease in the Modification of Diet in Renal Disease Study. Am J Kidney Dis 1996;27:652–666.

51. Milne RM, Mann JL, Chisholm AW, Williams SM. Long-term comparison of three dietary prescriptions in the treatment of NIDDM. Diabetes Care 1994;17:74–80.

52. Garg A. High-monounsaturated-fat diets for patients with diabetes mellitus: a meta-analysis. Am J Clin Nutr 1998;67(suppl 3):577S–582S.

53. Lichtenstein A. Dietary fat and cardiovascular disease risk: quantity or quality? J Women's Health 2003;12:109–114.

54. Christiansen E, Schnider S, Palmvig B, Tauber-Lassen E, Pederson O. Intake of a diet high in trans monounsaturated fatty acids or saturated fatty acids. Effects on postprandial insulinemia and glycemia in obese patients with NIDDM. Diabetes Care 1997;20:881–887.

55. Friedberg CE, Janssen MJ, Heine RJ, Grobbee DE. Fish oil and glycemic control in diabetes: a meta-analysis. Diabetes Care 1998;21:496–500.

56. Howard BV, Wylie-Rosett J. Sugar and cardiovascular disease (American Heart Association Scientific Advisory). Circulation 2002;106:523–527.

57. Brand Miller J, Hayne S, Petocz P, Colagiuri S. Low-glycemic index diets in the management of diabetes: a meta-analysis of randomized controlled trials. Diabetes Care 2003;26:2261–2267.

58. Sheard NF, Clark NG, Brand-Miller JC, et al. Dietary carbohydrate (amount and type) in the prevention and management of diabetes: a statement by the American Diabetes Association. Diabetes Care 2004;27:2266–2271.

59. US Department of Agriculture and US Department of Health and Human Services. 2005 Dietary Guidelines Advisory Committee Report. Dietary Guidelines for Americans 2005. Available at: http://www.health.gov/dietaryguidelines/Default.htm. Accessed January 14, 2005.

60. Vlassara H, Cai W, Crandall J, et al. Inflammatory mediators are induced by dietary glycotoxins, a major risk factor for diabetic angiopathy. Proc Natl Acad Sci USA 2002;99:15596–15601.

61. Goldberg T, Cai W, Peppa M, et al. Advanced glycoxidation end products in commonly consumed foods. J Am Diet Assoc 2004;104:1287–1291

62. Anderson JW, Randles KM, Kendall CW, Jenkins DJ. Carbohydrate and fiber recommendations for individuals with diabetes: a quantitative assessment and meta-analysis of the evidence. J Am Coll Nutr 2004;23:5–17.

63. Salmeron J, Manson JE, Stampfer MJ, Colzitz GA. Wing AL, Willett WC. Dietary fiber, glycemic load, and risk of non-insulin-dependent diabetes mellitus in women. JAMA 1997;277:472–477.

64. Salmeron J, Aacherio A, Rimm EB, et al. Dietary fiber, glycemic load, and risk of NIDDM in men. Diabetes Care 1997;20:545–550.

65. Frost F, Leeds A, Trew G, Margara R, Dornhorst A. Insulin sensitivity in women at risk of coronary heart disease and the effect of a low glycemic diet. Metabolism 1998;47:1245–1251.

66. Jarvi AE, Karlstrom BE, Franfiedt YE, Bjorck IE Asp NG, Vessby BO. Improved glycemic control and lipid profile and normalized fibrinolytic activity on a low-glycemic index diet in type 2 diabetic patients. Diabetes Care 1999;22:10–18.

67. Brand-Miller J, Wolever TMS, Foster-Powell K, Colagiuri S. The Glucose Revolution. New York: Avalon Press, 1999.

68. US Department of Agriculture, Food Safety and Inspection Service (FSIS), Office of Policy and Program Development. FSIS statement of interim policy on carbohydrate labeling statements: labeling and consumer protection. Available at: http://www.fsis.usda.gov/OPPDE/larc/Policies/CarbLabel.htm. Accessed October 7, 2005.

69. Wylie-Rosett J. Fat substitutes and health: an advisory from the Nutrition Committee of the American Heart Association. Circulation 2002;105:2800–2804.

70. Emmanuele NV, Swade TF, Emanuele MA. Consequences of alcohol use in diabetics. Alcohol Health Res World 1998;22:211–219.

71. Barringer TA, Kirk JK, Santaniello AC, Foley KL, Michielutte R. Effect of a multivitamin and mineral supplement on infection and quality of life. A randomized, double-blind, placebo-controlled trial. Ann Intern Med 2003;138:365–371.

72. Anderson RA, Cheng N, Bryden NA, Polansky MM, Cheng N, Chi J, Feng J. Elevated intakes of supplemental chromium improves glucose and insulin variables in individuals with type 2 diabetes. Diabetes 1997;46:1786–1791.

73. Ravina A, Slezak L, Mirsky N, Bryden NA, Anderson RA. Reversal of corticosteroid-induced diabetes with supplemental chromium. Diabetes Med 1999;16:164–267.

74. Cunningham JJ. Micronutrients as nutriceutical interventions in diabetes mellitus. J Am Coll Nutr 1998;17:7–10.

75. Anderson RA, Roussel AM, Zouari N, Mahjoub S, Matheau JM, Kerkeni A. Potential antioxidant effects of zinc and chromium supplementation in people with type 2 diabetes mellitus. J Am Coll Nutr 2001;20 212–218.

76. Brusell SE, Clermont AC, Aiello LP, et al. High dose vitamin E supplementation normalized retinal blood flow and creatinine clearance in patients with type 1 diabetes. Diabetes Care 1999;22:1245–1251.

77. Ford ES, Will JC, Bowman BA, Narayan KM. Diabetes mellitus and serum carotenoids: findings from the Third National Health and Nutrition Examination Survey. Am J Epidemiol 1999;149:168–176.

78. Will JC, Ford ES, Bowman BA. Serum vitamin C concentration and diabetes: findings from the Third National Health and Nutrition Examination Survey, 1988–1994. Am J Clin Nutr 1999;70:49–52.

79. Smulders YM, Rakic M, Slaats EH, et al. Fasting methionine and homocysteine levels in NIDDM. Determinants and correlations with retinopathy, albuminuria, and cardiovascular disease. Diabetes Care 1999;22:125–132.

80. Ford ES, Cogswell ME. Diabetes and serum ferritin concentration among US adults. Diabetes Care 1999;22:1978–1983.

81. Mull DS, Nguyen M, Mill JD. Vietnamese diabetic patients and their physicians: what ethnography can teach us. West J Med 2001;175:307–311.

82. McCarty MF. Nutraceutical resources for diabetes prevention—an update. Med Hypoth 2005;64:151–158.

83. Yeh GY, Eisenberg DM, Kaptchuk TJ, Phillips RS. Systematic review of herbs and dietary supplements for glycemic control in diabetes. Diabetes Care 2003;26:1277–1294.

84. Amato P, Morales AJ, Yen SS. Effects of chromium picolinate supplementation on insulin sensitivity, serum lipids, and body composition in healthy, nonobese, older men and women. J Gerontol A Biol Sci Med Sci 2000;55:M260–M263.

85. Kim DS, Kim TW, Kang JS. Chromium picolinate supplementation improves insulin sensitivity in Goto-Kakizaki diabetic rats. Trace Elem Med Biol 2004;17:243–247.

86. Khan A, Safdar M, Ali Khan MM, Khattak KN, Anderson RA. Cinnamon improves glucose and lipids of people with type 2 diabetes. Diabetes Care 2003;26:3215–3218.

87. Anderson RA, Broadhurst CL, Polansky MM, et al. Isolation and characterization of polyphenol type-A polymers from cinnamon with insulin-like biological activity. J Agric Food Chem 2004;52:65–70.

88. Hamdan II, Afifi FU. Studies on the in vitro and in vivo hypoglycemic activities of some medicinal plants used in treatment of diabetes in Jordanian traditional medicine. J Ethnopharmacol 2004;93:117–121.

89. Herrera-Arellano A, Aguilar-Santamaria L, Garcia-Hernandez B, Nicasio-Torres P, Tortoriello J. Clinical trial of Cecropia obtusifolia and Marrubium vulgare leaf extracts on blood glucose and serum lipids in type 2 diabetics. Phytomedicine 2004;11:561–566.

90. Hsia SH, Bazargan M, Davidson MB. Effect of pancreas tonic (an ayurvedic herbal supplement) in type 2 diabetes mellitus. Metabolism 2004;53:1166–1173.

91. Ludvik B, Neuffer B, Pacini G. Efficacy of Ipomoea batatas (Caiapo) on diabetes control in type 2 diabetic subjects treated with diet. Diabetes Care 2004;27:436–440.

92. Gonzalez MJ, Ricart CM, Miranda-Massari J. A vitamin, mineral, herb dietary supplement effect on blood glucose in uncontrolled type II diabetic subjects. PR Health Sci J 2004;23:119–120.

93. Mondal DK, Yousuf BM, Banu LA, Ferdousi R, Khalil M, Shamim KM. Effect of fenugreek seeds on the fasting blood glucose level in the streptozotocin induced diabetic rats. Mymensingh Med J 2004;13:161–164.

94. Al-Saeedi M, Elzubier AG, Bahnassi AA, Al-Dawood KM. Patterns of belief and use of traditional remedies by diabetic patients in Mecca, Saudi Arabia. East Mediterr Health J 2003;9:99–107.

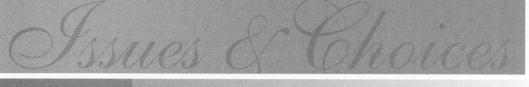

EMERGING ISSUES IN CANCER CARE
AND NUTRITION

Cynthia A. Thomson

In the United States, it is estimated that approximately 1.39 million people will be diagnosed with and treated for cancer in 2006.[1] Cancer treatments over the past several decades have focused on surgery, radiation, and/or chemotherapy as well as immunotherapy, used singly or in combination. Advances in treatment have resulted in less aggressive surgical approaches, reduced duration of radiation therapy, and improved control of chemotherapy-related toxicity. Despite these advancements, a large number of patients diagnosed with cancer will experience significant changes in nutrition status, ranging from single, correctable micronutrient deficiencies to full-fledged cancer cachexia. In addition, the increased incidence of cancer, coupled with improved survival rates, has resulted in a large cancer-survivor population who demonstrate their own unique nutrition problems. In 2001, the National Cancer Institute estimated that 9.8 million Americans had been previously diagnosed with cancer, and 5-year survival rates for all cancers are estimated at 65%.[2] The variable nutrition factors associated with cancer treatment, as well as long-term survival, suggest that medical nutrition therapy must be dynamic and responsive to the individual patient's nutrition needs throughout the continuum of care. Thus, the role of the dietetics professional in the care of oncological patients remains paramount.

It has been estimated that 30% of all cancers are modifiable through dietary change.[3,4] The World Cancer Research Fund and the American Institute for Cancer Research estimate that cancer rates would decrease by 20% nationally if the only change made to the American diet were increasing fruit and vegetable consumption to an average of five or more servings per day.[5] It is also now more clearly understood that carcinogenesis is a multistep, multiyear biological process during which diverse coexisting events likely compound to initiate abnormal cells, promote their growth, and eventually (if unchecked) allow the progression and spread of these damaged cells within the body. Multiple dietary factors have been shown to prevent cancer, although others have been associated with the development of this same disease. Modulating exposure to nutrients and dietary constituents has been postulated, and in some cases has been demonstrated, to reduce cancer.[6–8]

Despite these advances, gaps remain in our knowledge, hindering our ability to fully document and appreciate the role of diet in preventing cancer. For example, limitations in our ability to accurately measure dietary intake remain despite years of efforts to develop new tools and methodology.[9] Without reliable dietary intake data, it is extremely difficult to identify significant diet-cancer associations and to develop effective intervention strategies. When associations do exist, limitations in the accuracy of measurement also make it difficult to assess the specific level of intake necessary to maximize risk reduction. Further, there is a tendency to suggest that specific food groups are the panacea for reducing cancer risk based on ecological studies indicating that cancer rates vary considerably across countries where dietary selections are also extremely variable. The classic example of this is the reduced rates of breast cancer in Asian countries, which has been suggested to be attributable to reduced intake of dietary fat as well as increased intake of soy foods. Although protective associations may be identified in Asia, it may be unrealistic to expect to see similar associations in the United States, where exposure to dietary fat (particularly animal fat) is much greater and to soy much lower, especially when one considers exposure over a lifetime.

The lack of accuracy in the assessment of dietary intake exposure could potentially be overcome if highly reliable biomarkers of dietary intake were available that could provide insight as to both short- and long-term exposure to specific dietary constituents. To date, however, only a handful of such biomarkers exist (i.e., carotenoids—fruit/vegetables; isoflavones—soy foods; dithiocarbamates—cruciferous vegetables), and correlation coefficients between dietary intake and the exposure marker remain weak (0.2 at low levels of intake; 0.7 at highest levels of intake).

The field of diet and cancer might also see significant advancement if specific and sensitive preclinical biomarkers of cancer progression could be identified. Once these were available, short-term, cost-effective dietary interventions could then be implemented to evaluate the effects of specific nutrients, dietary constituents, or dietary patterns on cancer. Currently, for most cancers, we do not have adequate early disease biomarkers; therefore we must conduct longer-term studies that rely on cancer events for testing our diet-cancer hypotheses. Given the cost of such long-term trials, their numbers are limited. To some extent scientists have tried to overcome this limitation by describing what are believed to be intermediate biomarkers of cancer, including markers of immune dysfunction, oxidative damage, or even hormonal alterations, but there is seldom clear evidence that modulation of these biomarkers correlates with cancer endpoints.[10] Finally, as knowledge of genetics evolves, it is clear that the efficacy of dietary interventions must be considered in the context of an individual's genetic profile. Understanding the genetic polymorphisms that are associated with an increased or decreased response to diet will be a critical next step in the quest to understanding the link between diet and cancer.

Regardless of these limitations, progress is being made. This chapter focuses on the role of diet and specific dietary constituents, whether given as food or supplement, in cancer treatment. Many of the issues discussed have application to prevention and/or long-term survival. Several contemporary issues important to nutrition/dietetics professionals working in oncology are addressed. These issues include the use of fatty acids to modulate cancer cachexia, the use of antioxidant supplementation during cancer treatment, the relationship between diet and immunity, the control of oxidative damage, and the use of dietary intervention to prevent long-term effects on bone health. The chapter provides an up-to-date reference list but is augmented with professional opinion as to the appropriate application of current knowledge. The answers are not all in, but essential steps are being taken.

GOALS OF DIETARY INTERVENTION DURING CANCER

The ultimate goal for dietary intervention during cancer treatment is to optimize nutrition status and treatment efficacy. To achieve this goal, the dietetics professional must consider not only the baseline nutrition status of the individual but also the potential for the development of nutrient deficiencies as a result of cancer care. In addition, treatment-related side effects can pose significant challenges in meeting daily nutrition goals. Finally, nutrition modulation is increasingly recognized for its role in optimizing individual response to oncology care and potentially to long-term survival from this disease. The primary goals of nutrition in the care of oncology patients are highlighted in Table 18-1.

ASSESSMENT OF NUTRITION STATUS

As with other chronic diseases, the cancer patient must be evaluated nutritionally. Chapter 9 provides a discussion of nutrition status assessment and its use and interpretation in select practice settings. A few unique issues should be considered, however, in assessing patients diagnosed with cancer. Specifically, cancer patients may manifest biochemical abnormalities related to their diagnosis and treatment. These abnormalities are not generally responsive to nutrition intervention (Table 18-2). The Patient-Generated Subjective Global Assessment (PG-SGA; Fig 18-1) is a validated nutrition assessment tool developed for the unique and specific assessment issues of oncology patients and is widely used by oncology dietetics practitioners.[11,12] Unique to oncology care, it is also important for dietetics professionals to assess the patient's functional status (Karnofsky or Eastern Cooperative Oncology Group score) because loss of functional status is highly correlated with nutrition compromise in cancer.[13,14] In addition, several cancer-specific instruments have been developed by Cella and colleagues to objectively quantify functional and quality of life status at various stages of the cancer-care continuum (FACT-G, FAACT).[15,16]

TABLE 18-1	Goals of Nutrition Intervention
Maintain a healthy body composition; body weight.	
Maintain lean protein stores as assessed by serum albumin, prealbumin, total protein.	
Along with other health care professionals, work to minimize and control treatment-associated morbidity such as nausea, emesis, anorexia, xerostomia, mucositis, dehydration, constipation, etc.	
Reduce or prevent fatigue associated with cancer therapies.	
Reduce micronutrient deficiencies associated with either changes in eating patterns and/or medications and/or cancer therapies.	
Promote adequate fiber and fluid intake to prevent anesthesia- or treatment-related bowel dysfunction.	
Provide an increase in omega-3 versus omega-6 fatty acids to reduce the proinflammatory response, particularly postoperatively.	
Promote adequate (but not excess) intake of antioxidant nutrients and biologically active food constituents to reduce oxidative stress (including DNA damage or DNA adduct formation), understanding that supplementation during therapy is not currently recommended and that antioxidant exposure and its association with cancer is likely "U-shaped," in that either very low or very high intake during and after treatment may increase risk for cancer recurrence.	
Provide specific nutrient supplementation in the form of improved diet (whole foods) or supplementation to augment the healing process postoperatively (including vitamin A, zinc, vitamin C, fluids).	
Reduce risk for long-term cancer-associated comorbidity such as obesity, cardiovascular disease, insulin resistance, immunosuppression, loss of cognitive function, and/or depression.	
Promote quality of life.	

Scored Patient-Generated Subjective Global Assessment (PG-SGA)

Patient ID Information

History (Boxes 1–4 are designed to be completed by the patient.)

1. Weight (See Worksheet 1)

In summary of my current and recent weight:

I currently weigh about _____ pounds
I am about _____ feet _____ tall

One month ago I weighed about _____ pounds
Six months ago I weighed about _____ pounds

During the past two weeks my weight has:

☐ decreased (1)   ☐ not changed (0)   ☐ increased (0)

Box 1 ☐

2. Food Intake: As compared to my normal intake, I would rate my food intake during the past month as:

☐ unchanged (0)
☐ more than usual (0)
☐ less than usual (1)
   I am now taking:
   ☐ normal food but less than normal amount (1)
   ☐ little solid food (2)
   ☐ only liquids (3)
   ☐ only nutritonal supplements (3)
   ☐ very little of anything (4)
   ☐ only tube feedings or only nutrition by vein (0)

Box 2 ☐

3. Symptoms: I have had the following problems that have kept me from eating enough during the past two weeks (check all that apply):

☐ no problems eating (0)

☐ no appetite, just did not feel like eating (3)

☐ nausea (1)   ☐ vomiting (3)
☐ constipation (1)   ☐ diarrhea (3)
☐ mouth sores (2)   ☐ dry mouth (1)
☐ things taste funny or have no taste (1)   ☐ smells bother me (1)
☐ problems swallowing (2)   ☐ feel full quickly (1)
☐ pain; where? (3)_____
☐ other** (1) _____

** Examples: depression, money, or dental problems

Box 3 ☐

4. Activities and Function: Over the past month, I would generally rate my activity as:

☐ normal with no limitations (0)

☐ not my normal self, but able to be up and about with fairly normal activities (1)

☐ not feeling up to most things, but in bed or chair less than half the day (2)

☐ able to do little activity and spend most of the day in bed or chair (3)

☐ pretty much bedridden, rarely out of bed (3)

Box 4 ☐

Additive Score of the Boxes 1–4 ☐ A

The remainder of this form will be completed by your doctor, nurse, or therapist. Thank you.

5. Disease and its relation to nutritional requirements (See Worksheet 2)

All relevant diagnoses (specify) _____

Primary disease stage (circle if known or appropriate)   I   II   III   IV   Other _____

Age _____

Numerical score from Worksheet 2 ☐ B

6. Metabolic Demand (See Worksheet 3)

Numerical score from Worksheet 3 ☐ C

7. Physical (See Worksheet 4)

Numerical score from Worksheet 4 ☐ D

Global Assessment (See Worksheet 5)

☐ Well-nourished or anabolic (SGA-A)
☐ Moderate or suspected malnutrition (SGA-B)
☐ Severely malnourished (SGA-C)

Total PG-SGA score

(Total numerical score of A+B+C+D above) ☐
(See triage recommendations below)

Clinician Signature _____ RD RN PA MD DO Other _____   Date _____

Nutritional Triage Recommendations: Additive score is used to define specific nutritional interventions including patient & family education, symptom management including pharmacologic intervention, and appropriate nutrient intervention (food, nutritional supplements, enteral, or parenteral triage). First line nutrition intervention includes optimal symptom management.

0–1	No intervention required at this time. Re-assessment on routine and regular basis during treatment.
2–3	Patient & family education by dietitian, nurse, or other clinician with pharmacologic intervention as indicated by symptom survey (Box 3) and laboratory values as appropriate.
4–8	Requires intervention by dietitian, in conjunction with nurse or physician as indicated by symptoms survey (Box 3).
≥ 9	Indicates a critical need for improved symptom management and/or nutrient intervention options.

© FD Ottery, 2001   email: fdottery@savientpharma.com or noatpres1@aol.com

FIGURE 18-1 *Subjective global assessment (SGA) form.*

TABLE 18-2	Biochemical Abnormalities Associated with Cancer and Cancer Treatment
BIOCHEMICAL CHANGE	**ASSOCIATED FACTORS**
Depressed albumin levels	Fluid overload postchemotherapy; cancer cachexia
Anemia, decreased iron	Chronic disease
Neutropenia, decreased white cell count	Chemotherapy
Hypocalcemia	Decreased albumin (could respond to protein supplement)
Hypercalcemia	Metastatic disease with bone calcium mobilization
Hypomagnesemia	Severe diarrhea/prolonged enteritis
Hyponatremia	Fluid overload
Hypocholesterolemia	Decreased endogenous production of cholesterol

361

TREATMENT-ASSOCIATED SIDE EFFECTS RESULTING IN DIETARY INADEQUACY

It has been well established that oncology treatments can reduce nutrition status. This includes the effects of surgery, radiation therapy, and chemotherapy as well as hormone-ablation/receptor modulation therapies. Therapies are often done consecutively, increasing the severity of nutrition-related side effects. These side effects include such problems as nausea, emesis, weight loss, anorexia, dyspepsia, irritable bowel, early satiety, gastrointestinal (GI) bloating, flatulence, and altered taste perception (dysguesia) as well as others. To help reduce the detrimental effects of these treatments on the nutrition status of the host, dietetics professionals, along with professional organizations and meal-replacement/supplement manufacturers, have developed tips one can employ. To access these tips for patient education and assess potential components of the individual patient's nutrition care plan, the author recommends the following resources:

- American Cancer Society: http://www.cancer.org
- American Institute for Cancer Research: http://www.aicr.org
- Arizona Cancer Center: Nutrition Ways http://www.azcc.arizona.edu
- University of Nevada Reno – PG-SGA Online Calculator: http://www.unr.edu/nerp/pgsga.html
- http://www.involuntaryweightloss.org

BODY WEIGHT

ASSESSMENT OF BODY WEIGHT

Body weight takes on new importance in oncology care. Close monitoring for changes in body weight throughout cancer therapy is necessary to optimize cancer outcomes. For most patients with cancer, the focus is on the prevention of weight loss during treatment. The first line of treatment for most cancers is surgery, however, and surgery-related weight loss is to be expected. Efforts to reduce the extent of weight loss and/or to promote restoration of lean body tissue postoperatively should be included in any medical nutrition therapy plan. It has been well established that the weight loss associated with surgery is unique in that there is a predominant loss of lean mass, followed secondarily by loss of adipose stores. To the extent possible, it is important that patients optimize lean body stores, both pre- and postoperatively. Dietetics professionals are advised to assess lean mass prior to surgery to determine if a diet higher in protein and/or energy, along with increased physical activity, is warranted prior to surgery. In addition, protein status should be evaluated longitudinally following surgery to assess the individual response to dietary intervention and, as possible, physical activity.[17,18] Assessment should include routine measurement of body composition. Although dual x-ray absorptometry (DXA) is considered among the most reliable tools to accomplish this, several handheld bioimpedance monitors have been calibrated against DXA and provide sufficiently reliable measures, particularly when assessing the status of the same individual over time. In recent years, the term "anabolic competence" has been used to describe the desired metabolic state for optimal cancer outcomes. Specifically, it has been defined as "the state that optimally supports protein synthesis and lean body mass, as well as global aspects of muscle and organ function, and immune competence,"[19] suggesting that macro- and micronutrient intake, utilization, and hormonal and endocrine influences on nutrient substrates are all of importance to optimizing nutrition health in cancer patients.

Following surgery, many patients are treated with radiation and chemotherapy as well. Radiation therapy can have significant impact on dietary intake and, in turn, on body weight if the radiation field includes any portion of the GI system, including the head and neck. It is estimated that as much as 40% of cancer mortality is associated with malnutrition. In these instances, dietetics professionals are advised to be proactive in reestablishing normal protein stores and body weight (within 10% of usual body weight) to reduce the likelihood of immunosuppression, which would contribute to delayed healing, opportunistic infections, and/or reduced quality of life.[20]

BREAST CANCER: A UNIQUE WEIGHT RESPONSE

In patients being treated for breast and possibly prostate cancer, there may be an exception to the rule when it comes to body weight. Although surgery can result in weight loss, many patients receiving chemotherapy for breast cancer experience undesirable weight gain.[21] In the early and mid-1990s this was particularly apparent; however, by the late 1990s, it appeared evident that weight among women being treated with chemotherapy for breast cancer remained stable for the most part, generally as a result of less frequent use of steroids as well as the use of more cytotoxic chemotherapeutic regimes. Yet more recently, new therapeutic agents, such as docetaxel (Taxotere), have been introduced that again may be associated with undesirable weight gain in certain patients. In addition, women with estrogen-receptor positive cancers will be placed on tamoxifen or other selective estrogen-receptor modulators (SERMs)—agents that, although not conclusively associated with weight gain, do seem to be associated with weight gain in some women who use these medications. Thus, individualized attention to weight status throughout therapy is needed. Premorbid obesity and weight gain during treatment have both been associated with reduced survival and increased overall morbidities.[22,23] Efforts to prevent weight gain during therapy using energy restriction and physical activity interventions have proven successful and have been shown to reduce treatment-related fatigue; however, a large percentage of participants enrolled in such interventions during treatment drop out prior to completion of chemotherapy.[24] One reason for the treatment-related weight gain may be the reduction in resting energy expenditure that has been described during chemotherapy.[25,26] The Arizona Cancer Center has initiated a trial to evaluate the efficacy of regular green tea consumption to increase resting energy expenditure among breast cancer survivors. If effective, green tea may hold promise for also modulating body weight and/or body composition.[27–30]

EMERGING APPROACHES FOR WEIGHT-LOSS PREVENTION IN CANCER

As discussed, the majority of cancer patients, particularly those with advanced-stage disease, will experience undesirable weight loss during treatment accompanied by rapid lysis of protein tissue for energy utilization. Historically, dietetics professionals have focused on a high-energy, high-fat, high-protein diet to reduce treatment-associated weight loss. Many investigators have been somewhat uncomfortable with this approach in that dietary fats, more specifically omega-6 fatty acids, have been shown to increase cell proliferation in several cancer cell lines in vivo.[31] In recent years, new nutrition approaches have been evaluated to reduce this treatment-associated adverse effect. Adding omega-3 fatty acids, including eicosapentaenoic acid and/or fish oil, to the diet, usually in the form of a nutrient-dense beverage, has been shown to reduce weight loss and sustain lean body mass but has not been shown to be more effective than energy-dense beverages alone.[32–35] However, an oral supplement containing β-hydroxy-β-methylbutyrate, arginine, and glutamine has been shown to be effective in increasing fat-free mass in the context of advanced solid-tumor cancers. [36]

An additional nutrition approach to reducing cancer-related weight loss involves the potential efficacy of macronutrient manipulation. It has been well established that dietary fat intake at the point of gastric digestion increases reported satiety. Early satiety is thought to play a role in reducing caloric intake among cancer patients. To avoid this, clinicians should consider not only smaller, more frequent meals but also the possibility of feeding low-fat, lean protein, and carbohydrate food sources earlier in the meal, followed by fat-dense foods at the end of the meal. Although this has not been tested scientifically, physiological measures of satiety, including serum cholescystokinen and ghrelin concentrations, are now available to advance our understanding of this potential therapeutic approach. In addition, there are an increasing number of studies that utilize medications in combination with nutrition therapy to promote optimal weight and body composition[37]; these approaches include the use of nonsteroidal anti-inflammatory drugs (NSAIDs), thalidomide,[38,39] and melatonin.[40]

ROLE OF INSULIN-LIKE GROWTH FACTORS AND DIET IN CONTROLLING CANCER CACHEXIA

Cancer cachexia is characterized by weight loss, anorexia, futile cycling, and increased energy expenditure. Cancer patients experiencing cachexia, however, do not always demonstrate a reduction in energy intake, yet all demonstrate weight loss and, more importantly, a substantial loss of lean body mass. Crown and colleagues showed growth hormone resistance in cancer patients and proteolysis of IGFBP-3, which appears to be related to a rise in interleukin-6 levels (IL-6). In addition, C-reactive protein (CRP), which, like IL-6, is an inflammatory biomarker, is also elevated in advanced cancer. In cardiovascular disease, CRP levels have been shown to be reduced with antioxidant therapy. Similar approaches may be of benefit in cancer cachexia, but to date no data have been reported.[41] In an innovative approach to reducing the morbidity associated with cancer cachexia among patients with variable sites of advanced metastatic disease, Mantovani and colleagues administered a diet high in polyphenols (400 mg), with an omega-3 fatty acid–enriched nutrition supplement beverage (two cans per day), medroxyprogesterone acetate (500 mg), alpha-lipoic acid (300 mg), carbocysteine lysine salt (2.7 g), vitamin E (400 mg), vitamin A (30,000 IU), vitamin C (500 mg), and a cyclooxygenase-2 (COX-2) inhibitor (200 mg) daily for 16 weeks.[42] An interim analysis of the study results suggests that approximately 25 to 30% of subjects showed a clinical response, but all demonstrated improved inflammatory profiles, lean body mass, performance status, and quality-of-life measures. As clinicians continue monitoring the findings of this and other studies for peer-reviewed publications, our approach to care among patients with cancer cachexia may be altered.

Maintaining Gut Integrity

Aside from body weight, a second leading issue in the nutrition care of the cancer patient is sustaining healthy GI function. This can be challenging, particularly among patients who undergo GI surgery, who may remain without food for several days, and even more so in patients receiving bone marrow transplants, which results in prolonged parenteral feedings and limited gut use. Evidence suggests that it is critical to expeditiously reintroduce food, with close monitoring of patient tolerance. Historically, the solidity of the food offered is gradually increased, but there is little evidence that this is a necessary approach and, in fact, the high osmolarity of clear liquids may contribute to poor tolerance in some individuals. The need to promote solid food intake is of particular relevance in patients whose GI tract is within the radiation field.

The Role of L-Glutamine

Glutamine is a nonessential amino acid found predominantly in protein-rich foods. It is also synthesized in the body from glutamic acid. L-Glutamine supplementation has been offered as a therapeutic approach to the maintenance of gut integrity for almost 20 years. In fact, it has been well documented that, although glutamine is a nonessential amino acid, it is the preferential small bowel fuel during times of gut stress. Despite this, glutamine supplementation is not yet the standard of care for cancer patients who experience limited gut use due to oncological therapies. One reason is likely the paucity of clinical trial evidence to support its use in this setting. In a recent double-blind study of glutamine versus placebo for the prevention of radiation-induced diarrhea, patients in the glutamine group and the placebo group reported similar GI complaints and essentially identical numbers of bowel movements per day.[43] A second reason for the resistance to glutamine supplementation is early in vitro work suggesting that glutamine had a proliferative effect on tumor growth,[44] which was later dismissed by in vivo modeling.[45] Although conflicting evidence exists, a recent crossover study evaluating the potential therapeutic benefit of glutamine supplementation on oral mucositis indicated that supplementation of 1 g/m^2 was beneficial.[46] A separate study evaluating changes in GI mucosa using endoscopy showed favorable effects on gut villi; however, these effects did not translate to improved clinical response or reduced diarrhea.[47] Studies assessing the efficacy of glutamine in stem cell transplant have generally been unsuccessful in reducing days or severity of mucositis, length of stay, or infection rates.[48–50]

Probiotics and Gut Health

A significant number of cancer patients undergoing treatment for their disease will experience undesirable side effects related to suboptimal gut function. Although dietary modulation using such approaches as reducing caffeine intake, modifying dietary fat content, and/or avoidance of highly seasoned foods may prove effective in individual cases, many patients are seeking more definitive answers. One idea that has received growing attention over the past several years is the use of probiotic supplements. Probiotics are living microorganisms such as *Lactobacillus*, *Clostridium butyricum*, or *Bacillus mesentericus*, which form part of the colonic flora upon ingestion. Probiotic supplementation has shown promise for Crohn's disease and ulcerative colitis, thus initiating interest in these supplements to reduce the GI toxicity associated with cancer therapies. Limited data are available to assess the role of probiotic supplementation in cancer; however, dietetics professionals working in oncology have anecdotally used these supplements to restore gut health in patients undergoing GI surgery for cancer.[51,52]

Probiotics should not be mistaken for fermentable prebiotics, such as fructo-oligosaccharides, inulin, and/or soy oligosaccharide supplements, which have been used to stimulate growth of select bacteria in the gut. These fermentable prebiotics are associated with flatulence, bloating, and abdominal distention, side effects that would be strongly contraindicated in patients undergoing cancer therapy. Of new interest in dealing with treatment-related GI distress is the herbal supplement turmeric. Curcumin, the yellow pigment in turmeric, has been shown to reduce inflammatory response via a COX-2 inhibitory pathway.[53,54]

ONCOLOGY THERAPIES: POTENTIAL ROLE FOR ANTIOXIDANT NUTRIENTS

It is well recognized that chemotherapy and radiation induce toxicity in the host, but we are willing to accept these toxicities given the risk-benefit ratio. Efforts to reduce toxicity using dietary modification have predominantly focused on the use of antioxidant nutrient supplements. This approach is further justified by evidence suggesting that cancer patients, at the time of diagnosis, frequently present with micronutrient deficiencies, and that plasma antioxidant levels are depressed during chemotherapy.[55] A major concern is that supplementation that reduces toxicity may also interfere with the clinical efficacy of therapy, because most chemotherapeutic agents, as well as radiation therapy, produce high levels of reactive oxygen species (ROS) targeted at the tumor. Evidence suggests that although chemotherapy induces free radical formation, chemotherapy-related tumor cell death is not dependent on the formation of ROS[56,57]; however, this is likely to be highly dependent on the chemotherapeutic agent administered. Anthracyclines, platinum-based agents, alkylating agents, camptothecins, and epipodsophyllotoxins have all been shown to elicit oxidant effects on tumors, while taxanes, antimetabolites, vinca alkaloids, and purine/pyrimidine-based agents do not.[58] Much of the evidence in support of antioxidant use has been the work of Prasad and colleagues, who previously published a review of the controversy.[59] Despite this evidence, a recent NIH conference focusing on antioxidants and health confirmed this concern by restating the current clinical judgment to avoid high-dose antioxidant supplementation during cancer therapy.[60] One consideration, in reviewing the evidence, is the increasing realization that for many antioxidants, there may be an amount or a range of moderate exposure associated with optimal responsiveness to therapy and health status; below or above this "optimal range of exposure" exposure levels may be associated with increased risk. Efforts to measure plasma antioxidant levels as part of routine nutrition monitoring of cancer patients undergoing radiation or chemotherapy should be considered if only to provide the necessary epidemiological data to test the "U-shaped exposure" hypothesis.

Several reports have shown promise for antioxidant supplementation as a potential therapy for reducing treatment-related toxicity. For example, supplementation with 300 mg of alpha-tocopherol per day among patients receiving cisplatin therapy was associated with a significant decrease in both the incidence (31 versus 86%) and severity of cisplatin-associated neurotoxicity.[61] Mixed antioxidant supplementation (selenium, vitamins C and E, and beta-carotene) significantly reduced treatment-associated side effects in women with ovarian cancer.[62] In a study of dietary intake (not supplementation) in children being treated for leukemia, higher vitamin C intake at 6 months was associated with reduced delays in chemotherapy, higher vitamin E intakes were associated with reduced secondary infections, and greater beta-carotene intake was associated with reduced treatment toxicity.[63] Supplemental alpha-lipoic acid has also been shown to ameliorate docetaxel/cisplatin neurotoxicity; however, the study's sample size was insufficient to alter clinical care.[64] Similar protective effects in the form of cardiotoxicity have been described in patients taking antioxidant supplements along with doxorubicin (Adriamycin) therapy. Despite efficacy in reducing treatment-associated toxicity, clinicians agree that such effects may not be beneficial to the long-term therapeutic benefit of the chemotherapy in terms of cancer remission, as the reduction in toxicity is associated with a reduced capacity to achieve therapeutic levels of certain chemotherapy agents and in turn with reduced efficacy. A systematic review of this topic was recently published, giving clinicians guidance in evaluating the evidence and informing their patients.[58]

Radiotherapy-induced fibrosis (RIF) may be the exception to the rule in regard to current recommendations for the use of antioxidant supplements during cancer therapy. Although RIF has been shown to regress for up to 12 months after therapy, this is not always the case. In a study of 43 patients with RIF who were treated with pentoxifylline (400 mg) and vitamin E (500 IU) twice daily for 6 months,[65] supplementation was associated with a significant reduction in the skin surface area affected by RIF, which was further improved with extended time of treatment. While promising, given that no other effective treatments exist, a placebo-controlled trial is warranted before significant changes in clinical approaches should be made.

IMMUNE MODULATION THROUGH NUTRITION

One aspect of patient wellness that is known to be responsive to diet/nutrition intervention is immunity. Chandra and others have shown that patient populations with borderline micronutrient deficiencies demonstrate suboptimal immune function that is responsive to a diet high in fruits and vegetables and/or multivitamin-mineral supplementation.[66–68] Patients undergoing cancer treatment are clearly at risk for suboptimal micronutrient status, particularly those of advanced age. Dietary adequacy of selenium, zinc, copper, and vitamins A, C, and E, as well as protein, should be evaluated in all cancer patients. Once assessed, appropriate dietary interventions, including possible supplementation, should be provided to individual patients.

A more controversial approach to immune modulation for cancer patients is the use of medicinal mushrooms. Basic science investigations indicate that some mushrooms and mushroom extracts (such as reishi, shiitake, and mittake) may enhance immune response even among cancer patients. However, controlled clinical trials are lacking.

Another cornerstone association between cancer and immunity has to do with the potential to modulate the inflammatory response. Increasing evidence suggests that omega-3 fatty acids can reduce the inflammatory response and thus may be a viable approach to reduce cancer recurrence among patients previously treated for their disease. Although a theoretical basis for consuming an anti-inflammatory diet to prevent cancer recurrence exists, no randomized clinical controlled trials have yet been published. In addition, recent genetic research suggests that there is individual variability in response to anti-inflammatory agents. It is likely that a similar pattern of responsiveness would be demonstrated in studies using anti-inflammatory dietary intervention. Foods that could potentially increase or decrease inflammation are listed in Table 18-3, and the biochemical pathways associated with the inflammatory response, as well as the specific foods that may modulate response toward either pro- or anti-inflammatory endpoints, are illustrated in Figure 18-2.

MODULATING OXIDATIVE DAMAGE THROUGH DIET

Oxidative damage to DNA has been proposed as a primary biological mechanism for the development of cancer. Dietary intake consistent with lower total and saturated fat intake, as well as a higher intake of vegetables, fruit, and their constitutive antioxidant nutrients and phytochemicals, have each been associated with improved oxidative damage profiles.[69–71] Specifically, controlled feeding studies have shown a reduction in oxidative DNA damage biomarkers as well as reduced lipid peroxidation. Of importance, the efficacy of these types of dietary manipulations appears to be dependent on the baseline oxidative stress profile of the patient in that there appears to be a lower-end threshold beyond which added improvements in diet toward more fruits and vegetables and less fat is unlikely to reduce oxidant damage further. In addition, there is concern that some antioxidant food constituents consumed at high levels may actually increase oxidative stress by acting as prooxidants. This physiological response has been suggested for several biologically active food constituents, including beta-carotene, quercetin, and vitamin C.

Although oxidative damage markers are frequently elevated during and immediately after cancer therapy, cancer patients who are several months past treatment and who consume a relatively "healthy" diet may present with reduced oxidative damage levels even when compared to age- and gender-matched controls without a previous cancer diagnosis.[72] Thus, those who stand to benefit most in terms of reductions in oxidative damage are those with demonstrated micronutrient deficiencies and/or a regular intake of a diet high in fats and low in vegetables and

TABLE 18-3	Inflammatory Response Foods	
ELIMINATE FROM DIET	**ADD TO DIET**
Polyunsaturated fats	Fruits and vegetables in general
Partially hydrogenated fats	Citrus fruits
Hydrogenated fats	Monounsaturated oils such as olive oil
Trans fatty acids	Salmon and sardines
	Flax seed
	Walnuts
	Turmeric (spice)

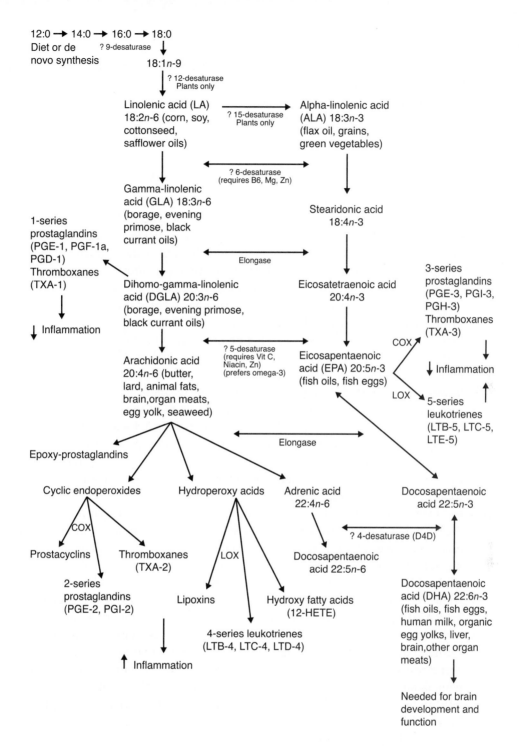

FIGURE 18-2 *The metabolic pathway of omega-3 and omega-6 fatty acids. Dietary omega-3 and omega-6 essential fatty acids compete for several enzymes for conversion into their respective metabolites. The major metabolite of the omega-6 fatty acid pathway is arachidonic acid (AA), which leads to the formation of proinflammatory compounds such as 2-series prostaglandins and thromboxanes (via the enzyme cyclooxygenase) and 4-series leukotrienes and lipoxins (via the enzymes 15- and 5-lipoxigenase). The major metabolite of the omega-3 fatty acid pathway is eicosapentaenoic acid (EPA), which is a precursor for the synthesis of anti-inflammatory 3-series prostaglandins and thromboxanes (via cyclooxigenase) and 5-series leukotrienes (via 5-lipoxigenase). EPA is also further metabolized to docosapentaenoic acid (DHA), necessary for development and function of the brain, retina, and testis. The production of inflammatory products can be reduced by shifting the balance toward synthesis of EPA over AA through the regular intake of food sources of omega-3 fatty acids such as flax, select nuts and whole grains, and fish oils or coldwater fatty fish.*

fruits. In addition, moderate daily physical activity has been shown to reduce oxidative damage, while intense physical activity (such as running marathons) can significantly increase oxidative damage.[73–76] Last, although data are limited, there is some evidence that probiotic supplementation may reduce oxidative damage.[77]

MODULATION OF HORMONES THROUGH DIET

Another area of active research relates to the potential for diet interventions to modulate hormone responses in hormone-dependent cancers. One example that has been well described is the reduction in free and bioavailable estradiol in response to diets high in dietary fiber (> 25 g/day). Thus, high-fiber diets should be routinely employed among breast cancer patients whose tumors express estrogen receptors.[78] A second dietary constituent with the potential to alter hormone levels is phytoestrogens. The majority of research in this area has focused on the role of soy foods in modulating estrogen and androgen response. Currently, the evidence suggests that diets high in soy foods during the prepubescent and adolescent periods of life may reduce breast cancer events; among men, a diet high in soy throughout life may have similar protective effects in regard to prostate cancer. Little evidence exists, however, to support diets high in soy posttherapy for these hormone-associated cancers, and at this time dietetics professionals are cautious to recommend limited soy food intake among women with known hormone-related disease. Given that serum estrogen receptor modulators (SERMs) that block estrogen receptors are now a front-line therapy for estrogen receptor–positive breast cancer, research to evaluate the combined effects of soy foods (or other phytoestrogens, such as flaxseed) and these medications is warranted.[79]

One additional food constituent shown to modulate estrogen levels is indole-3-carbinol, a biologically active food constituent found in high concentrations in cruciferous vegetables, particularly broccoli. Evidence suggests that daily supplementation with indole-3-carbinol or broccoli sprouts results in a significant and beneficial shift in the 2:16 hydroxyestradiol levels.[80,81] In addition to hormone receptor status, breast cancer patients also may have tumors that express a protein called HER2. The presence of this protein may actually improve long-term survival in that effective drugs (e.g., trastuzumab or Herceptin) can block the activity of this protein. Of interest, a recent clinical trial published in the *Journal of the National Cancer Institute* suggests that daily supplementation with evening primrose oil. a source of gamma-linolenic acid, further enhances the efficacy of this drug. Although results need to be replicated, this study supports the notion that dietary interventions may have additive effects and thus serve as adjuvant therapy in select cancer cases.[82]

DIETARY INTERVENTIONS TO REDUCE LONG-TERM SEQUELAE OF CANCER TREATMENT

WEIGHT CONTROL

Increasing evidence suggests that obesity plays a central role in cancer recurrence, particularly for hormone-related cancers. The mechanisms by which this may occur include suppression of immune response, micronutrient-deficient diets, altered hormone levels, increased oxidative damage, and insulin resistance. The majority of evidence associating excess body weight/fat with cancer recurrence comes from the study of breast cancer; however, similar patterns of association are being shown with other cancers. Both overweight status (body mass index, or BMI, 25 to 30 kg/m^2) and obesity (> 30 kg/m^2) have been associated with reduced disease-free survival and increased comorbidities among breast cancer survivors. Thus, dietetics professionals should consider weight loss for overweight cancer survivors a primary outcome for optimal care. Efforts to reduce weight should include a dietary plan that is energy-restricted while also adequate in micronutrients. Physical activity should be included as an essential component for weight-loss success. Intermediate endpoints—such as reductions in oxidative damage, improvements in immune response, or, more importantly, reduced insulin resistance—should be closely monitored throughout the intervention process. Although the optimal macronutrient composition to reduce body weight among cancer survivors remains inconclusive, mechanistic research suggests that a significant reduction in caloric intake is needed. A low-fat-diet intervention (< 20% total energy) was associated with improved progression-free survival among postmenopausal, estrogen receptor–negative breast cancer patients in a recent multicenter trial (Women's Intervention Nutrition Study) independent of weight loss. This protection was not demonstrated among women with estrogen receptor–positive cancer, however, and preliminary data would suggest that a low-carbohydrate diet that restricts refined sugars may be advantageous for modulation of estrogen receptor–positive breast cancer survival given the significant reduction in insulin resistance associated with these eating plans.[83–85] Other dietary constituents that may promote favorable insulin and insulin growth factor profiles include green tea,[86] fiber, beans, and other low-glycemic-index foods (Figure 18-3).

BONE HEALTH AND DIET

A year 2000 consensus report addressing the effects of cancer therapy on the bone health of cancer patients indicated that reduced bone health is a common occurrence. To this end, and in particular among overweight survivors requiring long-term weight-loss interventions, efforts to improve bone health through diet should be standard of care.[87,88] Evidence suggests

Issues to Ponder

- Does cancer induce malnutrition or is malnutrition a preclinical state that leads to the development of cancer? Or both?
- Is there a role for select nutrient supplementation during cancer therapy as an adjuvant that would enhance therapeutic response?
- Is weight loss the primary goal in reducing risk for cancer recurrence among overweight and/or obese patients or should the goal of nutrition therapy focus on intermediate health indicators, such as fasting insulin levels, adiponectin, or correction of dyslipidemia?
- If diet and/or nutrient intake can modulate oxidative damage, does this assure a decreased risk for cancer?
- If cancer patients are given cyclooxygenase inhibitors (1 and 2), is there a therapeutic need for an anti-inflammatory diet? Can we expect an additive effect that might be beneficial in modulating cancer outcomes?
- What is the optimal exposure to specific nutrients during each phase of cancer therapy?
- How can we define the "optimal" exposure level of micronutrients and biologically active food constituents during cancer care? Should we move toward routine measures of "exposure" levels in plasma, urine, etc.?

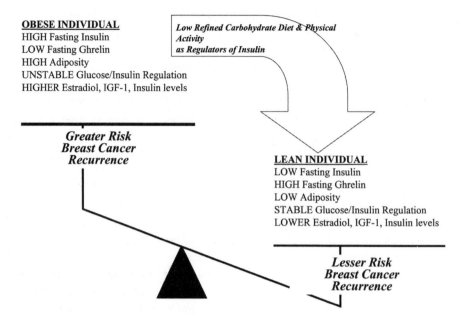

FIGURE 18-3 *Impact of dietary intervention on breast cancer promoters. Courtesy of P. Thompson, PhD, University of Arizona Cancer Center, 2005. Used with permission.*

that a large percentage of adults in the United States do not achieve the recommended daily intake of calcium. Thus, assessment of dietary calcium intake, along with instruction on how to improve calcium intake through both diet and supplementation, should be routinely provided. In addition, particularly among elderly cancer patients, vitamin D intake is frequently inadequate. Again, efforts to assess intake and status as well as to correct deficiencies through diet and supplementation should be undertaken with all cancer survivors. Although the evidence is less supportive, efforts to evaluate and address other dietary practices, such as intakes of vitamins A and K (or vitamin status), caffeine, or phytoestrogens, should also be addressed.[85–93]

SUMMARY

Diet and nutrition play a central role in the care of patients diagnosed and treated for cancer. Every cancer patient should ideally receive nutrition evaluation prior to and throughout his or her cancer experience. Efforts to improve immunity, reduce oxidative damage, and optimize overall health status can be enhanced only by a focused diet-nutrition intervention plan prior to, during, and after cancer treatment. Each individual will present unique challenges. Suggestions to counteract treatment-related side effects have been widely disseminated. Optimizing nutrition care requires thinking outside the box and applying nutrition therapies and approaches that have demonstrated mechanistic support, possibly limited evidence in terms of randomized clinical trials, and no indication of harm.

REFERENCES

1. American Cancer Society. Cancer Facts and Figures 2005. Atlanta, GA: American Cancer Society, 2005. Available at: http://www.cancer.org/downloads/STT/CAFF2006PWSecured.pdf. Accessed March 20, 2006.
2. Ries LAG, Eisner MP, Kosary CL, et al., eds. SEER Cancer Statistics Review, 1975-2002. Bethesda, MD: National Cancer Institute, 2005. Available at: http://seer.cancer.gov/csr/1975_2002/, based on November 2004 SEER data submission, posted to the SEER web site 2005. Accessed October 3, 2005.
3. Doll R, Peto R. The causes of cancer: quantitative estimates of avoidable risks of cancer in the United States today. J Natl Cancer Inst 1981;66:1191–1308.
4. Willett WC, Trichopoulos D. Nutrition and cancer: a summary of the evidence. Cancer Causes Control 1996;7:178–180.
5. World Cancer Research Fund. Food Nutrition and the Prevention of Cancer: A Global Perspective. Hong Kong: World Cancer Research Fund, 2003. Summary. Available at: http://www.aicr.org/research/report_summary.lasso. Accessed October 3, 2005.
6. Martinez ME, Giovannucci E. Diet and the prevention of cancer. Cancer Metast Rev 1997;16:357–376.
7. Cotugna N. Dietary factors and cancer risk. Semin Oncol Nurs 2000;16:99–105.
8. Gerber M. The comprehensive approach to diet: a critical review. J Nutr 2001;131:3051S–3055S.
9. Thompson FE, Subar AF. Dietary assessment methodology. In: Coulston AM, Rock CL, Monsen ER, eds. Nutrition in the Prevention and Treatment of Disease. San Diego, CA: Academic Press, 2001:3–30.
10. Wild CP, Andersson C, O'Brien NM, Wilson L, Woods JA. A critical evaluation of the application of biomarkers in epidemiological studies on diet and health. Br J Nutr 2001;86(suppl 1):S37–S53.
11. Ottery FD. Rethinking nutrition support of the cancer patient: the new field of nutrition oncology. Semin Oncol 1994;21:770–778.
12. Ottery FD. Definition of standardized nutrition assessment and interventional pathways in oncology. Nutrition 1996;12:S15–S19.
13. Schag CC, Heinrich RL, Ganz PA. Karnofsky performance status revisited: reliability, validity, and guidelines. J Clin Oncol 1984;2:187–193.
14. Oken MM, Creech RH, Tormey DC, et al. Toxicity and response criteria of the Eastern Cooperative Oncology Group. Am J Clin Oncol 1982;5:649–655.
15. FACIT.org. The Functional Assessment of Chronic Illness Therapy (FACIT). Elmhurst, IL: FACIT.org. Available at: http://www.facit.org/about/overview_measure.aspx. Accessed October 28, 2005.
16. Brucker PS, Yost K, Cashy J, Webster K, Cella D. General population and cancer patient norms for the Functional Assessment of Cancer Therapy—General (FACT-G). Eval Health Prof 2005;28:192-211.
17. Delmore, G. Assessment of nutrition status in cancer patients: widely neglected? Support Care Cancer 1997;5:376–380.
18. Strasser F, Bruera ED. Update on anorexia and cachexia. Hematol Oncol Clin North Am 2002;16:589–617.
19. Langer CJ, Hoffman JP, Ottery FD. Clinical significance of weight loss in cancer patients: rationale for the use of anabolic agents in the treatment of cancer-related cachexia. Nutrition 2001;17:S1–20.
20. Bozzetti F, Cozzaglio L, Gavazzi C, et al. Nutrition support in patients with cancer of the esophagus: impact on nutrition status, patient compliance to therapy, and survival. Tumori 1998;84:681–686.
21. Rock CL, Flatt SW, Newman V, et al. Factors associated with weight gain in women after diagnosis of breast cancer. Women's Healthy Eating and Living Study Group. J Am Diet Assoc 1999;99:1212–1221.
22. Chlebowski RT, Aiello E, McTiernan A. Weight loss in breast cancer patient management. J Clin Oncol 2002;20:1128–1143.
23. Demark-Wahnefried W, Rock CL. Nutrition-related issues for the breast cancer survivor. Semin Oncol 2003;30:789–798.
24. Del Rio G, Zironi S, Valeriani L, et al. Weight gain in women with breast cancer treated with adjuvant cyclophosphomide, methotrexate and 5-fluorouracil. Analysis of resting energy expenditure and body composition. Breast Cancer Res Treat 2002;73:267–273.
25. Demark-Wahnefried W, Peterson BL, et al. Changes in weight, body composition, and factors influencing energy balance among premenopausal breast cancer patients receiving adjuvant chemotherapy. J Clin Oncol 2001;19:2381–2389.

26. McInnes JA, Knobf MT. Weight gain and quality of life in women treated with adjuvant chemotherapy for early-stage breast cancer. Oncol Nurs Forum 2001;28:675–684.

27. Rumpler W, Seale J, Clevidence B, et al. Oolong tea increases metabolic rate and fat oxidation in men. J Nutr 2001;131:2848–2852.

28. Dulloo AG, Seydoux J, Girardier L, Chantre P, Vandermander J. Green tea and thermogenesis: interactions between catechin-polyphenols, caffeine and sympathetic activity. Int J Obes Rel Metab Disord 2000;24:252–258.

29. Bell SJ, Goodrick GK. A functional food product for the management of weight. Crit Rev Food Sci Nutr 2002;42:163–178.

30. Chantre P, Lairon D. Recent findings of green tea extract AR25 (Exolise) and its activity for the treatment of obesity. Phytomedicine 2002;9:3–8.

31. Nixon DW. Cancer, cancer cachexia, and diet: lessons from clinical research. Nutrition 1996;12:S52–S56.

32. Costelli P, Llovera M, Lopez-Soriano J, et al. Lack of effect of eicosapentaenoic acid in preventing cancer cachexia and inhibiting tumor growth. Cancer Lett 1995:97:25–32.

33. Bruera E, Strasser F, Palmer JL, et al. Effect of fish oil on appetite and other symptoms in patients with advanced cancer and anorexia/cachexia: a double-blind, placebo-controlled study. J Clin Oncol 2003;21:129–134.

34. Fearon KC, Von Meyenfeldt MF, Moses AG, et al. Effect of a protein and energy dense N-3 fatty acid enriched oral supplement on loss of weight and lean tissue in cancer cachexia: a randomised double blind trial. Gut 2003;52:1479–1486.

35. Jatoi A. Fish oil, lean tissue, and cancer: is there a role for eicosapentaenoic acid in treating the cancer anorexia/weight loss syndrome? Crit Rev Oncol Hematol 2005;55:37–43.

36. May PE, Barber A, D'Olimpio JT, Hourihane A, Abumrad NN. Reversal of cancer-related wasting using oral supplementation with a combination of beta-hydroxy-beta-methylbutyrate, arginine, and glutamine. Am J Surg 2002;183:471–479.

37. McQuellon RP, Moose DB, Russell GB, et al. Supportive use of megestrol acetate (Megace) with head/neck and lung cancer patients receiving radiation therapy. Int J Radiat Oncol Biol Phys 2002;52:1180–1185.

38. Bruera E, Neumann CM, Pituskin E, Calder K, Ball G, Hanson J. Thalidomide in patients with cachexia due to terminal cancer: preliminary report. Ann Oncol 1999;10:857–859.

39. Khan ZH, Simpson EJ, Cole AT, et al. Oesophageal cancer and cachexia: the effect of short-term treatment with thalidomide on weight loss and lean body mass. Aliment Pharmacol Ther 2003;17:677–682.

40. Lissoni P, Chilelli M, Villa S, Cerizza L, Tancini G. Five years survival in metastatic non-small cell lung cancer patients treated with chemotherapy alone or chemotherapy and melatonin: a randomized trial. J Pineal Res 2003;35:12–15.

41. Crown AL, Cottle K, Lightman SL, et al. What is the role of the insulin-like growth factor system in the pathophysiology of cancer cachexia, and how is it regulated? Clin Endocrinol (Oxf) 2002;56:723–733.

42. Mantovani G, Madeddu C, Maccio A, et al. Cancer-related anorexia/cachexia syndrome and oxidative stress: an innovative approach beyond current treatment. Cancer Epidemiol Biomarkers Prev 2004;13:1651–1659.

43. Kozelsky TF, Meyers GE, Sloan JA, et al. North Central Cancer Treatment Group. Phase III double-blind study of glutamine versus placebo for the prevention of acute diarrhea in patients receiving pelvic radiation therapy. J Clin Oncol 2003;21:1669–1674.

44. Kang YJ, Feng Y, Hatcher EL. Glutathione stimulates A549 cell proliferation in glutamine-deficient culture: the effect of glutamate supplementation. J Cell Physiol 1994;161:589–596.

45. Bartlett DL, Charland S, Torosian MH. Effect of glutamine on tumor and host growth. Ann Surg Oncol 1995;2:71–76.

46. Anderson PM, Schroeder G, Skubitz KM. Oral glutamine reduces the duration and severity of stomatitis after cytotoxic cancer chemotherapy. Cancer 1998;83:1433–1439.

47. Decker-Baumann C, Buhl K, Frohmuller S, von Herbay A, Dueck M, Schlag PM. Reduction of chemotherapy-induced side-effects by parenteral glutamine supplementation in patients with metastatic colorectal cancer. Eur J Cancer 1999;35:202–207.

48. Anderson PM, Ramsay NK, Shu XO, et al. Effect of low-dose oral glutamine on painful stomatitis during bone marrow transplantation. Bone Marrow Transplant 1998;22:339–344.

49. Coghlin Dickson TM, Wong RM, et al. Effect of oral glutamine supplementation during bone marrow transplantation. J Parenter Enteral Nutr 2000;24:61–66.

50. Buchman AL. Glutamine: commercially essential or conditionally essential? A critical appraisal of the human data. Am J Clin Nutr 2001;74:25–32.

51. Sullivan A, Nord CE. The place of probiotics in human intestinal infections. Int J Antimicrob Agents 2002;20:313–319.

52. Horie H, Zeisig M, Hirayama K, Midtvedt T, Moller L, Rafter J. Probiotic mixture decreases DNA adduct formation in colonic epithelium induced by the food mutagen 2-amino-9H-pyrido[2,3-b]indole in a human-flora associated mouse model. Eur J Cancer Prev 2003;12:101–107.

53. Huang MT, Lysz T, Ferraro T, Abidi TF, Laskin JD, Conney AH. Inhibitory effects of curcumin on in vitro lipoxygenase and cyclooxygenase activities in mouse epidermis. Cancer Res 1991;51:813–819.

54. Zhang F, Altorki NK, Mestre JR, Subbaramaiah K, Dannenberg AJ. Curcumin inhibits cyclooxygenase-2 transcription in bile acid- and phorbol ester-treated human gastrointestinal epithelial cells. Carcinogenesis 1999;20:445–451.

55. Weijl NI, Hopman GD, Wipkink-Bakker A, et al. Cisplatin combination chemotherapy induces a fall in plasma antioxidants of cancer patients. Ann Oncol 1998;9:1331–1337.

56. Senturker S, Tschirret-Guth R, Morrow J, Levine R, Shacter E. Induction of apoptosis by chemotherapeutic drugs without generation of reactive oxygen species. Arch Biochem Biophys 2002;397:262–272.

57. Drisko JA, Chapman J, Hunter VJ. The use of antioxidant therapies during chemotherapy. Gynecol Oncol 2003;88:434–439.

58. Ladas EJ, Jacobson JS, Kennedy DD, Teel K, Fleischauer A, Kelly KM. Antioxidants and cancer therapy: a systematic review. J Clin Oncol 2004;22:517–528.

59. Prasad KN, Cole WC, Kumar B, Prasad KC. Scientific rationale for using high-dose multiple micronutrients as an adjunct to standard and experimental cancer therapies. J Am Coll Nutr 2001;20:450S–463S.

60. Seifried HE, Anderson DE, Sorkin BC, Costello RB. Free radicals: the pros and cons of antioxidants. Executive summary report. J Nutr 2004;134:3143S–3163S.

61. Pace A, Savarese A, Picardo M, et al. Neuroprotective effect of vitamin E supplementation in patients treated with cisplatin chemotherapy. J Clin Oncol 2003;21:927–931.

62. Sieja K. Protective role of selenium against the toxicity of multi-drug chemotherapy in patients with ovarian cancer. Pharmazie 2000;55:958–959.

63. Kennedy DD, Tucker, KL, Ladas ED, Rheingold SR, Blumberg J, Kelly KM. Low antioxidant vitamin intakes are associated with increases in adverse effects of chemotherapy in children with acute lymphoblastic leukemia. Am J Clin Nutr 2004;79:1029–1036.

64. Gedlicka C, Kornek GV, Schmid K, Scheithauer W. Amelioration of docetaxel/cisplatin induced polyneuropathy by alpha-lipoic acid. Ann Oncol 2003;14:339–340.

65. Delanian S, Balla-Mekias S, Lefaix JL. Striking regression of chronic radiotherapy damage in a clinical trial of combined pentoxifylline and tocopherol. J Clin Oncol 1999;17:3283–3290.

66. Bendich A. Antioxidant vitamins and their functions in immune responses. Adv Exp Med Biol 1990;262:35–55.

67. Bogden JD, Oleske JM, Lavenhar MA, et al. Effects of one year of supplementation with zinc and other micronutrients on cellular immunity in the elderly. J Am Coll Nutr 1990;9:214–225.

68. Chandra RK. Effect of vitamin and trace-element supplementation on immune responses and infection in elderly subjects. Lancet 1992;340:1124–1127.

69. Loft S, Poulsen HE. Cancer risk and oxidative DNA damage in man. [erratum appears in J Mol Med 1997;75:67–68]. J Mol Med 1996;74:297–312.

70. Djuric Z, Depper JB, Uhley V, Smith D, Lababidi S, Martino S, Heilbrun LK. Oxidative NA damage levels in blood from women at high risk for breast cancer are associated with dietary intakes of meats, vegetables, and fruits. J Am Dietet Assoc 1998;98:524–528.

71. Thompson HJ, Heimendinger J, Haegele A, et al. Effect of increased vegetable and fruit consumption on markers of oxidative cellular damage. Carcinogenesis 1999;20:2261–2266.

72. Thomson CA, Giuliano AR, Shaw JW, et al. Diet and biomarkers of oxidative damage in women previously treated for breast cancer. Nutr Cancer 2005;51:146–154.

73. Niess AM, Hartmann A, Grunert-Fuchs M, Poch B, Speit G. DNA damage after exhaustive treadmill running in trained and untrained men. Int J Sports Med 1996;17:397–403.

74. Asami S, Hirano T, Yamaguchi R, Itoh H, Kasai H. Reduction of 8-hydroxyguanine in human leukocyte DNA by physical exercise. Free Radic Res 1998;29:581–584.

75. Radak Z, Apor P, Pucsok J, et al. Marathon running alters the DNA base excision repair in human skeletal muscle. Life Sci 2003;72:1627-1633.

76. Wang JS, Huang YH. Effects of exercise intensity on lymphocyte apoptosis induced by oxidative stress in men. Eur J Appl Physiol 2005;95:290–297.

77. Horie H, Zeisig M, Hirayama K, Midtvedt T, Moller L, Rafter J. Probiotic mixture decreases DNA adduct formation in colonic epithelium induced by the food mutagen 2-amino-9H-pyrido[2,3-b]indole in a human-flora associated mouse model. Eur J Cancer Prev 2003;12:101–107.

78. Rock CL, Flatt SW, Thomson CA, et al. Effects of a high-fiber, low-fat diet intervention on serum concentrations of reproductive steroid hormones in women with a history of breast cancer. J Clin Oncol 2004;22:2379–2387.

79. Messina MJ, Loprinzi CL. Soy for breast cancer survivors: a critical review of the literature. J Nutr 2001;131:3095S–3108S.

80. Fowke JH, Longcope C, Hebert JR. Brassica vegetable consumption shifts estrogen metabolism in healthy postmenopausal women. Cancer Epidemiol Biomarkers Prev 2000;9:773–779.

81. Auborn KJ, Fan S, Rosen EM, et al. Indole-3-carbinol is a negative regulator of estrogen. J Nutr 2003;133:2470S–2475S.

82. Menendez JA, Vellon L, Colomer R, Lupu R. Effect of γ-linolenic acid on the transcriptional activity of the Her-2/neu (erbB-2) oncogene. J Natl Cancer Inst 2005;97:1611.

83. McAuley KA, Hopkins CM, Smith KJ, et al. Comparison of high-fat and high-protein diets with a high-carbohydrate diet in insulin-resistant obese women. Diabetologia 2005;48:8–16.

84. McTiernan A. Obesity and cancer: the risks, science, and potential management strategies. Oncology (Williston Park) 2005;19:871–81; discussion 881–882, 885–886.

85. Chelbowski R, Blackburn G, Elashoff, Thomson C et al. Proc Amer Soc Clin Oncol 2005;24:10. In press

86. Kao Y-H, Hiipakka RA, Liao S. Modulation of endocrine systems and food intake by green tea epigallocatechin gallate. Endocrinology 2000;141:980–987.

87. Nguyen TV, Center JR, Eisman JA. Association between breast cancer and bone mineral density: the Dubbo Osteoporosis Epidemiology Study. Maturitas 2000;36:27–34.

88. Pfeilschifter J, Diel IJ. Osteoporosis due to cancer treatment: pathogenesis and management. J Clin Oncol 2000;18:1570–1593.

89. Kleerekoper M, Mendlovic DB. Sodium fluoride therapy of postmenopausal osteoporosis. [erratum appears in Endocr Rev 1993;14:479]. Endocr Rev 1993;14:312–323.

90. Barrett-Connor E, Chang JC, Edelstein SL. Coffee-associated osteoporosis offset by daily milk consumption. The Rancho Bernardo Study. JAMA 1994;271:280–283.

91. Melhus H, Michaëlsson K, Kindmark A, et al. Excessive dietary intake of vitamin A is associated with reduced bone mineral density and increased risk for hip fracture. Ann Intern Med 1998;129:770–778.

92. Morabito N, Crisafulli A, Vergara C, et al. Effects of genistein and hormone-replacement therapy on bone loss in early postmenopausal women: a randomized double-blind placebo-controlled study. J Bone Min Res 2002;17:1904–1912.

93. Rico H, Canal ML, Manas P, Lavado JM, Costa C, Pedrera JD. Effects of caffeine, vitamin D, and other nutrients on quantitative phalangeal bone ultrasound in postmenopausal women. Nutrition 2002;18:189–193.

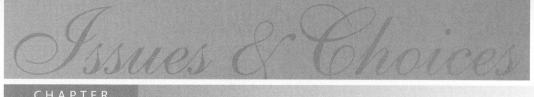
FOOD-DRUG INTERACTIONS

June H. McDermott and Carol J. Rollins

Advice related to food-drug interactions has become an important part of the professional scope of practice for many nutrition care providers. As reliance on prescription and nonprescription drugs to maintain laboratory and clinical parameters within prescribed ranges (often referred to as "health") has increased in the United States, so to has the prevalence of drug use and the complexity of the regimens. A telephone survey conducted in 1998 and 1999 that gathered data on drug use among an ambulatory population during the prior week indicated that for those 65 years of age or older, 57% of women and 44% of men had taken five or more drugs and 12% of both women and men had taken 10 or more drugs.[1] Among all participants 18 years of age or older, 50% had taken a prescription drug and 7% had taken five or more prescription drugs. Older individuals (65 years of age and up) had the highest prevalence of prescription drug use, with 81% of women and 71% of men taking at least one and 23% of women and 19% of men taking five or more prescription drugs. This high prevalence of drug use translates into an increased incidence of adverse drug reactions, including food-drug interactions, since some drugs have real or potential interactions with nutrition supplements and with the foods that we eat. In addition, diet is an important adjunct to drug therapy, and sometimes a primary therapy to maintain health. According to the survey, several of the most common reasons drugs were taken included hypertension, heart problems, diabetes mellitus, and hypercholesterolemia. Thus, it is obvious that nutrition care providers are now more likely to be presented with food-drug interaction issues, including a greater potential for serious interactions and multiple interactions that present more difficult choices for the sound dietary counseling of patients and appropriate advice to other healthcare professionals. How well nutrition care providers manage these complex issues will depend on their understanding of the problem.

Several handbooks related to food and nutrient interactions with drugs are published and widely used by nutrition care providers. Unfortunately, most of the handbooks provide little or no information on the strength of evidence for such interactions, mechanism of interaction, or severity of interaction; they simply list the drug and the food or nutrient that interact. For instance, a handbook may list potassium/hypokalemia as a nutrient interaction with digoxin. Does this mean digoxin causes hypokalemia? Should dietary counseling automatically include signs and symptoms (s/sx) of hypokalemia? Should advice on increased potassium intake be included in dietary counseling? Will there be an additive or synergistic effect on serum potassium if the patient is taking another drug listed as interacting with potassium in the opposite way (hypokalemia)? Does dietary advice change for the patient with renal insufficiency or the patient taking another drug that has been associated with hyperkalemia? Should laboratory monitoring of serum potassium be recommended, and if so, how often? What priority does counseling a patient with this food-drug interaction require when there is not enough time to see all the patients who have been referred for nutrition care? Would counseling on this interaction take priority over counseling on potassium/hypokalemia and furosemide (Lasix) if only one of the patients can be seen? In fact, the interaction between potassium and digoxin is probably a relatively low-priority item for nutrition care providers most of the time. Hypokalemia increases the risk of digoxin toxicity; digoxin does not cause potassium wasting. Therefore counseling on s/sx of digoxin toxicity is typically more important than s/sx of hypokalemia. Advice on high-potassium foods might still be relevant, although it cannot be assumed that increased potassium intake will be needed. In contrast, furosemide increases potassium losses through the kidneys, and hypokalemia will likely occur unless potassium intake increases. A notable exception is when the patient fails to respond to furosemide; with no increase in urine output, there is no increase in potassium losses. These examples illustrate the need to understand mechanisms behind listed interactions if the most appropriate advice is to be provided for a patient or another healthcare professional regarding the food-drug interaction. Other issues not illustrated in these examples include those related to the drug's dosage form and route of administration. Do all dosage forms [capsules, tablets, liquids (suspensions, solutions), sustained-action products] interact with the food or nutrient? Does a listed interaction occur if a drug is given via a route other than by mouth (injection, sublingual, transdermal, rectal)? By understanding the interaction, the choices that a nutrition care provider must make are often less difficult; it is easier to prioritize the risk level to the patient and customize dietary recommendations. It is also easier for the advanced practice nutrition care provider to teach and mentor others when food-drug interactions can be classified into logical groups based on mechanisms of interaction or similar dietary modifications rather than using a random, individual food-drug interaction approach to this very large topic. Unfortunately, most food-drug interactions are not adequately studied at this time.

Only recently have food-drug interactions come under close scrutiny, and while the knowledge base is expanding, much remains to be discovered in this area. Interactions can be complicated and difficult to sort out, since foods, like drugs, are "chemicals" that can have complex structures, various types of electrostatic and chemical bonds, sites designed to bind with specific compounds or chemical moieties, and other features that determine when and how interactions occur. Certain foods can induce or inhibit enzyme systems responsible for drug metabolism, just as other drugs do, and the method of cooking may influence enzyme activity. Transporter activity can also be enhanced or inhibited by certain foods. Therefore, methods that prevent or mitigate effects of one food-drug interaction can be ineffective with another despite the interactions appearing to be similar. The challenge for nutrition care providers is to recognize that limited data are available for many food-drug interactions and that decisions are often based on assumptions that may be erroneous rather than being evidenced based.

Two examples, both in patients receiving tube feeding, serve as cautionary notes regarding assumptions for the management of food-drug interactions. The warfarin–tube feeding interaction is the first example. Well known is the warfarin–green leafy vegetables interaction due to vitamin K content. Therefore it was assumed that "warfarin resistance" in tube-fed patients must be related to vitamin K in the feeding formula; most manufacturers therefore reduced the vitamin K content of formulas. Reports of subtherapeutic anticoagulation continued to occur despite relatively low vitamin K intake, suggesting that another mechanism must be involved in the interaction. No systematic evaluation of the problem was ever reported, but one small study found that warfarin binds to some component in enteral formula, most likely protein.[2] Larger studies are needed to confirm the binding of warfarin to protein as the mechanism responsible for warfarin resistance with formulas low in vitamin K, but this mechanism seems reasonable given that warfarin is highly protein bound in serum. Acceptance of this mechanism of interaction between warfarin and enteral formula requires a shift in management techniques. Separating warfarin administration from formula administration by 1 or 2 hours would not prevent an interaction mediated by vitamin K; however, a "binding" interaction would likely be prevented by the separation, as has been reported in practice.[3]

To follow the warfarin discussion another step, questions that must be asked are whether the interaction can be avoided by the use of hydrolyzed enteral formulas and whether all highly protein-bound drugs are at risk of interaction with enteral feeding formulas. Theoretically, protein binding is not expected with a hydrolyzed formula, since free amino acids and small peptides lack the complex structure typically associated with protein-binding sites. Studies to confirm or refute the effect of hydrolyzed formula on warfarin resistance are lacking. As to whether all highly protein-bound drugs are at risk, the answer is possibly yes, but specific binding characteristics might also be important. Unfortunately, a systematic investigation of the interactions with enteral formula and drugs has never occurred.

The second cautionary note comes from the interaction between fluoroquinolone antibiotics and tube feeding. This interaction highlights the potential complexity of interactions as well as an assumption related to mechanism of interaction. Fluoroquinolones (the "quinolones") are known to form nonabsorbable complexes with divalent cations, including calcium and magnesium; therefore, loss of drug from the formation of cation-drug complexes was assumed to be responsible for decreased serum concentrations of quinolones reported in patients receiving tube feeding. Separating quinolones administration from formula administration by 1 or 2 hours would mitigate such a binding-type interaction. An in vitro study reporting a wide range of fluoroquinolone recovery after mixing of antibiotic with enteral formula, however, suggested that the interaction may be more complex.[4] Recovery was lowest for ciprofloxacin (17.5%), intermediate for levofloxacin (39%), and highest for ofloxacin (54%); it was correlated with the hydrophilic character of the drug. Mixing with calcium and magnesium solutions had minimal effect on recovery of the antibiotics. A legitimate question was whether such in vitro data were supported by in vivo studies, which has proved to be the case. Differences in bioavailability have been reported between ofloxacin (90%) and ciprofloxacin (72%) in healthy volunteers receiving an enteral formula.[5] Whether this difference in bioavailability is the same for actual patients is more difficult to determine and has not been reported.

Interactions between quinolones and tube feeding are further complicated by issues related to the site of absorption. Tube feeding can deliver a drug into the stomach, duodenum, or jejunum, depending on tube placement. Most drugs are absorbed by passive absorption throughout the small bowel; however, degradation or preferential absorption may occur based on acidity along the gastrointestinal (GI) tract. Ciprofloxacin shows interesting absorption characteristics. About 40% of an oral ciprofloxacin dose is absorbed in the duodenum, and drug concentrations in both healthy volunteers and intensive care patients are higher after administration into the duodenum compared to the stomach due to drug degradation by stomach acid.[6,7] Administration through a jejunal feeding tube results in lower ciprofloxacin serum concentrations than oral administration, despite the drug's sensitivity to gastric acid.[8] The clinical significance of this difference in absorption depends on the site of infection and the necessary minimum inhibitory concentration (MIC) for eradication of the microorganism, which is beyond the scope of practice for a nutrition care provider. As part of a healthcare team, however, it is the nutrition care provider's responsibility to be aware of such interactions and make other members of the team aware of the potential problem. Absorption data are not necessarily consistent for all drugs within a class (i.e., for all fluoroquinolones); thus data from ciprofloxacin cannot be extrapolated to other floxacins.

The data on ciprofloxacin absorption raise an important consideration for reported food-drug interactions; that is, under what conditions has an interaction been reported? Do all reports involve healthy volunteers, or are sick patients included? Are subjects consuming a normal diet or an investigator-controlled diet? If the diet is controlled, is it realistic for patients to follow such a diet for the duration of their drug therapy? Do reports differ between ambulatory patients and critically ill patients or between those with a specific condition (such as diabetes mellitus which slows gastric emptying) and those without? Are studies based on single doses of the drug or on multiple doses, as would be seen with normal applications of the drug for therapeutic benefit? When the interaction involves enteral feeding, is there a feeding tube in place, and where does the tube empty? The ongoing controversy regarding phenytoin and tube feeding illustrates the potential problem of healthy subjects, single-dose studies, and the need to carefully evaluate the literature.

Phenytoin is a widely prescribed antiseizure drug with a narrow therapeutic index. This means that serum concentrations must remain within a relatively small range to be effective without being toxic. Any food-drug interaction that alters absorption can result in subtherapeutic or toxic concentrations, depending on the direction of change in absorption. Numerous reports related to an enteral formula's interaction with phenytoin can be found in the literature, including four prospective, randomized, placebo-controlled studies that did not find evidence of an interaction.[9] Countering this are many reports and studies (at least 25) indicating that an interaction does occur, but none are prospective, randomized, and placebo-controlled. Without further analysis of the data, the nutrition care provider must choose between the results from small yet well-designed studies or a larger number of reports with poorer designs. Closer scrutiny of the studies and reports indicates an important difference: studies using healthy subjects and single doses do not find an interaction, while reports in actual patients typically do find that an interaction occurs.[9] The interaction results in low serum phenytoin concentrations despite high doses of the drug, thereby increasing the risk of seizures.

The examples presented in the previous paragraphs serve to emphasize the complex nature of food-drug interactions and the necessity of knowing more than the food and the drug involved. Although most of these examples have been interactions with enteral feeding, this is not to imply that such interactions are more prevalent or more important than other food-drug interactions. There are many known food-drug interactions, including those that occur with the use of diuretics, antibiotics, anticoagulants, antihypertensive agents, antiretroviral drugs, antidepressants, thyroid compounds, and alcohol.[10] Some interactions have little impact on the patient, while others can cause significant health effects. In recent years, several serious interactions involving grapefruit juice have been reported. Considering the variability in food intake and the number of factor that can influence interactions, the difficulty lies in determining which interactions are most likely to result in clinically significant problems for a given patient. The more nutrition care providers learn about food-drug interactions, the better prepared they are to offer appropriate advice to patients and other healthcare providers. For this reason, a brief overview of food-drug interactions follows.

TYPES OF INTERACTIONS

Interactions between foods and drugs can be divided into two categories: pharmacokinetic and pharmacodynamic. At least theoretically, an interaction can affect the drug, the food, or both. Realistically, data related to drug effects on foods or nutrients other than food intake are nearly nonexistent, making effects on drugs the focus of food-drug interactions. Pharmacokinetic interactions include changes in the absorption, distribution, metabolism, or elimination of a drug, and are much more common than pharmacodynamic interactions. Pharmacodynamic interactions affect the activity of drugs at the site of action, presumably at the receptor level—for example, by having the same mechanism of action.

The interactions between food and drugs can either increase or decrease the effects of drugs. These changes may cause toxicity from the drug or, at the other extreme, a complete loss of therapeutic effect. In addition, the seasonal changes in diet, environmental factors including smoking and toxins, and periods of starvation for whatever reason will induce or inhibit metabolic enzymes and affect how the body absorbs and metabolizes drugs.[10] Many factors, therefore, make it difficult to predict with any precision the extent of food-drug interactions in a given person. Pharmacokinetic studies of these interactions in humans in the fed and fasting states are necessary.[11,12] Food is known to have significant effects on gastric emptying, and this, in turn, can greatly influence drug absorption.[13]

VARIABLES OF FOOD-DRUG INTERACTIONS

CHARACTERISTICS OF THE DRUG

Both the physical and chemical properties of the drug play a role in the likelihood of an interaction between the drug and food. Since drugs vary in their acidity or alkalinity, their rates of dissolution and absorption vary. Drugs in the same category can have different chemical characteristics and thus different effects and possible interactions.[13] Even the same drug, formulated differently, either with different binders and fillers or in a different dosage form altogether (capsule versus tablet or suspension), can have different chemical characteristics and therefore different interactions.

For the nutrition care provider, this can make it difficult to translate from research data, or even case reports, to practice. Advice from a pharmacist may help decide the risk of an interaction in this situation.

CHARACTERISTICS OF THE MEAL

Food-drug interactions are dependent on when the drug is taken in relation to the meal as well as the size of the meal and its composition (Table 19-1).[14] For example, taken on an empty stomach, most antibiotics will have increased absorption, resulting in higher blood levels and increased effects. On the other hand, the presence of food often decreases the absorption. Does this translate into ineffective treatment if the patients take the antibiotic with food because they experience nausea and vomiting when taking it without food? Obviously, absorption cannot be adequate if the antibiotic is lost in emesis. Is one food better than another if the patient must take the antibiotic with food to avoid vomiting? With antibiotics having a narrow therapeutic index, reduced absorption in the presence of food may prevent the MIC of an antibiotic from being reached, thus reducing its effectiveness, particularly if the infection is in a difficult-to-treat site (e.g., meningitis). An alternative antibiotic may need to be selected. More often the antibiotic has a wide effective range and an adequate MIC will be obtained despite slightly lower absorption when taken with food. The food consumed with the antibiotic could, however, influence the degree of antibiotic absorption.

The composition of the meal can alter the absorption of drugs. Foods and beverages can cause physiologic changes that alter the rate and extent of drug absorption. In some cases, foods or compounds in food will bind to the drug and decrease its absorption. Food may alter absorption by changing gastric motility. A high-fat meal will increase the absorption and thus the bioavailability of lipophilic drugs. This may be due in part to the increased secretion of bile, with a concomitant increase in drug dissolution and solubility in the intestinal tract.[13,15,16] Acid-labile drugs, on the other hand, are degraded in the presence of gastric acid and may not achieve therapeutic concentrations if they remain in the stomach for an extended time.

The clearance of drugs may be decreased by foods.[16] Food can compete for enzymes for metabolism and thus reduce the first-pass metabolism, again potentially increasing serum drug concentrations.[15] To minimize the known and unknown effects of food on the blood concentrations of the drugs, drugs should be taken consistently either with or without food.[15] It is probably better to take the drug with food than to have it lost in emesis or not taken at all. If the patient cannot tolerate the drug without food despite a need for it to be taken on an empty stomach, a therapeutic alternative should be discussed with the patient's primary healthcare provider.

PHARMACOKINETIC CHANGES

The changes in the bioavailability of a drug are important factors in pharmacokinetic food-drug interactions. Bioavailability is dependent on the absorption of the drug, presystemic metabolism, and first-pass metabolism. Alterations in presystemic metabolism appear to alter absorption, since the metabolism occurs before the drug reaches the bloodstream, which is the usual measurement pool to determine absorption. First-pass metabolism occurs in the liver before orally administered drugs reach

TABLE 19-1	Drug–Food Interactions with High Clinical Relevance	
DRUG	**DIETARY RECOMMENDATION**	**CONSEQUENCES OF THE INTERACTION WITH FOOD**
Albendazole	With a fatty meal.	Increases solubility and important if systemic infection.
Alendronic acid	Without food or milk.	Decreases effect of drug due to chelation.
Ampicillin	Without food.	Risk of treatment failure if low dose is given.
Atovaquone	With a fatty meal.	Increases solubility and likelihood of achieving target blood levels.
Azithromycin capsules	Without food.	Risk of treatment failure.
Ciprofloxacin	Without food.	Risk of treatment failure due to chelation.
Clodronic acid	Without food or milk.	High risk of treatment failure due to chelation.
Didanosine	Without food.	Risk of treatment failure in adults only.
Digoxin	With a consistent dietary fiber intake.	Change in dietary fiber intake may require dosage adjustment.
Erythromycin	Without food.	Risk of treatment failure.
Etidronic acid	Without food or milk.	High risk of treatment failure due to chelation.
Griseofulvin	With a fatty meal.	Taking with food increases absorption and avoids treatment failure, especially in children.
Halofantrine	Without food.	Taking with food increases absorption and may result in severe toxicity.
Indinavir	Without food.	High risk of treatment failure.
Isotretinoin	With a consistent relationship to meals since fat increases solubility.	Avoids fluctuations in drug effects.
Itraconazole capsules	With a meal.	Needs low pH for solubility and better clinical response.
Itraconazole solution	Without food.	Food increases first-pass metabolism and lowers effects.
Lovastatin	With a low-fiber meal.	High fiber may result in treatment failure.
Monoamine oxidase inhibitors (MAOIs)	With tyramine-restricted diet.	Increased risk of hypertensive crisis.
Melphalan	Without food.	Risk of treatment failure.
Mercaptopurine	Without food.	Risk of treatment failure due to oxidation into inactive metabolites.
Norfloxacin	Without milk.	Risk of treatment failure due to chelation.
Penicillamine	Without food or milk.	Risk of treatment failure due to chelation.
Perindopril	Without food.	Decreased effects since food inhibits conversion to active metabolite.
Phenytoin	Without enteral feedings.	High risk of treatment failure.
Saquinavir	With a meal.	High risk of treatment failure.
Spironolactone	Avoid excessive potassium intake.	Risk of hyperkalemia; pharmacodynamic interaction.
Tacrolimus	With a consistent relationship to meals.	Avoids fluctuations in drug effects since increased solubility with fat intake.
Tetracycline	Without food or milk.	High risk of treatment failure due to chelation.
Warfarin	Avoid excessive vitamin K intake.	Continuous daily ingestion of vitamin K–rich foods antagonizes drug effects.

Source: Adapted with permission from Schmidt and Dalhoff.[14]

systemic circulation, but they can be separated from absorption and presystemic metabolism in research studies by measuring drug concentrations in the portal vein.

CHANGES IN ABSORPTION

Among the pharmacokinetic parameters, food has the greatest effect on apparent absorption, which is the net effect of actual absorption and presystemic drug metabolism mediated by enzymes and drug transporters in gastric and intestinal epithelial cells. The presence of food in the stomach slows gastric emptying and alters the absorption of drugs. With slower entry into the small bowel, absorption processes may not be saturated and more drug may ultimately be absorbed, although this will take longer to occur.[15,17] Peak serum concentrations of the drug may not get as high even when total absorption is not changed or is slightly higher. Faster rates of absorption are needed to reach higher concentrations. With some drugs, as with certain antibiotics, where a MIC must be reached to treat the infection, the peak concentration is important. On the other hand, slower rates of absorption of some drugs (e.g., misoprostol and nifedipine capsules) result in lower peaks and potentially less toxic side effects.[14]

Foods can chelate or bind drugs in the GI tract, thus decreasing their absorption. Cations such as calcium, magnesium, and iron as well as antacids are important chelators. For example, the bioavailability of tetracycline and ciprofloxacin is decreased when taken with food, dairy products, iron, or antacids.[14] Even the small amount of milk that is put into tea or coffee can significantly decrease the bioavailability of tetracycline, possibly resulting in treatment failure or the development of resistant organisms. High-fiber foods bind some drugs before they can be absorbed, thereby decreasing serum concentrations. For example, the absorption of digoxin is decreased by 16 to 32% when taken with fiber.[14] Soluble fibers may be more problematic, as they form gels which can bind drugs and minerals in the fiber matrix.

Fat in a meal will increase the absorption of lipophilic drugs while possibly decreasing the absorption and/or maximum concentration of less lipophilic drugs. For example, atovaquone should be taken with a fatty meal to increase absorption and therefore the effects of the drug. On the other hand, the maximum serum concentration of cycloserine is decreased when it is administered with a high-fat meal, while the time it takes to reach maximum concentration is increased.[18]

CHANGES IN METABOLISM

Interactions affecting the systemic metabolism, distribution, or elimination of drugs by food are not as common as those affecting absorption and presystemic metabolism. Until the cytochrome P450 (CYP450) enzyme system was identified and studied, little was known about presystemic metabolism; effects appeared as part of absorption in pharmacokinetic studies unless portal vein drug concentrations were measured. Presystemic metabolism is mediated by CYP450 and its isoenzymes as well as by drug transporters.[13,10] About 60% of available drugs are metabolized by the CYP3A isoenzymes, and nearly 50% by the 3A4 subset.[19] Another major CYP450 isoenzyme is CYP2D6; together, CYP3A4 and CYP2D6 are responsible for many of the metabolic interactions reported.[20,21] CYP3A4 is found in the gut wall and metabolizes orally administered substrate drugs before they are absorbed,[22] thus decreasing the amounts available for absorption. Inhibition of CYP3A4 results in more drug being available for absorption, since normal loss to presystemic metabolism does not occur;

thus, the risk of toxicity is increased.[17,22] Drugs administered by routes other than the GI tract (intravenous, transdermal, rectal) are not absorbed via the portal vein and do not undergo presystemic metabolism by these gut wall enzymes and transporters.

The best-known food affecting CYP3A4 is grapefruit and its juice; such interactions can be life-threatening. Inhibition of CYP3A by grapefruit juice appears to be more than competitive inhibition; irreversible loss of intestinal CYP3A appears to occur while there is little loss of hepatic CYP3A activity.[23] Even a single glass of grapefruit juice can increase the effects of a drug, resulting in enhanced therapeutic efficacy or increased toxicity.[17] This effect is not short-lived. It may take at least 3 full days after the last glass (300 mL) of grapefruit juice for full enzyme activity to recover, since de novo synthesis of the enzyme is required to restore such activity.[24,25] The irreversible loss of activity explains why separating grapefruit juice intake from drug administration by 1 to 2 hours is not effective in preventing an interaction. It is important for nutrition care providers to realize that all citrus fruits are not equal in terms of this type of interaction, since orange juice does not appear to reduce CYP3A activity; thus patients do not need to avoid all citrus fruit to avoid this interaction.

As a general rule, the greater the concentration of CYP3A4 in intestinal cells and the greater the metabolism of a drug before it is absorbed, the more bioavailable the drug is likely to be after the ingestion of grapefruit.[26] There is variability in the concentration of enzymes from one person to another. In addition, there is considerable variability in the interaction of drugs with grapefruit, including significant interactions with some drugs in a given class but not with others. For instance, grapefruit inhibits the metabolism of certain cholesterol-lowering drugs (HMG-CoA reductase inhibitors, or "statins"), including simvastatin, lovastatin, and atorvastatin, but it has no effect on pravastatin. Seville oranges have a similar effect compared to grapefruit on CYP3A4. However, Seville orange juice, but not grapefruit juice, increased indinavir blood levels in healthy volunteers,[27] suggesting that other compounds may come into play, potentially transporters. The exact compound(s) in grapefruit and Seville oranges that inhibit the metabolic enzymes are not known. The flavanoids naringin and naringenin as well as the franocoumarin bergamotin are no longer thought to be the cause.[22]

Garlic supplements may also affect the CYP3A4 isoenzyme. When garlic tablets (GarliPure, Madimum Allicin Formula; Natrol) were coadministered with saquinavir, the mean maximum saquinivar plasma concentration (C_{max}) decreased by 54% and the area under the curve (AUC), representing concentration versus time, decreased by a mean of 51%. These decreases were still evident 10 days after the garlic tablets were discontinued.[28] On the other hand, the Kwai garlic supplement (Lichtwer Pharma, Eatontown, NJ) had little effect on CYP2D6 and CYP3A4 after 14 days of exposure.[29] The potential of a similar interaction with fresh, whole garlic is not known. The effect of garlic on the transporter P-glycoprotein was not measured.

Red wine is yet another food shown to inhibit CYP3A4 in vitro and may interact with drugs in a manner similar to grapefruit juice.[30] The interaction between red wine (250 mL) and cisapride was studied in 12 healthy males. There was only a minor increase in cisapride levels in most subjects, but there was a doubling of levels in one.[30] This significant patient variability can be problematic, especially since it is not predictable.

In animal studies, honey has recently been found to increase the clearance of several compounds, including diltiazem, carbamazepine and naringin. Additionally, there is a significant decrease in the plasma time-concentration curve (AUC), signifying an overall decrease in the amount of drug absorbed.[31–33] The effect of honey on the bioavailability of drugs in humans has not been investigated.

Presystemic drug metabolism may be affected by drug transporters as well as the CYP450 enzymes. The best known transporter, P-glycoprotein, is associated with efflux of drugs from the enterocyte back into the intestinal lumen, thereby limiting net drug absorption. Inhibition of P-glycoprotein results in increased drug absorption, since drug is not lost into the intestinal lumen. The juice of Seville oranges has been reported to inhibit P-glycoprotein in the GI tract.[34] Grapefruit juice has similar effects in some studies, including a doubling of the maximum plasma concentration of talinolol in an in vivo model.[35] On the other hand, in humans, grapefruit juice had no effect on the maximum plasma drug concentration during 48 hours following a single dose of digoxin 0.5 mg, a known P-glycoprotein substrate. Only a slight 9% increase in the area under the curve of digoxin occurred from 0 to 24 hours.[36] Based on these results, the author of the latter study concluded that grapefruit juice was not an important inhibitor of P-glycoprotein; however, in many studies, it is difficult to distinguish effects of CY3A4 from those of P-glycoprotein. The opposing results of these studies require an individual review of any drug known to be a P-glycoprotein substrate, as interactions are possible. Uptake transporters, specifically organic anion–transporting polypeptides (OATPs), usually balance efflux by increasing drug uptake from the intestinal lumen into enterocytes. Grapefruit juice does appear to inhibit OATPs, as do both orange and apple juice.[23]

PHARMACODYNAMIC EFFECTS

The anticoagulant effects of warfarin can be antagonized by foods rich in vitamin K. These include cabbage, broccoli, and liver. A single meal of vitamin K–rich foods has little clinical effect. On the other hand, daily ingestion of vitamin K–rich foods for a week can have significant effects, requiring a dosage adjustment of warfarin.[14] Avocado, even though it is low in vitamin K, also significantly antagonizes the effects of warfarin.[37]

Angiotensin converting enzyme (ACE) inhibitors (e.g., captopril, enalapril, cilazapril, lisinopril) are known to cause hyperkalemia. Foods high in potassium or the salt substitutes can potentiate this effect.[38]

Tyramine-rich foods, including draught beer, should be avoided by patients who take monoamine oxidase inhibitors (MAOIs), including phenelzine, tranylcypromine. and isocarboxazid. MAOIs inhibit the metabolism of the monoamines, putting the patient at risk for hypertensive crisis.

CONCLUSIONS

Foods are complex substances containing many active compounds capable of interacting with the drugs so frequently prescribed and taken. It is important for the nutrition care provider to be aware of the known food-drug interactions. It is also important to be suspicious of interactions when drugs are not producing the expected outcomes and to question methods of controlling or mitigating interactions when these methods are not producing the desired results. Our understanding of food-drug interactions, although still limited, is growing; thus it is important to recognize the changing knowledge base. Caution is needed in extrapolating from one food to all foods within that category (i.e., from grapefruit and Seville oranges to all citrus fruits). The more nutrition care providers understand about food-drug interactions, the better prepared they are to offer appropriate advice to patients and other healthcare providers regarding prevention or mitigation of the interaction. Taking drugs consistently with food may help prevent wide fluctuations in drug response and is reasonable advice for most patients, since the dose of the drug can be adjusted to account for many food effects. Serious interactions, however, may require discontinuation of a specific drug or tight dietary control of an interacting food/nutrient.

Issues to Ponder

The following are several questions pertinent to food-drug interactions that have no definitive answer but pose interesting dilemmas.

- When is a drug-nutrient interaction significant?
- Should a patient's drug regimen be changed from the "drug of choice" to an alternate, potentially less effective or more expensive drug due to drug-nutrient interactions?
- Is extrapolation of data related to enzyme and transporter activity relative to food-drug interactions valid across ethnic and gender lines?
- What do you tell the patient when a drug is to be taken on an empty stomach but he or she vomits every time it is taken without food?
- Does it matter that a different dosage form was used in the study compared to what the patient is receiving?
- For tube feeding interactions with drugs, does it matter that the components of an enteral formula have changed from those used in the original studies, even when the name has not changed?
- Is drinking an enteral formula the same as administering the formula via nasogastric or gastrostomy tube relative to food-drug interactions?
- Can data be extrapolated for studies in healthy subjects to sick patients?
- Should dietitians and other advanced practice healthcare providers be required to obtain formal training in food-drug interactions and the mechanisms of interaction?

REFERENCES

1. Kaufman DW, Kelly JP, Rosenberg L, Anderson TE, Mitchell AA. Recent patterns of medication use in the ambulatory adult population of the United States: the Slone survey. JAMA 2002;287:337–344.
2. Penrod LE, Allen JB, Cabacungan LR. Warfarin resistance and enteral feedings: 2 case reports and a supporting in vitro study. Arch Phys Med Rehabil 2001;82:1270–1271.
3. Petretich DA, Reversal of osmolite-warfarin interaction by changing warfarin administration time (letter). Clin Pharm 1990;9:93.
4. Wright DH, Pietz SL, Konstantinides MT, Rotschafer JC. Decreased in vitro fluoroquinolone concentrations after admixture with an enteral feeding formulation. J Parenter Enteral Nutr 2000;24:42–48.
5. Mueller BA, Brierton DG, Abel S, Bowman L. Effects of enteral feeding with Ensure on oral bioavailabilities of ofloxacin and ciprofloxacin. Antimicrob Agents Chemother 1994;38:2101–2105.
6. Staib AH, Beerman D, Harder S, Fuhr U, Lierman D. Absorption differences in ciprofloxacin along the human gastrointestinal tract using a remote-control drug delivery device. Am J Med 1989; 87(suppl 5A):66S–69S.
7. Yuk JH, Nightingale CH, Quintiliani R, et al. Absorption of ciprofloxacin administered through a nasogastric or a nasoduodenal tube in volunteers and patients receiving enteral nutrition. Diagn Microbiol Infect Dis 1990;13:99–102.

8. Healy DP, Brodbeck MC, Clendening CE. Ciprofloxacin absorption is impaired in patients given enteral feedings orally and via gastrostomy and jejunostomy tubes. Antimicrob Agents Chemother 1996;40:6–10.

9. Au Yeung SC, Ensom MHH. Phenytoin and enteral feedings: does evidence support an interaction? Ann Pharmacother 2000;34:896–905.

10. Sorensen JM. Herb-drug, food-drug, nutrient-drug and drug-drug interactions: mechanisms involved and their medical implications. J Alt Comp Med 2002;8; 293–308.

11. Charman WN, Porter CJ, Mithani S, et al. Physicochemical and physiological mechanisms for the effects of food on drug absorption: the role of lipids and pH. J Pharm Sci 1997;82:269–282.

12. al-Behaisi S, Antal I, Morovjan G, et al. Study of the acid buffering capacity of dietary components regarding food-drug interactions (abstr). Acta Pharm Hung 2002;72:A185–A190.

13. Singh BN. Effects of foods on clinical pharmacokinetics. Clin Pharmacokinet 1999;37:213–255.

14. Schmidt LE, Dalhoff K. Food-drug interactions. Drugs 2002;62:1481–1502.

15. Zimmerman JJ, Ferron GM, Lim, HK, Parker V. The effect of a high-fat meal on the oral bioavailability of the immunosuppressant sirolimus (rapamycin). J Clin Pharmacol 1999;39:1155–1161.

16. Brocks DR, Wasan KM. The influence of lipids on stereoselective pharmacokinetics of halofantrine: important implications in food-effect studies involving drugs that bind to lipoproteins. J Pharm Sci 2002;91:1817–1826.

17. Evans AM. Influence of dietary components on the gastrointestinal metabolism and transport of drugs. Ther Drug Monit 2000;22:131–136.

18. Zhu M, Nix DE, Adam RD, et al. Pharmacokinetics of cycloserine under fasting conditions and with high-fat meal, orange juice, and antacids. Pharmacotherapy 2001;21:891–897.

19. Zhou S, Chan SY, Goh BC, Chan E, Duan W, Huang M, McLeod HL. Mechanism-based inhibition of cytochrome P450 3A4 by therapeutic drugs. Clin Pharmacokinet 2005;44:279–304.

20. Zanger U, Eichelbaum M. CyP2D6. In: Levy H, Thummel KE, Trager W, Hansten PD, Eichelbuam M., eds. Metabolic Drug Interactions. New York: Lippincott Williams & Wilkins; 2000:87–94.

21. Wrighton SA, Thummel KE. CYP3A. In: Levy H, Thummel KE, Trager W, Hansten PD, Eichelbuam M., eds. Metabolic Drug Interactions. New York: Lippincott Williams & Wilkins; 2000:115–134.

22. Aronson JK. Forbidden fruit. Nature Med 2001;7:29–30.

23. Dresser GK, Bailey DG. The effects of fruit juices on drug disposition: a new model for drug interactions. Eur J Clin Invest 2003;33(suppl 2):10–16.

24. Greenblatt DJ, Moltke LL, Harmatz JS, et al. Time course of recovery of cytochrome P450 3A function after single doses of grapefruit juice. Clin Pharmacol Ther 2003;74:121–129.

25. Lilja JJ, Kivisto KT, Neuvonen PJ. Duration of effect of grapefruit juice on the pharmacokinetics of the CYP3A4 substrate simvastatin. Clin Pharmacol Ther 2000;68:384–390.

26. Transwell AS. The power of grapefruit (editorial). Nutr Diet 2003;60:6–8.

27. Penzak SR, Acosta EP, Turner M, et al. Effect of Seville orange juice and grapefruit juice on indinavir pharmcokinetics. J Clin Pharmacol 2002;42:1165–1170.

28. Piscitelli SC, Burstein AH, Welden N, Gallicano KD, Falloon J. The effect of garlic supplements on the pharmacokinetics of saquinavir. Clin Infect Dis 2002;34:234–238.

29. Markowitz JS, DeVane CL, Chavin KD, et al. Effects of garlic (Allium sativum L) supplementation on cytochrome P450 2D6 and 3A4 activity in healthy volunteers. Clin Pharmacol Ther 2003;74:170–177.

30. Chan KW, Nguyen LT, Miler VP, Harris RZ. Mechanism-based inactivation of human cytochrome P450 3A4 by grapefruit juice and red wine. Life Sci 1998;62:135–142.

31. Koumaravelou K, Adithan C, Shashindran CH, et al. Influence of honey on orally and intravenously administered diltiazem kinetics in rabbits. Indian J Exp Biol 2002a;40:1164–1168.

32. Koumaravelou K, Adithan C, Shashindran CH, Asad M, Abraham BK. Effect of honey on carbamazepine kinetics in rabbits. Indian J Exp Biol 2002;40:560–563.

33. Hou YC, Hsiu SL, Huang TY, Yang C, Tsai SY, Chao PD. Effect of honey and sugars on the metabolism and disposition of naringin in rabbits. Planta Med 2001;67:538–541.

34. Di Marco MP, Edwards DJ, Wainer IW, Ducharme MP. The effect of grapefruit juice and Seville orange juice on the pharmacokinetics of dextromethorphan: the role of gut CYP3A and P-glycoprotein. Life Sci 2002;71:1149–1160.

35. Spahn-Langguth H, Langguth P. Grapefruit juice enhances intestinal absorption of the P-glycoprotein substrate talinolol. Eur J Pharm Sci 2001;12:361–367.

36. Becquemont L, Verstuyft C, Kerb R, et al. Effect of grapefruit juice on digoxin pharmacokinetics in humans. Clin Pharmacol Ther 2001;70:311–316.

37. Blichstein D, Shaklai M, Inbal A. Warfarin antagonism by avocado. Lancet 1991;337:914–915.

38. Reardon LC, Macpherson DS. Hyperkalaemia due to the concomitant use of salt substitutes and ACE inhibitors in hypertension: a potentially life threatening interaction. J Hum Hypertens 1999;13:717–720.

CHAPTER

20

ISSUES WITH ALTERNATIVE/ COMPLEMENTARY NUTRITION THERAPIES: THEIR ROLE IN CLINICAL PRACTICES

Diane Rigassio Radler and Adam Perlman

Complementary and alternative medicine (CAM) involves therapeutic practices that are not routinely within the scope of conventional, mainstream medicine in the United States. CAM practices extend to a wide range of approaches and may be used to maintain wellness and prevent and manage disease. Although many CAM practices are indigenous to cultures outside the United States and may have been part of their traditional healthcare practices for centuries, CAM theory and practice have recently had a rapid and profound effect in the United States. The increasing use of CAM practices within the United States has been documented since the early 1990s, but little is known about their efficacy or long-term safety, which fosters a sense of uncertainty. The U.S. healthcare system is challenged to evaluate the safety and efficacy of a variety of CAM modalities and to integrate conventional and unconventional therapies where appropriate. Healthcare professionals and CAM providers must understand a common language, recognize diversity, and be prepared to counsel and provide guidance to patients.

WHAT IS CAM?

The leading agency for scientific research of CAM in the United States is the National Center for Complementary and Alternative Medicine (NCCAM) within the National Institutes of Health. NCCAM defines CAM as "a group of diverse medical and healthcare systems, practices, and products that are not presently considered to be part of conventional medicine."[1] Practices considered CAM may evolve over time when therapies that are proven safe and effective are adopted into conventional healthcare.[1] "Complementary" refers to practices that are adjunctive to conventional practice. "Alternative" refers to practices that are used instead of conventional practices. "Integrative," a term increasingly used, refers to a merging of allopathic approaches and CAM therapies for which evidence on safety and efficacy exists, to deliver healthcare that is superior to that of any one modality alone.[1]

NCCAM groups CAM practices into five domains: (1) alternative medical systems, (2) mind-body interventions, (3) biologically based treatments, (4) manipulative and body-based methods, and (5) energy therapies.[1] This chapter focuses on the role of the dietetics practitioner with regards to nutrition and dietary supplements in biologically based therapies; examples of each CAM domain are provided in Table 20-1.

TABLE 20-1	Five Domains of Complementary and Alternative Medicine Practice
TYPE	**CHARACTERISTICS**
I. Alternative medical systems include approaches such as homeopathy, natural medicine, and traditional Oriental medicine.	
Homeopathy[21,22]	• Developed in the late 18th century by Samuel Hahnemann, a German physician. • Based on the "law of similars," a concept of curing like with like. • One single remedy administered at a time. • Minimum dose given; side effects rare.
Natural medicine[23,24]	• Introduced in Western medicine in the late 19th century. • Holistic system of healthcare combining elements of allopathic philosophy with emphasis on clinical nutrition, acupuncture, botanical medicine, and psychology.
Traditional Oriental medicine (TOM)[25,26]	• Encompasses the ancient medical practices of Far Eastern countries such as China and Japan. • A holistic practice in which the body is viewed as being in a state of harmony and balance. • The body and mind are unified, and a universal life force of *chi* (pronounced "chee" in Chinese and "kee" in Japanese) flows throughout the body along specific channels or "meridians." • *Chi* flow or blockage is attributed to health or disease, respectively. • TOM practitioners use a combination of acupressure and acupuncture, herbal remedies, and meditative exercise to achieve balance.
II. Mind-body interventions[27,28] involve the mind's ability to influence the body's function and symptoms and include approaches such as meditation, hypnosis, yoga, progressive muscle relaxation, biofeedback, and music therapy.	
Meditation	• Involves deep breathing exercises and focused attention to attain muscle relaxation. Dr. Herbert Benson introduced the concept of the "relaxation response" in the early 1970s, incorporating several types of relaxation and meditation techniques to reduce heart rate, blood pressure, breathing rate, brainwave patterns, and pain.
Hypnosis	• Hypnosis is a state between sleep and wakefulness that allows for relaxation and deep concentration.
Yoga	• Yoga may be considered the "science of the spirit." Yoga incorporates postures, breathing exercises, and meditation and has recently become popular in the United States.
Biofeedback	• Biofeedback is a process of monitoring the tension in the body in response to thoughts, feelings, and sensations. Electrodes are attached to the body area that is tense, and the monitoring equipment provides feedback to the patient through an audible or visual signal. The patient is told to use thoughts and feelings to affect the amount of tension in the area being monitored. As muscles contract, the signal is rapid; as muscles relax, the signal is slowed. With training, patients learn to slow the signal through thoughts, feelings, and actions.

PREVALENCE OF CAM USE IN THE UNITED STATES

CAM use has been increasing in popularity in the United States for the past two decades. Eisenberg and colleagues were pioneers in uncovering the rampant increase in usage when they reported findings of a survey conducted in 1990.[2] The researchers disclosed that one in three Americans who participated in the survey had used at least one CAM therapy during the past year, visits to CAM providers ex-

TYPE	CHARACTERISTICS
TABLE 20-1 Five Domains of Complementary and Alternative Medicine Practice (*cont*)	
III. Biologically based treatments include special diets, herbal and other dietary supplements, and orthomolecular therapy (use of vitamin regimens at levels significantly greater than the daily recommended intake).	
Special diets[29]	• Dietary regimens that incorporate comprehensive alterations in eating patterns. Examples include the macrobiotic diet, raw foods diet, and the Gerson diet for cancer.
Dietary supplements[30]	• Dietary supplements can be logically divided into botanicals, which include herbs and other plant materials with potential health benefits, and nutritionals, which are essentially all other dietary supplements, such as vitamins, minerals, amino acids, fatty acids, and metabolites.
IV. Manipulative and body-based methods include methods involved in the manipulation or movement of the body, such as chiropractic, osteopathy, and massage.	
Chiropractic[31,32]	• Chiropractic, developed in the late 1800s by Daniel David Palmer, is rooted in the belief that proper alignment of the spine affects the health of the body. • Wellness and prevention are the guiding principles in chiropractic. Chiropractors manually manipulate the body to promote optimal functioning of the nervous system by aligning the spine properly and relieving muscle tension. • The chiropractic philosophy is based on two fundamental precepts: the importance of the influence that the structure and condition of the body have on its physiological functioning and the importance of the mind-body connection in promoting healing and maintaining health.
Osteopathy[32]	• Osteopathy is a holistic healing system introduced by Andrew Taylor Still in the late 1800s. Osteopathy is similar to chiropractic in that it includes a form of therapeutic manipulation to restore flexibility and mobility, relieve pain, and promote well-being. Originally osteopaths used long-lever manipulation, which involves the arms and legs as fulcrums for bending and twisting the body. Chiropractic, in contrast, used short-lever manipulation focused on the protruding parts of the spinal vertebrae. Today, however, osteopathic medicine training is essentially the same as that of medical doctors except that osteopaths receive additional training in the musculoskeletal system. Doctors of osteopathy (DOs) are fully trained and licensed physicians who may prescribe drugs, perform surgery, and utilize all accepted modalities to maintain and restore health. Many osteopaths serve as primary care physicians because of their commitment to treating the whole person. Rather than being an alternative therapy per se, osteopathy is a conventional medical system that includes the alternative practice of therapeutic manipulation.
Massage	• Massage is an ancient practice commonly used in Chinese, Greek, and Roman cultures. Massage therapists use fingers and palms to knead and manipulate soft tissues to relax sore, tired muscles, dispel tension from the body, and improve lymphatic circulation.
V. Energy therapies involve energy fields that may originate within the body (biofields) or those that originate outside the body (electromagnetic fields).	

Source: National Center for Complementary and Alternative medicine. Available at; www.nccam.nih.gov. Accessed November 12, 2004.

ceeded the number of visits to all U.S. primary care physicians that year, and most of the expenses associated with the use of CAM therapy were paid out of pocket. Additionally, the majority of those who used CAM therapies for serious medical conditions also sought care from their conventional physicians, but most (72%) did not disclose their CAM activities to their physicians.

When Eisenberg and colleagues conducted a follow-up survey in 1997, they found that a greater number of participants had used a CAM modality (42%, versus 34% in 1990), out-of-pocket expenditures were similar, and a similar percentage of users (60%) did not share information of their CAM use with their conventional physicians.[3] Other recent research[4,5] reported continued interest and popularity among Americans in using dietary supplements. CAM use remains a significant issue in current healthcare practice. Data from the Centers for Disease Control and Prevention (CDC) are presented in Figure 20-1; the full CDC report is available at http://www.cdc.gov/nchs/data/ad/ad343.pdf.

IMPLICATIONS FOR DIETETICS PROFESSIONALS: APPLICATION TO PRACTICE

Given the recent surge in CAM interest and the consumer-driven healthcare environment, all healthcare providers must be cognizant of the prevalent use of CAM and be familiar with the efficacy, limitations, and safety of CAM modalities. The dietetics professional is well poised to interact with patients regarding CAM, particularly with the use of dietary supplements and nutrition patterns. Although it may be debated as to which nutrition regimens are considered "conventional" versus "alternative" or "complementary," dietetics professionals must develop an awareness of such therapies to provide the best conventional care while guiding the judicious use of CAM. Such interaction with patients may be on various levels; dietetics professionals may inquire on their use during a nutrition screening process, discuss the use and limitations of diets or supplements during counseling, and document the recommendation for use or for discontinuation accordingly in a written nutrition assessment. Dietetics practitioners must be knowledgeable about common dietary supplements used in their patient populations; they are encouraged to seek continuing education opportunities in those areas. The goal of this chapter is to provide the logistics in information gathering and patient counseling regarding CAM, not to cover the gamut of specific dietary supplements for maintaining wellness and treating disease.

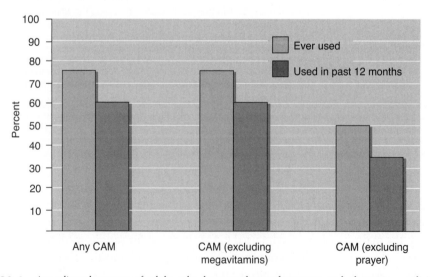

FIGURE 20-1 *Age-adjusted percent of adults who have used complementary and alternative medicine (CAM): United States, 2002. Data source: National Health Interview Survey, 2002. Reprinted from Barnes, Powell-Griner, McFann, & Nahin. Complementary and alternative medicine use among adults: United States, 2002. Advance data from vital and health statistics; no343. Hyattsville, MD: National Center for Health Statistics; 2004.*

The dietetics practitioner has a professional responsibility to the patient to protect, permit, promote, and partner for comprehensive healthcare. To protect the patient is "to do no harm" and avert patient interest in toxic or ineffective therapies that would be used in place of efficacious treatments. The practitioner should, however, also permit the patient to choose safe and adjunctive treatments with no adverse side effects as long as the therapy is accessible, not prohibitive in cost, and does not displace proven remedies. Questionable practices, which are those that lack evidence of safety or efficacy, should be approached with caution. These practices may be considered under the condition that the patient is continuously monitored for effectiveness of the therapy and that the therapy is free of adverse reactions.[6] Dietetics practitioners may engage in dialogue regarding the interest in CAM use and help consumers discern good information and reputable, safe, and effective therapies, products, and therapists. Finally, practitioners should partner with their patients to comanage illness, provide direction to resources and evidence, and offer professional input into the decision process. Partnership also is advisable for monitoring progress and response to treatment if a patient makes an informed decision to engage in CAM.

An open dialogue with all patients is essential and should be part of routine care. Salient questions to ask include "what, why, when, where, and how." The first step is to pose an open-ended question, such as "What are you taking?" or "What type of diet are you following?" This approach may indicate to the patient that you are receptive to an open discussion. A thorough discussion might include any CAM modality, but particularly for the dietetics practitioner, must include the use of any vitamins, minerals, botanicals, or other dietary supplements or regimens. If the patient discloses the use of supplements, the practitioner must ask, "What dosage do you take?" This should include how much per tablet or capsule or how much of an herb is brewed in tea; it should also include the frequency with which the patient consumes the supplement or participates in treatment. If possible, patients should bring their supplements in for review, as different brands may be standardized to different active ingredients. Nutrition recommendations and health implications may differ for the patient who takes ginger tea occasionally for nausea versus the one who takes concentrated ginger in capsules twice a day.

Query the reason for use by asking, "Why are you taking it?" or "Why are you following such a diet?" Is it to remedy a symptom, to treat a disease, or for disease prevention? A practitioner who discovers that a patient is taking garlic might question whether he is taking it in the interest of preventing colorectal cancer or cardiovascular disease, both of which would convey insight to the practitioner regarding the patient's health concerns.

To find out how long the patient has been on the regimen ask, "When did you start taking it?" (or, in the case of a treatment, "How long ago did you start using it?"). In the case of dietary supplements, symptom relief or the results of treatment may not appear noticeable for several months. If, however, the patient indicates that he has taken the supplement for several months without any relief, it may be advisable to discontinue the regimen and try another approach. Another important consideration is to ask "When in the day do you take it?" This will help to determine whether there are potential pharmacokinetic interactions with food or medications or whether the patient takes a remedy at a particular time when symptoms seem most severe.

Also during the interview, the practitioner should ask, "Where did you obtain your information and where do you buy the product?" These are important questions to determine whether the patient regularly sees a CAM provider or if the information was obtained from advertising or testimonials. The point of purchase will disclose whether the patient is buying directly from the person making recommendations or selecting a product independently, without guidance.

Finally the practitioner should ask, "How is it working?" Is the patient receiving the results that she thought she would? Have the symptoms been completely alleviated or just diminished? Are there any side effects attributable to the treatment?

These questions may at first seem daunting to a practitioner who is not fully knowledgeable about various dietary regimens or supplements. It is intimidating to consider starting a dialogue about CAM therapies when one has a limited knowledge base. The first step is to learn about the common diets and supplements most likely to be used by the population you serve. Familiarity with terminology may ease any tension in the discussion. Inquiry to the patient can also be educational, helping the practitioner to understand the patient's rationale for using a treatment. Additionally and perhaps most importantly, to increase the likelihood of honest responses, be sure that your patients understand at the onset why a discussion about CAM use is important in providing comprehensive healthcare.

Dietetics professionals may incorporate conversations about CAM use with patients in all phases of the nutrition care process. Nutrition screening, assessments, and counseling sessions, either in the inpatient or outpatient setting, are key opportunities to inquire about the use of CAM, specifically dietary patterns and dietary supplements. Done correctly, these conversations offer an opportunity to strengthen the dietetic professional–patient relationship (Table 20-2).

TABLE 20-2   Sample Questions to Elicit CAM Use by Patients

QUESTION	RATIONALE
What • What type of diet do you follow? • What dietary supplements or herbs do you use? • What is the dose of the dietary supplement?	Use open-ended approach; be receptive to a dialogue. Determine how much of the supplement; determine how much the patient knows about what he is taking.
Why • Why did you start taking it (dietary supplement)?	Determine if it is for disease prevention or treatment.
When • When did you start taking it? • When in the day do you take it?	Determine the course of treatment. Is this a new item to a regimen?
Where • Where did you get the information regarding the supplement?	Determine if the patient is acting on advice from a reputable source.
How • How is it working?	Evaluate efficacy of the supplement and assess for adverse effects.

CONCERNS ABOUT THE EFFICACY AND SAFETY OF CAM THERAPIES

Among the key issues concerning healthcare professionals regarding CAM use is the uncertainty over the efficacy and safety of many CAM practices. Many CAM modalities are inherent in other cultures; however, in the United States, a CAM practice may be used in a manner not intended (on the assumption that "more is better") and, in the case of botanicals, may differ from those of other regions due to species, soil, water, and growing conditions or may have interactions with conventional medications, either prescribed or over-the-counter varieties (Table 20-3). Through NCCAM, researchers have set the foundation for investigating the efficacy and

TABLE 20-3	Documented Herbal Supplement–Drug Interactions	
HERBAL INGREDIENT	**DRUG**	**COMMENT**
Betel nut (*Areca catechu*)	Antipsychotics[a]	↑Drug toxicity
Boldo (*Peumus boldus*)	Warfarin	↑Drug effect
Capsicum (*Capsicum annuum*)	Theophylline	↑Drug absorption
Danshen (*salvia miltiorrhiza*)	Warfarin	↑Drug effect
Devil's claw (*Harpagophytum procumbens*)	Warfarin	↑Drug effect
Dong quai (*Angelica sinensis*)	Warfarin	↑Drug effect
Fenugreek (*trigonella sp.*)	Warfarin	↑Drug effect
Garlic (*Allium sativum*)	Protease inhibitors[b]	↓Drug concentrations
	Warfarin	↑Drug effect
Ginger (*Zingiber sp.*)	Phenprocoumon	↑Bleeding risk
Ginkgo (*Gingko biloba*)	Trazodone	↑Drug effect
	Antiplatelet agents[c]	↑Bleeding risk
	Nifedipine	↑Drug effect
	Omeprazole	↓Drug effect
Ginseng (*Panax ginseng, P. quinquefolius*)	Warfarin	↓Drug effect
	Phenelzine	↑Drug effect
Green tea (*Camellia sinensis*)	Warfarin	↓Drug effect
Kava (*Piper methysticum*)	Alprazolam	↑Drug effect
	Levodopa	↓Drug effect
Licorice (*Glycyrrhiza glabra*)	Spironolactone	↓Drug effect
Milk thistle (*Silybum marianum*)	Indinavir	↓Drug concentrations
Papaya (*Carica papaya*)	Warfarin	↑Drug effect
Psyllium (*Plantago spp*)	Lithium	↓Drug levels
St. John's wort (*Hypericum perforatum*)	Numerous	Various
Valerian (*Valeriana officinalis*)	Barbiturates	↑Drug effect

↓, Decreased; ↑, Increased.

[a]Fluphenazine.

[b]Amprenavir, indinavir, nelfinavir, ritonavir, saquinavir.

[c]Aspirin, clopidogrel.

Source: Adapted from Boullata J. Natural health product interactions with medication. Nutr Clin Pract 2005;20:33–51, with permission from the American Society for Parenteral and Enteral Nutrition (ASPEN). ASPEN does not endorse the use of this material in any form other than its entirety.

safety of various CAM modalities. NCCAM's mission is to subject CAM practices to rigorous scientific scrutiny, train CAM researchers, and provide credible information to both consumers and healthcare professionals.[7] For those CAM modalities that are found to be health-promoting, efficacious, and safe, the expectation is that they will be integrated into mainstream medicine. Until then, the rise in demand and availability, ease of obtaining products, and limited proof of efficacy and safety are causes for concern (Table 20-3).

REGULATION OF DIETARY SUPPLEMENTS AND GUIDELINES FOR MANUFACTURERS

The rising interest in CAM by U.S. consumers has been fueled in part by the explosion in the number of dietary supplements that have been made available with relative ease to meet the demand since the passage of the Dietary Supplement Health and Education Act (DSHEA, pronounced "De-shay") of 1994. An amendment to the federal Food, Drug, and Cosmetic Act, DSHEA stipulated that dietary supplements and dietary supplement ingredients are exempt from the usual regulations that apply to food and drugs.[8] It defined "dietary supplement," established a new framework for assuring safety, provided guidelines for the use of claims that could be made about dietary supplements and for literature that was displayed where supplements were sold, established labeling requirements for dietary supplements, and granted the U.S. Food and Drug Administration (FDA) the authority to establish Good Manufacturing Practices (GMPs) for the production of dietary supplements.

Additionally, all dietary supplements must be labeled as such and must carry the following disclaimer: "This statement has not been evaluated by the Food and Drug Administration. This product is not intended to diagnose, treat, cure, mitigate or prevent any disease." This disclaimer is mandatory, whether or not the supplements are effective in improving health. Of concern to healthcare practitioners is the fact that it conveys no judgment on the part of the FDA as to whether the supplement is effective or safe. In contrast to drugs, dietary supplements are not subjected to premarket approval for safety and efficacy, nor are there, as yet, widespread stringent manufacturing standards for these products. The FDA, however, has the authority to implement quality standards in manufacturing and to remove from the market any products that are found to be unsafe.

The main difference between how dietary supplements and drugs (both prescription and over-the-counter) are made available to consumers relates to the degree of FDA scrutiny that products are given prior to being released to the market. Drugs undergo extensive safety and efficacy testing, which form the basis of FDA approval of a drug's entry into the marketplace; dietary supplements do not routinely undergo this level of premarket testing and approval. As a result, there is considerably more room for an unscrupulous supplement manufacturer to market an impure or ineffective product than for a drug manufacturer to do so and, indeed, several reports of such problems have been documented.[9] Information on dietary supplements with adverse effects can be found at the FDA website at http://www.fda.gov. Potential adverse reactions can be reported to the FDA at http://www.fda.gov/medwatch.

In addition to safety concerns, there is often limited scientific documentation that a particular supplement is effective for its intended purpose. The present adage of "buyer beware" applies to the natural products industry. Numerous high-quality manufacturers, however, have voluntarily adopted GMPs similar to those of the pharmaceutical industry and are producing excellent products based on the scientific literature and tested in clinical studies. Further, the supplement industry has instituted protocols in which a company subjects its products, facilities, and manufacturing procedures to evaluation by independent third parties. Among the more rigorous certification programs are those offered by U.S. Pharmacopeia (http://www.usp.org), NSF International (http://www.nsf.org), ConsumerLab.com (http://www.consumerlab .com), and Shuster Labs (http://www.shusterlabs.com). Table 20-4 provides a sample of independent agencies that assess quality of dietary supplements.

WHAT TO DO WHEN PATIENTS CHOOSE TO USE SUPPLEMENTS

If a patient's interest in dietary regimens and supplements persists after an evaluation of their safety and efficacy, both the patient and healthcare practitioner should also consider the mechanism of action, available research, adverse effects, legality of use, and professional ethics.[10] If patients make an informed decision to take dietary supplements, they should be advised to buy from well-known, reputable companies to reduce the risk of supplement adulteration and contamination.[11] Dietetics professionals are encouraged to review and follow the "Guidelines Regarding the Recommendation and Sale of Dietary Supplements" set forth by the American Dietetic Association.[12] Consumers should be educated to look for quality-control standards. One example is the Dietary Supplement Verification Program (DSVP) set up in 2000 by U.S. Pharmacopeia (USP), an independent, nongovernmental organization, to respond to the need to assure consumers that dietary supplements contain the types

TABLE 20-4	Sample of Independent Agencies Assessing Quality of Dietary Supplements	
AGENCY	**URL**	**QUALITY SEAL**
ConsumerLab	http://www.consumerlab.com	
NSF International	http://www.nsf.org	
Shuster Labs	http://www.shusterlabs.com	Technically Advanced Quality Assurance (TAQA®) program
US Pharmacopeia	http://www.usp.org	

and amounts of ingredients listed on the label.[13] Manufacturers of dietary supplements participate voluntarily in this rigorous program. The regimen subjects products to testing for purity, accuracy of ingredient labeling, and quality manufacturing practices. A product that passes the USP standards may bear the Dietary Supplement Verification Program (DSVP) certification mark.

Another similar voluntary certification program for dietary supplements is offered by NSF International.[14] The certification process includes product testing, GMP inspections, and ongoing monitoring in exchange for the NSF mark.

The USP and NSF International certifications are rigorous and ensure quality at all levels of the manufacturing process. Another independent and potentially useful source of information is ConsumerLab.com. This company investigates whether the label accurately reflects what is in the product container, whether the product is free of contaminates, whether the product disintegrates in a reasonable amount of time so that it can be absorbed by the body, and whether there is consistency among each unit (such as a tablet or capsule) within the product. If a product successfully meets these criteria, ConsumerLab.com awards its CL Seal of Approval to that product. Test results are available at http://www.consumerlab.com. Summaries of the findings are available free; full reports are available by subscription for a fee.[15]

These types of certifications are useful to consumers and healthcare practitioners. They help to identify quality products and increase confidence in the product selected. Patient and practitioner collaboration will be critical to safe and rational use of supplements.[16]

EVALUATING A PRACTITIONER

The NCCAM website contains a page (http://nccam.nih.gov/health/decisions/index.htm) offering a number of tips for consumers interested in exploring CAM therapies. Topics include selecting complementary and alternative therapies, examining the practitioner's expertise, considering the cost, partnering with your healthcare provider, and finding credible sources of information about complementary and al-

TABLE 20-5	Resources for Associations of CAM Practitioners
ASSOCIATION	**WEBSITE**
Academy for Guided Imagery	http://www.healthy.net/agi
American Association of Oriental Medicine	http://www.aaom.org
American Chiropractic Association	http://www.americhiro.org
American College of Rheumatology	http://www.rheumatology.org
American Massage Therapy Association	http://www.amtamassage.org
Association for Applied Psychophysiology and Biofeedback	http://www.aaph.org
National Certification Commission for Acupuncture and Oriental Medicine	http://www.nccaom.org
National Certification Board for Therapeutic Massage and Bodywork	http://www.ncbtmc.com

ternative therapies. Additionally, therapies requiring licenses for practice, such as natural medicine, will have a credentialing organization that may include a referral system or a process to check the qualifications of a particular therapist. A sample of such agencies and their websites are listed in Table 20-5. Dietetics practitioners should familiarize themselves with local CAM practitioners to get to know the resources likely used by patients and to establish rapport for future consultation with these practitioners. Additional information can be found at the websites listed in Table 20-6.

LEGAL ISSUES

All healthcare practitioners must advise patients of the potential harm or risk involved with any therapy, whether it is considered conventional or CAM. "Malpractice" refers to treatment that deviates from the accepted standards of care, which in dietetics are based on scientific knowledge, research, and proven practice. CAM may eventually prove to be scientifically valid and accepted into mainstream practice, but many of the therapies are not thoroughly studied at this time. Although there may be a legal distinction between a healthcare practitioner initiating the CAM referral and one who responds to a patient's request for advice on a CAM therapy, risk in either situation should be evaluated to avoid liability.[6] Figure 20-2 shows potential malpractice liability risks associated with CAM therapies.

Cohen and Eisenberg advocate five strategies to reduce the risk for potential malpractice liability.[6] First, determine the clinical risk level by reviewing the medical literature, including evidence-based practice databases. Second, document the literature supporting the therapy by noting the findings in the medical record and, if possible, including a copy of the appropriate articles. Third, provide adequate informed consent. Discuss the risks and benefits of any treatment, CAM or conventional, with the patient. Be sure to document in writing the essence of the discussion and the patient's assent. Fourth, continue to monitor the patient to prevent him or

TABLE 20-6	Electronic Resources
ORGANIZATION / AGENCY	**URL**
American Botanical Council	http://www.herbalgram.org
CAM on PubMed	http://www.nlm.nih.gov/nccam/camonpubmed.html
Dietary Supplement Health and Education Act (DSHEA)	http://vm.cfsan.fda.gov/~dms/dietsupp.html
Institute of Medicine	http://www.iom.edu
Medwatch	http://www.fda.gov/medwatch
National Center on Complementary and Alternative Medicine (NCCAM)	http://nccam.nih.gov
NCCAM tips for consumers	http://nccam.nih.gov/health/decisions/index.htm
Natural Medicines Comprehensive Database	http://www.naturaldatabase.com
Natural Standards	http://www.naturalstandards.com
Office on Dietary Supplements	http://dietary-supplements.info.nih.gov/index.aspx

B. *Evidence supports safety, but evidence regarding efficacy is inconclusive.*

Therapeutic posture:
Tolerate, provide caution, and closely monitor effectiveness.

Clinical examples:
Acupuncture for chronic pain; homeopathy for seasonal rhinitis; dietary fat reduction for certain types of cancer; mind-body techniques for metastatic cancer; massage therapy for low-back pain; self-hypnosis for pain from metastatic cancer.

Potential liability risk:
Conceivably liable but probably acceptable.

A. *Evidence supports both safety and efficacy.*

Therapeutic posture:
Recommend and continue to monitor.

Clinical examples:
Chiropractic care for acute low-back pain; acupuncture for chemotherapy-induced nausea and dental pain; mind-body techniques for chronic pain and insomnia.

Potential liability risk:
Probably not liable.

━━ Efficacy ━━

D. *Evidence indicates serious risk or inefficacy.*

Therapeutic posture:
Avoid and actively discourage.

Clinical examples:
Injections of unapproved substances; use of toxic herbs or substances; dangerous delay or replacement of curative conventional treatments; inattentive to known herb-drug interactions (for example, St. John's wort and indinavir or cyclosporine).

Potential liability risk:
Probably liable.

C. *Evidence supports efficacy, but evidence regarding safety is inconclusive.*

Therapeutic posture:
Consider tolerating, provide caution, and closely monitor safety.

Clinical examples:
St. John's wort for depression; saw palmetto for benign prostatic hyperplasia; chondroitin sulfate for osteoarthritis; *Ginkgo biloba* for cognitive function in dementia; acupuncture for breech presentation.

Potential liability risk:
Conceivably liable but more than likely acceptable.

Safety

FIGURE 20-2 *Potential malpractice liability risk associated with complementary and integrative medical therapies. Reprinted with permission from Cohen and Eisenberg.*[6]

her from deteriorating in health status and assigning liability. Keep regularly scheduled appointments to assess the CAM therapy or need for a different intervention. Fifth, in providing CAM referrals, inquire about the competence of the provider. Assessment of the integrity of the CAM provider may minimize the liability risk of the referring practitioner in the event of litigation. The dietetics practitioner is faced with keeping up with contemporary findings in CAM research and use, communicating the risks and benefits of the therapy or of the lack of standard care if the patient should choose only the alternative therapy, and obtaining and documenting informed consent from a competent patient.[17] Working together for the optimal solution should provide the patient with the best options from which to choose and the best outcomes in patient care.

RESEARCH ISSUES

While evaluating harm or risk and the legalities of clinical practice, dietetic professionals may feel the need for guidance and be faced with inconclusive research evidence. That a therapy or supplement has been in use in ethnic cultures for centuries does not necessarily mean that the active ingredient or the mechanism of action has been identified, that the therapy is safe, or that the therapy is used appropriately today. Research in CAM therapies proves challenging for several reasons, including developing controls, using placebos, and conducting ethical interventions.[18] As more research on CAM is published, the dietetics professional should evaluate current literature for the safety and efficacy of treatments by evaluating the strength of the findings. It may be useful to evaluate the literature according to a "levels of evidence" hierarchy in which the study design and quality is assessed and graded best to worst on a scale of one to five.[19] The best overall evidence for efficacy would come from a systematic review of multiple randomized controlled trials (RCT); next would be evidence from at least one RCT; third would be nonrandomized or case-controlled trials, fourth would be nonexperimental designs; and finally, the least convincing evidence would come from opinions and descriptive studies.[19]

Issues to Ponder

- To what extent should CAM be integrated into the practice of dietetics?
- What is the role of the dietetics practitioner in counseling patients in CAM? Should it be limited to dietary supplements and functional foods?
- How should CAM education effectively be integrated into the education of dietetics practitioners? At what level should it be introduced: undergraduate, preprofessional, graduate?
- How has the increased interest in CAM affected the dietetics profession? How might CAM impact the role of the dietetics practitioner in the future? How might the dietetics practitioner impact the use of dietary supplements in the future?
- What should the role be of the American Dietetic Association with regards to CAM?

SUMMARY AND FUTURE DIRECTIONS OF CAM

The medical marketplace is growing, with options including complementary therapies. Comprehensive healthcare compels dietetics professionals to heighten their awareness of the possible interest in CAM therapies by patients and their potential for use in the treatment or prevention of disease.

Recently the Institute of Medicine (IOM) issued a report on complementary and alternative medicine in the United States,[20] available online at http://www.iom.edu. At the conclusion of this comprehensive report, IOM notes that:

> The healthcare profession is in the midst of an exciting time of discovery, a time when an evidence-based approach to health care delivery brings opportunities for the incorporation of the best options from all sources of care, be it conventional medicine or CAM. The challenge is to avoid parochial bias and to approach each possibility with an appropriate degree of skepticism or belief. Only then will it be possible to ensure that informed, reasoned, and knowledge-based decisions are being made.

REFERENCES

1. National Center for Complementary and Alternative Medicine. What Is Complementary and Alternative Medicine (CAM)? Available at: http://nccam.nih.gov/health/whatiscam/. Accessed November 12, 2004.

2. Eisenberg DM, Kessler RC, Foster C, Norlock FE, Calkins DR, Delbanco TL. Unconventional medicine in the United States. Prevalence, costs, and patterns of use. N Engl J Med 1993;328:246–252.

3. Eisenberg DM, Davis RB, Ettner SL, et al. Trends in alternative medicine use in the United States, 1990–1997: results of a follow-up national survey. JAMA 1998;280:1569–1575.

4. Barnes PM, Powell-Griner E, McFann K, Nahin RL. Complementary and alternative medicine use among adults: United States, 2002. Advance data from vital and health statistics; no343. Hyattsville, MD: National Center for Health Statistics, 2004.

5. Kelly JP, Kaufman DW, Kelley K, Rosenberg L, Anderson TE, Mitchell AA. Recent trends in use of herbal and other natural products. Arch Intern Med 2005;165:281–286.

6. Cohen MH, Eisenberg DM. Potential physician malpractice liability associated with complementary and integrative medical therapies. Ann Intern Med 2002;136:596–603.

7. National Center for Complementary and Alternative Medicine. About the National Center for Complementary and Alternative Medicine. Available at: http://nccam.nih.gov/about/aboutnccam/index.htm. Accessed November 12, 2004.

8. US Food and Drug Administration Center for Food Safety and Applied Nutrition. Dietary Supplement Health and Education Act of 1994. Available at: http://vm.cfsan.fda.gov/~dms/dietsupp.html. Accessed November 13, 2004.

9. US Food and Drug Administration. MedWatch: 2002 Safety Information. Available at: http://www.fda.gov/medwatch/SAFETY/2004/safety04.htm. Accessed November 13, 2004.

10. Stephens MB. Ergogenic aids: powders, pills and potions to enhance performance. Am Fam Physician 2001;63:842–843.

11. Scott GN, Elmer GW. Update on natural product–drug interactions. Am J Health Syst Pharm 2002;59:339–347.

12. Thomson C, Diekman C, Fragakis A, Meerschaert C, Holler H, Devlin C. Guidelines regarding the recommendation and sale of dietary supplements. J Am Diet Assoc 2002;102:1158–1164.

13. US Pharmacopeia. USP-Dietary Supplement Verification Program. Available at: http://www.uspverified.org/. Accessed December 16, 2004.

14. NSF International. Dietary Supplements Certification. Available at: http://www.nsf.org/business/dietary_supplements/more_info_components.asp?program=DietarySups. Accessed December 16, 2004.

15. ConsumerLab.com. Independent tests of herbal, vitamin, and mineral supplements. Available at: http://www.consumerlab.com. Accessed December 16, 2004.

16. Bauer BA. Herbal therapy: what a clinician needs to know to counsel patients effectively. Mayo Clin Proc 2000;75:835–841.

17. Ernst E, Cohen MH. Informed consent in complementary and alternative medicine. Arch Intern Med 2001;161:2288–2292.

18. Smith WB. Research methodology: implications for CAM pain research. Clin J Pain 2004;20:3–7.

19. Bandolier. Types and strength or evidence. Available at: http://www.jr2.ox.ac.uk/bandolier/band6/b6-5.html. Accessed December 29, 2004.

20. Committee on the Use of Complementary and Alternative Medicine by the American Public. Complementary and Alterative Medicine in the United States. Institute of Medicine. Available at: http://www.nap.edu/catalog/11182.html. Accessed February 18, 2005.

21. National Center for Homeopathy. Introduction to homeopathy. Available at: http://www.homeopathic.org/. Accessed November 13, 2004.

22. Vickers A, Zollman C. ABC of complementary medicine. Homoeopathy. BMJ. 1999;319:1115–1118.

23. American Association of Naturopathic Physicians. What is naturopathic medicine? Available at: http://www.naturopathic.org/. Accessed November 13, 2004.

24. Smith MJ, Logan AC. Naturopathy. Med Clin North Am 2002;86:173–184.

25. Ergil KV. Chinese medicine: China's traditional medicine. In: Micozzi MS, ed. Fundamentals of Complementary and Alternative Medicine. New York: Churchill Livingstone, 1996:183–230.

26. Fugh-Berman A. Alternative Medicine: What Works. Tucson, AZ: Odonian Press, 1996.

27. Jacobs GD. The physiology of mind-body interactions: the stress response and the relaxation response. J Alt Comp Med 2001;7(suppl 1):S83–S92.

28. Benson H. The Relaxation Response. New York: Outlet Books, 1993.

29. Vickers A, Zollman C. ABC of complementary medicine. Unconventional approaches to nutritional medicine. BMJ 1999;319:1419–1422.
30. Office of Dietary Supplements. Dietary Supplements: Background Information. Available at: http://ods.od.nih.gov/Health_Information/Health_Information.aspx. Accessed December 29, 2004.
31. Redwood D. Chiropractic. In: Micozzi MS, ed. Fundamentals of Complementary and Alternative Medicine. New York: Churchill Livingstone, 1996:91–110.
32. Vickers A, Zollman C. ABC of complementary medicine. The manipulative therapies: osteopathy and chiropractic. BMJ 1999;319:1176–1179.

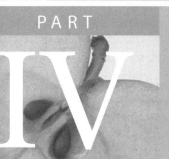

INTERNATIONAL TABLES AND GLOBAL NUTRITION STANDARDS AND GUIDELINES

Editor: Abby S. Bloch

IMPLEMENTING NUTRIENT-BASED

RECOMMENDATIONS AND

DIETARY GUIDELINES

Ricardo Uauy and Abby S. Bloch

During the preliminary stages of developing the concept for this book, the question about different management strategies, approaches to nutritional management, and dietary practices was the overriding theme. Although many healthcare professionals practicing in an insular environment have no reason to view the nutrient recommendations or dietary guidelines from other countries, it is of interest to note the similarities as well as the differences among different populations and to ponder the possibility and/or feasibility of global dietary recommendations.

As this section was being developed and material from around the globe began to be collected, several observations became apparent. Many countries had not updated their information for many years. Numerous countries were using recommendations created by other organizations or countries such the World Health Organization or the American or British nutrient recommendations. Most countries appear to have a dietary guideline available reflecting their specific public health and nutrition concerns, be they excess or insufficiency, as well as food availability and access. Table 21-1 compiles web links for international dietary guidelines and resources. In addition, the most recent edition of *Modern Nutrition in Health and Disease*[1] presents an excellent discussion (in part VI, Diet and Nutrition in Health of Populations) for those who would like more in-depth coverage of this topic. In this chapter, excerpted sections as well as several tables and figures from chapter 107 of that title are used to address some of the issues surrounding international nutrition recommendations, also addressing the question of whether it is possible to create standard guidelines and recommendations for all countries.

The remainder of this chapter is excerpted from *Modern Nutrition in Health and Disease*.[1]

BASIC CONSIDERATIONS IN DEFINING NUTRITIONAL REQUIREMENTS AND FOOD-BASED DIETARY GUIDELINES

... The quantitative definitions of nutrient needs and their expression as recommended nutrient intakes (RNIs) or dietary reference intakes have been important instruments of food and nutrition policy in many countries and have focused the attention of international bodies on necessary nutrient intakes. RNIs are customarily defined as the intake of energy and specific nutrients necessary to satisfy the requirements of a group of healthy individuals. This nutrient-based approach has served well to advance science

TABLE 21-1	International Dietary Guidelines and Resources

DIETARY GUIDELINES[a]

Australia. National Health and Medical Research Council.
Available at: http://www.nhmrc.gov.au/publications/_files/n33.pdf.

Asian Food Information Center (AFIC). Available at: http://www.afic.org/search.asp?ID=1.

Canada. Canada's Guide to Healthy Eating and Physical Activity.
Available at: http://www.phac-aspc.gc.ca/guide/index_e.html.

Caribbean Food & Nutrition Institute. Available at: http://www.paho.org/english/cfni/home.htm.

Finland. KTL National Public Health Institute/Nutrition Unit. Available at: http://www.ktl.fi/nutrition/finnutrec98.pdf.

Fun-in-Seven.
Available at: http://www.bch.cuhk.edu.hk/fns/fun-in-seven/english/primary-Breastfeeding-background.html.

Germany. German Nutrition Society.
Available at: http://www.dge.de/modules.php?name=Content&pa=showpage&pid=16.

Ireland. Food Safety Authority of Ireland.
Available at: http://www.fsai.ie/publications/reports/recommended_dietary_allowances_ireland_1999.pdf.

Malaysia. Nutrition Society of Malaysia. Available at: http://www.nutrition.com.sg/he/hepyr.aspPyramid.

Mexico. NutriPac. Available at: http://www.nutripac.com.mx/software/rec-mex.pdf.

Singapore. Nutrition.com.sg. Available at: http://www.nutrition.com.sg/he/hepyr.asp.

United Kingdom. Department of Health and Department for Education and Skills.
Available at: http://www.wiredforhealth.gov.uk/doc.php?docid=7267.

INTERNATIONAL RESOURCES[b]

Chinese Food Composition Tables. Available at:
https://www.ntis.gov/search/product.asp?ABBR=PB92500644&starDB=GRAHIST.

Food Composition in Denmark. Available at: http://www.foodcomp.dk/fcdb_default.asp.

International Network of Food Data Systems Project. Available at: http://www.fao.org/infoods/index_en.stm.

United States Department of Agriculture Food Composition Data.
Available at: http://www.nal.usda.gov/fnic/foodcomp/Data/index.html.

[a] Adapted from the Food and Nutrition Information Center. Available at: http://www.nal.usda.gov/fnic/etext/xtocid2381833.
[b] Adapted from the Food and Nutrition Information Center. Available at: http://www.nal.usda.gov/fnic/etext/000020.html.

but has not always fostered the establishment of nutritional and dietary priorities consistent with broad public health interests at national and international levels.[2]

In contrast, food-based dietary guidelines (FBDGs) as instruments of policy are more closely linked to the diet-health relationships of relevance to the particular country or region of interest.[3] FBDGs address health concerns related to dietary insufficiency, excess, or imbalance with a broader perspective, considering the totality of the effects of a given dietary pattern.[4] A clear definition of nutritional requirements of the population has its role as a fundamental component of food and nutrition policy goals along with the priorities embodied in the FBDGs for improved nutrition, health, and well-being. In this setting, RNIs are used as a basic criteria to assess whether the proposed diet is sufficient to meet established nutrient recommendations. RNIs can also be used to support educational efforts in the implementation of dietary guidelines and to provide a basis for consumer information on the nutritional adequacy of specific foods. ...

The main approaches used in establishing international recommendations are as follows:

1. The clinical approach is based on the need to correct or prevent nutrient-specific diseases associated with deficient intake. ...This methodology is a highly specific but, for ethical reasons, clearly inappropriate method for establishing nutrient dose responses...

2. Functional indicators of nutritional sufficiency (molecular, cellular, biochemical, physiologic) can be used to assess nutritional normalcy and to define the limits for deficit and excess of specific nutrients. The approach is based on a defined set of biomarkers that are sensitive to changes in nutritional state and are specific in terms of identifying subclinical deficiency conditions. ...The set of biomarkers that can be used to define requirements includes measures of nutrient stores, nutrient turnover, or critical tissue/organ pools.

3. The habitual consumption levels of "healthy" populations serve as a basis to establish a range of adequate intakes. In the absence of quantitative estimates based on the clinical or functional indicators of sufficiency, this criterion remains the first approximation to establishing requirements.

4. More recently, the concept of optimal nutrient intake has emerged and has influenced both scientists and the general public. The idea of optimal nutrient intake is based on the quest for improved functionality, be it in terms of muscle strength, immune function, or intellectual ability. The question "Optimal for what?" is usually answered by the suggestion that diet or specific nutrients can improve or enhance a given function, ameliorate the age-related decline in function, or decrease the burden of illness associated with loss of function. The goal is to add healthy life years and to prevent disability, in line with the use of disability-adjusted life years as a measure of health. ...

...RNIs serve as the basis to establish nutrient intake goals that correspond to the desired target intakes that will achieve better health and nutrition for a given population within an ecologic setting. Their purpose is to promote overall health and/or to control specific nutritional disease induced by excess or deficit, as well as to reduce health risks considering the multifactorial nature of disease. Once nutrient intake goals are defined, FBDGs can be established, by taking into account the customary dietary pattern, the foods available, and the factors that determine the consumption of foods and by indicating what aspects should be modified (Figure 21-1). FBDGs consider the ecologic setting, socioeconomic and cultural factors, and the biologic and physical environments that affect the health and nutrition of a given population or community.

...The purpose of nutrient intake goals is to promote overall health, to prevent specific nutritional disease, and to reduce the risk of diet-related diseases. Dietary guidelines represent a practical way to reach the nutritional goals for a given population.

FBDGs are an instrument and an expression of food and nutrition policy and should be based directly on diet and disease relationships of particular relevance to individual countries. Priorities in establishing dietary guidelines will thereby address the relevant public health concerns whether they are related to dietary insufficiency or excess. ...

TABLE 21-2	Key Factors in Developing National Food-Based Dietary Guidelines, According to the Joint Food and Agriculture Organization/World Health Organization Consultation on Preparation and Use of Food-Based Dietary Guidelines

Scientific evidence concerning diet-health relationships

Prevalence of diet-related public health problems

Food consumption patterns of the population

Nutritional requirements

Potential food supply

Composition of foods, including consideration of food preparation practices

Bioavailability of nutrients, supplied by the mixed local diet

Sociocultural factors that relate to food choices and accessibility

Food costs

Data from Food and Agriculture Organization/World Health Organization Consultation (FAO/WHO). Preparation and Use of Food-Based Dietary Guidelines. Report of a joint FAO/WHO Expert Consultation, Nicosia, Cyprus. WHO/NUT/96.6. Geneva: World Health Organization, 1996. Reprinted from Uauy et al.[1]

Importantly, FBDGs must facilitate choices for consumers that are consistent with their preferences, food culture, and economic resources. Typically, such guidelines recommend a minimum number of servings from each of four to seven basic food groups. FBDGs also commonly suggest the need to limit intake of certain components of foods, such as saturated and trans-fatty acids, added sugars, and salt.

Food-based strategies also offer many benefits that go beyond the prevention and control of nutrient deficiencies (Table 21-2). For example, FBDGs:

- Help prevent and control both macronutrient and micronutrient deficiencies by addressing underlying causes.
- Support health promotion and preventive health.
- Should be cost-effective and sustainable.
- Can be adapted to different cultural and dietary traditions and to strategies that are feasible at the local level.
- Address multiple nutrition problems simultaneously.
- Minimize the risk of toxicity and adverse nutrient interactions because the amounts of nutrients consumed are within usual physiologic levels. ...

VARIATIONS IN NATIONAL FOOD-BASED DIETARY GUIDELINES

Many nations have developed FBDGs for their populations (Table 21-3). Dietary guidelines across countries tend to be similar in their purposes, development, and uses. They are intended for use by health professionals but also by members of the general population and thus are mostly worded in simple, concrete terms. The similarity among the guidelines of many nations is striking: they all place an emphasis on balance, moderation, (especially with regard to fat, sugar, salt, and alcohol) and variety, and they all highlight the importance of consuming sufficient portions of fruits, vegeta-

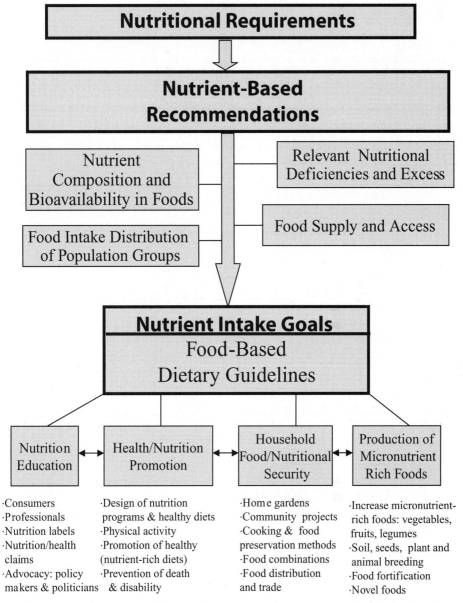

Nutritional Requirements

Nutrient-Based Recommendations

Nutrient Composition and Bioavailability in Foods

Relevant Nutritional Deficiencies and Excess

Food Intake Distribution of Population Groups

Food Supply and Access

Nutrient Intake Goals
Food-Based Dietary Guidelines

| Nutrition Education | Health/Nutrition Promotion | Household Food/Nutritional Security | Production of Micronutrient Rich Foods |

·Consumers
·Professionals
·Nutrition labels
·Nutrition/health claims
·Advocacy: policy makers & politicians

·Design of nutrition programs & healthy diets
·Physical activity
·Promotion of healthy (nutrient-rich diets)
·Prevention of death & disability

·Home gardens
·Community projects
·Cooking & food preservation methods
·Food combinations
·Food distribution and trade

·Increase micronutrient-rich foods: vegetables, fruits, legumes
·Soil, seeds, plant and animal breeding
·Food fortification
·Novel foods

FIGURE 21-1 *This schematic representation summarizes the process of defining food-based dietary guidelines (FBDGs). The bottom panel presents the end uses of FBDGs and provides specific examples. Reprinted with permission from Uauy et al,[1] p. 1703.*

bles, and grains. However, there are also several differences among guidelines, including the following:

- Total number of guidelines: They range from 5 to 15.
- Food groupings: The greatest variance is in the grouping of starchy foods.
- Difference in emphasis on particular foods, food groups, or nutrients...
- Specificity of recommendation...
- Substantial differences in the approach to the fat intake recommendation...

TABLE 21-3	Comparison of Dietary Guidelines Among Countries*	
DIETARY GUIDELINE	**COUNTRIES HAVING SIMILAR GUIDELINES**	**COUNTRIES MAKING DISTINCT VARIATIONS**
Keep a healthy weight	Argentina (eat enough for adequate weight), Australia, Canada, China, Japan, Korea, Malaysia, Mexico, the Netherlands, New Zealand, Panama, Philippines, Singapore, Thailand, United Kingdom, United States, Venezuela	France: Weigh yourself every month
Engage in physical activity each day	Australia, Canada, China, France, Indonesia, Japan, Malaysia, Mexico, Philippines, South Africa, United States	Many combine weight and physical activity, mentioning balance
Use the pyramid as a guide for food choices	Variety: Argentina, Australia, Canada, Chile, China, Costa Rica, France, Germany, Guatemala, Hungary, Indonesia, Korea, Malaysia, Mexico (mentions Health Pyramid), New Zealand, Panama, Philippines, Singapore, South Africa, Sri Lanka, Thailand, United Kingdom, United States, Venezuela Five Steps to Healthy Eating: India	Japan (>30 different kinds of foods/d)
Eat a variety of grains daily (whole grains)	Argentina, Australia, Canada, Denmark, Germany, Guatemala (in all meals, including potatoes), Hungary (choose potatoes over rice), Mexico (preferably with legumes), Norway, Panama (includes roots), Singapore, South Africa (starchy foods), Thailand, United States	United Kingdom: Eat plenty of foods rich in starch and fiber
Consume a variety of fruits and vegetables	Argentina, Australia, Chile (increase your intake, mentions legumes), Denmark, France, Germany, Guatemala (green leafy, other vegetables, any fruit), Hungary (includes salads), India, Malaysia, Mexico, Norway, Panama (eating enough), Singapore, South Africa, Sri Lanka (leafy greens daily), Thailand, United States	Thailand: Eat fiber-rich foods regularly Venezuela: Eat the fiber that your body needs from daily consumption of vegetables
Be concerned with food safety	Argentina, China, Costa Rica (practice good hygiene), Indonesia, Philippines, Thailand, United States, Venezuela	

- Different approach to selection of types of fats…
- Guidelines also differ in their emphases on the following: limiting foods or ingredients such as sugar, salt, alcohol, food additives; actions necessary for weight maintenance and the need for physical activity; chemical and microbiologic food safety; the positive and pleasurable aspects of food…

GLOBAL FOOD-BASED DIETARY GUIDELINES: ARE THEY POSSIBLE, DESIRABLE, AND ACHIEVABLE?

The possibility of defining one set of dietary guidelines is indeed attractive, considering the need for uniformity in the global village. Why should the optimal diet be different from one population to the next? Cultural and/or

TABLE 21-3	Comparison of Dietary Guidelines Among Countries* *(cont)*	
DIETARY GUIDELINE	**COUNTRIES HAVING SIMILAR GUIDELINES**	**COUNTRIES MAKING DISTINCT VARIATIONS**
Select a diet low in saturated fat and cholesterol and moderate in total fat	Australia (but low-fat diets not suitable for children), Canada, Japan, the Netherlands, Mexico, New Zealand, Panama (total fat not mentioned), Singapore, South Africa, United States	Argentina: limit animal fat Chile: as above (prefer meats such as fish, turkey or chicken), prefer vebetable oils China: as above, eat "light" diet Costa Rica, Thailand: moderate amounts of fat Denmark: only small amounts of butter, margarine and oil, choose low-fat dairy and meat products Germany, Hungary, United Kingdom: avoid too much fat India: fat eat least Malaysia: minimize fat in foods, choose prepared foods that are low in fat and cholesterol Norway: similar to Denmark Thailand: see Costa Rica Venezuela: consume moderate amounts of animal products; avoid excess animal fats
Moderate intake of free sugars	Argentina, Australia, Chile, Costa Rica, Denmark, Germany, Hungary, India, Malaysia, Mexico, Panama, Singapore, Thailand, United Kingdom, United States	New Zealand (preprepared foods, drinks and snacks)
Limit salt intake	Argentina, Australia, Canada, Chile, China, Costa Rica, Denmark, Germany, Hungary, India, Japan, Korea, Malaysia, Mexico, the Netherlands, Panama, Singapore, South Africa, Thailand, United States, Venezuela	New Zealand (preprepared foods, drinks and snacks)
If you drink alcohol, do so in moderation	Argentina, Canada, China, France, Germany, Indonesia (avoid), Hungary (forbidden for pregnant women and children), Korea, Mexico, the Netherlands, New Zealand, Singapore, South Africa, United Kingdom, United States, Venezuela (alcohol not part of a healthy diet)	

*Most countries omit mention of cholesterol.

Data from Argentina, 1998; Australia, 1992; Canada, 1992; Chile, 1997; China, 1997; Costa Rica, 1997; Guatemala, 1998; Indonesia, 1995; Hungary, 1988; Japan, 1985; Korea, 1986; Malaysia, 1996; Mexico, 1993; the Netherlands, 1985; New Zealand, 1991; Panama, 1995; Philippines, 1990; Singapore, 1989; South Africa, 1998; preliminary; Sri Lanka, 1994; Thailand, 1991; United Kingdom, 1990; United States, 2000; Venezuela, 1990. Editor's note: Newer guidelines are available for several of these countries. Reprinted from Uauy et al.[1]

ethnic differences may result in the selection of population-specific foods to meet human nutritional needs but do not necessarily imply different dietary guidelines. The only justification for this would be a solid genetic basis for nutritional individuality. Indeed, present knowledge on genomics indicates that close to 30,000 genes encode the biologic basis of what makes us Homo sapiens, and around 3,000 of these are key for most organic functions. Mutations in these 3,000 genes occur infrequently (1 to 0.01 per 1,000 births), but some will result in changed requirements to meet individual nutritional needs. ... However, because these mutations are rare and occur similarly across different regions of the world, we need not establish specific recommendations for different populations. ...[5-7]

At this stage, we are just beginning to discover the implications of genetic and epigenetic influences on nutritional needs of individuals and population groups. It remains to be seen whether biochemical or genomic individuality leads to nutritional individuality, and if this is the case, we may need to redefine the approach used to establish dietary recommendations. ...

Are global guidelines desirable? Undoubtedly, the answer must be "yes." However, universal guidelines present new problems and novel challenges. A single unified set of guidelines will fail to address cultural diversity and the complex social, economic, and political interactions between humans and their food supply. Present user-needs of FBDGs have changed. It is no longer sufficient to prevent disease of mind and body; we now want to extend our healthy life years and minimize the loss of function associated with aging. The bottom panel of the scheme presented in Figure 21-1 serves to exemplify the different uses of dietary guidelines and also the expectations that may be associated with these different groups.

Are unified guidelines achievable? The answer to this is that for some guidelines this is certainly possible. ... However, ... we cannot have a one-size-fits-all approach. Guidelines can most likely be harmonized following a unified approach to defining them, but there must be room to accommodate nutritional individuality. Global guidelines will fail unless they provide the necessary options for individuals and societies to select the foods they prefer and to combine them in the way that best suits their tastes and other sensory requirements. Most consumers will agree that food is far too important to be left solely in the hands of the experts.

....

REFERENCES
....

1. Uauy R, Hertrampf E, Dangour AD. Food-based dietary guidelines for healthier populations: international considerations. In: Shils ME, Shike M, Ross AC, et al., eds. Modern Nutrition in Health and Disease. 10th Ed. Baltimore: Lippincott Williams & Wilkins, 2006:1702–1714.
2. Food and Agriculture Organization/World Health Organization (FAO/WHO). International Conference on Nutrition. World Declaration and Plan of Action for Nutrition. Rome: Food and Agriculture Organization and World Health Organization, 1992:1–50.
3. Food and Agriculture Organization/World Health Organization (FAO/WHO). Preparation and Use of Food-Based Dietary Guidelines. Report of a joint FAO/WHO Expert Consultation, Nicosia, Cyprus. WHO/NUT/96.6. Geneva: World Health Organization, 1996.
4. Uauy R, Hertrampf E. Food-based dietary recommendations: possibilities and limitations. In: Bowman B, Russell R, eds. Present Knowledge in Nutrition. 8th Ed. Washington, DC: ILSI Press, 2001:636–649.
5. Risch NJ. Searching for genetic determinants in the new millennium. Nature 2000;405:847–856.
6. Davey Smith G, Ebrahim S. "Mendelian randomization": can genetic epidemiology contribute to understanding environmental determinants of disease? Int J Epidemiol 2003;32:1–22.
7. Stover PJ. Nutritional genomics. Physiol Genom 2004;16:161–165.

CHAPTER

22

GLOBAL NUTRIENT RECOMMENDATIONS
AND FOOD-BASED DIETARY GUIDELINES:
TABLES

Abby S. Bloch

I n introducing global nutrition recommendations and guidelines, the World
Health Organization (WHO) Technical Report Series 916, *Diet, Nutrition and
the Prevention of Chronic Diseases*, "Developments in the Availability of
Dietary Energy,"[1] states:

> Food consumption expressed in kilocalories (kcal) per capita per day is a
> key variable used for measuring and evaluating the evolution of the global
> and regional food situation. A more appropriate term for this variable
> would be "national average apparent food consumption" since the data
> come from national Food Balance Sheets rather than from food consump-
> tion surveys. ...[D]ietary energy measured in kcals per capita per day has
> been steadily increasing on a worldwide basis; availability of calories per
> capita from the mid-1960s to the late 1990s increased globally by approx-
> imately 450 kcal per capita per day and by over 600 kcal per capita per day
> in developing countries.... This change has not, however, been equal across
> regions. The per capita supply of calories has remained almost stagnant in
> sub-Saharan Africa and has recently fallen in the countries in economic
> transition. In contrast, the per capita supply of energy has risen dramati-
> cally in East Asia (by almost 1000 kcal per capita per day, mainly in China)
> and in the Near East/North Africa region (by over 700 kcal per capita per
> day).

This chapter provides tables with dietary and nutrient recommendations for
various populations worldwide. As several countries are in the process of revising
their nutritional information, websites are included where available, so that the
reader may obtain updated or more in-depth information.

Table 22-1 provides a comparison of international dietary guidelines. Tables
22-2 through 22-5 are from the WHO Technical Report cited above. Table 22-6 is
the European recommendation for nutrition and diet for healthy lifestyle. Tables
22-7 and 22-8 are from the 2005 USDA dietary guidelines for Americans.[2] Figure
22-1 and Tables 22-9 through 22-25 are from the six volumes of the most recent
Dietary Reference Intakes (DRIs) published by the Institute of Medicine (IOM),
Food and Nutrition Board, through a joint effort between the United States and
Canada.[3] These tables have been excerpted with permission from *Modern Nutrition
in Health and Disease*.[4] Tables 22-26 through 22-40 present dietary values for select
countries, also excerpted with permission from *Modern Nutrition*.[4]

| TABLE 22-1 | International Dietary Guidelines |

COUNTRY OR ORGANIZATION	PUBLISHED	POPULATION DIETARY GOALS	ENERGY (KCAL)	PROTEIN	TOTAL FAT	SATURATED FATS	TRANS FATS	PUFA	MUFA
European Heart Network	2002	Yes			< 30% E	< 10% E	< 2% E		
Eurodiet	2000	Yes		− 15% E	< 30% E	< 10% E	< 2% E		
WHO/FAO				10–15% E	15–30%	< 10% E	< 1%	6–10%	Remainder
US FNB/NAS[a]	2000			10–35%	20–35%	< 10% E		12–19 g/d[b]	
Australia	2003	Yes			20–30%				
Austria	2000	Yes	2,000	− 20% E	< 30% E	< 10% E		7% E	Remainder
Belgium	2000	Yes		− 15% E	< 30% E	< 10% E		3–7% E	
Brazil		Yes	US-based						
Canada		Yes		10–35% E	< 30% E	< 10% E			
China		Yes	1,800–2,000		25 g				
Denmark	1996	Yes		10–15% E	<30% E	< 10% E		5–10% E	10–15% E
Finland	1998	Yes		10–15% E	30% E	< 10% E		5–10% E	10–15% E
France	2001	Yes		10–20% E	30–35% E	8% E		4% E	20% E
Germany	2000	Yes		?–20% E	30% E	10% E	< 1% E	2.5% E	> 10% E
Greece	1993 EU	FBDG[e] and EU-based							
Ireland	1995	Yes			U	U	U	2% E	
Italy	1996	Yes		15–20% E	25% E	< 10% E	< 5 g	< 15% E	10–15% E
Korea									
Malaysia				50g					
Mexico		Yes	1,850–3,100	10–14% E	< 30% E	< 10% E			
Netherlands	2001	Yes			20–40% E	< 10% E	< 1% E	< 12% E	
Norway	1997	Yes		10–15% E	30% E	10% E		5–10% E	10–15% E
Philippines									
Portugal									
Puerto Rico									
Singapore	1993	Yes	1,800–2,550/		20–30%				
Slovenia	No								
Spain	2001	Yes		10–20% E	< 30–35% E	7–8% E		5% E	15–20% E
Sweden	1997	Yes		10–15% E	< 30% E	< 10% E		5–10% E	10–15% E
Switzerland	2000	Yes		?–20% E	30% E	< 10% E	< 1% E	7–10% E	> 10% E
UK	1991	Yes		20% E	33% E	10% E	2% E	6% E	12% E

[a]For adults. [b]Linoleic & linolenic only. [c]USDA/HHS. [d]Not quantified, but exists. [e]Food-Based Dietary Guidelines. [f]RDA.

| TABLE 22-1 | International Dietary Guidelines (cont) |

CHOLESTEROL	TOTAL CHO	TOTAL SUGARS	DIETARY FIBER	SALT	FRUITS & VEGETABLES	BREADS, CEREALS, GRAINS	SUGARY FOODS	PHYSICAL ACTIVITY
	> 55% E		> 25 g per day	< 6 g	> 400 g		< 4/day	25 min 3 per week
	> 55% E		> 25 g	< 6 g	> 400 g		< 4/day	
< 300 mg	55–75% E	< 10%	> 25 g	< 5 g	> 400 g			
< 300 mg	45–65% E	≤ 25% E	21–38 g		5–10 servings	6–11 servings[c]		30 min per day
					5 veg per day 2 fruit per day	4–9 servings		
< 300 mg	> 50% E	< 10% E	30 g	< 6 g	> 400 g	500–750 g	2X week	> 25 min 3 per week
< 300 mg	> 55% E	NQ[d]	15–22 g / 1000 kcal	< 5 g	> 240 g	U	U	> 30 min per day
	55% E			U		300–500 g		
					500–700 g	300–500 g		
< 300 mg	55–60% E	< 10% E	25–35 g	< 5 g	660 g			30 min per day
< 300 mg	55–60% E	< 10% E	25–25 g	< 5 g	500 g	U	U	> 30 min per day
300 mg	50–55% E	< 10% E	25–30 g	6–8 g	600 g	400–500 g		
< 300 mg	> 50% E	U	> 30 g	< 6 g	800 g	U	U	PAL of 1.75
				U	320 g	U	U	U
< 300 mg	55–60% E	10–12% E	30 g	< 6 g	240–400 g	2–4/day	U	20 min 3–4 per week
≤ 300 mg	60–70%		18–24 g				< 7	
< 300 mg	> 40% E		> 3 g/MJ	< 9 g	400 g	8–12/day	< 7	> 30 min
300 mg	55–60% E	10% E	22–35 G	5 g	750 g			> 30 min
< 300 mg	– 50%			< 5 g				
< 300 mg	50–55% E		> 25 G	< 6 g	700 g	6–11/day	< 4	PAL 1.75
	55–60% E	< 10% E	> 25–35 G	< 6 g	> 500 g	U	< 4	30 min per PAL 1.75
< 300 mg	> 50% E	< 10% E	> 30 G	< 6 g	500 g	3/day	U	30 min
< 335 mg	47%	10% E	18 G	6 g	400 g	U	U	30 min 5–6 per week

| **TABLE 22-2** | Global and Regional per Capita Food Consumption (kcal per capita per day) |

REGION	1964–1966	1974–1976	1984–1986	1997–1999	2015	2030
World	2,358	2,435	2,655	2,803	2,940	3,050
Developing countries	2,054	2,152	2,450	2,681	2,850	2,980
Near East and North Africa	2,290	2,591	2,953	3,006	3,090	3,170
Sub-Saharan Africa[a]	2,058	2,079	2,057	2,195	2,360	2,540
Latin America and the Caribbean	2,393	2,546	2,689	2,824	2,980	3,140
East Asia	1,957	2,105	2,559	2,921	3,060	3,190
South Asia	2,017	1,986	2,205	2,403	2,700	2,900
Industrialized countries	2,947	3,065	3,206	3,380	3,440	3,500
Transitional countries	3,222	3,385	3,379	2,906	3,060	3,180

[a]Excludes South Africa

Source: WHO Technical Report Series 916, Diet, Nutrition and the Prevention of Chronic Diseases. Report of a Joint WHO/FAO Expert Consultation. Geneva: World Health Organization, 2003. Available at: http://www.who.int/nut/documents/trs_916.pdf.

| **TABLE 22-3** | Ranges of Population Nutrient Intake Goals |

DIETARY FACTOR	GOAL (% OF TOTAL ENERGY, UNLESS OTHERWISE STATED)
Total fat	15–30%
Saturated fatty acids	< 10%
Polyunsaturated fatty acids (PUFAs)	6–10%
n-6 Polyunsaturated fatty acids (PUFAs)	5–8%
n-3 Polyunsaturated fatty acids (PUFAs)	1–2%
Trans fatty acids	< 1%
Monounsaturated fatty acids (MUFAs)	By difference[a]
Total carbohydrate	55–75%[b]
Free sugars[c]	< 10%
Protein	10–15%[d]
Cholesterol	< 300 mg/day
Sodium chloride (sodium)[e]	< 5 g/day (<2 g/day)
Fruits and vegetables	≥ 400 g/day
Total dietary fiber	From foods[f]
Non-starch polysaccharides (NSP)	From foods[f]

[a] This is calculated as total fat (saturated fatty acids + polyunsaturated fatty acids + trans fatty acids).
[b] The percentage of total energy available after taking into account that consumed as protein and fat, hence the wide range.
[c] The term "free sugars" refers to all monosaccharides and disaccharides added to foods by the manufacturer, cook, or consumer, plus sugars naturally present in honey, syrups and fruit juices.
[d] The suggested range should be seen in the light of the Joint WHO/FAO/UNU Expert Consultation on Protein and Amino Acid Requirements in Human Nutrition, held in Geneva from April 9 to 16, 2002.
[e] Salt should be iodized appropriately. The need to adjust salt iodization, depending on observed sodium intake and surveillance of iodine status of the population, should be recognized.
[f] See page 58, under "Non-starch polysaccharides," in original text.

Source: WHO Technical Report Series 916, Diet, Nutrition and the Prevention of Chronic Diseases. Report of a Joint WHO/FAO Expert Consultation. Geneva: World Health Organization, 2003. Available at: http://www.who.int/nut/documents/trs_916.pdf.

TABLE 22-4	Summary of Strength of Evidence on Lifestyle Factors and Risk of Developing Cardiovascular Diseases		
EVIDENCE	**DECREASED RISK**	**NO RELATIONSHIP**	**INCREASED RISK**

Convincing	Regular physical activity
	Linoleic acid
	Fish and fish oils (EHA and DHA)
	Vegetables and fruits
	  (including berries)
	Potassium
	Low to moderate alcohol intake
	  (for coronary heart disease)
		Vitamin E
		  supplements
			Myristic and palmitic acids
			Trans fatty acids
			High sodium intake
			Overweight
			High alcohol intake (for stroke)

Probable	α-Linoleic acid Oleic acid NSP Whole-grain cereals Nuts (unsalted) Plant sterols/stanols	Stearic acid	Dietary cholesterol Unfiltered boiled coffee
Possible	Folate Flavonoids Soy products		Fats rich in lauric acid Impaired fetal nutrition Beta-carotene supplements Carbohydrates Iron
Insufficient	Calcium Magnesium Vitamin C		

DHA, docosahexaenoic acid; EPA, eicosapentaenoic acid; NSP, nonstarch polysaccharides.

Source: WHO Technical Report Series 916, Diet, Nutrition and the Prevention of Chronic Diseases. Report of a Joint WHO/FAO Expert Consultation. Geneva: World Health Organization, 2003. Available at: http://www.who.int/nut/documents/trs_916.pdf.

TABLE 22-5 Summary of the Strength of Evidence for Obesity, Type 2 Diabetes, Cardiovascular Disease (CVD), Cancer, Dental Disease, and Osteoporosis[a]

	OBESITY	TYPE 2 DIABETES	CVD	CANCER	DENTAL DISEASE	OSTEOPOROSIS
Energy and fats						
High intake of energy-dense foods	C↑					
Saturated fatty acids		P↑	C↑[b]			
Trans fatty acids			C↑			
Dietary cholesterol			P↑			
Myristic and palmitic acid			C↑			
Linoleic acid			C↓			
Fish and fish oils (EPA and DHA)			C↓			
Plant sterols and stanols			P↓			
α-Linolenic acid			P↓			
Oleic acid			P↓			
Stearic acid			P-NR			
Nuts (unsalted)			P↓			
Carbohydrate						
High intake of NSP (dietary fiber)	C↓	P↓		P↓		
Free sugars (frequency and amount)					C↑[c]	
Sugar-free chewing gum					P↓[c]	
Starch[d]					C-NR	
Whole-grain cereals				P↓		
Vitamins						
Vitamin C deficiency					C↑[e]	
Vitamin D					C↓[f]	C↓[g]
Vitamin E supplements			C-NR			
Folate				P↓		
Minerals						
High sodium intake			C↑			
Salt-preserved foods and salt				P↑[h]		
Potassium			C↓			
Calcium						C↓[g]
Fluoride, local					C↓[c]	
Fluoride, systemic					C↓[c]	P-NR[g]
Fluoride, excess					C↑[f]	
Hypocalcemia					P↑[f]	
Meat and fish						
Preserved meat				P↑[i]		
Chinese-style salted fish				C↑[j]		

C↑, convincing increasing risk; C↓, convincing decreasing risk; C-NR, convincing, no relationship; P↑, probable increasing risk; P↓, probable decreasing risk; P-NR, probable, no relationship; EPA, eicosapentaenoic acid; DHA, docosahexaenoic acid; NSP, nonstarch polysaccharides.

[a] Only convincing (C) and probable (P) evidence is included in this summary table.

[b] Evidence also summarized for selected specific fatty acids; see myristic and palmitic acid.

[c] For dental caries.

[d] Includes cooked and raw starchy foods, such as rice, potatoes, and bread. Excludes cakes, biscuits, and snacks with added sugar.

[e] For periodontal disease.

[f] For enamel developmental defects.

[g] In populations with high fracture incidents only; applies to men and women more than 50–60 years old.

[h] For stomach cancer.

[i] For colorectal cancer.

[j] For nasopharyngeal cancer.

TABLE 22-5	Summary of the Strength of Evidence for Obesity, Type 2 Diabetes, Cardio-vascular Disease (CVD), Cancer, Dental Disease, and Osteoporosis[q] (cont)					
	OBESITY	**TYPE 2 DIABETES**	**CVD**	**CANCER**	**DENTAL DISEASE**	**OSTEOPOROSIS**
Fruits (including berries) and vegetables						
Fruits (including berries) and vegetables	C↓[k]	P↓[k]	C↓	P↓[l]		
Whole fresh fruits					P-NR[o]	
Beverages, non-alcoholic						
Sugar-sweetened soft drinks and fruit juices	P↑				P↑[m]	
Very hot (thermally) drinks and food				P↑[n]		
Unfiltered boiled coffee			P↑			
Beverages, alcoholic						
High alcohol intake			C↑[o]	C↑[p]		C↑[g]
Low to moderate alcohol intake			C↓[q]			
Other food-borne						
Alfatoxins				C↑[r]		
Weight and physical activity						
Abdominal obesity		C↑				
Overweight and obesity		C↑	C↑	C↑[s]		
Voluntary weight loss in overweight and obese people		C↓				
Low body weight						C↓[g]
Physical activity, regular	C↓	C↓	C↓	C↓[t] P↓[t]		C↓[g]
Physical inactivity/sedentary lifestyle	C↑	C↑				
Other factors						
Exclusive breast-feeding	P↓					
Maternal diabetes		C↑				
Intrauterine growth retardation		P↑				
Good oral hygiene/absence of plaque					C↓[e]	
Hard cheese					P↓[c]	
Environmental variables						
Home and school environments that support healthy food choices for children	P↓					
Heavy marketing of energy-dense foods, and fast-food outlets	P↑					
Adverse socioeconomic conditions	P↑					

[k] Based on the contributions of fruits and vegetables to nonstarch polysaccharides.

[l] For cancer of the oral cavity, esophagus, stomach, and colorectum.

[m] For dental erosion.

[n] For cancer of the oral cavity, pharynx, and esophagus.

[o] For stroke.

[p] For cancer of the oral cavity, pharynx, larynx, esophagus, liver, and breast.

[q] For coronary heart disease.

[r] For liver cancer.

[s] For cancer of esophagus, colorectum, breast (in postmenopausal women), endometrium, and kidney.

[t] For breast cancer.

Source: WHO Technical Report Series 916, Diet, Nutrition and the Prevention of Chronic Diseases. Report of a Joint WHO/FAO Expert Consultation. Geneva: World Health Organization, 2003 (summary in original document). Available at: http://www.who.int/nut/documents/trs_916.pdf.

TABLE 22-6	Population Goals for Nutrients and Features of Lifestyle Consistent with the Prevention of Major Public Health Problems in Europe.[a]

COMPONENT	POPULATION GOALS	LEVELS OF EVIDENCE[b]
Physical activity level (PAL)	PAL > 1.75[c]	++
Adult body weight as BMI	BMI 21–22	++
Dietary fat, % E	< 30[c]	++
Fatty acids, % total E		
Saturated	< 10	++++
Trans	< 2	++
Polyunsaturated (PUFA)		
n-6	4–8	+++
n-3	2 g linolenic + 200 mg very long chain	++
Carbohydrates, total % E	> 55	+++
Sugary food consumption, occasions per day[d]	≤ 4	++
Fruit and vegetables (g/day^{-1})	> 400	++
Folate from food (mg/day^{-1})	> 400	+++
Dietary fiber (g/day^{-1})	> 25 (or 3 g/MJ)	++
Sodium (expressed as sodium chloride) (g/day^{-1})	< 8	+++
Iodine (µg/day)	150 (infants, 50) (pregnancy, 200)	+++
Exclusive breast-feeding	About 6 months	+++

BMI, body mass index.

[a] Other nutrient goals, e.g., on iron, calcium, alcohol, water and vitamin D, are important and are included in the text.

[b] Levels of evidence are based on those used in several guideline systems, e.g., the Cochrane System, The U.S. Academy of Science scheme, and the systems used in the assessment of diet in relation to cancer by WCRF (1997) and member state expert bodies. These other systems are included because it is often difficult to undertake dietary studies in a double-blind placebo-controlled manner as for drug trials. Thus the best evidence is considered convincing by these expert groups when integrating meta-analyses of different types of study but are nevertheless classified as either ++ or only +.

++++ Multiple double-blind placebo-controlled trials.

+++ Single study of double-blind analyses or, for breast-feeding, a series of non-double-blind analyses.

++ Ecological analyses compatible with non-double-blind intervention and physiological studies.

+ Integration of multiple levels of evidence by expert groups.

These trials and other analyses do not prove that only the precise values in Table 22-6 are correct but the evidence from dietary change or differences support these values.

[c] Sedentary societies will probably need to be on a lower fat intake, e.g., 20–25%, to avoid excessive weight gain. The PAL value is equivalent to 60–80 min. of walking daily to avoid weight gain on high fat intakes; this includes the 30-min. goal for preventing cardiovascular diseases and diabetes..

[d] An occasion includes any episode of food and drink consumption in the day. This limited intake is compatible with many member states' limits on total sugar intake and the Nordic concern to limit the intake of children and those adults on low-energy intakes to no more than 10%.

Those wishing to pursue general issues or particular themes raised in this core report in greater depth are referred to two publications on (1) the *EURODIET Reports and Proceedings* and (2) the *EURODIET Evidence . Public Health Nutrition Vol 4. 2(A) and 2(B) 2001*. The Working Party reports are also currently available on the project website, http://eurodiet.med.uoc.gr.

Source: http://eurodiet.med.uoc.gr/ © 2000.

TABLE 22-7	Comparison of Selected Nutrients in the Dietary Approaches to Stop Hypertension (DASH) Eating Plan,[a] the USDA Food Guide,[b] and Nutrient Intakes Recommended per Day by the Institute of Medicine (IOM)[c]

NUTRIENT	DASH EATING PLAN (2,000 kcal)	USDA FOOD GUIDE (2,000 kcal)	IOM RECOMMENDATIONS FOR FEMALES 19–30 YEARS OF AGE
Protein, g	108	91	RDA: 46
Protein, % kcal	21	18	AMDR: 10–35
Carbohydrate, g	288	271	RDA: 130
Carbohydrate, % kcal	57	55	AMDR: 45–65
Total fat, g	48	65	—
Total fat, kcal	22	29	AMDR: 20–35
Saturated fat, g	10	17	—
Saturated fat, % kcal	5	7.8	ALAP[d]
Monounsaturated fat, g	21	24	—
Monounsaturated fat, % kcal	10	11	—
Polyunsaturated fat, g	12	20	—
Polyunsaturated fat, % kcal	5.5	9.0	—
Linoleic acid, g	11	18	AI: 12
Alpha-linoleic acid, g	1	1.7	AI: 1.1
Cholesterol, mg	136	230	ALAP[d]
Total dietary fiber, g	30	31	AI: 28[e]
Potassium, mg	4,706	4,044	AI: 4,700
Sodium, mg	2,329[f]	1,779	AI: 1,500, UL: < 2,300
Calcium, mg	1,619	1,316	AI: 1,000
Magnesium, mg	500	380	RDA: 310
Copper, mg	2	1.5	RDA: 0.9
Iron, mg	21	18	RDA: 18
Phosphorous, mg	2,066	1,740	RDA: 700
Zinc, mg	14	14	RDA: 8
Thiamine, mg	2.0	2.0	RDA: 1.1
Riboflavin, mg	2.8	2.8	RDA: 1.1
Niacin equivalents, mg	31	22	RDA: 14
Vitamin B_6, mg	3.4	2.4	RDA: 1.3
Vitamin B_{12}, µg	7.1	8.3	RDA: 2.4
Vitamin C, mg	181	155	RDA: 75
Vitamin E (AT)[g]	16.5	9.5	RDA: 15.0
Vitamin A, mg (RAE)[h]	851	1,052	RDA: 700

[a] DASH nutrient values are based on a 1-week menu of DASH Eating Plan. NIH publication No. 03-4082. www.nhlbi.nih.gov.

[b] USDA nutrient values are based on population-weighted averages of typical food choices within each food group or subgroup.

[c] Recommended intakes for adult females19–30; RDA, recommended dietary allowance; AI, adequate intake; AMDR, acceptable macronutrient distribution range; UL, upper limit.

[d] As low as possible while consuming nutritionally adequate diet.

[e] Amount listed based on a 14-g dietary fiber/1,000 kcal.

[f] The DASH Eating Plan also can be used to follow at 1,500 mg sodium per day.

[g] AT = mg d-α-tocopherol.

[h] RAE = Retinol activity equivalents.

Source: U.S. Department of Health and Human Services (HHS) and U.S. Department of Agriculture (USDA). 2005 Dietary Guidelines for Americans (Table 2 in original document). Available at: http://www.health.gov/dietaryguidelines/dga2005/document/default.htm.

TABLE 22-8	Estimated Calorie Requirements (in kilocalories) for Each Gender and Age Group at Three Levels of Physical Activity[a]		

		ACTIVITY LEVEL[b,c,d]		
GENDER	AGE (YEARS)	SEDENTARY[b]	MODERATE ACTIVITY[c]	ACTIVE[d]
Child	2–3	1,000	1,000–1,400 [e]	1,000–1,400 [e]
Female	4–8	1,200	1,400–1,600	1,400–1,800
	9–13	1,600	1,600–2,000	1,800–2,200
	14–18	1,800	2,000	2,400
	19–30	2,000	2,000–2,200	2,400
	31–50	1,800	2,000	2,200
	51+	1,600	1,800	2,000–2,200
Male	4–8	1,400	1,400–1,600	1,600–2,000
	9–13	1,800	1,800–2,200	2,000–2,600
	14–18	2,200	2,400–2,800	2,800–3,200
	19–30	2,400	2,600–2,800	3,000
	31–50	2,200	2,400–2,600	2,800–3,000
	51+	2,000	2,200–2,400	2,400–2,800

[a] These levels are based on estimated energy requirements (EER) from the Institute of Medicine Dietary Reference Intakes macronutrients report, 2002, calculated by gender, age, and activity level for referenced-sized individuals. "Reference size," as determined by IOM, is based on median height and weight for ages up to age 18 years and median height and weight for that height to give a BMI of 21.5 for adult females and 22.5 for adult males. The estimates are rounded to the nearest 200 calories and were determined using the Institute of Medicine equation.

[b] "Sedentary" means a lifestyle that includes only light physical activity associated with typical day-to-day life.

[c] "Moderate activity" means a lifestyle that includes physical activity equivalent to walking about 1.5 to 3 miles per day at 3 to 4 miles per hour in addition to the light physical activity associated with typical day-to-day life.

[d] "Active" means a lifestyle that includes physical activity eqivalent to walking more than 3 miles per day at 3 to 4 miles per hour in addition to the light physical activity associated with typical day-to-day life.

[e] The caloric ranges shown are to accomodate needs of different ages within the group. For children and adolescents, more calories are needed at older ages. For adults, fewer calories are needed at older ages.

Source: U.S. Department of Health and Human Services (HHS) and U.S. Department of Agriculture (USDA). 2005 Dietary Guidelines for Americans (Table 3 in original document). Available at: http://www.health.gov/dietaryguidelines/dga2005/document/default.htm

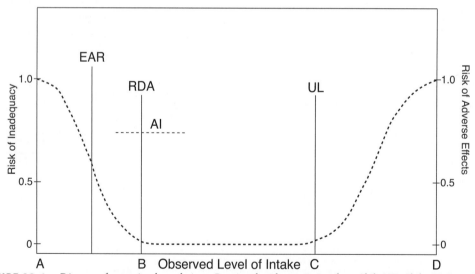

FIGURE 22-1   *Dietary reference intakes relations. Reprinted with permission from Shils ME, Shike M, Ross AC, et al. Modern Nutrition in Health and Disease. 10th Ed. Baltimore: Lippincott Williams & Wilkins, 2006:1854.*

TABLE 22-9 Dietary Reference Intakes: Definitions

Recommended dietary allowance (RDA): the average daily dietary nutrient intake level sufficient to meet the nutrient requirement of nearly all (97–98%) healthy individuals in a particular life stage and gender group.

Adequate intake (AI): the recommended average daily intake level based on observed or experimentally determined approximations or estimates of nutrient intake by a group (or groups) of apparently healthy people that are assumed to be adequate—used when an RDA cannot be determined.

Tolerable upper intake level (UL): the highest average daily nutrient intake level that is likely to pose no risk of adverse health effects to almost all individuals in the general population. As intake increases above the UL, the potential risk of adverse effects may increase.

Estimated average requirement (EAR): the average daily nutrient intake level estimated to meet the requirement of half the healthy individuals in a particular life stage and gender group.[a]

[a] In the case of energy, an estimated energy requirement (EER) is provided; it is the average dietary energy intake that is predicted to maintain energy balance in a healthy adult of a defined age, gender, weight, height, and level of physical activity consistent with good health. In children and pregnant and lactating women, the EER is taken to include the needs associated with the deposition of tissues or the secretion of milk at rates consistent with good health.

Source: Shils ME, Shike M, Ross AC, et al. Modern Nutrition in Health and Disease. 10th Ed. Baltimore: Lippincott Williams & Wilkins, 2006:1853.

TABLE 22-10 Uses of Dietary Reference Intakes for Healthy Individuals and Groups

TYPE OF USE	FOR AN INDIVIDUAL[a]	FOR A GROUP[b]
Assessment	**EAR:** Use to examine the probability that usual intake is inadequate.	**EAR:** Use to estimate the prevalence of inadequate intakes within a group.
	EER[d]: Use to examine the probability that usual energy intake is inadequate.	**EER:** Use to estimate the prevalence of inadequate energy intakes within a group.
	RDA: Usual intake at or above this level has a low probability of inadequacy.	**RDA:** Do not use to assess intakes of groups.
	AI[c]: Usual intake at or above this level has a low probability of inadequacy.	**AI[c]:** Mean usual intake at or above this level implies a low prevalence of inadequate intakes.
	UL: Usual intake above this level may place an individual at risk of adverse effects from excessive nutrient intake.	**UL:** Use to estimate the percentage of the population at potential risk of adverse effects from excess nutrient intake.
Planning	**RDA:** Aim for this intake.	**EAR:** Use to plan an intake distribution with a low prevalence of inadequate intakes.
		EER: Use to plan an energy intake distribution with a low prevalence of inadequate intakes.
	AI[c]: Aim for this intake.	**AI[c]:** Use to plan mean intakes.
	UL: Use as a guide to limit intake; chronic intake of higher amounts may increase the potential risk of adverse effects.	**UL:** Use to plan intake distributions with a low prevalence of intakes potentially at risk of adverse effects.

AI, adequate intake; EAR, estimated average requirement; RDA, recommended dietary allowance; UL, tolerable upper level

[a] Evaluation of true status requires clinical, biochemical, and anthropometric data.
[b] Requires statistically valid approximation of distribution of usual intakes.
[c] For the nutrients in this report, AIs are set for infants for all nutrients, and for other age groups for fiber, n-6, and n-3 fatty acids. The AI may be used as a guide for infants, as it reflects the average intake from human milk. Infants consuming formulas with the same nutrient composition as human milk are consuming an adequate amount after adjustments are made for differences in bioavailability. When the AI for a nutrient is not based on mean intakes of healthy populations, this assessment is made with less confidence.
[d] Estimated energy requirement (EER) may be used as the EAR for these applications.

Source: Shils ME, Shike M, Ross AC, et al. Modern Nutrition in Health and Disease. 10th Ed. Baltimore: Lippincott Williams & Wilkins, 2006:1856.

HEIGHT, M (INCHES)	PAL[b]	WEIGHT[c] FOR BMI OF 18.5 KG/M², KG (LB)	WEIGHT[c] FOR BMI OF 24.99 KG/M², KG (LB)	EER, MEN (KCAL/DAY)		EER, WOMEN (KCAL/DAY)	
				BMI OF 18.5, KG/M²	BMI OF 24.99, KG/M²	BMI OF 18.5, KG/M²	BMI OF 24.99, KG/M²
1.45 (57)	Sedentary	38.9 (86)	52.5 (116)	1,777	1,994	1,564	1,691
	Low active			1,931	2,172	1,734	1,877
	Active			2,127	2,399	1,946	2,108
	Very active			2,450	2,771	2,201	2,386
1.50 (59)	Sedentary	41.6 (92)	56.2 (124)	1,848	2,080	1,625	1,762
	Low active			2,009	2,267	1,803	1,956
	Active			2,215	2,506	2,025	2,198
	Very active			2,554	2,898	2,291	2,489
1.55 (61)	Sedentary	44.4 (98)	60.0 (132)	1,919	2,167	1,688	1,834
	Low active			2,089	2,365	1,873	2,037
	Active			2,305	2,615	2,104	2,290
	Very active			2,660	3,027	2,382	2,593
1.60 (63)	Sedentary	47.4 (104)	64.0 (141)	1,993	2,257	1,752	1,907
	Low active			2,171	2,464	1,944	2,118
	Active			2,397	2,727	2,185	2,383
	Very active			2,769	3,160	2,474	2,699
1.65 (65)	Sedentary	50.4 (111)	68.0 (150)	2,068	2,349	1,816	1,982
	Low active			2,254	2,566	2,016	2,202
	Active			2,490	2,842	2,267	2,477
	Very active			2,880	3,296	2,567	2,807
1.70 (67)	Sedentary	53.5 (118)	72.2 (159)	2,144	2,442	1,881	2,057
	Low active			2,338	2,670	2,090	2,286
	Active			2,586	2,959	2,350	2,573
	Very active			2,992	3,434	2,662	2,917
1.75 (69)	Sedentary	56.7 (125)	76.5 (169)	2,222	2,538	1,948	2,134
	Low active			2,425	2,776	2,164	2,372
	Active			2,683	3,078	2,434	2,670
	Very active			3,108	3,576	2,758	3,028
1.80 (71)	Sedentary	59.9 (132)	81.0 (178)	2,301	2,635	2,015	2,211
	Low active			2,513	2,884	2,239	2,459
	Active			2,782	3,200	2,519	2,769
	Very active			3,225	3,720	2,855	3,141
1.85 (73)	Sedentary	63.3 (139)	85.5 (188)	2,382	2,735	2,083	2,290
	Low active			2,602	2,994	2,315	2,548
	Active			2,883	3,325	2,605	2,869
	Very active			3,344	3,867	2,954	3,255
1.90 (75)	Sedentary	66.8 (147)	90.2 (199)	2,464	2,836	2,151	2,371
	Low active			2,693	3,107	2,392	2,637
	Active			2,986	3,452	2,693	2,971
	Very active			3,466	4,018	3,053	3,371
1.95 (77)	Sedentary	70.3 (155)	95.0 (209)	2,547	2,940	2,221	2,452
	Low active			2,786	3,222	2,470	2,729
	Active			3,090	3,581	2,781	3,074
	Very active			3,590	4,171	3,154	3,489

[a]For each year below 30, add 7 kcal/day for women and 10 kcal/day for men. For each year above 30, subtract 7 kcal/day for women and 10 kcal/day for men.
[b]PAL, physical activity level.
Where PA is the physical activity coefficient:
PA = 1.00 if PAL is estimated to be ≥ 1.0 < 1.4 (sedentary)
PA = 1.12 if PAL is estimated to be ≥ 1.4 < 1.6 (low active)
PA = 1.27 if PAL is estimated to be ≥ 1.6 < 1.9 (active)
PA = 1.45 if PAL is estimated to be ≥ 1.9 < 2.5 (very active)
c Addendum from text:

Because of the direct impact of deviations from energy balance on body weight and of changes in body weight, body weight data represent critical indicators of the adequacy of energy intake. Energy requirements are defined as the amounts of energy that need to be consumed by individuals to sustain stable body weights in the range desired for good health (BMI from 18.5 up to 25 kg/m2) while maintaining lifestyles that include adequate levels of physical activity. Since any energy intakes above the EER would be expected to result in weight gain and a likely increased risk of morbidity, the UL method is not applicable to energy. If weight gain was identified as the hazard, the lowest-observed-adverse-effect level (LOAEL) would be any intake above the EER for adults and the uncertainty factor would be one, as there is no uncertainty in the fact that overconsumption of energy leads to weight gain. Thus, because of the adverse effects of excess weight gain, a UL for energy is not established (Jony, 2002: 5–83).

od and Nutrition Board, Institute of Medicine, Dietary Reference Intakes for Energy, Carbohydrate, Fiber, Fat, Fatty Acids, Cholesterol, Protein, and s. Washington, DC: National Academy Press, 2002.

| TABLE 22-12 | Criteria and Dietary Reference Intake Values for Carbohydrate by Life-Stage Group | | | | | |

LIFE-STAGE GROUP	CRITERION	EAR (G/DAY)[a]		RDA (G/DAY)[b]		AI (G/DAY)[c]
		MALE	FEMALE	MALE	FEMALE	
0–6 months	Average content of human milk					60
7–12 months	Average intake from human milk plus complementary foods					95
1–3 years	Extrapolation from adult data	100	100	130	130	
4–8 years	Extrapolation from adult data	100	100	130	130	
9–13 years	Extrapolation from adult data	100	100	130	130	
14–18 years	Extrapolation from adult data	100	100	130	130	
>18 years	Brain glucose utilization	100	100	130	130	
Pregnancy						
14–18 years	Adolescent female EAR plus fetal brain glucose utilization		135		175	
19–50 years	Adult female EAR plus fetal brain glucose utilization		135		175	
Lactation						
14–18 years	Adolescent female EAR plus average human milk content of carbohydrate		160		210	
19–50 years	Adult female EAR plus average human milk content of carbohydrate		160		210	

[a] EAR, estimated average requirement. The intake that meets the estimated nutrient needs of half of the individuals in a group.

[b] RDA, recommended dietary allowance. The intake that meets the nutrient need of almost all (97–98%) of individuals in a group.

[c] AI, adequate intake. The observed average or experimentally determined intake by a defined population or subgroup that appears to sustain a defined nutritional status, such as growth rate, normal circulating nutrient values, or other functional indicators of health. The AI is used if sufficient scientific evidence is not available to derive an EAR. For healthy infants receiving human milk, the AI is the mean intake. The AI is not equivalent to an RDA.

Source: Food and Nutrition Board, Institute of Medicine, Dietary Reference Intakes for Energy, Carbohydrate, Fiber, Fat, Fatty Acids, Cholesterol, Protein, and Amino Acids. Washington, DC: National Academy Press, 2002.

TABLE 22-13	Criteria and Dietary Reference Intake Values for Total Fiber by Life-Stage Group		
		AI (G/DAY)[a]	
LIFE-STAGE GROUP	CRITERION	MALE	FEMALE
0–6 months		ND[b]	ND
7–12 months		ND	ND
1–3 years	Intake level shown to provide the greatest protection against coronary heart disease (14 g/1,000 kcal) × median energy intake level (kcal/1,000 kcal/day)	19	19
4–8 years	Intake level shown to provide the greatest protection against coronary heart disease (14 g/1,000 kcal) × median energy intake level (kcal/1,000 kcal/day)	25	25
9-13 years	Intake level shown to provide the greatest protection against coronary heart disease (14 g/1,000 kcal) × median energy intake level (kcal/1,000 kcal/day)	31	26
14–18 years		38	36
19–30 years	Intake level shown to provide the greatest protection against coronary heart disease (14 g/1,000 kcal) × median energy intake level (kcal/1,000 kcal/day)	38	25
31–50 years	Intake level shown to provide the greatest protection against coronary heart disease (14 g/1,000 kcal) × median energy intake level (kcal/1,000 kcal/day)	38	25
51–70 years	Intake level shown to provide the greatest protection against coronary heart disease (14 g/1,000 kcal) × median energy intake level (kcal/1,000 kcal/day)	30	21
>70 years	Intake level shown to provide the greatest protection against coronary heart disease (14 g/1,000 kcal) × median energy intake level (kcal/1,000 kcal/day)	30	21
Pregnancy			
14–18 years	Intake level shown to provide the greatest protection against coronary heart disease (14 g/1,000 kcal) × median energy intake level (kcal/1,000 kcal/day)		28
19–50 years	Intake level shown to provide the greatest protection against coronary heart disease (14 g/1,000 kcal) × median energy intake level (kcal/1,000 kcal/day)		28
Lactation			
14–18 years	Intake level shown to provide the greatest protection against coronary heart disease (14 g/1,000 kcal) × median energy intake level (kcal/1,000 kcal/d)		29
19–50 years	Intake level shown to provide the greatest protection against coronary heart disease (14 g /1,000 kcal) × median energy intake level (kcal/1,000 kcal/day)		29

[a] AI, adequate intake. Based on 14 g/1,000 kcal of required energy.

[b] ND, not determined. The observed average or experimentally determined intake by a defined population or subgroup that appears to sustain a defined nutritional status, such as growth rate, normal circulating nutrient values, or other functional indicators of health. The AI is used if sufficient scientific evidence is not available to derive an estimated average requirement (EAR). For healthy infants receiving human milk, the AI is the mean intake. The AI is not equivalent to an RDA.

Source: Food and Nutrition Board, Institute of Medicine, Dietary Reference Intakes for Energy, Carbohydrate, Fiber, Fat, Fatty Acids, Cholesterol, Protein, and Amino Acids. Washington, DC: National Academy Press, 2002.

TABLE 22-14 Criteria and Dietary Reference Intake Values for Total Fat by Life-Stage Group

		AI (G/DAY)[a]	
LIFE-STAGE GROUP	CRITERION	MALE	FEMALE
0–6 months	Average consumption of total fat from human milk	31	31
7–12 months	Average consumption of total fat from human milk and complementary foods	30	30
1–3 years		ND[b]	ND
4–8 years		ND	ND
9–13 years		ND	ND
14–18 years		ND	ND
>18 years		ND	ND
Pregnancy		ND	ND
14–18 years		ND	ND
19–50 years		ND	ND
Lactation		ND	ND
14–18 years		ND	ND
19–50 years		ND	ND

[a] AI, adequate intake.

[b] ND, not determined. The observed average or experimentally determined intake by a defined population or subgroup that appears to sustain a defined nutritional status, such as growth rate, normal circulating nutrient values, or other functional indicators of health. The AI is used if sufficient scientific evidence is not available to derive an estimated average requirement (EAR). For healthy infants receiving human milk, the AI is the mean intake. The AI is not equivalent to an RDA.

Source: Food and Nutrition Board, Institute of Medicine, Dietary Reference Intakes for Energy, Carbohydrate, Fiber, Fat, Fatty Acids, Cholesterol, Protein, and Amino Acids. Washington, DC: National Academy Press, 2002.

TABLE 22-15 Criteria and Dietary Reference Intake Values for n-6 Polyunsaturated Fatty Acids (Linoleic Acid) by Life-Stage Group

		AI (G/DAY)[a]	
LIFE-STAGE GROUP	CRITERION	MALE	FEMALE
0–6 months	Average consumption of total n-6 fatty acids from human milk	4.4	4.4
7–12 months	Average consumption of total n-6 fatty acids from human milk and complementary foods	4.6	4.6
1–3 years	Median intake of linoleic acid from CSFII[b]	7	7
4–8 years	Median intake of linoleic acid from CSFII	10	10
9–13 years	Median intake of linoleic acid from CSFII	12	10
14–18 years	Median intake of linoleic acid from CSFII	16	11
19–30 years	Median intake of linoleic acid from CSFII	17	12
31–50 years	Median intake of linoleic acid from CSFII	17	12
51–70 years	Median intake of linoleic acid from CSFII	14	11
>70 years	Median intake of linoleic acid from CSFII	14	11
Pregnancy			
14–18 years	Median intake of linoleic acid from CSFII		13
19–50 years	Median intake of linoleic acid from CSFII		13
Lactation			
14–18 years	Median intake of linoleic acid from CSFII		13
19–50 years	Median intake of linoleic acid from CSFII		13

[a] AI, adequate intake. The observed average or experimentally determined intake by a defined population or subgroup that appears to sustain a defined nutritional status, such as growth rate, normal circulating nutrient values, or other functional indicators of health. The AI is used if sufficient scientific evidence is not available to derive an estimated average requirement (EAR). For healthy infants receiving human milk, the AI is the mean intake. The AI is not equivalent to an RDA.

[b] CSFII, Continuing Survey of Food Intake by Individuals.

Source: Food and Nutrition Board, Institute of Medicine, Dietary Reference Intakes for Energy, Carbohydrate, Fiber, Fat, Fatty Acids, Cholesterol, Protein, and Amino Acids. Washington, DC: National Academy Press, 2002.

TABLE 22-16 Criteria and Dietary Reference Intake Values for n-3 Polyunsaturated Fatty Acids (α-Linolenic Acid) by Life-Stage Group

LIFE-STAGE GROUP	CRITERION	AI (G/DAY)[a] MALE	AI (G/DAY)[a] FEMALE
0–6 months	Average consumption of total n-3 fatty acids from human milk	0.5	0.5
7–12 months	Average consumption of total n-3 fatty acids from human milk and complementary foods	0.5	0.5
1–3 years	Median intake of α-linolenic acid from CSFII[b]	0.7	0.7
4–8 years	Median intake of α-linolenic acid from CSFII	0.9	0.9
9–13 years	Median intake of α-linolenic acid from CSFII	1.2	1.0
14–18 years	Median intake of α-linolenic acid from CSFII	1.6	1.1
19–30 years	Median intake of α-linolenic acid from CSFII	1.6	1.1
31–50 years	Median intake of α-linolenic acid from CSFII	1.6	1.1
51–70 years	Median intake of α-linolenic acid from CSFII	1.6	1.1
>70 years		1.6	1.1
Pregnancy			
14–18 years	Median intake of α-linolenic acid from CSFII		1.4
19–50 years	Median intake of α-linolenic acid from CSFII		1.4
Lactation			
14–18 years	Median intake of α-linolenic acid from CSFII		1.3
19–50 years	Median intake of α-linolenic acid from CSFII		1.3

[a] AI, adequate intake. The observed average or experimentally determined intake by a defined population or subgroup that appears to sustain a defined nutritional status, such as growth rate, normal circulating nutrient values, or other functional indicators of health. The AI is used if sufficient scientific evidence is not available to derive an estimated average requirement (EAR). For healthy infants receiving human milk, the AI is the mean intake. The AI is not equivalent to an RDA.
[b] CSFII, Continuing Survey of Food Intake by Individuals.

Source: Food and Nutrition Board, Institute of Medicine, Dietary Reference Intakes for Energy, Carbohydrate, Fiber, Fat, Fatty Acids, Cholesterol, Protein, and Amino Acids. Washington, DC: National Academy Press, 2002.

TABLE 22-17 Criteria and Dietary Reference Intake Values for Protein by Life-Stage Group

LIFE-STAGE GROUP	CRITERION	AI OR RDA FOR REFERENCE INDIVIDUAL (G/DAY) MALE	AI OR RDA FOR REFERENCE INDIVIDUAL (G/DAY) FEMALE	EAR (G/KG/DAY)[a] MALE	EAR (G/KG/DAY)[a] FEMALE	RDA (G/KG/DAY)[b] MALE	RDA (G/KG/DAY)[b] FEMALE	AI (G/KG/DAY)[c]
0–6 months	Average consumption of protein from human milk	9.1 (AI)	9.1 (AI)					1.52
7–12 months	Nitrogen equilibrium + protein deposition	13.5	13.5	1.1	1.1	1.5	1.5	
1–3 years	Nitrogen equilibrium + protein deposition	13	13	0.88	0.88	1.10	1.10	
4–8 years	Nitrogen equilibrium + protein deposition	19	19	0.76	0.76	0.95	0.95	
9–13 years	Nitrogen equilibrium + protein deposition	34	34	0.76	0.76	0.95	0.95	
14–18 years	Nitrogen equilibrium + protein deposition	52	46	0.73	0.71	0.85	0.85	
>18 years	Nitrogen equilibrium	56	46	0.66	0.66	0.80	0.80	

[a] EAR, estimated average requirement. The intake that meets the estimated nutrient needs of half of the individuals in a group.
[b] RDA, recommended dietary allowance. The intake that meets the nutrient need of almost all (97–98%) of individuals in a group.
[c] AI, adequate intake. The observed average or experimentally determined intake by a defined population or subgroup that appears to sustain a defined nutritional status, such as growth rate, normal circulating nutrient values, or other functional indicators of health. The AI is used if sufficient scientific evidence is not available to derive an EAR. For healthy infants receiving human milk, the AI is the mean intake. The AI is not equivalent to an RDA.
[d] The EAR and RDA for pregnancy are only for the second half of pregnancy. For the first half of pregnancy the protein requirements are the same as those of the nonpregnant woman.
[b] In addition to the EAR and RDA of the nonlactating adolescent or woman.

Source: Food and Nutrition Board, Institute of Medicine, Dietary Reference Intakes for Energy, Carbohydrate, Fiber, Fat, Fatty Acids, Cholesterol, Protein, and Amino Acids. Washington, DC: National Academy Press, 2002.

TABLE 22-18 Criteria and Dietary Reference Intake Values[a] for Total Water[b]

LIFE-STAGE GROUP	CRITERION	AI[c] (L/DAY)L		
		FROM FOODS	FROM BEVERAGES	TOTAL WATER
Males				
0–6 months	Average consumption of water from human milk	0	0.7	0.7
7–12 months	Average consumption of water from human milk and complementary foods	0.2	0.6	0.8
1–3 years	Median total water intake from NHANES III	0.4	0.9	1.3
4–8 years	Median total water intake from NHANES III	0.5	1.2	1.7
9–13 years	Median total water intake from NHANES III	0.6	1.8	2.4
14–18 years	Median total water intake from NHANES III	0.7	2.6	3.3
>19 years	Median total water intake from NHANES III	0.7	3.0	3.7
Females				
0–6 months	Median total water intake from NHANES III	0	0.7	0.7
7–12 months	Median total water intake from NHANES III	0.2	0.6	0.8
1–3 years	Median total water intake from NHANES III	0.4	0.9	1.3
4–8 years	Median total water intake from NHANES III	0.5	1.2	1.7
9–13 years	Median total water intake from NHANES III	0.5	1.6	2.1
14–18 years	Median total water intake from NHANES III	0.5	1.8	2.3
>19 years	Median total water intake from NHANES III	0.5	2.2	2.7
Pregnancy				
14–50 years	Median total water intake from NHANES III	0.7	2.3	3.0
Lactation				
14–50 years	Median total water intake from NHANES III	0.7	3.1	3.8

[a] No UL established; however, maximal capacity to excrete excess water in individuals with normal kidney function approximately 0.7 L/hour.
[b] Total water represents drinking water, other beverages, and water from food.
[c] AI, adequate intake. The observed average or experimentally determined intake by a defined population or subgroup that appears to sustain a defined nutritional status, such as growth rate, normal circulating nutrient values, or other functional indicators of health. The AI is used if sufficient scientific evidence is not available to derive an EAR. The AI is not equivalent to an RDA.

Source: Food and Nutrition Board, Institute of Medicine, Dietary Reference Intakes for Water, Potassium, Sodium, Chloride, and Sulfate. Washington, DC: National Academy Press, 2004.

TABLE 22-19 Criteria and Dietary Reference Intake Values[a] for Potassium by Life-Stage Group

LIFE-STAGE GROUP	CRITERION	AI[c] (L/DAY)L	
		MALE	FEMALE
0–6 months	Average consumption of potassium from human milk	0.4	0.4
7–12 months	Average consumption of potassium from human milk and complementary foods	0.7	0.7
1–3 years	Extrapolation of adult AI based on energy intake	3.0	3.0
4-8 years	Extrapolation of adult AI based on energy intake	3.8	3.8
9-13 years	Extrapolation of adult AI based on energy intake	4.5	4.5
14-18 years	Extrapolation of adult AI based on energy intake	4.7	4.7
>18 years	Intake level to lower blood pressure, reduce the extent of salt sensitivity, and minimize the risk of kidney stones	4.7	4.7
Pregnancy			
14–50 years	Intake level to lower blood pressure, reduce the extent of salt sensitivity, and minimize the risk of kidney stones		4.7
Lactation			
14–50 years	Intake level to lower blood pressure, reduce the extent of salt sensitivity, and minimize the risk of kidney stones plus replace the amount of potassium in breast milk (0.4 g/day)		5.1

[a] No UL (tolerable upper intake level) is established; however, caution is warranted given concerns about adverse effects when individuals consume excess amounts of potassium from potassium supplements while on drug therapy or in the presence of undiagnosed chronic disease.
[b] AI, adequate intake. The observed average or experimentally determined intake by a defined population or subgroup that appears to sustain a defined nutritional status, such as growth rate, normal circulating nutrient values, or other functional indicators of health. The AI is used if sufficient scientific evidence is not available to derive an EAR. The AI is not equivalent to an RDA.

Source: Food and Nutrition Board, Institute of Medicine, Dietary Reference Intakes for Water, Potassium, Sodium, Chloride, and Sulfate. Washington, DC: National Academy Press, 2004.

TABLE 22-20   Criteria and Dietary Reference Intake Values for Sodium

LIFE-STAGE GROUP	CRITERION FOR AI	AI[a] (G/DAY)		UL[b] (G/DAY)	
		MALE	FEMALE	MALE	FEMALE
0–6 months	Average consumption of sodium from human milk	0.12	0.12	ND[c]	ND
7–12 months	Average consumption of sodium from human milk and complementary foods	0.37	0.37	ND	ND
1–3 years	Extrapolation of adult AI based on energy intake	1.0	1.0	1.5	1.5
4–8 years	Extrapolation of adult AI based on energy intake	1.2	1.2	1.9	1.9
9–13 years	Extrapolation of adult AI based on energy intake	1.5	1.5	2.2	2.2
14–18 years	Extrapolation of adult AI based on energy intake	1.5	1.5	2.3	2.3
19–50 years	Intake level to cover possible daily losses, provide adequate intakes of other nutrients, and maintain normal function	1.5	1.5	2.3	2.3
51–70 years	Extrapolated from younger adults based on energy intake	1.3	1.3	2.3	2.3
>70 years	Extrapolated from younger adults based on energy	1.2	1.2	2.3	2.3
Pregnancy					
14–50 years	Same as nonpregnant women		1.5		2.3
Lactation					
14–50 years	Same as nonlactating women		1.5		2.3

[a] AI, adequate intake. The observed average or experimentally determined intake by a defined population or subgroup that appears to sustain a defined nutritional status, such as growth rate, normal circulating nutrient values, or other functional indicators of health. The AI is used if sufficient scientific evidence is not available to derive an EAR. The AI is not equivalent to an RDA.
[b] UL, tolerable upper intake level. Based on prevention of increased blood pressure.
[c] ND, not determined. Intake should be from food or formula only.

Source: Food and Nutrition Board, Institute of Medicine, Dietary Reference Intakes for Water, Potassium, Sodium, Chloride, and Sulfate. Washington, DC: National Academy Press, 2004.

TABLE 22-21   Criteria and Dietary Reference Intake Values for Chloride

LIFE-STAGE GROUP	AI[a] (G/DAY)		TOLERABLE UPPER LIMIT (UL) (G/DAY)
	MALE	FEMALE	
0–6 months	0.18		Not set
7–12 months	0.57		Not set
1–3 years	1.5		2.3
4–8 years	1.9		2.9
9–13 years	2.3	2.3	3.4
14–18 years	2.3	2.3	3.6
19–30 years	2.3	2.3	3.6
31–50 years	2.3	2.3	3.6
51–70 years	2.0	2.0	3.6
>70 years	1.8	1.8	3.6
Pregnancy			
14–50 years		2.3	3.6
Lactation			
14–50 years		2.3	3.6

[a] AI, average intake.

Source: Food and Nutrition Board, Institute of Medicine, Dietary Reference Intakes for Water, Potassium, Sodium, Chloride, and Sulfate. Washington, DC: National Academy Press, 2004.

TABLE 22-22   Recommended Intakes for Individuals, Vitamins: Dietary Reference Intakes from the Food and Nutrition Board, Institute of Medicine, National Academy of Sciences[a]

LIFE-STAGE GROUP	VITAMIN A (μg/DAY)[b]	VITAMIN C (MG/DAY)	VITAMIN D (μg/DAY)[c,d]	VITAMIN E (MG/DAY)[e]	VITAMIN K (μg/DAY)	THIAMIN (MG/DAY)	RIBOFLAVIN (MG/DAY)	NIACIN (MG/DAY)[f]	VITAMIN B6 (MG/DAY)	FOLATE (μg/DAY)[g]	VITAMIN B12 (μg/DAY)	PANTOTHENIC ACID (MG/DAY)	BIOTIN (μg/DAY)	CHOLINE (MG/DAY)[h]
Infants														
0–6 months	400*	40*	5*	4*	2.0*	0.2*	0.3*	2*	0.1*	65*	0.4*	1.7*	5*	125*
7–12 months	500*	50*	5*	5*	2.5*	0.3*	0.4*	4*	0.3*	80*	0.5*	1.8*	6*	150*
Children														
1–3 years	300	15	5*	6	30*	0.5	0.5	6	0.5	150	0.9	2*	8*	200*
4–8 years	400	25	5*	7	55*	0.6	0.6	8	0.6	200	1.2	3*	12*	250*
Males														
9–13 years	600	45	5*	11	60*	0.9	0.9	12	1.0	300	1.8	4*	20*	375*
14–18 years	900	75	5*	15	75*	1.2	1.3	16	1.3	400	2.4	5*	25*	550*
19–30 years	900	90	5*	15	120*	1.2	1.3	16	1.3	400	2.4	5*	30*	550*
31–50 years	900	90	5*	15	120*	1.2	1.3	16	1.3	400	2.4	5*	30*	550*
51–70 years	900	90	10*	15	120*	1.2	1.3	16	1.7	400	2.4[i]	5*	30*	550*
>70 years	900	90	15*	15	120*	1.2	1.3	16	1.7	400	2.4[i]	5*	30*	550*
Females														
9–13 years	600	45	5*	11	60*	0.9	0.9	12	1.0	300	1.8	4*	20*	375*
14–18 years	700	65	5*	15	75*	1.0	1.0	14	1.2	400[j]	2.4	5*	25*	400*
19–30 years	700	75	5*	15	90*	1.1	1.1	14	1.3	400[j]	2.4	5*	30*	425*
31–50 years	700	75	5*	15	90*	1.1	1.1	14	1.3	400[j]	2.4	5*	30*	425*
51–70 years	700	75	10*	15	90*	1.1	1.1	14	1.5	400	2.4[i]	5*	30*	425*
>70 years	700	75	15*	15	90*	1.1	1.1	14	1.5	400	2.4[i]	5*	30*	425*
Pregnancy														
≤18 years	750	80	5*	15	75*	1.4	1.4	18	1.9	600[j]	2.6	6*	30*	450*
19–30 years	770	85	5*	15	90*	1.4	1.4	18	1.9	600[j]	2.6	6*	30*	450*
31–50 years	770	85	5*	15	90*	1.4	1.4	18	1.9	600[j]	2.6	6*	30*	450*
Lactation														
≤18 years	1,200	115	5*	19	75*	1.4	1.6	17	2.0	500	2.8	7*	35*	550*
19–30 years	1,300	120	5*	19	90*	1.4	1.6	17	2.0	500	2.8	7*	35*	550*
31–50 years	1,300	120	5*	19	90*	1.4	1.6	17	2.0	500	2.8	7*	35*	550*

[a] This table (taken from the DRI reports, see www.nap.edu) presents recommended dietary allowances (RDAs) in bold type and adequate intakes (AIs) in ordinary type followed by an asterisk (*). RDAs and AIs may both be used as goals for individual intake. RDAs are set to meet the needs of almost all (97–98%) individuals in a group. For healthy breast-fed infants, the AI is the mean intake. The AI for other life-stage and gender groups is believed to cover needs of all individuals in the group, but lack of data or uncertainty in the data prevents being able to specify with confidence the percentage of individuals covered by this intake.

[b] As retinol activity equivalents (RAEs). 1 RAE = 1 μg retinol, 12 μg α-carotene, 24 μg β-carotene, or 24 μg β-cryptoxanthin. To calculate RAEs from REs of provitamin A carotenoids in foods, divide the REs by 2. For preformed vitamin A in foods or supplements and for provitamin A carotenoids in supplements, 1 RE = 1 RAE.

[c] Calciferol. 1 μg calciferol = 40 IU vitamin D.

[d] In the absence of adequate exposure to sunlight.

[e] As α-tocopherol. α-Tocopherol includes *RRR*-α-tocopherol, the only form of α-tocopherol that occurs naturally in foods, and the 2R-stereoisomeric forms of α-tocopherol (*RRR*-, *RSR*-, *RRS*-, and *RSS*-α-tocopherol) that occur in fortified foods and supplements. It does not include the 2S-stereoisomeric forms of α-tocopherol (*SRR*-, *SSR*-, *SRS*-, and *SSS*-α-tocopherol), also found in fortified foods and supplements.

[f] As niacin equivalents (NE). 1 mg of niacin = 60 mg of tryptophan; 0–6 months = preformed niacin (not NE).

[g] As dietary folate equivalents (DFE). 1 DFE = 1 μg food folate = 0.6 μg of folic acid from fortified food or as a supplement consumed with food = 0.5 μg of a supplement taken on an empty stomach.

[h] Although AIs have been set for choline, there are few data to assess whether a dietary supply of choline is needed at all stages of the life cycle, and it may be that the choline requirement can be met by endogenous synthesis at some of these stages.

[i] Because 10–30% of older people may malabsorb food-bound B12, it is advisable for those older than 50 years to meet their RDA mainly by consuming foods fortified with B12 or a supplement containing B12.

[j] In view of evidence linking folate intake with neural tube defects in the fetus, it is recommended that all women capable of becoming pregnant consume 400 μg from supplements or fortified foods in addition to intake of food folate from a varied diet.

Source: Shils ME, Ross AC, et al. Modern Nutrition in Health and Disease.10th Ed. Baltimore: Lippincott Williams & Wilkins, 2006:1868.

TABLE 22-23 Tolerable Upper Intake Levels (UL^a), Vitamins: Dietary Reference Intakes from the Food and Nutrition Board, Institute of Medicine, National Academy of Sciences

LIFE-STAGE GROUP	VITAMIN A EL_G/DAY)^b	VITAMIN C (MG/DAY)	VITAMIN D (µG/DAY)	VITAMIN E (MG/DAY)^{a,d}	VITAMIN K	THIAMIN	RIBOFLAVIN	NIACIN (MG/DAY)^d	VITAMIN B$_6$ (MG/DAY)	FOLATE (µG/DAY)D	VITAMIN B$_{12}$	PANTOTHENIC ACID	BIOTIN	CHOLINE (G/D)	CAROTENOIDS^e
Infants
0–6 months	600	ND^f	25	ND	ND	ND	ND	ND	ND	ND	ND	ND	ND	ND	ND
7–12 months	600	ND	25	ND	ND	ND	ND	ND	ND	ND	ND	ND	ND	ND	ND
Children
1–3 years	600	400	50	200	ND	ND	ND	10	30	300	ND	ND	ND	1.0	ND
4–8 years	900	650	50	300	ND	ND	ND	15	40	400	ND	ND	ND	1.0	ND
Males, Females
9–13 years	1,700	1,200	50	600	ND	ND	ND	20	60	600	ND	ND	ND	2.0	ND
14–18 years	2,800	1,800	50	800	ND	ND	ND	30	80	800	ND	ND	ND	3.0	ND
19–70 years	3,000	2,000	50	1,000	ND	ND	ND	35	100	1,000	ND	ND	ND	3.5	ND
>70 years	3,000	2,000	50	1,000	ND	ND	ND	35	100	1,000	ND	ND	ND	3.5	ND
Pregnancy
≤18 years	2,800	1,800	50	800	ND	ND	ND	30	80	800	ND	ND	ND	3.0	ND
19–50 years	3,000	2,000	50	1,000	ND	ND	ND	35	100	1,000	ND	ND	ND	3.5	ND
Lactation
≤18 years	2,800	1,800	50	800	ND	ND	ND	30	80	800	ND	ND	ND	3.0	ND
19–50 years	3,000	2,000	50	1,000	ND	ND	ND	35	100	1,000	ND	ND	ND	3.5	ND

^{a} UL = The maximum level of daily nutrient intake that is likely to pose no risk of adverse effects. Unless otherwise specified, the UL represents total intake from food, water, and supplements. Due to lack of suitable data, ULs could not be established for vitamin K, thiamin, riboflavin, vitamin B, pantothenic acid, biotin, or carotenoids. In the absence of ULs, extra caution may be warranted in consuming levels above recommended intakes.

^{b} As preformed vitamin A only.

^{c} As α-tocopherol; applies to any form of supplemental α-tocopherol.

^{d} The ULs for vitamin E, niacin, and folate apply to synthetic forms obtained from supplements, fortified foods, or a combination of the two.

^{e} β-Carotene supplements are advised only to serve as a provitamin A source for individuals at risk of vitamin A deficiency.

^{f} ND = Not determinable due to lack of data of adverse effects in this age group and concern with regard to lack of ability to handle excess amounts. Source of intake should be from food only to prevent high levels of intake.

TABLE 22-24 Recommended Intakes for Individuals, Elements: Dietary Reference Intakes from the Food and Nutrition Board, Institute of Medicine, National Academy of Sciences[a]

LIFE-STAGE GROUP	CALCIUM (MG/DAY)	CHROMIUM (μG/DAY)	COPPER (μG/DAY)	FLUORIDE (MG/DAY)	IODINE (μG/DAY)	IRON (MG/DAY)	MAGNESIUM (MG/D)	MANGANESE (MG/D)	MOLYBDENUM (μG/D)	PHOSPHORUS (MG/DAY)	SELENIUM (μG/DAY)	ZINC (MG/DAY)
Infants												
0–6 months	210*	0.2*	200*	0.01*	110*	0.27*	30*	0.003*	2*	100*	15*	2*
7–12 months	270*	5.5*	220*	0.5*	130*	11	75*	0.6*	3*	275*	20*	3
Children												
1–3 years	500*	11*	340	0.7*	90	7	80	1.2*	17	460	20	3
4–8 years	800*	15*	440	1*	90	10	130	1.5*	22	500	30	5
Males												
9–13 years	1,300*	25*	700	2*	120	8	240	1.9*	34	1,250	40	8
14–18 years	1,300*	35*	890	3*	150	11	410	2.2*	43	1,250	55	11
19–30 years	1,000*	35*	900	4*	150	8	400	2.3*	45	700	55	11
31–50 years	1,000*	35*	900	4*	150	8	420	2.3*	45	700	55	11
51–70 years	1,200*	30*	900	4*	150	8	420	2.3*	45	700	55	11
>70 years	1,200*	30*	900	4*	150	8	420	2.3*	45	700	55	11
Females												
9–13 years	1,300*	21*	700	2*	120	8	240	1.6*	34	1,250	40	8
14–18 years	1,300*	24*	890	3*	150	15	360	1.6*	43	1,250	55	9
19–30 years	1,000*	25*	900	3*	150	18	310	1.8*	45	700	55	8
31–50 years	1,000*	25*	900	3*	150	18	320	1.8*	45	700	55	8
51–70 years	1,200*	20*	900	3*	150	8	320	1.8*	45	700	55	8
>70 years	1,200*	20*	900	3*	150	8	320	1.8*	45	700	55	8
Pregnancy												
≤18 years	1,300*	29*	1,000	3*	220	27	400	2.0*	50	1,250	60	13
19–30 years	1,000*	30*	1,000	3*	220	27	350	2.0*	50	700	60	11
31–50 years	1,000*	30*	1,000	3*	220	27	360	2.0*	50	700	60	11
Lactation												
≤18 years	1,300*	44*	1,300	3*	290	10	360	2.6*	50	1,250	70	14
19–30 years	1,000*	45*	1,300	3*	290	9	310	2.6*	50	700	70	12
31–50 years	1,000*	45*	1,300	3*	290	9	320	2.6*	50	700	70	12

[a]This table presents Recommended Dietary Allowances (RDAs) in bold type and Adequate Intakes (AIs) in ordinary type followed by an asterisk (*). RDAs and AIs may both be used as goals for individual intake. RDAs are set to meet the needs of almost all (97 to 98 percent) individuals in a group. For healthy breastfed infants, the AI is the mean intake. The AI for other life stage and gender groups is believed to cover needs of all individuals in the group, but lack of data or uncertainty in the data prevent being able to specify with confidence the percentage of individuals covered by this intake.

Source: Dietary Reference Intakes for Calcium, Phosphorus, Magnesium, Vitamin D, and Fluoride (1997); Dietary Reference Intakes for Thiamin, Riboflavin, Niacin, Vitamin B_6, Folate, Vitamin B_{12}, Pantothenic Acid, Biotin, and Choline (1998); Dietary Reference Intakes for Vitamin C, Vitamin E, Selenium, and Carotenoids (2000); and Dietary Reference Intakes for Vitamin A, Vitamin K, Arsenic, Boron, Chromium, Copper, Iodine, Iron, Manganese, Molybdenum, Nickel, Silicon, Vanadium, and Zinc (2001). These reports may be accessed at http://www.nap.edu. © 2001 by The National Academies of Sciences. All rights reserved.

TABLE 22-25   Tolerable Upper Intake Levels (UL^a), Elements: Dietary Reference Intakes from the Food and Nutrition Board, Institute of Medicine, National Academy of Sciences

LIFE-STAGE GROUP	ARSENIC[b]	BORON (MG/DAY)	CALCIUM (G/DAY)	CHROMIUM	COPPER (μG/DAY)	FLUORIDE (MG/DAY)	IODINE (μG/DAY)	IRON (MG/DAY)	MAGNESIUM (MG/DAY)[c]	MANGANESE (MG/DAY)	MOLYBDENUM (μG/DAY)	NICKEL (MG/DAY)	PHOSPHORUS (G/DAY)	SELENIUM (μG/DAY)	SILICON[d]	VANADIUM (MG/DAY)[a]	ZINC (MG/DAY)
Infants																	
0–6 months	ND[f]	ND	ND	ND	ND	0.7	ND	40	ND	ND	ND	ND	ND	45	ND	ND	4
7–12 months	ND	ND	ND	ND	ND	0.9	ND	40	ND	ND	ND	ND	ND	60	ND	ND	5
Children																	
1–3 years	ND	3	2.5	ND	1,000	1.3	200	40	65	2	300	0.2	3	90	ND	ND	7
4–8 years	ND	6	2.5	ND	3,000	2.2	300	40	110	3	600	0.3	3	150	ND	ND	12
Males, Females																	
9–13 years	ND	11	2.5	ND	5,000	10	600	40	350	6	1,100	0.6	4	280	ND	ND	23
14–18 years	ND	17	2.5	ND	8,000	10	900	45	350	9	1,700	1.0	4	400	ND	ND	34
19–70 years	ND	20	2.5	ND	10,000	10	1,100	45	350	11	2,000	1.0	4	400	ND	1.8	40
> 70 years	ND	20	2.5	ND	10,000	10	1,100	45	350	11	2,000	1.0	3	400	ND	1.8	40
Pregnancy																	
≤ 18 years	ND	17	2.5	ND	8,000	10	900	45	350	9	1,700	1.0	3.5	400	ND	ND	34
19–50 years	ND	20	2.5	ND	10,000	10	1,100	45	350	11	2,000	1.0	3.5	400	ND	ND	40
Lactation																	
≤ 18 years	ND	17	2.5	ND	8,000	10	900	45	350	9	1,700	1.0	4	400	ND	ND	34
19–50 years	ND	20	2.5	ND	10,000	10	1,100	45	350	11	2,000	1.0	4	400	ND	ND	40

[a] UL = the maximum level of daily nutrient intake that is likely to pose no risk of adverse effects. Unless otherwise specified, the UL represents total intake from food, water, and supplements. Due to lack of suitable data, ULs could not be established for arsenic, chromium, and silicon. In the absence of ULs, extra caution may be warranted in consuming levels above recommended intakes.

[b] Although the UL was not determined for arsenic, there is no justification for adding arsenic to food or supplements.

[c] The ULs for magnesium represent intake from a pharmacological agent only and do not include intake from food and water.

[d] Although silicon has not been shown to cause adverse effects in humans, there is no justification for adding silicon to supplements.

[e] Although vanadium in food has not been shown to cause adverse effects in humans, there is no justification for adding vanadium to food and vanadium supplements should be used with caution. The UL is based on adverse effects in laboratory animals and these data could be used to set a UL for adults but not children and adolescents.

[f] ND = not determinable due to lack of data of adverse effects in this age group and concern with regard to lack of ability to handle excess amounts. Source of intake should be from food only to prevent high levels of intake.

Source: Dietary Reference Intakes for Calcium, Phosphorus, Magnesium, Vitamin D, and Fluoride (1997); Dietary Reference Intakes for Thiamin, Riboflavin, Niacin, Vitamin B₆, Folate, Vitamin B₁₂, Pantothenic Acid, Biotin, and Choline (1998); Dietary Reference Intakes for Vitamin C, Vitamin E, Selenium, and Carotenoids (2000); and Dietary Reference intakes for Vitamin A. Vitamin K, Arsenic, Boron, Chromium, Cooper, Iodine, Iron, Manganese, Molybdenum, Nickel, Silicon, Vanadium, and Zinc (2001). These reports may be accessed at http://www.nap.edu. © 2001 by The National Academy of Sciences. All rights reserved.

DIETARY REFERENCE VALUES FOR FOOD ENERGY AND NUTRIENTS FOR THE UNITED KINGDOM

Tables 22-26 through 22-31 provide dietary reference values for food energy and nutrients for the United Kingdom They are reprinted with permission from the Appendix of the 10th edition of Modern Nutrition in Health and Disease, 2006.

TABLE 22-26	Estimated Average Requirements (EARS) for Energy, United Kingdom[a]	
	EARS **MJ/DAY (KCAL/DAY)**	
AGE	**MALES**	**FEMALES**
0–3 months	2.28 (545)	2.16 (515)
4–6 months	2.89 (690)	2.69 (645)
7–9 months	3.44 (825)	3.20 (765)
10–12 months	3.85 (920)	3.61 (865)
1–3 years	5.15 (1,230)	4.86 (1,165)
4–6 years	7.16 (1,715)	6.46 (1,545)
7–10 years	8.24 (1,970)	7.28 (1,740)
11–14 years	9.27 (2,220)	7.72 (1,845)
15–18 years	11.51 (2,755)	8.83 (2,110)
19–50 years	10.60 (2,550)	8.10 (1,940)
51–59 years	10.60 (2,550)	8.00 (1,900)
60–64 years	9.93 (2,380)	7.99 (1,900)
65–74 years	9.71 (2,330)	7.96 (1,900)
75+ years	8.77 (2,100)	7.61 (1,810)
Pregnancy		+ 0.80[b] (200)
Lactation		
1 month		+ 1.90 (450)
2 month		+ 2.20 (530)
3 month		+ 2.40 (570)
4–6 month (group 1)[c]		+ 2.00 (480)
4–6 month (group 2)		+ 2.40 (570)
> 6 month (group 1)		+ 1.00 (240)
> 6 month (group 2)		+ 2.30 (550)

[a] See paragraph 1.5 in Table 11-A-4-a.
[b] Last trimester only.
[c] See original text for comments.

Source: Report on Health and Social Subjects: no. 41, Dietary Reference Values for Food Energy and Nutrients for the United Kingdom. Report of the Panel on Dietary Reference Values of the Committee on Medical Aspects of Food Policy. London: Her Majesty's Stationery Office, 1991. This is the UK's Report Table 1.1.

TABLE 22-27 — Reference Nutrient Intakes (RNI) for Protein, United Kingdom[a]

AGE	REFERENCE NUTRIENT INTAKE[b] (G/DAY)
0–3 months	12.5[c]
4–6 months	12.7
7–9 months	13.7
10–12 months	14.9
1–3 years	14.5
4–6 years	19.7
7–10 years	28.3
Males	
11–14 years	42.1
15–18 years	55.2
19–50 years	55.5
50+ years	53.3
Females	
11–14 years	41.2
15–18 years	45.0
19–50 years	45.0
50+ years	46.5
Pregnancy[d]	+ 6
Lactation[d]	
0–4 months	+ 11
4+ months	+ 8

[a] See paragraph 1.7 in Table 11-A-4-a.
[b] These figures, based on egg and milk protein, assume complete digestibility.
[c] No values for infants 0–3 months of age are given by WHO. The RNI is calculated from the recommendations of Committee on Medical Aspects of Food Policy (COMA).
[d] To be added to adult requirement through all stages of pregnancy and lactation.

Source: Report on Health and Social Subjects: no. 41, Dietary Reference Values for Food Energy and Nutrients for the United Kingdom. Report of the Panel on Dietary Reference Values of the Committee on Medical Aspects of Food Policy. London: Her Majesty's Stationery Office, 1991. This is the UK's Report Table 1.3.

TABLE 22-28 — Reference Nutrient Intakes for Vitamins, United Kingdom[a]

AGE	THIAMIN (MG/DAY)	RIBOFLAVIN (MG/DAY)	NIACIN (NICOTINIC ACID EQUIVALENT) (MG/DAY)	VITAMIN B_6 (MG/DAY)[b]	VITAMIN B_{12} (µG/DAY)	FOLATE (µG/DAY)	VITAMIN C (MG/DAY)	VITAMIN A (µG/DAY)	VITAMIN D (µG/DAY)
0–3 months	0.2	0.4	3	0.2	0.3	50	25	350	8.5
4–6 months	0.2	0.4	3	0.2	0.3	50	25	350	8.5
7–9 months	0.2	0.4	4	0.3	0.4	50	25	350	7
10–12 months	0.3	0.4	5	0.4	0.4	50	25	350	7
1–3 years	0.5	0.6	8	0.7	0.5	70	30	400	7
4–6 years	0.7	0.8	11	0.9	0.8	100	30	400	—
7–10 years	0.7	1.0	12	1.0	1.0	150	30	500	—
Males									
11–14 years	0.9	1.2	15	1.2	1.2	200	35	600	—
15–18 years	1.1	1.3	18	1.5	1.5	200	40	700	—
19–50 years	1.0	1.3	17	1.4	1.5	200	40	700	—
50+ years	0.9	1.3	16	1.4	1.5	200	40	700	—[c]
Females									
11–14 years	0.7	1.1	12	1.0	1.2	200	35	600	—
15–18 years	0.8	1.1	14	1.2	1.5	200	40	600	—
19–50 years	0.8	1.1	13	1.2	1.5	200	40	600	—
50+ years	0.8	1.1	12	1.2	1.5	200	40	600	—[c]
Pregnancy	+ 0.1[d]	+ 0.3	—[e]	—[e]	—[e]	+ 100	+ 10d	+ 100	10
Lactation									
0–4 months	+ 0.2	+ 0.5	+ 2	—[e]	+ 0.5	+ 60	+ 30	+ 350	10
4+ months	+ 0.2	+ 0.5	+ 2	—[e]	+ 0.5	+ 60	+ 30	+ 350	10

[a] See paragraph 11-A-4-a for definition.
[b] Based on protein providing 14.7% of EAR for energy.
[c] After age 65 the RNI is 10 _g/day for men and women.
[d] For last trimester only.
[e] No increment.

Source: Report on Health and Social Subjects: no. 41. Dietary Reference Values for Food Energy and Nutrients for the United Kingdom. Report of the Panel on Dietary Reference Values of the Committee on Medical Aspects of Food Policy. London: Her Majesty's Stationery Office, 1991. This is the UK's Report Table 1.4.

TABLE 22-29	Reference Nutrient Intakes for Minerals (SI Units), United Kingdom[a]										
AGE	CALCIUM (MMOL/DAY)	PHOSPHORUS[b] (MMOL/DAY)	MAGNESIUM (MMOL/DAY)	SODIUM[c] (MMOL/DAY)	POTASSIUM[d] (MMOL/DAY)	CHLORIDE[e] (MMOL/DAY)	IRON (μMOL/DAY)	ZINC (μMOL/DAY)	COPPER (μMOL/DAY)	SELENIUM (μMOL/DAY)	IODINE (μMOL/DAY)
0–3 months	13.1	13.1	2.2	9	20	9	30	60	5	0.1	0.4
4–6 months	13.1	13.1	2.5	12	22	12	80	60	5	0.2	0.5
7–9 months	13.1	13.1	3.2	14	18	14	140	75	5	0.1	0.5
10–12 months	13.1	13.1	3.3	15	18	15	140	75	5	0.1	0.5
1–3 years	8.8	8.8	3.5	22	20	22	120	75	6	0.2	0.6
4–6 years	11.3	11.3	4.8	30	28	30	110	100	9	0.3	0.8
7–10 years	13.8	13.8	8.0	50	50	50	160	110	11	0.4	0.9
Males											
11–14 years	25.0	25.0	11.5	70	80	70	200	140	13	0.6	1.0
15–18 years	25.0	25.0	12.3	70	90	70	200	145	16	0.9	1.0
19–50 years	17.5	17.5	12.3	70	90	70	160	145	19	0.9	1.0
50+ years	17.5	17.5	12.3	70	90	70	160	145	19	0.9	1.0
Females											
11–14 years	20.0	20.0	11.5	70	80	70	260f	140	13	0.6	1.0
15–18 years	20.0	20.0	12.3	70	90	70	260f	110	16	0.8	1.1
19–50 years	17.5	17.5	10.9	70	90	70	260f	110	19	0.8	1.1
50+ years	17.5	17.5	10.9	70	90	70	160	110	19	0.8	1.1
Pregnancy	c,f,e	—f	—f	—f	—f	—f	*	*	*	*	*
Lactation											
0–4 months	+14.3	+14.3	+2.1	*	*	*	*	+90	+5	+0.2	*
4+ months	+14.3	+14.3	+2.1	*	*	*	*	+40	+5	+0.2	*

* Indicates no increment.
[a] See paragraph A-4-a for definition.
[b] Phosphorus RNI is set equal to calcium in molar terms.
[c] 1 mmol sodium = 23 mg.
[d] 1 mmol potassium = 39 mg.
[e] Corresponds to sodium 1 mmol = 35.5 mg.
[f] Insufficient for women with high menstrual losses where the most practical way of meeting iron requirements is to take iron supplements (see Table 28-2 in original report).

Source: Report on Health and Social Subjects: no. 41. Dietary Reference Values for Food Energy and Nutrients for the United Kingdom. Report of the Panel on Dietary Reference Values of the Committee on Medical Aspects of Food Policy. London: Her Majesty's Stationery Office, 1991. This is the UK's Report Table 1.5.

| TABLE 22-30 | Reference Nutrient Intakes for Minerals (Traditional Units), United Kingdom[a] |

AGE	CALCIUM (MG/DAY)	PHOSPHORUS[b] (MG/DAY)	MAGNESIUM (MG/DAY)	SODIUM[c] (MG/DAY)	POTASSIUM[d] (MGL/DAY)	CHLORIDE[e] (MG/DAY)	IRON (MG/DAY)	ZINC (MG/DAY)	COPPER[f] (MG/DAY)	SELENIUM (µG/DAY)	IODINE (µG/DAY)
0–3 months	525	400	55	210	800	320	1.7	4.0	0.2	10	50
4–6 months	525	400	60	280	850	400	4.3	4.0	0.3	13	60
7–9 months	525	400	75	320	700	500	7.8	5.0	0.3	10	60
10–12 months	525	400	80	350	700	500	7.8	5.0	0.3	10	60
1–3 years	350	270	85	500	800	800	6.9	5.0	0.4	15	70
4–6 years	450	350	120	700	1,100	1,100	6.1	6.5	0.6	20	100
7–10 years	550	450	200	1,200	2,000	1,800	8.7	7.0	0.7	30	110
Males											
11–14 years	1,000	775	280	1,600	3,100	2,500	11.3	9.0	0.8	45	130
15–18 years	1,000	775	300	1,600	3,500	2,500	11.3	9.5	1.0	70	140
19–50 years	700	550	300	1,600	3,500	2,500	8.7	9.5	1.2	75	140
50+ years	700	550	300	1,600	3,500	2,500	8.7	9.5	1.2	75	140
Females											
11–14 years	800	625	280	1,600	3,100	2,500	14.8f	9.0	0.8	45	130
15–18 years	800	625	300	1,600	3,500	2,500	14.8f	7.0	1.0	60	140
19–50 years	700	550	270	1,600	3,500	2,500	14.8f	7.0	1.2	60	140
50+ years	700	550	270	1,600	3,500	2,500	8.7	7.0	1.2	60	140
Pregnancy	—*	—*	—*	—*	—*	—*	—*	—*	—*	—*	—*
Lactation											
0–4 months	+ 550	+ 440	+ 50	—*	—*	—*	*	+ 6.0	+ 0.3	+ 15	—*
4+ months	+ 550	+ 440	+ 50	—*	—*	—*	*	+ 2.5	+ 0.3	+ 15	—*

* Indicates no increment.
[a] See paragraph II-A-4-a for definition.
[b] Phosphorus RNI is set equal to calcium in molar terms.
[c] 1 mmol sodium = 23 mg.
[d] 1 mmol potassium = 39 mg.
[e] Corresponds to sodium 1 mmol = 35.5 mg.
[f] Insufficient for women with high menstrual losses where the most practical way of meeting iron requirements is to take iron supplements (see Table 28.2 in original report).

Source: Report on Health and Social Subjects: no. 41. Dietary Reference Values for Food Energy and Nutrients for the United Kingdom. Report of the Panel on Dietary Reference Values of the Committee on Medical Aspects of Food Policy. London: Her Majesty's Stationery Office, 1991. This is the UK's Report Table 1.5.

TABLE 22-31	Safe Intakes, United Kingdom[a]
NUTRIENT	**SAFE INTAKE[b]**
Vitamins	
Pantothenic acid	
Adults	3–7 mg/day
Infants	1.7 mg/day
Biotin	10–200 µg/day
Vitamin E	
Men	Above 4 mg/day
Women	Above 3 mg/day
Infants	0.4 mg/g polyunsaturated fatty acids
Vitamin K	
Adults	1 µg/kg/day
Infants	10 µg/day
Minerals	
Manganese	
Adults	Above 1.4 mg (26 µmol)/day
Infants and children	Above 16 µg (0.3 µmol)/kg/day
Molybdenum	
Adults	50–400 µg/day
Infants, children, and adolescents	0.5–1.5 µg/kg per day
Chromium	
Adults	Above 25 µg (0.5 µmol)/day
Children and adolescents	0.1–1.0 µg (2–20 nmol)/kg per day
Fluoride	
Children over 6 years and adults	0.5 mg/kg per day (3 µmol/kg per day)
Children over 6 months	0.12 mg/kg per day (6 µmol/kg per day)
Infants under 6 months	0.22 mg/kg per day (12 µmol/kg per day)

a See paragraph II-A-4-a for definition.

b For some nutrients, which are known to have important functions in humans, the Panel found insufficient reliable data on human requirements and were unable to set any dietary reference values for these. However, they decided on grounds of prudence to set a safe intake, particularly for infants and children. The safe intake was judged to be a level or range of intake at which there is no risk of deficiency and below a level where there is risk of undesirable effects. They are not therefore intended as a "toxic level," and although exceeding these safe intakes would not necessarily result in undesirable effects, equally there is no evidence for any benefits. The Panel agreed that the safe range of intakes set for the nutrients need not be exceeded.

Source: Report on Health and Social Subjects: no. 41. Dietary Reference Values for Food Energy and Nutrients for the United Kingdom. Report of the Panel on Dietary Reference Values of the Committee on Medical Aspects of Food Policy. London: Her Majesty's Stationery Office, 1991. This is the UK's Report Table 1.6.

RECOMMENDED DIETARY ALLOWANCES FOR THE JAPANESE

Tables 22-32 through 22-35 provide recommended dietary allowances for the Japanese. They are reprinted with permission from the Appendix of the 10th edition of *Modern Nutrition in Health and Disease*. The 2005 tables are available but were not translated into English at the time of publication. See http://www.mhlw.go.jp/houdou/2004/11/h1122-2.html for updated documents.

TABLE 22-32	Recommended Dietary Allowances for the Japanese: Dietary Allowances for Growth Period and Moderate Level (II) of Physical Activity, Japan[a]

AGE	REFERENCE HEIGHT (CM) MALE	FEMALE	REFERENCE BODY WEIGHT (KG) MALE	FEMALE	ENERGY (KCAL) MALE	FEMALE	PROTEIN (G) MALE	FEMALE	FAT ENERGY RATIO (%)	CALCIUM (G) MALE	FEMALE
0 months					1,20/kg		3.0/kg		45	0.5	
2 months					1,10/kg		2.4/kg		45	0.5	
6 months					1,00/kg		2.8/kg		30–40	0.5	
1 year	80.2	79.1	10.57	10.07	960	920	30	30	⎫	⎫	
2 years	89.6	88.4	12.85	12.36	1,200	1,150	35	35			
3 years	97.6	96.4	15.00	14.57	1,400	1,350	40	40			
4 years	104.7	103.6	17.12	16.74	1,550	1,500	45	45		⎬ 0.5	
5 years	111.2	110.2	19.34	18.97	1,650	1,550	50	50			
6 years	117.2	116.2	21.70	21.25	1,700	1,600	55	50			
7 years	123.0	121.9	24.40	23.75	1,800	1,650	60	55			
8 years	128.6	127.5	27.42	26.60	1,900	1,750	65	60	⎭	⎭	
9 years	133.9	133.2	30.69	29.95	1,950	1,850	70	65	⎬ 25–30		
10 years	139.2	139.7	34.34	34.23	2,050	1,950	75	70		0.6 ⎫	0.6
11 years	145.4	146.5	38.73	39.28	2,200	2,100	80	75		0.7	
12 years	153.0	151.6	44.31	43.92	2,350	2,250	85	75		0.8	
13 years	160.5	154.7	50.39	47.60	2,550	2,300	90	75		0.9	
14 years	166.0	156.5	55.69	50.38	2,650	2,300	90	75		0.9	⎬ 0.7
15 years	169.3	157.4	59.62	52.08	2,700	2,250	90	70		0.8	
16 years	171.0	158.0	61.93	52.92	2,750	2,200	80	65		0.8	
17 years	171.9	158.3	63.15	52.95	2,700	2,150	75	65	⎭	0.7	
18 years	172.3	158.5	63.53	52.53	2,700	2,100	75	60	⎫	0.7 ⎭	
19 years	172.3	158.5	63.53	51.93	2,600	2,050	70	60			
20–29 years	171.3	158.1	64.69	51.31	2,550	2,000	70	60			
30–39 years	170.8	157.3	66.62	54.02	2,500	2,000	70	60			
40–49 years	168.8	155.9	66.19	55.49	2,400	1,950	70	60			
50–59 years	165.9	153.0	63.66	53.95	2,300	1,850	70	60	⎬ 20–25		
60–64 years	163.4	150.6	61.12	51.28	2,100	1,750	70	60		⎫ 0.6	⎬ 0.6
65–69 years	162.1	149.1	59.28	49.53	2,100	1,700	70	60			
70–74 years	160.7	147.6	57.28	47.69	1,850	1,600	70	60			
75–79 years	159.3	146.1	55.30	45.83	1,800	1,500	65	55			
>80 years	157.3	143.9	52.85	43.67	1,650	1,400	65	55	⎭	⎭	

[a] In 2005, the Japanese Ministry of Health, Labor and Welfare issued new dietary reference allowances. These were not available in English at the time of book publication. Those interested in the published version of the new guidelines can obtain them from the following websites:
http://www.mhlw.go.jp/houdou/2004/11/h1122-2.html
http://www.mhlw.go.jp/houdou/2004/11/h1122-2a.html
http://www.mhlw.go.jp/houdou/2004/11/d1/h1122-2b.pdf (full version of guidelines in PDF)

TABLE 22-32   Recommended Dietary Allowances for the Japanese: Dietary Allowances for Growth Period and Moderate Level (II) of Physical Activity, Japan[a] (cont)

IRON (MG) MALE	IRON (MG) FEMALE	VITAMIN A (IU) MALE	VITAMIN A (IU) FEMALE	VITAMIN B$_1$ (MG) MALE	VITAMIN B$_1$ (MG) FEMALE	VITAMIN B$_2$ (MG) MALE	VITAMIN B$_2$ (MG) FEMALE	NIACIN (MG) MALE	NIACIN (MG) FEMALE	VITAMIN C (MG)	VITAMIN D (IU)
6		1,300		0.2		0.3		4			
6		1,300		0.3		0.4		6			
6		1,000		0.4		0.5		6			
7	7	1,000	1,000	0.4	0.4	0.5	0.5	6	6		400
7	7	1,000	1,000	0.5	0.5	0.7	0.6	8	8		
8	8	1,000	1,000	0.6	0.5	0.8	0.7	9	9		
8	8	1,000	1,000	0.6	0.6	0.9	0.8	10	10	40	
8	8	1,000	1,000	0.7	0.6	0.9	0.9	11	10		
9	9	1,200	1,200	0.7	0.6	0.9	0.9	11	11		
9	9	1,200	1,200	0.7	0.7	1.0	0.9	12	11		
9	9	1,200	1,200	0.8	0.7	1.0	1.0	13	12		
10	10	1,500	1,500	0.8	0.7	1.1	1.0	13	12		
10	10	1,500	1,500	0.8	0.8	1.1	1.1	14	13		
10	10	1,500	1,500	0.9	0.8	1.2	1.2	15	14		
12	12	1,500	1,500	0.9	0.9	1.3	1.2	16	15		
12	12	2,000	1,800	1.0	0.9	1.4	1.3	17	15		
12	12	2,000	1,800	1.1	0.9	1.5	1.3	17	15		
12	12	2,000	1,800	1.1	0.9	1.5	1.2	18	15		
12	12	2,000	1,800	1.1	0.9	1.5	1.2	18	15		
12	12	2,000	1,800	1.1	0.9	1.5	1.2	18	14		100
12	12	2,000	1,800	1.1	0.8	1.5	1.2	18	14		
12	12	2,000	1,800	1.0	0.8	1.4	1.1	17	14		
10	12	2,000	1,800	1.0	0.8	1.4	1.1	17	13	50	
10	12	2,000	1,800	1.0	0.8	1.4	1.1	17	13		
10	12	2,000	1,800	1.0	0.8	1.3	1.1	16	13		
10	12	2,000	1,800	0.9	0.7	1.3	1.0	15	12		
10	10	2,000	1,800	0.8	0.7	1.2	1.0	14	12		
10	10	2,000	1,800	0.8	0.7	1.2	1.0	14	12		
10	10	2,000	1,800	0.8	0.7	1.2	1.0	14	12		
10	10	2,000	1,800	0.8	0.7	1.2	1.0	14	12		
10	10	2,000	1,800	0.8	0.7	1.2	1.0	14	12		

Source: Recommended Dietary Allowances for the Japanese, 5th rev. Supervised by Health and Nutrition Division, Health Service Bureau, Ministry of Health and Welfare, 1996. With permission. The dietary allowances shown in Tables 22-32 through 22-35 are not to be applied to individuals without modification. Reference should be made to original report for application. As for determination of the intensity of living activity, reference should be made to the "classification" for intensities of living activities as viewed from daily life (standards). Those falling under "I (light)" in the degree of intensity of living activities are recommended to expend calories equivalent to "II (moderate)" degree of intensity as listed in Table 22-32 by either changing the daily activities or engaging in additional physical activities. The daily salt intake is recommended to be 10 g/day/person or less as previously. Vitamin E (α-tocopherol equivalent) intake should preferably be 8 mg for adult males and 7 mg for adult females.

TABLE 22-33 Recommended Dietary Allowances for the Japanese: Dietary Allowances for Light Level (I) of Physical Activity[a]

AGE	ENERGY (KCAL) MEN	WOMEN	PROTEIN (G) MEN	WOMEN	FAT ENERGY RATIO (%)	CALCIUM (G) MEN	WOMEN	IRON (MG) MEN	WOMEN
15 years	2,400	2,000	90	70		0.8		12	12
16 years	2,400	1,950	80	65	25–30	0.8	0.7	12	12
17 years	2,400	1,900	75	65		0.7		12	12
18 years	2,400	1,850	75	60		0.7		12	12
19 years	2,350	1,850	70	60				12	12
20–29 years	2,250	1,800	70	60				10	12
30–39 years	2,200	1,750	70	60				10	12
40–49 years	2,150	1,700	70	60				10	12
50–59 years	2,050	1,650	70	60	20–25	0.6	0.6	10	12
60–64 years	1,900	1,550	70	60				10	10
65–69 years	1,800	1,500	70	60				10	10
70–74 years	1,700	1,400	70	60				10	10
75–79 years	1,600	1,350	65	55				10	10
>80 years	1,500	1,250	65	55				10	10
Pregnancy 1–5 months		+ 150		+ 10			+ 0.3		+ 3
Additions 6–10 months		+ 350		+ 20	25–30		+ 0.3		+ 8
Lactation		+ 700		+ 20			+ 0.5		+ 8

[a] Additions for pregnant and lactating women are shown for convenience. Their levels of physical activity should not be regarded uniformly as falling subject to the light level (1).

Source: Recommended Dietary Allowances for the Japanese, 5th rev. Supervised by Health and Nutrition Division, Health Service Bureau, Ministry of Health and Welfare, 1996. With permission. The dietary allowances shown in Tables 22-32 through 22-35 are not to be applied to individuals without modification. Reference should be made to original report for application. As for determination of the intensity of living activity, reference should be made to the "classification" for intensities of living activities as viewed from daily life (standards). Those falling under "I (light)" in the degree of intensity of living activities are recommended to expend calories equivalent to "II (moderate)" degree of intensity as listed in Table 22-32 by either changing the daily activities or engaging in additional physical activities. The daily salt intake is recommended to be 10 g/day/person or less as previously. Vitamin E (α-tocopherol equivalent) intake should preferably be 8 mg for adult males and 7 mg for adult females.

TABLE 22-34 Recommended Dietary Allowances for the Japanese: Dietary Allowances for Light-Heavy Level (III) of Physical Activity

AGE	ENERGY (KCAL) MEN	WOMEN	PROTEIN (G) MEN	WOMEN	FAT ENERGY RATIO (%)	CALCIUM (G) MEN	WOMEN	IRON (MG) MEN	WOMEN
15 years	3,250	2,650	105	85		0.8		12	12
16 years	3,250	2,600	95	80		0.8	0.7	12	12
17 years	3,250	2,550	90	80		0.7		12	12
18 years	3,200	2,500	90	75		0.7		12	12
19 years	3,150	2,450	85	70				12	12
20–29 years	3,050	2,400	85	70	25–30			10	12
30–39 years	3,000	2,350	85	70				10	12
40–49 years	2,900	2,300	85	70		0.6	0.6	10	12
50–59 years	2,750	2,250	85	70				10	12
60–64 years	2,500	2,050	80	70				10	10
65–69 years	2,400	2,000	80	70				10	10

Source: Recommended Dietary Allowances for the Japanese, 5th rev. Supervised by Health and Nutrition Division, Health Service Bureau, Ministry of Health and Welfare, 1996. With permission. The dietary allowances shown in Tables 22-32 through 22-35 are not to be applied to individuals without modification. Reference should be made to original report for application. As for determination of the intensity of living activity, reference should be made to the "classification" for intensities of living activities as viewed from daily life (standards). Those falling under "I (light)" in the degree of intensity of living activities are recommended to expend calories equivalent to "II (moderate)" degree of intensity as listed in Table 22-32 by either changing the daily activities or engaging in additional physical activities. The daily salt intake is recommended to be 10 g/day/person or less as previously. Vitamin E (α-tocopherol equivalent) intake should preferably be 8 mg for adult males and 7 mg for adult females.

TABLE 22-33 Recommended Dietary Allowances for the Japanese: Dietary Allowances for Light Level (I) of Physical Activity[a] (continued)

VITAMIN A (IU)		VITAMIN B₁ (MG)		VITAMIN B₂ (MG)		NIACIN (MG)		VITAMIN C (MG)	VITAMIN D (IU)
MEN	WOMEN	MEN	WOMEN	MEN	WOMEN	MEN	WOMEN	(MG)	(IU)
2,000	1,800	1.0	0.8	1.3	1.1	16	13		
2,000	1,800	1.0	0.8	1.3	1.1	16	13		
2,000	1,800	1.0	0.8	1.3	1.0	16	13		
2,000	1,800	1.0	0.7	1.3	1.0	16	12		
2,000	1,800	0.9	0.7	1.3	1.0	16	12		
2,000	1,800	0.9	0.7	1.2	1.0	15	12		
2,000	1,800	0.9	0.7	1.2	1.0	15	12		
2,000	1,800	0.9	0.7	1.2	0.9	14	11	50	100
2,000	1,800	0.8	0.7	1.1	0.9	14	11		
2,000	1,800	0.8	0.6	1.0	0.9	13	10		
2,000	1,800	0.7	0.6	1.0	0.9	12	10		
2,000	1,800	0.7	0.6	0.9	0.9	12	10		
2,000	1,800	0.7	0.6	0.9	0.9	12	10		
2,000	1,800	0.7	0.6	0.9	0.9	12	10		
	+ 0		+ 0.1		+ 0.1		+ 1	+ 10	+ 300
	+ 200		+ 0.2		+ 0.2		+ 2	+ 10	+ 300
	+ 1400		+ 0.3		+ 0.4		+ 5	+ 40	+ 300

TABLE 22-34 Recommended Dietary Allowances for the Japanese: Dietary Allowances for Light-Heavy Level (III) of Physical Activity (continued)

VITAMIN A (IU)		VITAMIN B₁ (MG)		VITAMIN B₂ (MG)		NIACIN (MG)		VITAMIN C (MG)	VITAMIN D (IU)
MEN	WOMEN	MEN	WOMEN	MEN	WOMEN	MEN	WOMEN	(MG)	(IU)
2,000	1,800	1.3	1.1	1.8	1.5	21	17		
2,000	1,800	1.3	1.0	1.8	1.4	21	17		
2,000	1,800	1.3	1.0	1.8	1.4	21	17		
2,000	1,800	1.3	1.0	1.8	1.4	21	17		
2,000	1,800	1.3	1.0	1.7	1.3	21	16		
2,000	1,800	1.2	1.0	1.7	1.3	20	16	50	100
2,000	1,800	1.2	0.9	1.7	1.3	20	16		
2,000	1,800	1.2	0.9	1.6	1.3	19	15		
2,000	1,800	1.1	0.9	1.5	1.2	18	15		
2,000	1,800	1.0	0.8	1.4	1.1	17	14		
2,000	1,800	1.0	0.8	1.4	1.1	17	14		

TABLE 22-35	Recommended Dietary Allowances for the Japanese: Dietary Allowances for Heavy Level (IV) of Physical Activity

AGE	ENERGY (KCAL) MEN	ENERGY (KCAL) WOMEN	PROTEIN (G) MEN	PROTEIN (G) WOMEN	FAT ENERGY RATIO (%)	CALCIUM (G) MEN	CALCIUM (G) WOMEN	IRON (MG) MEN	IRON (MG) WOMEN
15 years	3,800	3,100	115	95		0.8		12	12
16 years	3,800	3,050	115	95		0.8	0.7	12	12
17 years	3,800	2,950	110	90		0.7		12	12
18 years	3,750	2,950	110	90		0.7		12	12
19 years	3,700	2,850	105	85				12	12
20–29 years	3,550	2,800	100	85	25–30			10	12
30–39 years	3,500	2,750	100	85				10	12
40–49 years	3,400	2,700	100	85		0.6	0.6	10	12
50–59 years	3,200	2,600	100	85				10	12
60–64 years	2,900	2,350	95	80				10	10
65–69 years	2,800	2,300	95	80				10	10

Source: Recommended Dietary Allowances for the Japanese, 5th rev. Supervised by Health and Nutrition Division, Health Service Bureau, Ministry of Health and Welfare, 1996. With permission. The dietary allowances shown in Tables 22-32 through 22-35 are not to be applied to individuals without modification. Reference should be made to original report for application. As for determination of the intensity of living activity, reference should be made to the "classification" for intensities of living activities as viewed from daily life (standards). Those falling under "I (light)" in the degree of intensity of living activities are recommended to expend calories equivalent to "II (moderate)" degree of intensity as listed in Table 22-32 by either changing the daily activities or engaging in additional physical activities. The daily salt intake is recommended to be 10 g/day/person or less as previously. Vitamin E (α-tocopherol equivalent) intake should preferably be 8 mg for adult males and 7 mg for adult females.

TABLE 22-35	Recommended Dietary Allowances for the Japanese: Dietary Allowances for Heavy Level (IV) of Physical Activity (*cont*)

| VITAMIN A (IU) | | VITAMIN B₁ (MG) | | VITAMIN B₂ (MG) | | NIACIN (MG) | | VITAMIN C (MG) (MG) | VITAMIN D (IU) (IU) |
MEN	WOMEN	MEN	WOMEN	MEN	WOMEN	MEN	WOMEN		
2,000	1,800	1.5	1.2	2.1	1.7	25	20		
2,000	1,800	1.5	1.2	2.1	1.7	25	20		
2,000	1,800	1.5	1.2	2.1	1.6	25	19		
2,000	1,800	1.5	1.2	2.1	1.6	25	19		
2,000	1,800	1.5	1.1	2.0	1.6	24	19		
2,000	1,800	1.4	1.1	2.0	1.5	23	18	50	100
2,000	1,800	1.4	1.1	1.9	1.5	23	18		
2,000	1,800	1.4	1.1	1.9	1.5	22	18		
2,000	1,800	1.3	1.0	1.8	1.4	21	17		
2,000	1,800	1.2	1.0	1.6	1.3	19	16		
2,000	1,800	1.1	1.0	1.6	1.3	19	16		

NUTRIENT REFERENCE VALUES FOR AUSTRALIA AND NEW ZEALAND

Tables 22-36 through 22-40 are draft tables providing nutrient reference values for Australia and New Zealand. They are reprinted with permission from the Appendix of the 10th edition of Modern Nutrition in Health and Disease, 2006. For 2005 final tables, see the NHMRC website, available at http://www.nhmrc.gov.au

TABLE 22-36 Nutrient Reference Values for Australia and New Zealand: Macronutrients and Water

Age/Gender Group		Energy[b], MJ/day (EER)	Protein, g/day (AI/EAR)	(RDI)	(UIL)	Dietary Fats[a] — Linoleic (n6), g/day (AI)	(UIL)	α-Linolenic (n3), g/day (AI)	(UIL)	VLC N3 (DHA/EPA/DPA), mg/day (AI)	(UIL)	Carbohydrate, g/day (AI)	(UIL)	Dietary Fibre, g/day (AI)	(UIL)	Total Water[a] (Fluids), L/day (AI)	(UIL)
Infants[c]	0–6 months	1.8–2.7	10		BM	4.4	BM	0.5[a]	BM	–		60	BM	NP	NP	0.7 (0.7)	NP.
	7–12 months	2.5–3.5	14		B/F	4.6	B/F	0.5[a]	B/F	–		95	B/F	NP	NP	0.8 (0.6)	NP
Children	1–3 years	3.2–5.5	12	14	NP	5	NP	0.5	NP	40	3000	None set for other ages		12	NP	1.4 (1.0)	NP
	4–8 years	5.5–7.4	16	20	NP	8	NP	0.8	NP	55	3000			16	NP	1.6 (1.2)	NP
Boys	9–13 years	7.8–10.0	31	40	NP	10	Np	1.0	Np	70	3000			21	NP	2.2 (1.6)	NP
	14–18 years	10.6–12.5	49	65	NP	12	NP	1.2	NP	125	3000			23	NP	2.7 (1.9)	NP
Girls	9–13 years	7.3–8.9	24	35	NP	8	NP	0.8	NP	70	3000			17	NP	1.9 (1.4)	NP
	14–18 years	9.2–9.7	35	45	NP	8	NP	0.8	NP	85	3000			18	NP	2.2 (1.4)	NP
Men	19–30 years	10.3–13.5	52	64	NP	13	NP	1.3	NP	190	3000			25	NP	3.4 (2.6)	NP
	31–50 years	10.2–12.6	52	64	NP	13	NP	1.3	NP	190	3000			25	NP	3.4 (2.6)	NP
	51–70 years	10.2–12.6	52	64	NP	13	NP	1.3	NP	190	3000			25	NP	3.4 (2.6)	NP
	>70 years	8.3–10.8	52	64	NP	13	NP	1.3	NP	190	3000			25	NP	3.4 (2.6)	NP
Women	19–30 years	8.2–11.1	37	46	NP	8	NP	0.8	NP	90	3000			20	NP	2.8 (2.1)	NP
	31–50 years	8.4–10.0	37	46	NP	8	NP	0.8	NP	90	3000			20	NP	2.8 (2.1)	NP
	51–70 years	8.4–10.0	37	46	NP	8	NP	0.8	NP	90	3000			20	NP	2.8 (2.1)	NP
	>70 years	7.4–9.2	37	46	NP	8	NP	0.8	NP	90	3000			20	NP	2.8 (2.1)	NP
Pregnant	14–18 years	2nd trimester + 1.4MJ	47[d]	58[d]	NP	10	NP	1.0	NP	110	3000			20	NP	2.4 (1.8)	NP
	19–30 years		49[d]	60[d]	NP	10	NP	1.0	NP	115	3000			22	NP	3.1 (2.3)	NP
	31–50 years	3rd trimester − 1.9MJ	49[d]	60[d]	NP	10	NP	1.0	NP	115	3000			22	NP	3.1 (2.3)	NP
Lactating	14–18 years	+ 2.0–2.1MJ	51	63	NP	12	NP	1.2	NP	140	3000			22	NP	3.5 (2.6)	NP
	19–30 years		54	67	NP	12	NP	1.2	NP	145	3000			24	NP	3.5 (2.6)	NP
	31–50 years		54	67	NP	12	NP	1.2	NP	145	3000			24	NP	3.5 (2.6)	NP

AI, adequate intakes; BM, amount normally received from breast milk for healthy women; B/F, amount in breast milk and food; EAR, estimated average requirement; NP, not possible to set (may be insufficient evidence or no clear level for adverse effects); RDI, recommended dietary intake; UIL—Upper Intake Limit.
[a] Recommendations for total n6 and total n3; total fat AI also set at 30–31 g/day for infants. Total water includes water from foods as well as fluids.
[b] Energy needs are dependent on body size and activity.
[c] AI recommendations for infants are based on amounts in breast milk.
[d] In second and third trimesters only.

Source: Shils ME, Shike M, Ross AC, et al. Modern Nutrition in Health and Disease. 10th Ed. Baltimore: Lippincott Williams & Wilkins, 2006:1884.

TABLE 22-37   Nutrient Reference Values for Australia and New Zealand: B Vitamins

Age/Gender Group		Thiamin, mg/day AI	EAR	RDI	UIL	Riboflavin, mg/day AI	EAR	RDI	UIL	Niacin[a] (niacin equivalents), mg/d AI	EAR	RDI	UIL	Vitamin B$_6$[b], mg/day AI	EAR	RDI	UIL	Vitamin B$_{12}$, µg/day AI	EAR	RDI	UIL	Folate (folate equivalents), mg/day AI	EAR	RDI	UIL	Pantothenate, mg/day AI	UIL	Biotin, µg/day AI	UIL
Infants[c]	0–6 months	0.2			NP	0.3			BM	2			BM	0.1			BM	0.4			BM	65			BM	1.7	BM	5	BM
	7–12 months	0.3			NP	0.4			B/F	4			B/F	0.3			B/F	0.5			B/F	80			B/F	2.2	B/F	6	B/F
Children	1–3 years		0.4	0.5	NP		0.4	0.5	NP		5	6	10		0.4	0.5	30		0.7	0.9	NP		120	150	300	3.5	NP	8	NP
	4–8 years		0.5	0.6	NP		0.5	0.6	NP		6	8	15		0.5	0.6	40		1.0	1.2	NP		160	200	400	4	NP	12	NP
Boys	9–13 years		0.7	0.9	NP		0.8	0.9	NP		9	12	20		0.8	1.0	60		1.5	1.8	NP		250	300	600	5	NP	20	NP
	14–18 years		1.0	1.2	NP		1.1	1.3	NP		12	16	30		1.1	1.3	80		2.0	2.4	NP		330	400	800	6	NP	30	NP
Girls	9–13 years		0.7	0.9	NP		0.8	0.9	NP		9	12	20		0.8	1.0	60		1.5	1.8	NP		250	300	600	4	NP	20	NP
	14–18 years		0.9	1.0	NP		0.9	1.0	NP		11	14	30		1.0	1.2	80		2.0	2.4	NP		330	400	800	4	NP	25	NP
Men	19–30 years		1.0	1.2	NP		1.1	1.3	NP		12	16	35		1.1	1.3	100		2.0	2.4	NP		320	400	1000	6	NP	30	NP
	31–50 years		1.0	1.2	NP		1.1	1.3	NP		12	16	35		1.1	1.3	100		2.0	2.4	NP		320	400	1000	6	NP	30	NP
	51–70 years		1.0	1.2	NP		1.1	1.3	NP		12	16	35		1.4	1.7	100		2.0	2.4	NP		320	400	1000	6	NP	30	NP
	>70 years		1.0	1.2	NP		1.3	1.6	NP		12	16	35		1.4	1.7	100		2.0	2.4	NP		320	400	1000	6	NP	30	NP
Women	19–30 years		0.9	1.1	NP		0.9	1.1	NP		11	14	35		1.1	1.3	100		2.0	2.4	NP		320	400	1000	4	NP	25	NP
	31–50 years		0.9	1.1	NP		0.9	1.1	NP		11	14	35		1.1	1.3	100		2.0	2.4	NP		320	400	1000	4	NP	25	NP
	51–70 years		0.9	1.1	NP		0.9	1.1	NP		11	14	35		1.3	1.5	100		2.0	2.4	NP		320	400	1000	4	NP	25	NP
	>70 years		0.9	1.1	NP		1.1	1.3	NP		11	14	35		1.3	1.5	100		2.0	2.4	NP		320	400	1000	4	NP	25	NP
Pregnant	14–18 years		1.2	1.4	NP		1.2	1.4	NP		14	18	30		1.6	1.9	80		2.2	2.6	NP		520	600	800	5	NP	30	NP
	19–30 years		1.2	1.4	NP		1.2	1.4	NP		14	18	35		1.6	1.9	100		2.2	2.6	NP		520	600	1000	5	NP	30	NP
	31–50 years		1.2	1.4	NP		1.2	1.4	NP		14	18	35		1.6	1.9	100		2.2	2.6	NP		520	600	1000	5	NP	30	NP
Lactating	14–18 years		1.2	1.4	NP		1.3	1.6	NP		13	17	30		1.7	2.0	80		2.4	2.8	NP		450	500	800	6	NP	35	NP
	19–30 years		1.2	1.4	NP		1.3	1.6	NP		13	17	35		1.7	2.0	100		2.4	2.8	NP		450	500	1000	6	NP	35	NP
	31–50 years		1.2	1.4	NP		1.3	1.6	NP		13	17	35		1.7	2.0	100		2.4	2.8	NP		450	500	1000	6	NP	35	NP

AI, adequate intakes; BM, amount normally received from breast milk for healthy women; B/F, amount in breast milk and food; EAR, estimated average requirement; NP, not possible to set (may be insufficient evidence or no clear level for adverse effects); RDI, recommended dietary intake; UIL, Upper Intake Limit.

[a] UIL for nicotinic acid. For supplement, nicotinamide UIL is 1,000 mg/day for men and 850 mg/day for nonpregnant women. Insufficient evidence for upper limits for nicotinamide in pregnancy and lactation or for children and adolescents.

[b] For Vitamin B$_6$, UIL set for phyridoxine. For folate, UIL is for intake from fortified foods and supplements as dietary folate equivalents.

[c] All infant AIs are based on estimates based on breast-milk concentrations in healthy women and average volumes.

Source: Shils ME, Shike M, Ross AC, et al. Modern Nutrition in Health and Disease. 10th Ed. Baltimore: Lippincott Williams & Wilkins, 2006:1884.

TABLE 22-38   Nutrient Reference Values for Australia and New Zealand: Vitamin A, C, D, E and K and Choline

AGE/GENDER GROUP		VITAMIN A (RETINOL EQUIVALENTS), µG/DAY			VITAMIN C, MG/DAY			VITAMIN D, µG/DAY		VITAMIN E (ALPHA-TOCOPHEROL EQUIVALENTS), MG/DAY		VITAMIN K, µG/DAY		CHOLINE, MG/DAY	
		AI		UIL	AI		UIL	AI	UIL	AI	UIL	AI	UIL	AI	UIL
Infants[c]	0–6 months	250 (as retinol)		600	25		BM	5	MB	4	BM	2	BM	125	BM
	7–12 months	430		600	30		B/F	5	B/F	5	B/F	2.5	B/F	150	B/F
		EAR	RDI	UIL	EAR	RDI	UIL	AI	UIL	AI	UIL	AI	UIL	AI	UIL
Children	1–3 years	210	300	600	25	35	NP	5	NP	5	70	25	NP	200	1,000
	4–8 years	275	400	900	25	35	NP	5	NP	6	100	35	NP	250	1,000
Boys	9–13 years	445	600	1,700	28	40	NP	5	NP	9	180	45	NP	375	1,000
	14–18 years	630	900	2,800	28	40	NP	5	NP	10	250	45	NP	375	1,000
Girls	9–13 years	420	600	1,700	28	40	NP	5	NP	8	180	45	NP	550	1,000
	14–18 years	485	700	2,800	28	40	NP	5	NP	8	250	55	NP	400	3,000
Men	19–30 years	625	900	3,000	30	45	NP	5	NP	10	300	70	NP	550	3,500
	31–50 years	625	900	3,000	30	45	NP	5	NP	10	300	70	NP	550	3,500
	51–70 years	625	900	3,000	30	45	NP	10	NP	10	300	70	NP	550	3,500
	> 70 years	625	900	3,000	30	45	NP	15	NP	10	300	70	NP	550	3,500
Women	19–30 years	500	700	3,000	30	45	NP	5	NP	7	300	60	NP	475	3,500
	31–50 years	500	700	3,000	30	45	NP	5	NP	7	300	60	NP	475	3,500
	51–70 years	500	700	3,000	30	45	NP	10	NP	7	300	60	NP	475	3,500
	> 70 years	500	700	3,000	30	45	NP	15	NP	7	300	60	NP	475	3,500
Pregnant	14–18 years	530	700	2,800	38	55	NP	5	NP	7	300	60	NP	420	3,000
	19–30 years	550	800	3,000	40	60	NP	5	NP	7	300	60	NP	450	3,500
	31–50 years	550	800	3,000	40	60	NP	5	NP	7	300	60	NP	450	3,500
Lactating	14–18 years	780	1,100	2,800	58	80	NP	5	NP	12	300	60	NP	525	3,000
	19–30 years	800	1,110	3,000	60	85	NP	5	NP	11	300	60	NP	550	3,500
	31–50 years	800	1,110	3,000	60	85	NP	5	NP	11	300	60	NP	550	3,500

EAR—Estimated Average Requirement. RDI—Recommended Dietary Intake. AI—Adequate Intakes. UIL—Upper Intake Limit. * Not possible to establish UIL for Vitamin C but 1000 mg/day would be a prudent limit. # One alpha-tocopherol equivalent is equal to 1 mg RRR alpha (or d-l) tocopherol; 2 mg beta tocopherol; 10 mg gamma tocopherol; 3 mg alpha decotrienol. The relevant figure for synthetic all-rac-alpha tocopherols (di-alpha tocopherol) is 14 mg.

Source: Shils ME, Shike M, Ross AC, et al. Modern Nutrition in Health and Disease. 10th Ed. Baltimore: Lippincott Williams & Wilkins, 2006:1885.

TABLE 22-39 Nutrient Reference Values for Australia and New Zealand: Minerals (EARs and RDIs)

Age/Gender Group		Calcium, mg/day				Phosphorus, mg/day				Zinc, mg/day				Iron, mg/day			
		EAR	AI	RDI	UIL	EAR	AI	RDI	UIL	EAR	AI	RDI	UIL	EAR	AI	RDI	UIL
Infants	0–6 months		210		BM		100		BM		2		4		0.27		20
	7–12 months		270		B/F		275		B/F	2.5	3.0		5	6.9		11.0	20
Children	1–3 years	360		500	2,500	380		460	3,000	2.5		3	7	4.1		9	20
	4–8 years	520		700	2,500	405		500	3,000	3		4	12	4.1		10	40
Boys	9–13 years	800/1,050		1,000/1,300	2,500	1,055		1,250	4,000	5.2		6	25	5.9		8	40
	14–18 years	1,050		1,300	2,500	1,055		1,250	4,000	10.5		13	35	7.7		11	45
Girls	9–13 years	800/1,050		1,000/1,300	2,500	1,055		1,250	4,000	5.2		6	25	5.7		8	40
	14–18 years	1,050		1,300	2,500	1,055		1,250	4,000	5.9		7	35	7.9		15	45
Men	19–30 years	840		1,000	2,500	580		1,000	4,000	11.7		14	40	6		8	45
	31–50 years	840		1,000	2,500	580		1,000	4,000	11.7		14	40	6		8	45
	51–70 years	840		1,000	2,500	580		1,000	4,000	11.7		14	40	6		8	45
	>70 years	1,100		1,300	2,500	580		1,000	3,000	11.7		14	40	6		8	45
Women	19–30 years	840		1,100	2,500	580		1,000	4,000	6.5		8	35	8		18	45
	31–50 years	840		1,100	2,500	580		1,000	4,000	6.5		8	35	8		18	45
	51–70 years	1,100		1,300	2,500	580		1,000	4,000	6.5		8	35	5		8	45
	>70 years	1,100		1,300	2,500	580		1,000	3,000	6.5		8	35	5		8	45
Pregnant	14–18 years	1,050		1,300	2,500	1,055		1,250	3,500	8.3		10	35	23		27	45
	19–30 years	840		1,000	2,500	580		1,000	3,500	8.9		11	40	22		27	45
	31–50 years	840		1,000	2,500	580		1,000	3,500	8.9		11	40	22		27	45
Lactating	14–18 years	1,050		1,300	2,500	1,055		1,250	4,000	9.1		11	35	7		10	45
	19–30 years	840		1,000	2,500	580		1,000	4,000	9.7		12	40	6.5		9	45
	31–50 years	840		1,000	2,500	580		1,000	4,000	9.7		12	40	6.5		9	45

Source: Shils ME, Shike M, Ross AC, et al. Modern Nutrition in Health and Disease. 10th ed. Baltimore: Lippincott Williams & Wilkins, 2006:1885.

TABLE 22-39   Nutrient Reference Values for Australia and New Zealand: Minerals (EARs and RDIs) (cont)

AGE/GENDER GROUP		MAGNESIUM, MG/DAY				IODINE, µG/DAY				SELENIUM, µG/DAY				MOLYBDENUM, µG/DAY			
		EAR	AI	RDI	UIL#	EAR	AI	RDI	UIL	EAR	AI	RDI	UIL	EAR	AI	RDI	UIL
Infants	0–6 months		30		BM		90		BM		12		45		2		BM
	7–12 months		75		B/F		110		B/F		15		60		3		B/F
Children	1–3 years	65		80	65	65		90	200	20		25	90	13		17	300
	4–8 years	110		130	110	65		90	300	25		30	150	17		22	600
Boys	9–13 years	200		240	350	73		120	600	40		50	280	26		34	1,100
	14–18 years	340		410	350	95		150	900	55		65	400	33		43	1,700
Girls	9–13 years	200		240	350	73		120	600	40		50	280	26		34	1,100
	14–18 years	300		360	350	95		150	900	55		65	400	33		43	1,700
Men	19–30 years	330		400	350	100		150	1,100	55		65	400	34		45	2,000
	31–50 years	350		420	350	100		150	1,100	55		65	400	34		45	2,000
	51–70 years	350		420	350	100		150	1,100	55		65	400	34		45	2,000
	> 70 years	350		420	350	100		150	1,100	55		65	400	34		45	2,000
Women	19–30 years	255		310	350	100		150	1,100	45		55	400	34		45	2,000
	31–50 years	265		320	350	100		150	1,100	45		55	400	34		45	2,000
	51–70 years	265		320	350	100		150	1,100	45		55	400	34		45	2,000
	> 70 years	265		320	350	100		150	1,100	45		55	400	34		45	2,000
Pregnant	14–18 years	335		400	350	160		220	900	47		57	400	40		50	1,700
	19–30 years	290		350	350	160		220	1,100	47		57	400	40		50	1,700
	31–50 years	300		360	350	160		220	1,100	47		57	400	40		50	1,700
Lactating	14–18 years	300		360	350	190		270	900	55		65	400	35		50	1,700
	19–30 years	255		310	350	190		270	1,100	55		65	400	36		50	2,000
	31–50 years	365		320	350	190		270	1,100	55		65	400	36		50	2,000

Source: Shils ME, Shike M, Ross AC, et al. Modern Nutrition in Health and Disease. 10th ed. Baltimore: Lippincott Williams & Wilkins, 2006:1885.

TABLE 22-40 Nutrient Reference Values for Australia and New Zealand: Minerals (Adequate Intakes)

AGE/GENDER GROUP		COPPER, MG/DAY		CHROMIUM, µG/DAY		MANGANESE, MG/DAY		FLUORIDE, MG/DAY*		SODIUM, MG/DAY*		POTASSIUM, MG/DAY	
		AI	UIL	AI	UIL	AI	UIL	AI	UIL	AI	UIL	AI	UIL
Infants	0–6 months	0.20	BM	0.2	NP	0.003	BM	0.01	0.7	120	700	400	NP
	7–12 months	0.22	B/F	5.5	NP	0.6	B/F	0.5	0.9	170	1,000	700	NP
Children	1–3 years	0.7	1	11	NP	2.0	2	0.7	1.3	200–400	1,400	3,000	NP
	4–8 years	1.0	3	15	NP	2.5	3	1	2.2	300–600	1,600	3,700	NP
Boys	9–13 years	1.3	5	25	NP	3.0	6	2	10	400–800	1,400	4,400	NP
	14–18 years	1.5	8	35	NP	3.5	9	3	10	460–920	1,600	4,700	NP
Girls	9–13 years	1.1	5	21	NP	2.5	6	2	10	400–800	1,600	4,400	NP
	14–18 years	1.1	8	24	NP	3.0	9	3	10	460–920	1,600	4,700	NP
Men	19–30 years	1.7	10	35	NP	5.5	11	4	10	460–920	1,600	4,700	NP
	31–50 years	1.7	10	35	NP	5.5	11	4	10	460–920	1,600	4,700	NP
	51–70 years	1.7	1	35	NP	5.5	11	4	10	460–920	1,600	4,700	NP
	>70 years	1.2	10	35	NP	5.5	11	4	10	460–920	1,600	4,700	NP
Women	19–30 years	1.2	10	25	NP	5.0	11	3	10	460–920	1,600	4,700	NP
	31–50 years	1.2	10	25	NP	5.0	1	3	10	460–920	1,600	4,700	NP
	51–70 years	1.2	10	25	NP	5.0	11	3	10	460–920	1,600	4,700	NP
	>70 years	1.2	10	25	NP	5.0	11	3	10	460–920	1,600	4,700	NP
Pregnant	14–18 years	1.2	8	30	NP	5.0	9	3	10	460–920	1,600	4,700	NP
	19–30 years	1.3	10	30	NP	5.0	11	3	10	460–920	1,600	4,700	NP
	31–50 years	1.3	10	30	NP	5.0	11	3	10	460–920	1,600	4,700	NP
Lactating	14–18 years	1.4	8	45	NP	5.0	9	3	10	460–920	1,600	4,700	NP
	19–30 years	1.5	10	45	NP	5.0	11	3	10	460–920	1,600	4,700	NP
	31–50 years	1.5	10	45	NP	5.0	11	3	10	460–920	1,600	4,700	NP

Source: Shils ME, Shike M, Ross AC, et al. Modern Nutrition in Health and Disease. 10th Ed. Baltimore: Lippincott Williams & Wilkins, 2006:1886.

REFERENCES

1. WHO Technical Report Series 916. Diet, nutrition and the prevention of chronic diseases. Available at: http://www.who.int/dietphysicalactivity/publications/trs916/en/gsfao_introduction.pdf. Accessed March 21, 2006.
2. US Department of Agriculture. 2005 dietary guidelines for Americans. Available at: http://www.health.gov/dietaryguidelines/dga2005/document. Accessed March 21, 2006.
3. National Academies Press. Dietary reference intakes. Available at: http://www.nap.edu. Accessed March 21, 2006.
4. Shils ME, Shike M, Ross AC, Caballero B, Cousins RJ. Modern Nutrition in Health and Disease. 10th Ed. Baltimore: Lippincott Williams & Wilkins, 2006:1852–1890.

Pages numbers in *italics* indicate figure. Page numbers followed by t indicate table.